LIVESTOCK ECONOMY OF INDIA

LIVESTOCK ECONOMY OF INDIA

P.C. Bansil

Techno Economic Research Institute
New Delhi

S.P. Malhotra

Ex-FAO Commodity Specialist

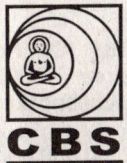

CBS

CBS PUBLISHERS & DISTRIBUTORS

New Delhi • Bangalore

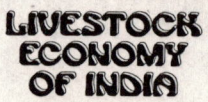

LIVESTOCK
ECONOMY
OF INDIA

Copyright © Authors and Publishers

ISBN : 81-239-1236-6

First Edition 2006

Production Director : Vinod K. Jain

Published by :
Satish Kumar Jain for CBS Publishers & Distributors,
4596/1-A, 11 Darya Ganj, New Delhi - 110 002 (India)
E-mail : cbspubs@vsnl.com
Website : www.cbspd.com

Branch Office :
Seema House, 2975, 17th Cross, K.R. Road,
Bansankari 2nd Stage, Bangalore - 560070
Fax : 080-6771680 • E-mail : cbsbng@vsnl.net

Typeset at CBS P&D Typesetting unit and printed at
Asia Printograph, Shahdara, Delhi - 110032 (India)

Preface

Livestock and rural economy in India have been intricately woven into each other since times immemorial. Not only have they have been coexisting in the same premises, but even food – left over of the household is being fed to animals. If you had asked a ruralite in the early fifties about the size of his family, he would include the number of animals along with those of humans. Role of the cow as *mother* is a reflection of the reverence with which livestock are worshiped. Indians have held milk in high esteem through the ages, considering it good enough as an offering to gods. Since childhood, it is drilled into their head that milk is the food par excellence. It provides 95 percent of animal proteins and almost 100 percent of animal fat in the daily diet. Despite all this, animal husbandry has all these years remained as an adjunct of agriculture without any individual identity of its own.

This would explain that even during the first twenty years of Indian Independence, there was hardly any visible development either in dairy or poultry—the two major sub-sectors of the livestock economy. A somewhat organised system of development under OPERATION FLOOD in dairy during the early seventies ushered what is popularly known as WHITE REVOLUTION. Introduction of broiler industry and commercial egg production more or less at the same time have brought Indian livestock on the world map, although village free range poultry continues to be backward. India has no doubt attained first place in the world production of milk, average productivity levels of indigenous animals which are still disproportionately large, remain very low.

A country study was undertaken by the Institute on behalf of Food and Agriculture Organisation of the United Nations. It formed a part of the Regional Study on Perspectives and Strategies for the Asian Livestock Sector in the next three decades. The purpose of the study was to equip decision-makers at the national and international level with baseline information and strategic assessment of the Asian livestock sector. The livestock sector encompasses livestock production, processing and distribution. It includes production on the traditional farms as well as production in industrial livestock facilities that are characterised by high capital–labour ratios. The time frame of the study was up to 2030. The discussions and the material presented covered short- and medium-term as well as the long-term developments. This book is the revised and expanded version of the original study. Most of the chapters have been revised and updated and as many as 18 new chapters have been added. The book covers livestock as well as fishery sectors.

The authors felt that there was a need for a comprehensive volume on livestock and fishery sectors in India, as the available material for these sectors is rather limited and scattered. We have tried to bring together material on all aspects of these two sectors at one place. It is hoped that it would serve as a useful reference material for planning, policy formulation, as well as for academic, research and extension workers.

Since basic data on livestock and fishery sector are inadequate and unreliable, we had to fall back on various published and unpublished sources of varied nature. We had also to make some assumptions and sometime use guess estimates. Every effort has, however, been made to maintain and ensure consistency. We are grateful to the Food and Agriculture Organization of the United Nations for having given us the opportunity to undertake an initial in-depth study on the important livestock sector and subsequently allowing us to get this revised and expanded version printed under our authorship. We would like to express our sincere thanks, especially to Dr. Wagner, Senior Animal Production and Health Officer, FAO Regional Office for Asia and the Pacific, Bangkok, and Dr. Henning Steinfed, Chief Animal Production Health Division, FAO, Rome.

A number of experts have provided us technical assistance, guidance and inputs during the preparation of this book. We would like to express special thanks to Dr. Pratap Birthal and Dr. Praduman Kumar, principal scientist, Divison of Agricultural Economics, Indian Research Institute, New Delhi, who have contributed a full chapter on 'emerging pattern of consumption of livestock products' in this book. TERI faculty members Dr. S.R. Mehnot and Dr. P.N. Radhakrishnan, and a number of other experts were helpful to provide various inputs and we benefited immensely from their contributions at every stage. We highly appreciate their valuable contribution. Mr. D.S. Negi, Joint Secretary, Ministry of Agriculture; Mr. B.K. Taimini, Former Secretary, Ministry of Food; and Prof. P.N. Bhat, former Animal Husbandry Commissioner; were all available for ready guidance on various ticklish problems. This study would not have been possible without their spontaneous help.

Our senior colleagues in the Institute Mr. K.R. Das Gupta and Mr. C.P. Sharma took full responsiblity in the organisation and finalisation of the study. Mr. Y.N. Arjuna, Publishing Director, CBS Publishers & Distributors, was actually the real motivator to bring the book to its final shape. But for his patience to cope with the frequent changes made in the various drafts of the book and his editorial improvements, this edition of the book would not have seen the light of the day. Many thanks to him. Last but not the least, our thanks are due to Mrs Ajitha Gangadharan and Mrs Vasantha R. Pillai who took charge of the most difficult task of typing the entire draft of the text.

P.C. Bansil
S.P. Malhotra

New Delhi

Contents

Chapter **5**

Dairy Industry in India

Chapter **6**

Poultry Development

Chapter **7**

Role of Sheep and Goat in Rural Economy

Chapter **8**

Meat Production and other Livestock Products

Chapter **9**

Government Policies

300

Chapter **10**

Animal Health Services and Impact of Livestock Sector on Public Health

350

Chapter **11**

Environmental Impact of Livestock Industry

388

Chapter **12**

Foreign Trade in Livestock Products

406

Chapter **23**

WTO's Trade Reforms and Livestock Sector
716

Chapter **24**

Strengths, Weaknesses, Opportunity and Threat (SWOT) Analysis for Livestock and Livestock Products
737

Chapter **25**

Future: Constraint Analysis: A Field Survey Processing Industry
746

Chapter **26**

Livestock Revolution—The World Scenario
759

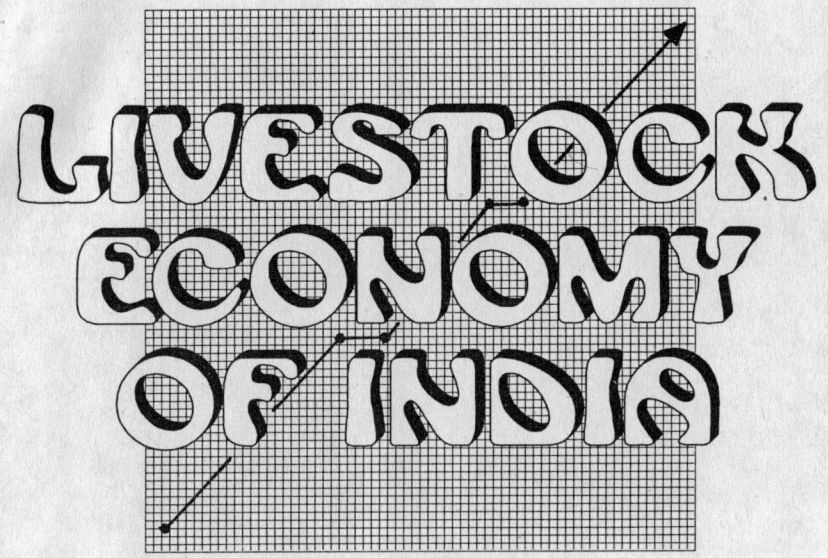

1

Introduction

India has had a mixed tradition regarding livestock. They are raised by some for milking them, by some for eating some of these while some worship a few. Most of them are held in good esteem for socioreligious considerations. For pastoral tribes it is their insurance against drought as well as a symbol of wealth: for the urban rich horse used to be a means of transportation in the era bygone and for the rural well-to-do as draught cattle for ploughing and other agricultural operations. Celebrated in our scriptures and folklore, its role in daily life of most of the people continues to be relevant albeit for entirely different and ever-changing reasons. All in all, it has been and continues to be part of our rural scene – be it perceived as part of personal wealth, status symbol or mode of transportation as draught cattle. Things are now changing for whose appreciation a peep into perspective shall be in order.

Domestication of cattle originated in pre-vedic, pre-Aryan India, among the civilizations that flourished in the Indus Valley. Terra-cotta relics from Mohenjodaro and Harappa have helped archaeologists and historians to reconstruct the history of a pre-Aryan civilization of some 5000 years ago, of a people living in sedentary agrarian settlements with domesticated animals: some for food, some for transport and work, and some as companions. Vedic Aryans were pastoralists: cows and oxen were their chief form of wealth. The cow had a special status even in the vedic era and figures prominently among other animals in the *Rigveda*, the oldest of the four *Vedas*. Cattle as an important source of food and farm power finds extensive mention in Kautilya's *Arthashastra* (1000-400 BC), *Manusmriti* (1-4th century AD) and the *Sukraniti* (9th century AD). Communities flourishing under the cumulative impact of the ancient India religions were, over the millennia, guided into a way of life harmonious with nature, with many complementarities between man, animals and nature. Livestock were an integral part of the ancient Indian farming systems and today's mixed crop-livestock farming system preponderant among the farming communities in India is the direct descendent of the ancient farming culture and practices, down through the millennia.

The Asian region is largest in the world both in terms of livestock population and growth rates of livestock industry. With around 1,300 breeds/strains, the region has over 30% of the known global farm animal genetic resources in terms of breed populations. The process of identification and characterization of breeds is still on and many more breeds may be added to the existing resource. Of the total buffalo and cattle breeds of the world, around 80 percent subsist in Asian region. These breeds of livestock and poultry in the region are essentially the product of long term natural selection under low input, harsh climatic conditions, parasitic load and diseases. The indigenous breeds are better adapted to withstand diseases and are efficient converters of low quality roughages. The need is to identify genes for prolificacy, resistance to diseases and fast growth in these breeds and use them for synthesis of new breeds/types for increasing production and productivity.

India has a large cattle wealth. It plays an important role in the socioeconomic life of people in general and in the villages in particular. Statistically, India has the largest number of cows and buffaloes (56.5 percent) in the world. The livestock sector plays an important role in the rural economy through its contribution to food, income and employment. Animals provide a diverse range of output varying from draught for cultivation, irrigation, transport; to fibre and leather goods and to manure for fertilizers and fuel in addition to milk and meat. The rural women constitute 71% of the labour force engaged in livestock farming and they are involved in all major operations like feeding, breeding, management and health care. As the ownership of livestock is more evenly distributed among small and marginal farmers, the progress in this sector will result in a more balanced growth of the rural economy and in poverty alleviation.

India with annual 85 million tonnes of milk and 34 billion eggs (2000-01) ranks 1st and 4th in the world. Annual growth rates of 4-5% for milk, meat and egg production have been achieved during the last 10 years. Increasing these growth rates further to 6-8% would call for higher investments and improved technological interventions. The value of output from Animal Husbandry and Dairying to Agriculture over the years has gone up and was 28% in 2000-01. This did not include draught animal power which was valued at between Rs. 40-95 billion. The value of output of milk (Rs. 1,020 billion) was higher than that of paddy (Rs. 811 billion), wheat (Rs. 471 billion), and Sugarcane (Rs. 275 billion). The higher output from livestock has been achieved despite poor investments relative to crop agriculture. The value of output from livestock to agriculture is likely to go to 50% by 2020.

Subsistence-based Production

The poorest of the world's poor people comprise hundreds of millions of families existing on less than $1 per day. Approximately 50% of these families own livestock and in some parts of the world will remain reliant for at least some more human generations on adapted genetic livestock resources that can cope with low-input, high-stress production systems to provide food, fibre and hides for home use and local sales; serve as a source of traction and fuel; meet cultural and religious needs and provide a reliable and readily convertible means of managing family resources. Low literacy rates and very real risks of hunger are common problems. Consequently, programmes and policies have to be adjusted to their needs.

Livestock sector plays a crucial role in sustaining rural economy and livelihood. In this sector, the poor contribute to growth directly instead of benefiting from growth generated elsewhere. The overall growth rate in livestock sector in India is steady at around 6%. Rural women play a significant role in animal husbandry, being directly involved in major operations like feeding, breeding, management and health care. Progress in this sector therefore can result in a more balanced development of the rural economy and contribute to reduction of poverty.

Livestock production systems mostly are based on low cost agro-by-products as nutritional input and use traditional technologies for producing milk, meat, egg, fibre. The holding size invariably is small. Medium to large herds of cattle and buffalo also exist in the periphery of large towns and cities mainly for supply of milk. Small ruminants and pigs are reared under extensive, semi-intensive and intensive systems of production. Although small farm production would continue to dominate animal production system, semi-intensive and intensive systems would also be adopted as commercial ventures. The livestock farming though is a major player in dry lands and hill regions, the focus of investment and developmental strategy still continues on crop agriculture. The priority in these regions should be on livestock production as more than 70% family income is derived from livestock. Such an approach will help to alleviate poverty and increase the family income of livestock owners in these regions.

Research and Technology

Commercial poultry production is often located in suburban areas and is supported by a large network of pure line performing layer and broiler breeding stocks, hatcheries and feed plants. Farm holdings with 1,000-10,000 birds for egg production and 100-500 birds for broiler production system after meeting household requirement, still contribute substantially, to the total egg and broiler production. It is this sector which needs to be addressed through research and technology.

The present trends indicate that animal protein requirement would rise faster than cereals in the consumption pattern mainly due to increase in income and need for quality food. Such a demand driven growth which is taking place mostly in developing countries will call for greater emphasis on harvesting, storing and processing facilities. Government and industry must prepare themselves for long term policies and investments that will satisfy consumer demand for foods of animal origin, improve nutrition, income and opportunities for employment. Productivity is the key to growth. We have no option but to improve productivity of our livestock through scientific breeding, feeding and management. Use of technological and marketing interventions in production, processing, and distribution of livestock products should be central theme of any future programme for livestock development. Technology support is imperative not only for enhancement of productivity but also for reduction of per unit cost. Generation and dissemination of appropriate technologies to enhance production and productivity should be given greater attention.

Sustainable Development Strategy

To meet this challenge, animals husbandry and dairying should receive a high priority. A sustainable and financially viable livestock and poultry farming, which will generate wealth and self-employment through entrepreneurship, is need of the day. The overall focus will have to be on four broad pillars, viz. (i) removing policy distortions that hinder the growth of livestock production; (ii) building participatory institutions for collective action by small scale farmers that allow them to get vertically integrated with livestock processors and input suppliers; (iii) creating an environment in which farmers increase investment for improved productivity in the livestock sector; and (iv) promoting effective regulatory institutions to deal with the threat of environmental and health crises stemming form livestock. For a financially viable livestock and poultry farming, technology support is imperative not only for enhancement of productivity but also reduction of unit cost. Technological and marketing interventions in production, processing and distribution of livestock products will be central to all future programmes for livestock development. Generation and dissemination of appropriate technologies for animal production and health care deserve high priority and particular attention of livestock owners, service providers, veterinarians and planners. All players in this sector will have to acquire the ability to absorb, assimilate and adopt the spectacular development in the animal and veterinary science and related technologies.

External markets are an extremely important source of demand and these need to be tapped much more aggressively. In order to encourage exports, licensing control for processing of livestock products/byproducts and restrictions on the export of livestock and its products need to be reviewed for devising liberal and pragmatic policies. Since animal disease eradication and quarantine is critical to exports, animal health systems will have to be strengthened and disease free zones created. After the successful eradication of rinderpest disease in most of Asia, the major thrust should now be to adopt a National Immunization Programme against the prevalent animal diseases. Some of the urgent action points which need consideration are:

(i) Conservation of threatened livestock breeds and improvement of draught animals.

(ii) Immunisation programme against important animal diseases and creation of disease free zones.

(iii) Enhancement of feed and fodder production using new bio-technologies and improvement of common property resources.

(iv) Building infrastructure for animal husbandry extension network (service providers):

(v) Biotechnologies which can bypass traditional genetics for improvement.

(vi) Broadening of Research and Educational base of scientists and farmers in new millennium.

Market-based Production

Opportunities for small to medium scale commercial animal production reflect global patterns of urbanization, economic development and globalization. These changes provide opportunities for farmers to move from subsistence production for primarily home use to market-oriented production with attendant demands for greater consistency of production, more reliable and predictable product quality, better producer organization, equitable price negotiations, reliable product delivery, access to credit, greater economic risk, and increasing competition for resources, markets, credit and political favours from outside the traditional agricultural sector. This system relies on increasing external inputs.

Livestock Production Inputs

Feeds and Fodder

Increasing livestock numbers, growing integration of farm households with both input and output markets over the past five decades; and the consequent increasing household income from livestock, have steadily pushed up the demand for production inputs and services in the livestock sector: feed, fodder, veterinary drugs, pharmaceuticals, vaccines, credit and insurance; as well as veterinary and AI services. There had also been matching increase in the supply of most of the inputs, except in the case of feed concentrates where critical shortages persist, if demand estimates based on nutritional requirements form the basis for balancing demand and supply. Over a third of the total dry matter intake of the large ruminants and almost 100 per cent in the case of the small ruminants, come from grazing in the common property resources, fallows and borders and boundaries of crop land. Common property resources, some 121 mln ha. (1989), had all been heavily overgrazed over decades of open access and are now in a state of denudation all over the country, with scanty biomass cover.

All livestock production in India is primarily based on crop residues and crop byproducts, as grain feeding for livestock production is seldom practiced, except for high yielding milch animals. In the commercial poultry industry however, grains form a substantial ingredient in the compounded poultry feeds. The commonly used crop residues are: straws, stalks, stovers, tops and crop thrush; and byproducts like: brans, husk, chunni, cotton seed, expeller cakes and solvent extracted meals of oil seeds/oil cakes. Demand estimates of feeds and fodder over the past five decades, consistently project huge deficits in the supply of all feed and fodder types: dry fodder 17 per cent, green 31 per cent and 47 per cent for concentrates (2000); while all species have increased in numbers (from 100 to over 400 per cent) and output of all livestock products have gone up by 300 to 400 per cent, over the same period. Demand estimates had all along been armchair exercises based on nutritional requirements (simplistic). Development of a methodology for estimating the effective/economic demand of feeds and fodder is long over due.

India has a growing animal feed milling industry, with a total compounded feed output of some 12 million mt in 2001 (some 25 per cent of the total raw feed ingredients available). The quality of the feed is highly variable, from very poor to extremely high quality. Even though there are standards for balanced animal feeds set up by the Bureau of Indian Standards, only a small percentage among the feed manufacturers conform to the standards. The feed milling infrastructure is made up of some 200 large feed milling plants of 100 to 500 mtpd, along with thousands of small and tiny milling plants of some 8 to 50 mtpd, scattered all over the country, particularly in clusters around the major grain markets in the country.

Not all the dry fodder available in the country is utilized for animal feed, some of it is used as industrial substrate (paper/packaging industry) and very large quantities are burnt *in situ* by farmers as a measure for disposal (millions of tons of wheat straw in Gujarat and rice straw in Punjab and Haryana). Application of industrial scale technologies (mechanical/ biotechnological) for enriching and pelletising/ briquetting straw are not attempted so far in the country, even though technologies exist and droughts accompanied by severe fodder shortage is rampant in some part or the other of the country, almost every year.

High–Input Production

High input production increasingly is becoming a global phenomenon. In the developed economies food costs are a relatively small percentage of disposable income, food security has been essentially achieved, and per capita consumption of animal products is stable or declining. In these economies issues of food quality, food safety and respect for animal welfare and the environment are of increasing importance. Farmers in developing nations must also address these issues if they aspire to market products in the most developed nations. High input livestock production is also becoming common in periurban areas of developing countries as urban populations expand and economic development leads to larger, more lucrative and more consistent markets for animal products. These systems often attract investments from outside traditional agricultural communities which do not contribute to facilitate rural development.

Policy makers must address the desired mix of systems including the need of each system as a part of comprehensive national development strategy. Moving away from the subsistence production is generally a development goal although the desired mix of households in other systems is much less clear, but will have a profound effect on the proportion of a nation's households involved in agriculture, and will likely differ among countries, depending on other, nonagricultural developments goals. It is within these three categories that scientists of this region have to interphase the technologies for alleviation of poverty, generation of wealth and employment.

Livestock production is an important source of income for the rural poor in developing countries. It enables poor and landless farmers to earn income using common-property resources, crop byproducts that would otherwise become waste; use land that has no other sustainable agricultural use. Livestock products are an important source of nutrients. The addition of milk and meat to the diet provides protein, calcium, vitamins, and other nutrients that are lacking in their usual diets. Besides providing food, the driving force behind increased livestock production, they have other valuable uses. Livestock remain the most important if not the sole form of nonhuman power available to poor farmers. The poor, in particular, use fertilizer from livestock operations. Livestock also act as a bank and provide insurance for people who have no other financial market available to them. Skins wool, fat and other resources are used as inputs in many industries. The rapid growth in livestock production is critical to designing policies that promote the incorporation of the rural poor into economically and environmentally sustainable growth patterns.

Employment

Animal Husbandry sector provides large self-employment to millions of households in rural areas both in principal status as well as in subsidiary status, this includes persons, employed in sale, reprocessing and transport of animal products at secondary market level. Apart from these, large manpower is involved in livestock related activities viz., manufacture of animal food products and beverages, manufacture of woolens, tanning and dressing of leather, farming of animals, production, processing and preserving meat and meat products, manufacture of dairy products, retail and wholesale trade of livestock products. Animal Husbandry and Dairying sector in India contributes about 22 percent of the value of the output from total agriculture and allied sector employment (1993-94) in animal husbandry sector was 9.8 million in principle status and 8.6 million in subsidiary status. Women constitute 71% of the labour force in livestock farming and 75% in dairying.

Thus rural women have a special place in this sector. They play a significant role in animal husbandry. Decisions in livestock production lie with men while those of feeding and milk production, breeding of animal and fodder cultivation lie with women. Although, women are involved in most livestock operations, their knowledge level is low. Therefore, in order to further increase income from livestock farming, knowledge level of women has to be increased. Special programmes need be taken up to move this employment growth to higher levels.

Increasing Demand

Population growth, urbanization and income growth in developing countries are fuelling a massive global increase in demand for food of animal origin, Twenty three percent of the world's population living in developed countries presently consume three to four times the meat and fish and five to six times the milk per capita as those in developing countries. A change has, however, taken place in the last few decades resulting in massive annual increases in the aggregate consumption of animal products in developing countries. From the early 1970s to the mid 1990s, consumption of meat in developing countries grew by 70 million metric tons, whereas consumption in developed countries grew by only 26 million metric tons. In value and caloric terms, meat consumption in developing countries increased by more than three times the increases in developed countries. Milk consumption in the developing world increased by more than twice as much as milk consumption in the developed world in terms of quantity, money value and calories. The consumption of food of animal origin is however still small, income increases would make people consume more of these items resulting in improved overall nutrition, export potential in this sector is immense which should be realized.

In India, food consumption pattern is gradually diversifying in favour of non-food-grain items like milk, meat and eggs. These changes in diets of millions of people will create a massive increase in demand for food of animal origin, which could provide income growth opportunities for many rural poor. But such demand driven growth will stretch the capacity of existing production and distribution systems. Rapid advances in feed improvement and genetic and reproductive technologies offer scope for overcoming many of the technical problems posed by increased livestock production. Productivity is the key to growth. We have no option but to raise the productivity of our livestock through scientific breeding, feeding and management. The goal should no longer be the farmer's share of the consumer's rupee; it should instead be a significant and sustained increase in farmer's income and employment. Government and industry must evolve long-term policies and make investments that will satisfy consumer demand, improve nutrition, direct income growth and create opportunities for those who need them most. All this will have to be done in a scenario that alleviates environmental and public health stress.

The demand for foods of animal origin comes from changes in the diets of billions of people and could provide income growth opportunities for many rural poor. This is what can be designated as "Livestock Revolution". The label is a simple and convenient expression that summarizes a complex series of interrelated processes and outcomes in production, consumption, and economic growth. As in the case of cereals, the stakes for the poor are enormous. Transformation has been brought in by new biology, which has changed the technologies and are knowledge intensive. The Green Revolution was supply-driven, whereas the Livestock Revolution is driven by demand. The demand driven 'Livestock Revolution' will stretch the capacity of existing production and distribution systems and exacerbate environmental and public health problems.

The rapid increases in this demand presents crucially important policy dilemmas that must be resolved for the well being of both rural and urban people in our country. These dilemmas involve complex environmental and public health issues in the context of weak regulatory environment. Taken together, many opportunities and dangers of the Livestock Revolution suggest that it would be foolish for us to adopt a "laissez faire" policy for livestock development. Technological progress in the production, processing, and distribution of livestock products will be central to the positive outcome of the Livestock Revolution. Rapid advances in feed improvement and genetic and reproductive technologies offer scope for overcoming many of the technical problems posed by increased livestock production. Institutional and regulatory development will also be critical to securing desirable environmental and public health outcomes.

Livestock and livelihood are closely interconnected in the country, since ownership of livestock is more egalitarian. Feed and fodder are the major limiting factors in enhancing farm animal productivity. Tamil Nadu has become a leader in egg and broiler production. There is therefore a growing demand for feed. We should establish a Livestock Feed Warehousing Corporation, which could support the establishment of feed and fodder banks operated by self-help groups (SHGs). Without such support, landless labour families will not be able to take up animal husbandry to supplement income.

Livestock Viability—Indian Scene

Livestock, as they are raised presently at subsistence farming level, is financially unviable but by increasing the unit size and using current technologies it has an opportunity of generating wealth and employment. Livestock enterprises with crossbred cattle and high yielding buffaloes have shown to be a remunerative business. Studies have shown that diary enterprise as against crops in rural areas has larger profit margins in marginal, small and medium holdings. Studies have also shown that dairying and crop production taken together by small farmers having irrigated land was more profitable than crop farming alone. On the macro level, prospects for the livestock sector look bright and is steadily marching to prepare-itself for the challenges in the next millennium. In India and many countries in South Asia, the land-man ratio is low and distribution of land is skewed; diversification of a crop based rural economy into an animal husbandry and or mixed farming system must be encouraged for rapid economic development and generating equitable income and employment in the country.

PERSPECTIVE

The country has largely been a vegetarian society and changed over from middle of last millennium to non-vegetarian, valid for a select group. Basically, it is the first fifty years or so which reflects a perceptible change in food habits. Customarily, families used to have goat/sheep meat once a weak, in the hinterland and hills, by certain castes, and fish on the seacoast. Now poultry and fish are the main dishes in well to do middle and upper level families. Pork has not been favorite dish of the majority except with a certain community particularly in the North East, while beef is a taboo among Hindus. No doubt demand for fish, milk and diary products are on the increase.

Food, Security now, is defined to mean Food and Nutrition Security, thus widening the scope to include consumption not only of cereals but also other non-cereal food items like meat, milk and eggs. This has given a new direction to the policy framers and the Administrators.

The growth in livestock sector in future is now being perceived not only in terms of food security but also in terms of income security. With about seventy percent of the population living in rural areas, of which, around fifty percent are landless agricultural labourers and a large number of small and marginal landholders being uneconomic holdings – many of these fall within the definition what is termed as living 'Below Poverty-Line' (BPL). It is essential to tackle the core problem of Poverty , i.e.. BPL families living in rural areas. But this dream shall remain where it has stayed so far a mere dream. Diversification is the answer and moving towards income generating activities like the one in livestock sector hold the key. The current stories of success in what is termed as White Revolution have been scripted by erstwhile landless and small/marginal farmers-be it in the sector of dairying, poultry or egg production. Lead in this sector was given by the hugely successful Cooperative sector followed by some Multinational Companies entering this sector-many establishing backward linkages thus profiting the small holders of the livestock assets including those families for whom this was a subsidiary occupation. Processing continued to be handled by a very large number of small-scale enterprises. This situation continues till date for the simple reason that the habitants of this country prefer fresh edible item—be it milk, meat fish, or fruits or vegetables.

With the highly ambitious yet attainable policy objective set by the Planners and Administrators, the country is factorizing the key inputs considered essential to reach these goals. Most essential among these include the factor of efficiencies, market development, market information, backward and forward linkages, i.e. livestock- business linkaging' as also Technological and more specifically the quality and hygiene parameters. Huge wastages and losses due to poor handling, absence of adequate cold chains are some of the other issues drawing the attention of the policy makers. It is realized that this sector ensures nutrition security as well as income security to a large number, yet the effort has to be balanced with its impact on environment and sensitivity associated with this sector in this country. The proposed policy on the subject and opening up of economy as part of the reform process and WTO related future trade-all bode well for the expansion and a much higher investment in this sector. This sector is likely to grow at a much faster and higher rate than its competitor – agriculture sector.

The objective of this study is to develop a clear understanding of the growth potential of livestock and livestock industry in India, identify challenges it faces and to develop a clear road map of its development. Poverty, Food and Nutrition security are the emerging threats in India as well as in south Asia. Part of the response to this 'challenge' lies perhaps in the developments in this sector. With the introduction of economic reforms, liberalization and opening up of economy the middle class is bound to be on high swell, demand for high value goods led by food, beverages, meat and other livestock products are also going to be on the rise as a result of rising income level, not a little part being contributed by major international players especially in view of the Import-Export Policy –2001 announced on 31st March 2001 opening the doors to milk, meat and poultry industry albeit within certain phyto-sanitary parameters.

India boasts success of Green Revolution, White Revolution (milk and dairy products), Yellow Revolution (oil seed-source of vegetable fat) and Blue Revolution (fish production) and leaders and administrators have started taking of a second Green revolution to touch the rainfed areas. It is time that livestock sector Revolution is also brought on the agenda of the policy makers and programme administrators with a view to developing an 'integrated' approach to Livestock sector including its 'processing', its effects on Health Environment, Income et al. Hence the importance and urgency of undertaking this Study which seems to be well timed.

Straws, stovers and agricultural by-product will continue to be the major input as livestock feed for ruminants. Unfortunately, the existing technologies for improving digestibility of straws have not been used by the farmer. The need is to use biotechnological techniques to develop the recombinant microbes to digest straws and make available energy for livestock feeding. Suitable investments in research and technology development need to be made. Efforts also need to be made to increase availability of green fodder and grasses through increasing area under fodder crops, agro-forestry, etc. The issue of shortage of fodder seeds needs to be addressed on priority basis. Feed quality standards need to be enforced and updated to ensure availability of quality compound feed to the livestock owners.

Animal husbandry and dairying should receive a high priority both in research and development efforts for generating employment and investment, increasing animal protein availability in the food basket and for generating exportable surpluses. A sustainable and financially viable livestock and poultry farming, which will generate wealth, and self-employment is need of the day. The overall focus should be on (i) removing policy distortions which are hindering the natural growth of livestock production; (ii) building participatory institutions of collective action especially for small farmers that allows them to get vertically integrated with livestock processors and input suppliers; (iii) creating environment for increased investment to improve productivity; and (iv) promoting effective regulatory institutions to deal with the environmental and health threats stemming from livestock.

Over the years, a wealth of experience and results of the livestock sector have been generated and parts of them have been written up, stored as hard copies in official records and some archives. They are, however, not readily accessible to outside. Some of the key information and results are only available from key sources persons who played an active role in the development programmes for the livestock sector.

Fortunately, the value of proper knowledge management has lately been recognized and efforts are being undertaken by some institutions to capitalize on past experience in order to improve future actions. In this spirit the authors have undertaken this compressive study to review past experience in the livestock sector and the future road map of this important sector. Livestock could play a strategic role in promoting rural growth and reducing rural poverty. The study identifies key issues and recommends policy directions and investments to promote the livestock's growth in all subsections including sheep, goats and poultry. Also the book comprehensively addresses the linkages between globalization/liberalization process to the future of livestock sector and rural poverty and offers solutions.

The study dwells on the current livestock systems, which are based on low cost agro-products as nutritional inputs, using traditional technologies for productivity. A number of suggestions are made to improve the production systems so as to make the sector more competitive and face the challenges posed by the gloabalisation.

A section is devoted to the role of livestock sector in the economy. A detailed review is provided on the wealth and growth of livestock population and their distribution among states and according to the size of land holdings. Livestock fulfills many roles in the rural economy. The sector plays a significant role in the welfare of India's rural population. The sector employed eight percent of the country's labour force including vast majority of small and marginal farmers, women and landless agricultural workers. Milk production involves more than 30 million small producers, each raising one or two cows or buffaloes. In additional to being an important source of supplying nutritious food, supplementary income and employment for poor households, livestock supply a significant portion of draft power and rural transportation. The organic fertilizers produced by the sector is an important input to crop production, and dung from livestock is widely used as fuel in rural areas. Livestock also serves as an insurance substitute especially for poor rural household, it can easily be sold during times of distress. The progress of processing of milk, poultry and leather is also reviewed and the challenges and opportunities in these sub-sectors are analyzed. An important aspect is the industrialization of livestock industries. Industrialization is a concept that may be defined in a number of ways. Typically industrialization occurs with large-scale operation that has high capital labour ratios. Vertical integration, involving production linkages with input suppliers and distribution firms, is usually of industrialized livestock production.

Industrialization of livestock raises many important issues including the effect on the environment, on small economically vulnerable farmers, human nutrition and health. The study deals with all these problems. Production performance of individual livestock products, i.e. milk and milk products, meat and meat products, eggs and poultry meat, hides and skins and wool and hairs, is reviewed and contributions of various factors in growth are analysed. Policy reforms are essential at both the central and state government levels for promoting growth and increasing marketing efficiency. The study identifies the most pressing issues facing the livestock sector.

Livestock development needs to be balanced with environmental conservation. Attempt is made to list environmental degradation caused by the livestock sector in India and also discusses the positive impact of livestock sector on environment. The growth in livestock populations, coupled with shrinking grazing areas, has put intense pressure on existing pastures, encouraged encroachment into forestland and contributed to the degradation of land resources. Moreover, livestock processing particularly leather processing also has been a major cause of industrial pollution. The study reviews the attempts made by various stakeholders to minimize the detrimental impact on environment by the livestock sector and suggests measures to balance the significant benefits generated by the livestock sector with environmental conservation.

The problems of marketing livestock and livestock products are discussed in detail. The study emphasizes that increasing livestock marketing efficiency is critical to meet future growth in demand for livestock products. The Operation Flood has been no doubt successful in spreading the diary cooperatives concept and providing an important demonstration effect on the potential for diary development in India. However, many cooperatives are performing poorly. The underlying causes and remedies for these are suggested. The cooperatives have considerable potential to improve their performance. Promoting marketing competition is needed to ensure development of a sustainable and efficient dairy industry. This implies ensuring a level playing for all participants and elimination of any barriers to entry to any firm. The creation of a level playing field for all market participants will require a package of reforms, which are dealt with in the study.

Ensuring an adequate supply of livestock inputs is essential. Currently national feed suppliers fall short of 20-30 percent of the requirement. This deficit is equivalent to about 250 million tones of dry feed per year. Future projections indicate a widening gap. The chapter on feed and fodder supplies reviews the current status and identifies constraints that hamper their development. Structural problems and public sector policies influencing the performance of the sector are examined. The challenge of improving the genetic base in India, which could increase the efficiency of feed use, is also discussed. Moreover, a comparative study of roughage production and utilization in India and selected Asian countries is presented in separate chapter.

The government livestock policy and livestock support services are reviewed. The Government policies covered scientific management and genetic upgradation of cattle and buffalo, expansion of existing infrastructure and delivery of breeding inputs and services to farmers, control animal disease, creation of disease free zones, development of processing and marketing facilities. The examination of the policies reveals a number of problem areas. Several crucial changes would have therefore to be introduced in the Government policy for livestock sector in the future. For instance the future strategies for development of livestock have to be based on a mixed approach of reduction in population number and vertical genetic improvement of livestock, For, hygienic meat production an implementation of pragmatic slaughter policy is important. The needed policy reforms are dealt with.

Food processing industry, which is nascent sector in the country, has enormous potential. To ascertain the reason for poor capacity utilization, a field study was carried out. The results of the field survey are presented in the study. The development of the sector so far has been primarily because of the positive perception of its potential at the Central Government level and not because of interest of domestic or overseas business community. The study recommends that maximum emphasis has to be laid on quality control in production and processing in order to improve quality and acceptability of finished products both in the domestic and international markets.

In addition to proper feed and production management, livestock health and breeding services are crucial in achieving the productive potential of livestock. For this a number of suggestions are made. To increase the availability of and access to animal health services, the state's focus should shift towards delivery partly of public services while the private sector should take over activities such as clinical treatment and noncompulsory vaccinations. Key steps required to promote private participation in animal services are dealt with. Impact of livestock sector on public health is also discussed.

A perspective of market opportunities and challenges, both in the domestic and international markets, is presented. The analyses cover Emerging Trends in Consumption of Livestock Products, Demand and Supply Projections to the year 2030 and performance of international trade and the future projections. The foreign trade Chapter discusses specifically the likely level of the trade for individual products and the likely trading partners for these. The detailed discussions in followed by SWOT analysis. These analyses identify Strengths. Weakness, Opportunities and Threats for various sub-sectors of livestock sector as well as for overall livestock sector. Goals and objectives of the governments contained in the Vision Statement and other documents form part of the discussion in these chapters.

The Study

Currently little reliable information is available on the level of employment in the livestock sector. In fact an estimation of employment in the sector is rather tricky job. While it is primarily a part time avocation, there is no holiday from the job, which has to be performed every day. We have tried to put together all the available information and provided an estimate of total employment relating to the maintenance of the livestock population. We have stressed that livestock employment under Indian conditions has its own peculiarities and have suggested the urgent need to evolve an appropriate methodology by a team of experts. This chapter also discusses the effect of the livestock sector development on women and children in India, who play an important role in this sector.

Current systems of data collection on livestock sector and implementation of various schemes in the animal husbandry and dairy statistics and livestock census are reviewed. Although considerable resources have been directed toward collecting and disseminating information on basic crops (cereals groundnuts and so on) less attention has been given to collecting, disseminating, and analyzing livestock and livestock product data. Timely information on prices, volumes produced, quantities traded, locational availability, and stocks are largely unavailable. Agricultural market information is vital, because such data are not only a key input for informed planning and decision making by agricultural market participants, but also for effective government policy formulation and administrative decision making. A number of recommendations are made to improve the data collection and its timely dissemination among all the stakeholders.

Economics of livestock enterprises are worked out separately for dairy cow and buffalo units, for goats, sheep and poultry. Livestock farming in general and the diary industry and poultry have undergone great changes, both in their structure and methods of production. A wide range of factors are involved in determining the ultimate profitability of these enterprises and much confused thinking persists on the relative importance of each factors. All these factors are discussed in detailed and samples of economic enterprises of the above-mentioned sub-sectors have been prepared. It is, however, essential to underline that these samples are based on limited data available and number of assumptions and these need to be improved further based on actual data. However, we hope that these samples will serve as a useful guide to research workers and financial institutions.

2

Livestock Population

First a few revealing quantitative approximations regarding the surprising but curiously little-noted biomass of domestic animals are presented — the rapidly growing zoomass of domestic animals has made dairy and meat mammals the dominant class of vertebrates on Earth. In 1900 there were some 1.3 billion large animals, including about 500 million head of cattle; a century later, after growing at about the same rate as humans, the count of large domestic animals surpassed 4.3 billion, including 1.65 billion head of cattle and water buffaloes and 900 million pigs. Calculations based on the best available head counts and on typical average body weights result in less than 180 mt of live weight of domesticated zoomass in 1900, and in no less than 620 mt in 2000, a nearly 3.5 fold increase during the twentieth century in contrast, the zoomass of wild terrestrial mammals is now most likely below 40 mt. or less than 10 percent of the biomass of domestical meat and dairy species.

The contrast is even greater for the largest herbivores. Bovine biomass is now almost 450 mt, while the zoomass of remaining African elephants, whose population was about 387,000 in 1995, even when using a high average body mass of 2,500 kg/elephant, was less than 1 mt or not even 0.2 percent of the worldwide mass of cows, bulls, calves, steers, and heifers. Moreover, the global cattle count has grown by some 130 million head since 1980, while African elephants, although prospering in some countries, now number only a fraction of their total a half-century ago. This is not an appealing thought: if sapient extraterrestrial visitors could get an instant census of mammalian biomass on the Earth in order to judge the importance of organisms simply by their abundance, they would conclude that life on the third solar planet is dominated by cattle.

LIVESTOCK WEALTH OF INDIA

In terms of population, India is the second largest in the world with over a billion people. Situated in the continent of Asia, it is well marked off from the rest of the Asian countries by mountains and seas and extends north—south between latitudes 68 and 99 degrees east. Consequently the country has regions lying in the tropical, sub-tropical and temperate zones. The agro-climatic variations range between extremes in respect of soils, temperature, rainfall etc. Widely varying climatic zones occur, such as high altitude Himalayan regions, the Indo-Gangetic plains, hot arid zones in Western India, the Deccan plateau in the south and hot humid coastal areas.

Agriculture development in India has almost reached a plateau, due to various reasons. It has, therefore, become necessary to diversify to improve the economic condition of the landless, small and marginal farmers, who form the bulk of the population of the country. Given the situation, livestock sector, which has a great potential for development, will be the main focus of development planners in the decades to follow. The agro-climatic diversity of the country with 15 agro-climatic regions, is a unique opportunity for the people to exploit the natural resources for the sustainable development of agriculture and livestock industry. Recent studies indicate that the northern, western, southern and some pockets of eastern regions of the country are best suited for dairy development and the north eastern areas, including tribal dominated regions of Jharkhand and Chhattisgarh have great scope for the development of monogastric animals, backyard poultry and small ruminants, primarily due to reasons of geography and socio-cultural traditions. However northeast and the other tribal dominated areas of the country lack basic infrastructure, essential inputs and marketing facilities. Each region therefore needs different development strategies and orchestration.

Historically India contributed significantly to world animal production: the Red Indian Jungle fowl is the progenitor of the modern commercial layer and broiler breeds, the Indian Runne duck is a source of the best breeds of ducks in the world. Jamanpari was the male parent of Anglo Nubian goats; Sindhi, Sahiwal, Ongole, Kankrej and Gir have contributed to the now famous tropical dairy and meat breeds of the world.[1]

LIVESTOCK CENSUS DURING PRE-INDEPENDENCE PERIOD

Cattle and buffaloes are occupying a pivotal position in the national life since time immemorial. The first livestock census in the country was undertaken in 1919-20 and till Independence, six such censuses were undertaken. The number of cattle and buffaloes under different broad classifications enumerated from the first to sixth Livestock Census (1919-20 to 1945) are given in Table 2.1. It would be observed that there had been a small but progressive increase in the number of male and female cattle from the year 1919-20 to 1929-30. The number of animals in each of the categories as well as of total cattle showed a progressive decrease

---

[1]Bhat, P.N. and Batobyal, Asim: Science and Technology in Animal Husbandry Development – A Key to Future. *Indian Journal of Animal Production*: Vol. 30: Nos. 1-4, January –December, 1998: p. 21.

Table 2.1: Cattle and Buffalo Population in Undivided India 1919-20 to 1944-45[A,1,2,3]

(In '000 nos.)

Category	1919-20	1924-25	1929-30	1934-35	1939-40	1944-45
Cattle:						
Bulls	5100	4,672	3980	48870	46856	47319
Bullocks	41642	43886	45372			
Sub- total	46742	48558	49352			
Cows	35863	36434	37295	37255	36445	35140
Youngstock (calves)	30138	30299	31119	34463	32216	28998
TOTAL CATTLE	112743	115291	117766	120588	115517	111457
Buffaloes :						
Male	5091	5054	5224	5473	4911	4979
Female	12968	13796	14376	15039	15131	15646
Youngstock(calves)	9385	10570	11001	12645	12053	11395
TOTAL BUFFALOES	27444	29420	30601	33157	32095	32020
Grand Total (Cattle and Buffaloes)	140187	144711	148367*	153745**	147612@	143477

* Exclusive of the two Agency districts of the NW Frontier Province (NWFP).

** Includes 1929-30 census figures for Bengal, Bihar and Orissa where no census was taken in 1934-35, but excludes those for the two Agency districts of the NWFP.

@Includes 1935-36 census figures for Orissa and 1934-35 census figures for U.P. where no census was taken in 1939-40 but excludes those for the two Agency districts of N.W.F.P.

[A]Relates to territories now constituted as Indian Union, Pakistan and Bangladesh.

[1]*Indian Agricultural Statistics*, Vol. I (Provinces) 1939-40 to 1942-43 (pages 2 and 3).

[2]*Agricultural Statistics of India*, Vol. I- 1919-20 (page 8).

[3]*Indian Agricultural Statistics* 1943-47, Vol. 1 (page 2).

between 1934-35 and 1944-45. There was a small but steady increase in the total buffalo population up to the year 1934-35. Thereafter there was a slight decline. The number of she-buffaloes, however, maintained a steady rise right upto 1945, registering an increase of about 4.5 million over 1919-20 population. These data call for two interesting observations. Death rate of livestock during this period must had been very high and secondly, the numbers would appear to be highly underestimated. Indian Union alone had 198.7 million bovine (1951) against 143.5 (1944-45) for united India. The National Commission on Agriculture (1976) pointed out that "for the census period 1919-1945 figures in respect of only the British Provinces have been taken into consideration as participation of the then Princely States in census enumeration was not regular".[2]

_____

[2]Report of the National Commission on Agriculture, 1976, Part VII, Animal Husbandry, p.3.

Kinds and Growth Pattern

The country is a treasure house of livestock animals with great diversity of germplasms, ranging from cattle, buffaloes, goats and sheep to mithuns and yaks of Himalaya. Livestock population increased from 293 million in 1951 to about 471 million in 1992. It was for the first time that there was a perceptible decline in livestock population to 452.4 million according to 1997 census (Table 2.2). Based on the statistical data available India has the second largest livestock population in the world, next to China which occupies the first place because of its largest number of pig, sharing almost 40 per cent of world pig population.

The absolute number of all the categories of livestock increased till 1992. Of the total livestock population, bovines account for the lion's share followed by ovine and pigs. Of the total bovine population, cattle outnumber buffaloes. Indian livestock economy is, therefore, often referred to as the cow economy. However, over the years there is a slow but perceptible change in favour of buffaloes. Estimates for the 1997 livestock Census

Table 2.2: Livestock Population – 1951 to 1997 All India Speciewise

(In million numbers)

Species	1951	1956	1961	1966	1972	1977	1982	1987	1992	1997
1. Cattle	155.30	158.70	175.60	176.20	178.30	180.00	192.45	199.69	204.58	174.97
2. Adult Female Cattle	54.40	47.30	51.00	51.80	53.40	54.60	59.21	62.07	64.36	N.A.
3. Buffaloes	43.40	44.90	51.20	53.00	57.40	62.00	69.78	75.97	84.21	84.02
4. Adult Female Buffalo	21.00	21.70	24.30	25.40	28.60	31.30	32.50	39.13	43.81	N.A.
5. Total Bovines	198.70	203.60	226.80	229.20	235.70	242.00	262.36	275.82	289.00	259.00
6. Sheep	39.10	39.30	40.20	42.00	40.00	41.00	48.76	45.70	50.78	55.30
7. Goat	47.20	55.40	60.90	64.60	67.50	75.60	95.25	110.21	115.28	102.26
8. Horses & Ponies	1.50	1.50	1.30	1.10	0.90	0.90	0.90	0.80	0.82	0.71
9. Camels	0.60	0.80	0.90	1.00	1.10	1.10	1.08	1.00	1.03	0.91
10. pigs	4.40	4.90	5.20	5.00	6.90	7.60	10.07	10.62	12.79	12.37
11. Mules	0.06	0.04	0.05	0.08	0.08	0.09	0.13	0.17	0.19	0.29
12. Donkeys	1.30	1.10	1.10	1.10	1.00	1.00	1.02	0.96	0.97	0.78
13. Yak	NC	NC	0.02	0.03	0.04	0.13	0.13	0.04	0.06	0.07
14. Total Livestock	292.80	306.60	335.40	344.10	353.40	369.00	419.50	445.28	470.86	452.45
15. Poultry	73.50	94.80	114.20	115.40	138.50	159.20	207.74	275.32	307.07	347.61
16. Dogs	NC	NC	NC	NC	NC	NC	18.54	17.95	21.77	20.3
17. Rabits	-	-	-	-	-	-	-	-	-	0.3

N.C. = Not Collected Total Livestock excludes Mules an Yaks.

Source:- Livestock Census Reports – Directorate of Economics and Statistics.

indicate that in absolute terms, the number of cattle has declined for the first time. Cattle accounted for 78.2 percent of total bovine population in 1951. It declined to 71 percent by 1992 and further to 67.5 percent in 1997. Similarly, of the total ovine population, goats outnumber sheep. Goats accounted for 55 percent of the total ovine population in 1951, which increased to 69 percent by 1992 but declined to 65 percent in 1997. The absolute number of poultry birds has increased manifold over this period. The pattern of livestock population statistics clearly reveals that cattle rearing still dominates the livestock sector (38.67 percent of the total) and the importance of buffalo, goat and poultry is increasing. The annual growth rate for total livestock was 1.14 percent, although it varied widely during different periods, ranging from as low as 0.53 percent during 1966 - 1972 to 2.6 percent during 1977-82 (Table 2.3). The state-wise livestock and poultry population in 1997 is given in Appendix I.

Annual Growth Rate

There have been significant variations in the nature and magnitude of growth rates in the population of different species of livestock during 1951 to 1997 (Table 2.3 and Graph 2.1). The rate of growth in buffalo population is almost thrice that of cattle. Similarly, goats grew at a faster rate than sheep. Notwithstanding annual slaughter rate of around 40%, goats are growing at the rate of 2.5 percent. Poultry witnessed spectacular growth and its number has increased by over fourfold i.e. from 73.5 million to 307 million during the period 1951 to 1992. The rapid annual growth rate in poultry husbandry may be attributed to the fact that amongst farm animals, poultry is one of the quickest and most efficient converters of plant products into food of high biological value. Further, requirement of small area, low initial capital investment, manageability with ease by women and children, use of various kinds of by-products unfit for human consumption as feed-stuff, quick returns and well distributed turnover throughout the year make poultry farming remunerative in both the rural and urban areas. Most of the livestock species recorded highest growth during 1977-82 inter census period, thereafter showing a declining trend. The growth rates are indicative of suitability of the species under present production system and preference of the farmers.

Since 1951 there is a steady growth in the bovine population in the country. Though the average annual growth rate is less than 1 per cent in respect of cattle population except during the period 1956-61 and 1977-82 when the growth rates were 2.04 and 1.35 per annum respectively the cattle population in the country has already become very large as the base itself was very large. In case of buffalo, the average annual growth rate exceeded 1 per cent. There had been a progressive increase in the number of cattle and buffaloes from 1951 onwards, but for 1992-97 when there was a sharp decline. The quality and productivity of the majority of this bovine population are very poor. There is also an adverse relationship between the number of cattle and buffalo population and land utilization pattern and·

Table 2.3: Growth Pattern of Livestock Population, India - 1951 to 1997

Species	Annual Growth Rates (%)								
	1951-56	1956-61	1961-66	1966-72	1972-77	1977-82	1982-87	1987-92	1992-97
1. Cattle	0.43	2.04	0.07	0.24	0.19	1.35	0.74	0.48	-2.89
2. Adult Female Cattle	-2.76	1.52	0.31	0.61	0.45	1.63	0.95	0.73	
3. Buffalo	0.68	2.66	0.69	1.61	1.55	2.39	1.71	2.08	-0.04
4. Adult Female Buffalo	0.66	2.29	0.89	2.40	1.82	0.76	3.78	2.28	
5. Total Bovines	0.49	2.18	0.21	0.56	0.53	1.63	1.01	0.94	-2.06
6. Sheep	0.10	0.45	0.88	-0.97	0.50	3.53	-1.29	2.13	1.78
7. Goats	3.26	1.91	1.19	0.88	2.29	4.73	2.96	0.90	-2.26
8. Horses & Ponies	0.00	-2.82	-3.29	-3.93	0.00	0.00	-2.33	0.49	-2.59
9. Camels	5.92	2.38	2.13	1.92	0.00	-0.37	-1.53	0.59	-2.37
10. Pigs	2.18	1.20	-0.78	6.65	1.95	5.79	1.07	3.79	-0.66
11. Mules	-7.79	4.56	9.86	0.00	2.38	7.63	5.51	2.25	9.64
12. Donkeys	-3.29	0.00	0.00	-1.89	0.00	0.40	-1.21	0.21	-3.91
13. Yaks	N.C.	N.C	8.45	5.92	26.58	0.00	-21.00	8.45	4.14
14. Total Livestock	0.93	1.81	0.51	0.53	0.87	2.60	1.20	1.12	-0.78
15. Poultry	5.22	3.79	0.21	3.72	2.82	5.47	5.79	2.21	13.2
16. Dogs	—	—	—	—	—	—	-0.64	3.93	-6.77

N.C. = Not Collected

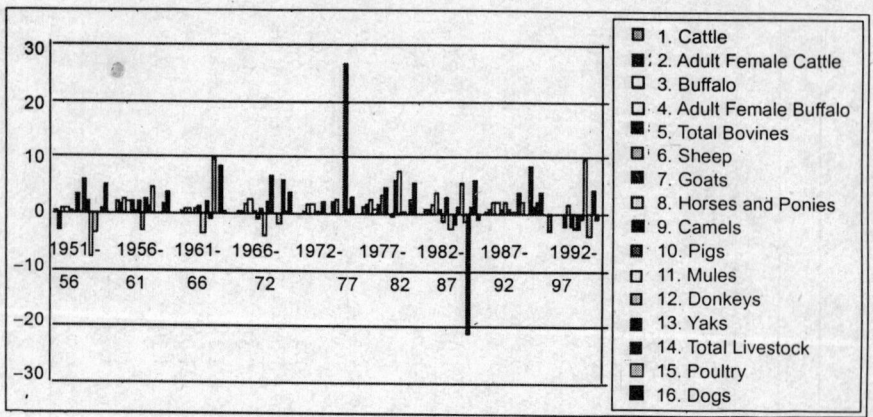

Graph 2.1: Growth Pattern of Livestock Population, India-1951-1992

the availability of feeds and fodder. The large number of cattle and bullocks in the country is the result of operation of a vicious circle causing degeneration in the quality of bovine animals. It is of utmost importance that the trend of future cattle and buffalo population in the country should show significant increase in the proportion of improved types with overall reduction in the total numbers.

NSSO Estimates

There is another source for estimates of livestock population. According to the NSSO data, during the period 1971/72 to 1991/92 the cattle population that declined (from 175 million to 169 million) during the first of the two decades was more than compensated by the rise in the following decade. Nevertheless according to the livestock census data, cattle population increased steadily from 178 million in 1971/72 to 204 million in 1991/92 (Table 2.3 A). The buffalo population during this period increased from 57 million to 84 million.

There has been a significant variation in the nature and magnitude of growth rates in the population of different species of livestock during 1971/72 to 1991/92. During the 1970s and 1980s, there was a fairly extensive growth of mechanization in agriculture. This reduced the importance of bullock power in crop cultivation and other allied activities. This was reflected in the fall in the stock of working cattle from 73 million in 1971/72 to 66 million in 1981/82 in rural areas. With the falling requirement of bullock power in cultivation, it appears likely that cattle rearing had slackened during this decade. As a result, the number of in-milk cattle too, declined from 27 million in 1971/72 to 19 million in 1981/82. However, by this time the campaign for Operation Flood were well under way[3]. The following decade saw a substantial expansion in the coverage of the campaign. Besides there was a growing demand for milk in the agriculturally advanced states like Punjab and Haryana. The consequent growth in dairy farming during the 1980s brought about an increase in the cattle population, with a shift in its composition towards in-milk cattle and away from working cattle in 1992.

Table 2.3 A: Number of Livestock in Different NSS Rounds: Rural and Urban

(No. in million)

Livestock/ poultry	Area	1971/72	1981/82	1991/92	Growth rate 1991/ 92 over 19881/82 (percent)
1. Cattle	Rural	169	161	169	0.5
	Urban	6	8	8	...
	Total	175	169	177	0.5
		(178)	(192)	(204)	(6.3)
2. Buffalo	Rural	48	64	73	1.4
	Urban	3	3 •	4	2.9
	Total	51	67	77	1.4
		(57)	(70)	(84)	(19.6)
3. Bovine	Rural	217	225	242	0.7
	Urban	9	11	12	0.9
	Total	226	236	262	1.1
		(236)	(262)	(288)	(9.9)
4. Poultry	Rural	79	135	193	3.6
	Urban	5	13	33	9.7
	Total	84	148	226	4.3
		(138)	(208)	(308)	(42.3)

Note: Figures in brackets are livestock census data of 1972, 1982 and 1992 respectively. *Source*: Sarvekshana: Summary Findings of NSSO Land and Livestock Holdings Survey: July-September 1998.

There is a strong positive association between in-milk bovine stock and size of household operational holdings. The larger sized holdings, endowed with greater resources for fodder supply, investments and human labour time, could naturally maintain a larger bovine stock. The landless, marginal and small holdings, on the other hand, with their limited resources, had fewer in-milk cattle and buffaloes on an average. The positive relationship in in-milk bovine stock, however, gradually weakened during the two decades since 1971/72. The ratio of in-milk bovine stock to 100 household in the marginal, small and semi-medium categories in each decade moved in the same direction as the all-categories ratio. The ratio for the medium and larger holdings, on the other hand, declined progressively during the period. With the marginal and smallholdings becoming less and less viable for crop production owing to rising costs of cultivation, the households with such holdings are turning to dairy farming in greater proportion (Table 2.3 B).

The share of marginal category in dairy farming has risen during the last two decades. The marginal and small categories form the core of the milk production sector. Taken together, they accounted for about 66 percent of

Table 2.3 B: Changes in the in-milk Bovine Stock Per 100 Households by Category of Household Operational Holdings

(Rural)

Category	In-milk bovine stock per 100 hhs		
	71-72 (26th Round)	*81-82 (37th Round)*	*91-92 (48th Round)*
Nil	16	7	6
Marginal	33	28	41
Small	64	48	69
Semi-medium	92	74	80
Medium	142	106	102
Large	225	153	130
All	54	37	46

Source: Sarvekshana: Summary findings of NSSO Livestock and Household and Household Operational Holdings survey : 76th Issue July Septemeber, 1998.

in-milk bovine stock in 1991/92. Also there has been a sharp increase in the percentage share of marginal category in the in-milk bovine population. This percentage increased steadily from 20 percent in 1971/72 to 44 percent in 1991/92. Buffalo, in dairy farming activity, yield higher returns as compared to the cattle stock. Buffaloes are used mainly for milk production. The in-milk stock accounted for substantially higher proportion of the population among the buffaloes (43 percent in 1991/92) than among the cattle (only 18 percent).

Besides the rise in the percentage of buffaloes in the in-milk bovine stock since 1971/72, the pattern and composition of in-milk bovine stock across the size-categories of holdings have undergone a considerable change. Changes in the in-milk cattle and buffalo stock per 100 households by categories of holdings during the last two decades are shown in Table 2.3 C. There has been increasing use of buffaloes in dairy farming, especially in the holdings of higher size-categories. In the marginal and small farmers categories, the number of in-milk cattle per 100 households was more than in-milk buffaloes. The medium and large holdings, on the other hand, have shown a clear preference for buffalo in dairy farming. In these two size-categories, while the number of in-milk cattle per 100 households has declined in both the decades, the number of in-milk buffaloes per 100 households, after having fallen in 1980, has increased substantially in 1990. However, in the first three categories the number of in-milk cattle had increased from 1980 to 1990. The preference for buffalo reflects the access to higher financial, feed and manpower resources by these two-categories of farmers and probably also due to higher income/ profit earned by buffalo from the sale of milk. The expansion of in-milk herds in 1990 serves as an anecdotal evidence that all groups of Indian rural society benefited from dairy farming.

Table 2.3 C: Changes in the in-milk Cattle Stock and Buffaloes Per 100 Households in Rural India

Category	No. of "in-milk" cattle			No. of "in-milk" buffalo		
	1971/72	1981/82	1991/92	1970/71	1981/82	1991/92
Nil	9	3	5	7	4	6
Marginal	23	15	25	10	13	16
Small	41	26	38	24	22	31
Semimedium	58	40	39	35	34	41
Medium	86	54	43	56	51	59
Large	140	86	43	85	67	87
All	34	20	26	20	17	20

Source: National Sample Survey: Sarvekshana: July-September 1998 op. cit.

The country ranked first in the case of cattle and buffalo population and accounted for 57 percent of the world buffalo and 16 percent of the cattle population (Table 2.4). In respect of goat, sheep population, India's share was 16 percent and 5.7 percent respectively in 2003 ranking second and third position respectively. Of all the livestock species in India, bovine (cattle and buffalo) alone accounted for about 64 percent. The percentage increase among different livestock species varied considerably. The total livestock population increased by 5.7 percent while buffalo population rose by 10.8 percent but number of cattle increased only by 2.4 percent between 1951 and 1992, but declined sharply by about 15 per cent in 1997. Total poultry birds increased by 11.5 percent.

Table 2.4: Livestock population in the World and India : 1998 and 2003

(In million nos.)

Livestock	World		India		India's share in the world (in percentage)	
	1998	2003	1998	2003	1998	2003
Cattle	1318.4	1368.0	209.5	226.1	15.9	16.5
Buffaloes	162.4	170.5	91.8	96.9	56.5	56.8
Sheep	1064.0	1028.6	56.5	59.0	5.3	5.7
Goats	699.9	764.5	120.6	124.5	17.2	16.3
Horses	60.9	56.3	0.9	0.8	1.6	1.4
Camels	19.1	18.4	1.0	0.9	5.4	4.9
Pigs	953.6	952.9	16.0	18.5	1.7	1.9

Source: FAO: Production Year Book and FAOSTAT online

LIVESTOCK COMPOSITION

The composition of livestock population has undergone significant transformation. First, the share of bovine population declined from about 68 percent in 1951 to less than 61 percent in 1992 and 57 percent in 1997.

However, the share of goats increased from 16 to 23 percent in 1997. Within the bovine population, there has been a significant shift towards buffaloes. The share of buffaloes, in the bovine population increased from 22 to 32 percent. Further, within cattle there has been a marked shift from work animals towards milch animals. Finally, within the milch cattle, the population of crossbred cows has grown at a much faster rate than the indigenous stock. For example, the population of crossbred cows increased at the rate of 7.2 percent during 1987-92, compared to 1.25 percent for indigenous cows. As a result, the number of crossbred cows increased from 7.5 million in 1987 to 10.6 million in 1992 (Table 2.5).

India has a very large, diverse and dynamic livestock genetic resource base, with many known and catalogued breeds among all species of livestock and poultry, though their population size varies and some of them are on the decline. There had so far been no worthwhile effort to develop the potential of indigenous breeds, even though there is a lot of rhetoric on conservation of biodiversity. As regards genetic diversity of cattle, there are 30 breeds of cattle, each having its own characteristics. These are: Amrit Mahal, Bachur, Bargur, Dangi, Deoni, Gaolao, and Gir. Hallikar, Hariana, Kangayam, Kankrej, Kenkantha, Khurugarh, Khillari, Krishna valley, Malvi, Mewati, Nagori, Nimari, Ongole, Ponwar, Punganur, Rathi, Red Kandhari, Red Sindi, Sahiwal, Siri, Tharparkar, Umbalachery and Vechur.

While some breeds are known for their high milk yield, others are known for producing quality bulls/bullocks. Many of the breeds have distinctive features. Some breeds can thrive well under cold and temperate conditions, whereas other thrives well under hot and humid conditions. In the present era of rapid advances in biotechnology particularly molecular biology, the genetic diversity available in respect of cows in India is a unique type of wealth. This may be a source of developing new breeds with higher potential.

Buffaloes are the main source of milk in India. They can thrive under hard conditions and on poor quality feeds and concentrates. In addition to providing milk, buffaloes are also a source of employment for the rural poor and landless families. In fact, the Government of India tried to create jobs by encouraging buffalo rearing in the rural areas under various programmes of poverty alleviation and employment generation in late 1970s. India possesses some of the best milk buffalo breeds in the world. These include Murah, Nili-Ravi and Surti. The other prominent breeds of buffaloes found in India are Bhadawari, Jaffarabadi, Marathawada, Mehsana, Nagpuri, Pandhar Puri and Toda. This kind of diversity is a great strength for the development of India's livestock sector. India with 83.5 million buffaloes (1992) accounts for 58% share in the global buffalo population. Though buffaloes are widely distributed throughout the country, their concentration is significant in a few states. Uttar Pradesh accounts for the first rank with 19.5 million with one forth of the country's share; followed by Andhra Pradesh (9.2 million), Madhya Pradesh (8.0 million),

Table 2.5: Cross Bred Cattle

(in thousand number)

Category	1987			1992			Annual Growth 1987-1992
	Rural	Urban	Total	Rural	Urban	Total	
CATTLE CROSSBRED							
1. Male							
Used for breeding only	390	21	415	156	19	175	-15.86
Total cross bred male cattle	3509	235	3951	4275	383	4658	3.35
2. Female							
(i) Under 1 year	1256	175	1490	1869	289	2158	7.69
(ii) Under 1-2.5 years	1144	142	1361	1681	225	1906	6.97
(iii) Over 2.5 years							
(a) in milk	2382	359	2878	3448	563	4011	6.86
(b) dry	1168	133	1235	1578	203	1781	7.60
(c) not yet calved	346	48	423	501	74	575	6.33
(d) others	66	8	74	110	16	126	11.23
Total cross-bred female cattle 6273	865	7462	9187	1369	10557	7.19	
Total cross-bred cattle	9782	1400	11413	13462	1753	15215	5.92
CATTLE INDIGENOUS							
1. Male							
a) Used for breeding only	13812	80	13911	9447	595	10042	-6.31
Total male indigenous	93908	2028	96981	93977	2961	96938	-0.01
2. Female							
(i) Under 1 year	13664	562	14413	14209	715	14924	0.70
(ii) 1.3 years	18651	555	19426	18852	787	19639	0.22
(iii) over 3 years							
(a) in milk	25387	1110	26940	26145	1406	27551	0.45
(b) dry	24110	678	25034	23590	860	24450	-0.47
(c) not yet calved	4163	163	4418	4145	167	4312	-0.48
(d) others	1034	31	1070	1507	48	1555	7.76
Total female indigenous	87009	3099	91301	88448	3983	92431	0.25
Total indigenous cattle	180917	5127	188282	182425	6944	189369	0.12
Total Cattle	190699	6227	199695	195887	8697	204584	0.48
II Buffalo							
2. Female							
(i) Under 1 year	10086	548	10709	11363	651	12014	2.33
(ii) 1.3 years	9746	431	10253	10528	507	11035	1.48
(iii) over 2.5 years							
(a) in milk	21480	1479	23150	24147	1745	25892	2.26
(b) dry	12127	508	12738	13762	621	14383	2.46
(c) not yet calved	2607	146	2778	2765	137	2902	0.88
(d) others	437	27	467	571	58	629	6.14
Total female buffaloes	56483	3140	60095	63136	3719	66855	2.15
Total buffaloes	71616	3787	75967	79915	4291	84206	2.08

Source: Government of India, Ministry of Agriculture, Department of Animal Husbandry and Dairying: Basic Animal Husbandry Statistics, 1999.

Rajasthan (7.7 million) and Punjab (6.0 million). These five major states together account for about 60% of the total country's buffaloes.

Buffalo population has been increasing at a steady growth rate over the year. From 51.2 million in 1961, it increased to 83.5 million in 1992 recording an overall growth rate of 63% over a period of 31 years. During the same period, cattle population has increased only by 13.7%. If these growth trends are any indication, buffalo would become the future Indian bovine animal in 21st century, because of its economic contribution even though their numbers are less compared to cattle. The major reason for growth rate in buffalo as compared to cattle is due to increasing demand for milk and milk products, coupled with the dairy development programmes.

There are forty breeds of sheep in India, which can be gainfully utilized to develop superior strains. Similarly, India has a rich biodiversity of goats. There are twenty well-defined breeds of goats in India.

LIVESTOCK POPULATION DENSITY

The state-wise per capita and per hectare livestock based on 1992 livestock census are given in Tables 2.6 and 2.7. It may be seen that per capita and per hectare cattle are quite high in the states of eastern region though there are wide variations between the states of the region. While for the region as a

Table 2.6: Per Capita Number of Livestock-Statewise

State/ Region	Rural (thousands)	Population 1991							
		Cattle		Buffaloes		Others		Total	
		(000 Nos)	Per capita No.	(000 Nos)	Per capita No.	(000 Nos)	Per capita No.	(000 Nos)	Per capita No.
Eastern Region									
Assam	19926	10120	0.51	958	0.05	4987	0.25	16065	0.81
Bihar	75021	22155	0.30	5353	0.07	20426	0.27	47934	0.64
Orissa	27425	13844	0.50	1539	0.06	7368	0.27	22751	0.83
West Bengal	49370	17454	0.35	1011	0.02	16625	0.34	35090	0.71
Arunachal Pradesh	754	327	0.43	9	0.01	518	0.69	854	1.13
Manipur	1332	717	0.54	115	0.09	458	0.34	1290	0.97
Meghalaya	1445	637	0.44	34	0.02	515	0.36	1186	0.82
Mizoram	372	61	0.16	6	0.02	141	0.38	208	0.56
Nagaland	1001	331	0.33	34	0.03	710	0.71	1075	1.07
Sikkim	369	200	0.54	3	0.01	188	0.51	391	1.06
Tripura	2335	950	0.41	20	0.01	623	0.27	1593	0.68
Total	179350	66796	0.37	9082	0.05	52559	0.29	128437	0.72
Northern Region									
Haryana	12409	2133	0.2	4373	0.4	2638	0.2	9144	0.7
Himachal Pradesh	4722	2165	0.5	703	0.1	2248	0.5	5116	1.1

Table 2.6: Per Capita Number of Livestock-Statewise (Contd.)

State/ Region	Rural (thousands)	Cattle (000 Nos)	Per capita No	Buffaloes (000 Nos)	Per capita No.	Others (000 Nos)	Per capita No.	Total (000 Nos)	Per capita No
Jammu & Kashmir	5880	3055	0.5	732	0.1	4919	0.8	8706	1.5
Punjab	14289	2911	0.2	5238	0.4	1305	0.1	9454	0.7
Uttar Pradesh	111506	25631	0.2	20086	0.2	19082	0.2	64799	0.6
Delhi	949	41	0.0	249	0.3	30	0.0	320	0.3
Chandigarh	66	8	0.1	23	0.3	8	0.1	39	0.6
Total	149821	35944	0.2	31404	0.2	30230	0.2	97578	0.7
Southern Region									
Andhra Pradesh	48621	10947	0.2	9153	0.2	12811	0.3	32911	0.7
Karnataka	31069	13175	0.4	4251	0.1	12144	0.4	29570	1.0
Kerala	21418	3529	0.2	296	0.0	2013	0.1	5838	0.3
Tamil Nadu	36781	9275	0.3	2814	0.1	12916	0.4	25005	0.7
A & N Island	206	53	0.3	14	0.1	93	0.5	160	0.8
Lakshadweep	23	2	0.1	-	0.0	17	0.7	19	0.8
Pondicherry	291	93	0.3	7	0.0	49	0.2	149	0.5
Total	138409	37074	0.3	16535	0.1	40043	0.3	93652	0.7
Western Region									
Gujarat	27064	6803	0.3	5268	0.2	6526	0.2	18597	0.7
Madhya Pradesh	50842	28687	0.6	7970	0.2	10085	0.2	46742	0.9
Maharashtra	48396	17441	0.4	5447	0.1	12504	0.3	36392	0.8
Rajasthan	33939	11632	0.3	7743	0.2	29038	0.9	48413	1.4
Goa	690	99	0.1	45	0.1	105	0.2	249	0.4
Dadra & Nagar Haveli	127	50	0.4	4	0.0	19	0.1	73	0.6
Daman & Diu	54	7	0.1	1	0.0	4	0.1	12	0.2
Total	161112	64719	0.4	26478	0.2	59281	0.4	150478	0.9
All-India	**628692**	**204533**	**0.3**	**83499**	**0.1**	**182113**	**0.3**	**470145**	**0.7**

Source: Prepared by the authors by taking data from Population Census, 1991 and Livestock Census 1992.

Table 2.7: Per Hectare Number of Livestock

State/ Region	Gross Sown 1992- 93 (000 hec.)	Cattle		Buffaloes		Others		Total	
		(000 Nos.)	Per hect No.	(000 Nos.)	Per hect No.	(000 Nos.)	Per hect No.	(000 Nos.)	Per hect No.
Eastern Region									
Assam	3837	10120	2.64	958	0.25	4987	1.30	16065	4.19
Bihar	9356	22155	2.37	5353	0.57	20426	2.18	·47934	5.12
Orissa	9416	13844	1.47	1539	0.16	7368	0.78	22751	2.42
West Bengal	8540	17454	2.04	1011	0.12	16625	1.95	35090	4.11
Arunachal Pradesh	255	327	1.28	9	0.04	518	2.03	854	3.35
Manipur	187	717	3.83	115	0.61	458	2.45	1290	6.90
Meghalaya	239	637	2.67	34	0.14	515	2.15	1186	4.96
Mizoram	102	61	0.60	6	0.06	141	1.38	208	2.04
Nagaland	228	331	1.45	34	0.15	710	3.11	1075	4.71
Sikkim	125	200	1.60	3	0.02	188	1.50	391	3.13
Tripura	440	950	2.16	20	0.05	623	1.42	1593	3.62
Total	32725	66796	2.04	9082	0.28	52559	1.61	128437	3.92
Northern Region									
Haryana	5852	2133	0.4	4373	0.7	2638	0.5	9144	1.6
Himachal Pradesh	973	2165	2.2	703	0.7	2248	2.3	5116	5.3
Jammu & Kashmir	1074	3055	2.8	732	0.7	4919	4.6	8706	8.1
Punjab	7552	2911	0.4	5238	0.7	1305	0.2	9454	1.3
Uttar Pradesh	25673	25631	1.0	20086	0.8	19082	0.7	64799	2.5
Delhi	56	41	0.7	249	4.4	30	0.5	320	5.7
Chandi- garh	4	8	2.0	23	5.8	8	2.0	39	9.8
Total	41184	35944	0.9	31404	0.8	30230	0.7	97578	2.4
Southern Region									
Andhra Pradesh	12754	10947	0.9	9153	0.7	12811	1.0	32911	2.6
Karnataka	12412	13175	1.1	4251	0.3	12144	1.0	29570	2.4
Kerala	3047	3529	1.2	296	0.1	2013	0.7	5838	1.9
Tamil Nadu	7067	9275	1.3	2814	0.4	12916	1.8	25005	3.5
A & N Island	38	53	1.4	14	0.4	93	2.4	160	4.2
Laksha- dweep	4	2	0.5	0	0.0	17	4.3	19	4.8
Pondi- cherry	47	93	2.0	7	0.1	49	1.0	149	3.2
Total	35369	37074	1.0	16535	0.5	40043	1.1	93652	2.6

Table 2.7: Per Hectare Number of Livestock (Contd.)

State/ Region	Gross Sown 1992-93 (000 hec.)	Cattle		Buffaloes		Others		Total	
		(000 Nos.)	Per hect No.	(000 Nos.)	Per hect No.	(000 Nos.)	Per hect No.	(000 Nos.)	Per hect No.
Western Region									
Gujarat	11003	6803	0.6	5268	0.5	6526	0.6	18597	1.7
Madhya Pradesh	23807	28687	1.2	7970	0.3	10085	0.4	46742	2.0
Maharashtra	21171	17441	0.8	5447	0.3	12504	0.6	36392	1.7
Rajasthan	20167	11632	0.6	7743	0.4	29038	1.4	48413	2.4
Goa	161	99	0.6	45	0.3	105	0.7	249	1.5
Dadra & Nagar Haveli	26	50	1.9	4	0.2	19	0.7	73	2.8
Daman & Diu	5	7	1.4	1	0.2	4	0.8	12	2.4
Total	76340	64719	0.8	26478	0.3	59281	0.8	150478	2.0
All-India	185618	204533	1.1	83499	0.4	182113	1.0	470145	2.5

Source: Prepared by the authors by taking data from Livestock Census, 1992 and area data from Directorate of Economics and Statistics, Ministry of Agriculture, Govt. of India.

whole, per capita cattle population is nearly 0.4 number, in the states of Assam, Orissa, Manipur and Sikkim the number is 0.5. On the other hand in Mizoram, Bihar, West Bengal and Nagaland, the number vary between 0.2 and 0.3. In all the states of the region the number of per capita buffalo is extremely small. For the region as a whole, the average is only 0.05, the largest being in Manipur (0.09 number) and least in Arunachal Pradesh, Sikkim and Tripura (0.01 number each). The number of other livestock like pigs, goats, sheep, etc. per capita is around 0.3. Thus, in the region as a whole, the per capita number of total livestocks is 0.7 which matches with that of all the other three regions, viz. northern, southern and western.

In the northern region, the average per capita number of both cattle, buffaloes and other livestocks is same being 0.2, though there are perceptible inter-state variations. On the other hand, in southern and western regions, while the average per capita number of cattle and other livestocks is 0.3 each, the number of buffaloes is only 0.1. In these regions too, there are wide inter-state variations in the per capita number of different livestocks. J & K and Rajasthan are the two very interesting cases where for every human population, the number of various categories of livestock is 1.5 and 1.4 respectively. Eastern States of Nagaland, Arunachal Pradesh and Sikkim are others along with Himachal Pradesh and Karnataka where livestock population is more than the human.

When looked into the density of different livestocks in the gross area sown of the states, the inter-state variations are found to be much wider. The density depended on size of the cultivated area in a state, level of urbanization, conditionality of the natural habitat of the animals and density of human population. For example, in the eastern region, in Mizoram and Arunachal Pradesh, per hectare buffalo population was negligible as both the states are sparsely populated and buffalo rearing is not in vogue among the inhabitants. The number of ·cattle population per hectare was also negligible being only 0.6 and 1.3 respectively. But in the region as a whole, the density of cattle population was highest being 2.04 number per hectare as against 0.96, 1.0 and 1.1 respectively in northern, southern and western regions indicating wide inter-state variations in the number of cattle.

In case of buffaloes, the density is least in eastern region being only 0.28 number per hectare and highest in northern region being 0.8 number per hectare. In southern and western regions their numbers are 0.5 and 0.4 per hectare respectively. On the whole, the per hectare number of livestock is highest in eastern region being 3.02, followed by 2.4 in northern region, 2.6 in southern region 2.5 in western region.

Distribution of Livestock among Zones and States

India can be broadly divided into 4 zones, viz. eastern, northern, southern and western. Gross area sown in each of these four zones is 33m, 47m, 35m and 19m hectares respectively. However, livestock population is highest in western zone (32%), followed by eastern zone (27%), northern zone (21%) and southern zone (20%). The disaggregated livestock population, however, depicts a slightly different picture. Concentration of cattle population is very high in eastern and western zones (33% and 32% respectively). The other two zones accounted for 18% each of the total cattle population. On the other hand, buffalo population is concentrated mainly in northern zone (38%) and western zone (32%). Eastern zone has the least number of buffalo population being only 11 per cent of the total (Table 2.8 and Graph 2.2).

The state-wise dispersal of the livestock population as indicated in Table 2.9 shows significant variations in the livestock population of different species from one state to another depending on geographical area, size of rural population, socio-economic status of the states, agro-climatic conditions, etc. For example, while cattle and buffaloes are by and large reared in almost all the states, camels are reared mostly in arid and desert states like Rajasthan (73%), Haryana (12%), Gujarat (6%). In Punjab, Uttar Pradesh and Madhya Pradesh too, a small percentages of camel population varying between 1 and 4 were recorded in 1992 census. Similarly, mithuns are predominantly available in Arunachal Pradesh where around 68 per cent of the country's mithun population is found. The rest of the mithuns are also in the two north-eastern states, namely Mizoram (17%) and Manipur (14%). On the other hand, Jammu & Kashmir state is the main habitat of yak where nearly 57 per cent of the country's yak population is found.

Table 2.8: Regional Distribution of Livestock Population in 1992 (in Thousand)

State/Region	Cattle	(%)	Buffaloes	(%)	Others	(%)	Total	(%)	% of BPL Population
Eastern Region									
Assam	10120	15.2	958	10.5	4987	9.5	16065	12.5	45.01
Bihar	22155	33.2	5353	58.9	20426	38.9	47934	37.3	58.21
Orissa	13844	20.7	1539	16.9	7368	14.0	22751	17.7	49.72
West Bengal	17454	26.1	1011	11.1	16625	31.6	35090	27.3	40.80
Arunachal Pradesh	327	0.5	9	0.1	518	1.0	854	0.7	45.01
Manipur	717	1.1	115	1.3	458	0.9	1290	1.0	45.01
Meghalaya	637	1.0	34	0.4	515	1.0	1186	0.9	45.01
Mizoram	61	0.1	6	0.1	141	0.3	208	0.2	45.01
Nagaland	331	0.5	34	0.4	710	1.4	1075	0.8	45.01
Sikkim	200	0.3	3	0.0	188	0.4	391	0.3	45.01
Tripura	950	1.4	20	0.2	623	1.2	1593	1.2	45.01
Total	66796 (32.7)	100.0	9082 (10.9)	100.0	52559 (28.9)	100.0	128437 (27.3)	100.0	
Northern Region									
Haryana	2133	5.9	4373	13.9	2638	8.7	9144	9.4	28.04
Himachal Pradesh	2165	6.0	703	2.2	2248	7.4	5116	5.2	30.34
Jammu & Kashmir	3055	8.5	732	2.3	4919	16.3	8706	8.9	30.34
Punjab	2911	8.1	5238	16.7	1305	4.3	9454	9.7	11.95
Uttar Pradesh	25631	71.3	20086	64.0	19082	63.1	64799	66.4	42.28
Delhi	41	0.1	249	0.8	30	0.1	320	0.3	1.90
Chandigargh	8	0.0	23	0.1	8	0.0	39	0.0	11.35
Total	35944 (17.6)	100.0	31404 (37.6)	100.0	30230 (16.6)	100.0	97578 (20.8)	100.0	
Southern Region									
Andhra Pradesh	10947	29.5	9153	55.4	12811	32.0	32911	35.1	15.92
Karnataka	13175	35.5	4251	25.7	12144	30.3	29570	31.6	29.88
Kerala	3529	9.5	296	1.8	2013	5.0	5838	6.2	25.76
Tamil Nadu	9275	25.0	2814	17.0	12916	32.3	25005	26.7	32.48
A & N Island	53	0.1	14	0.1	93	0.2	160	0.2	40.80
Lakshadweep	2	0.0	-	0.0	17	0.0	19	0.0	25.76
Pondicherry	93	0.3	7	0.0	49	0.1	149	0.2	32.48
Total	37074 (18.1)	100.0	16535 (19.8)	100.0	40043 (22.0)	100.0	93652 (19.9)	100.0	
Western Region									
Gujarat	6803	10.5	5268	19.9	6526	11.0	18597	12.4	22.18
Madhya Pradesh	28687	44.3	7970	30.1	10085	17.0	46742	31.1	40.84
Maharashtra	17441	26.9	5447	20.6	12504	21.1	36392	24.2	37.93
Rajasthan	11632	18.0	7743	29.2	29038	49.0	48413	32.2	26.46
Goa	99	0.2	45	0.2	105	0.2	249	0.2	5.34
Dadra & Nagar Haveli	50	0.1	4	0.0	19	0.0	73	0.0	
Daman & Diu	7	0.0	1	0.0	4	0.0	12	0.0	
Total	64719 (31.6)	100.0	26478 (31.7)	100.0	59281 (32.5)	100.0	150478 (32.0)	100.0	
All-India	204533	(100.0)	83499	(100.0)	182113	(100.0)	470145	(100.0)	

Source: Prepared by the authors from Livestock Census Data, 1992

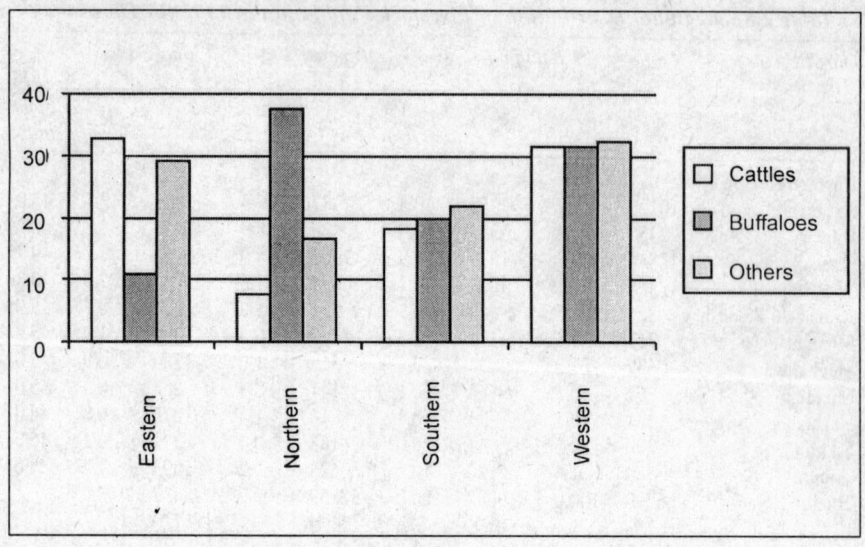

Graph 2.2: Regional Distribution of Livestock Population

Sikkim (17%), Arunachal Pradesh (15%) and Himachal Pradesh (9%) are the other important states where yaks are found. In Mizoram state also a small percentage (2%) of yak is available.

Distribution of various livestock species according to agroclimatic zones shows that while lower Gangetic Plains have the highest priority for cattle, goat and pig, buffalo falls in the lowest priority. At the same time buffalo comes under the highest category in the Trans Gangetic Plains where cattle and goat has low priority (Table 2.10).

Ownership Pattern

Traditionally farmers keep lifestock in proportion to the free crop residue and family labour available in their households. Livestock holdings are small and are made up of a mix of several species, with wide variations in the mix, between households and between regions. Cattle and buffalo are the widely held and the most interactive species: subsisting on crop resideues while contributing food, farm power and manure.

Land holdings in India are in general small and fragmented; medium and large holdings account for less than 10 per cent of the total holdings. Distribution of land, however, is highly iniquitous: marginal and small holdings account for over 78 per cent of the total holdings size had been declining over the decades: from 2.52 ha. per holding in 1961 to some 1.34 ha by 1992. Livestock holding too is small, a mix of various sepcies, except in the case of the large migratory herds in Gujarat, Rajasthan, and North-West India, where the herds are considerably larger from a few hundreds to a couple of thousands. Livestock holding is less iniquitous, with over 70 per cent of all species owned by the small holder group(marginal & small

Table 2.9: Percentage of Livestock and Poultry Population by State/UT-1992

State/UT	Cattle	Buffaloes	Sheep	Goats	Pigs	Horses & Ponies	Mules	Donkeys	Camels	Yaks	Mithuns	Total Livestock	Total Poultry
1. Andhra Pradesh	5.35	10.87	15.34	3.75	5.08	0.98	0.00	4.24	0.00	0.00	0.00	6.99	16.25
2. Arunachal Pradesh	0.16	0.01	0.06	0.11	1.85	0.61	0.00	0.00	0.00	15.52	68.18	0.18	0.39
3. Assam	4.95	1.14	0.29	3.00	10.67	2.20	0.00	0.00	0.00	0.00	0.00	3.41	5.34
4. Bihar	10.83	6.36	3.33	15.14	8.81	14.20	2.07	3.00	0.00	0.00	0.00	10.18	5.75
5. Gujarat	3.33	6.26	3.99	3.68	0.80	1.59	0.00	8.17	6.11	0.00	0.00	3.95	1.84
6. Goa	0.05	0.05	0.00	0.01	0.70	0.00	0.00	0.00	0.00	0.00	0.00	0.05	0.24
7. Haryana	1.04	5.19	2.05	0.69	4.04	6.12	12.95	7.55	12.42	0.00	0.00	1.94	2.79
8. Himachal Pradesh	1.06	0.83	2.12	0.97	0.04	1.59	8.29	0.72	0.00	8.62	0.00	1.08	0.24
9. J. & Kashmir	1.49	0.87	5.80	1.53	0.09	14.93	9.84	1.96	0.19	56.90	0.00	1.85	1.51
10. Karnataka	6.44	5.05	10.69	5.45	2.97	1.59	0.00	3.41	0.00	0.00	0.00	6.28	5.26
11. Kerala	1.72	0.35	0.06	1.60	1.06	1.06	0.00	0.00	0.00	0.00	0.00	1.24	7.13
12. Madhya Pradesh	13.97	9.46	1.65	7.26	5.70	8.94	4.15	6.00	1.16	0.00	0.00	9.93	3.84
13. Maharashtra	8.53	6.47	6.06	8.63	2.94	5.02	0.00	7.55	0.00	0.00	0.00	7.73	10.48
14. Manipur	0.35	0.14	0.03	0.03	2.99	0.00	0.00	0.00	0.00	0.00	14.29	0.27	1.06
15. Meghalaya	0.26	0.04	0.04	0.17	2.13	0.24	0.00	0.00	0.00	0.00	0.00	0.25	0.59
16. Mizoram	0.03	0.01	0.00	0.02	0.88	0.24	0.00	0.00	0.00	1.72	0.65	0.04	0.35
17. Nagaland	0.16	0.04	0.00	0.13	4.11	0.73	0.00	0.00	0.00	0.00	16.88	0.23	0.70
18. Orrisa	6.77	1.82	3.62	4.29	4.57	0.00	0.00	0.00	0.00	0.00	0.00	4.83	4.25
19. Punjab	1.42	7.13	1.04	0.47	0.79	4.77	8.29	3.72	4.07	0.00	0.00	2.17	5.97
20. Rajasthan	5.72	9.15	24.61	13.28	1.98	2.94	1.55	20.68	72.65	0.00	0.00	10.29	0.99
21. Sikkim	0.10	0.00	0.03	0.10	0.34	0.24	0.00	0.00	0.00	17.24	0.00	0.08	0.10

Table 2.9: Percentage of Livestock and Poultry Population by State/UT-1992 (Contd.)

State/UT	Cattle	Buffaloes	Sheep	Goats	Pigs	Horses & Ponies	Mules	Donkeys	Camels	Yaks	Mithuns	Total Livestock	Total Poultry
22. Tamil Nadu	4.54	3.34	11.52	5.50	5.25	1.10	0.00	4.45	0.00	0.00	0.00	5.31	8.00
23. Tripura	0.46	0.02	0.01	0.37	1.47	0.00	0.00	0.00	0.00	0.00	0.00	0.34	0.85
24. Uttar Pradesh	12.53	23.85	4.73	11.37	22.72	30.48	52.85	28.54	3.39	0.00	0.00	13.76	3.51
25. West Bengal	8.53	1.20	2.93	12.29	7.47	1.47	0.00	0.00	0.00	0.00	0.00	7.45	12.18
26. A & N Islands	0.02	0.02	0.00	0.05	0.27	0.00	0.00	0.00	0.00	0.00	0.00	0.03	0.20
27. Chandigarh	0.00	0.03	0.00	0.00	0.02	0.00	0.00	0.00	0.00	0.00	0.00	0.01	0.06
28. D & N Haveli	0.02	0.00	0.00	0.02	0.00	0.00	0.00	0.00	0.00	0.00	0.00	0.02	0.04
29. Delhi	0.02	0.29	0.00	0.01	0.08	0.00	0.00	0.00	0.00	0.00	0.00	0.07	0.01
30. Lakshadweep	0.00	0.00	0.00	0.01	0.00	0.00	0.00	0.00	0.00	0.00	0.00	0.00	0.02
31. Pondicherry	0.04	0.01	0.01	0.04	0.00	0.00	0.00	0.00	0.00	0.00	0.00	0.03	0.04
32. Daman & Diu	0.00	0.00	0.00	0.00	0.00	0.00	0.00	0.00	0.00	0.00	0.00	0.00	0.01
Total	100.00	100.00	100.00	100.00	100.00	100.00	100.00	100.00	100.00	100.00	100.00	100.00	100.00

Source: Prepared by the authors from Livestock census, 1992 data.

Table 2.10: Distribution of Livestock Species – Agro-Climatic Zones

Agro-Climatic Zones	Species Priority				Description	Products
	Very high	High	Low	Very low		
Western		S	CBG	P	Sheep-goat-cattle	Wool-meat
Eastern Himalayan		CP	G	BS	Cattle-goat-pig	Meat-draft
Lower Gangetic Plains	CGP	S	B		Cattle-goat-pig	Draft-meat
Middle Gangetic Plains	P	CBG	S		Pig-bovine-goat	Draft-meat
Upper Gangetic Plains	BP	G	CS		Buff-pig-goat	Milk-meat
Trans Gangetic Plains	B	SP	CG		Buff-sheep-goat	Milk-meat
Eastern Plateau & Hills		C	BSGP		Cattle-all others	Draft-meat
Central Plateau & Hills	SG	B	CP		Sheep-goat-buff	Wool-meat
Western Plateau & Hills			CBSG	All	All livestock	Supplementary
Southern Plateau & Hills	S		CBGP		Sheep-all others	Meat-supplementary
East Coast Plains & Hills		BS	CGP		Buff-sheep	Milk-supplementary
West Coast Plains & Hills	C	G	P	BS	Cattle-goat-pig	Draft-meat
Gujarat Plains & Hills			CBSG	P	All livestock	Supplementary
Western Dry	S		BG	CP	Sheep-others	Wool-meat
Islands			GP	CBS	Low livestock	Supplementary

C-cattle, B-buffalo, S-sheep, G-goat, P-pig

Source: Dr NSR Sastry, "Regional considerations for appropriate livestock development strategies in India, Journal of Indian Veterinary Association, Kerela, Vol.5, Issue 3

along with the landless): the Gini Coefficient (the index of inequity of ownership) for dairy stock had declined from 0.43 in 1961 to 0.28 by 1991.

National Sample Survey (NSSO) data for the 48th Round provides valuable information regarding the distribution of livestock population according to size of holdings. Both for Kharif and Rabi, no livestock or poultry is kept on holdings over 10 hectares in the Eastern Region. The position is more or less the same with regard to Northern Region with the exception of Punjab. Andhra Pradesh and Karnataka (Southern Region) and Gujarat, MP and Rajasthan (Western Region) have also a small number of livestock on large holdings. Interestingly poultry is more or less completely missing in the case of all holdings above 4 hectares. As against this, small and marginal holdings account for a major part of livestock and poultry (Table 2.11). Families owning milch animals are also concentrated among landless and small/marginal holders. Any development programme for livestock will thus primarily benefit the poorer sections of the society (Table 2.12). Latest information regarding distribution of size of holdings (1995-96) is shown in Table 2.13 and Graph 2.3.

Ownership pattern of livestock is much less skewed than in the case of arable land (Graph –2.3). A sizeable proportion of livestock owners are below the poverty line being either landless, marginal or small farmers (Table 2.12). Production Systems are based on low cost agro by- products as nutritional inputs, using traditional technologies for production. Gender equity is more pronounced in livestock sector with women constituting 71% of labour force in livestock sector as against 33% in crop farming.

SOME OTHER SPECIES

Sheep

India possesses 55 million sheep (1997) which is a little over 5 per cent of the world sheep population. There is a wide variation in the types of sheep found in different parts of the country. Taking into consideration the varying agro-climatic conditions and types of sheep found in different zones, the following regions can be distinguished:

(i)   The northern temperate region comprising Jammu and Kashmir, Himachal Pradesh and hilly parts of Uttar Pradesh (now Uttaranchal) has approximately six million sheep producing medium to fine wool. The region carries 12.6 per cent of the sheep population. The important breeds in the region are Gurez, Karnah, Bhakarwal, Gaddi, Kashmir Valley and Rampur Bushhair. Quite a sizeable proportion of the sheep population in this region especially in Jammu and Kashmir consists of crosses between the indigenous and exotic fine wool producing breeds.

(ii) The North Western region comprising Punjab, Haryana, plains of Uttar Pradesh, Rajasthan, Gujarat and Madhya Pradesh (including Chattisgarh) has 17 million sheep producing mostly coarse carpet quality wool. The region is mostly arid and semi-arid and carries about 34 per cent of the sheep population. Important sheep breeds of this region are Chokla, Nali, Magra, Pugal, Marwari, Jaisalmeri, Malpura, Sonadi, Lohi, Maunjal, Muzzaffaranagari, Pattanwadi (Kutchi) and Jalauni.

(iii) The southern peninsular region comprising Maharashtra, Andhra Pradesh, Karnataka and Tamil Nadu has 22 million or 44 per cent of the sheep, of which almost 50 per cent produce no wool and the

Table 2.11: *Percentage Distribution of Operational Holdings by Main Use of the Holding for Broad Size-Class of Operational Holdings for Kharif and Rabi Season*

| States/Region | Less than 0.002 | | 0.002-0.20 | | 0.21-0.50 | | 4.01-10.00 | | 10.01 & above | | All sizes | |
	(a) Livestock keeping	(b) Poultry raising	(a) Livestock keeping	(b) Poultry raising	(a) Livestock keeping	(b) Poultry raising	(a) Livestock keeping	(b) Poultry raising	(a) Livestock keeping	(b) Poultry raising	(a) Livestock keeping	(b) Poultry raising
(1)	(2)	(3)	(4)	(5)	(6)	(7)	(8)	(9)	(10)	(11)	(12)	(13)
					KHARIF							
Eastern Region												
Assam	22.10	20.74	6.50	6.47	2.22	1.36	0.00	0.00	0.00	0.00	2.94	2.10
Bihar	31.61	0.00	14.97	1.22	5.94	0.30	8.37	0.00	0.00	0.00	9.81	0.71
Orrisa	77.63	11.80	19.11	6.82	4.61	0.00	1.86	0.00	0.00	0.00	5.47	1.32
West Bengal	24.98	44.45	17.56	13.92	0.78	0.56	4.91	0.00	0.00	0.00	7.94	6.04
Arunachal Pradesh	0.00	0.00	0.00	2.31	0.00	0.00	0.00	0.00	0.00	0.00	0.78	0.07
Manipur	0.00	0.00	2.70	4.50	0.00	0.00	0.00	0.00	0.00	0.00	3.21	3.19
Meghalaya	0.00	23.30	8.85	9.47	2.89	1.55	0.00	0.00	0.00	0.00	2.02	3.59
Mizoram	0.00	0.00	0.00	9.13	6.93	1.73	0.00	0.00	0.00	0.00	2.45	2.52
Nagaland	63.84	26.50	18.42	3.22	0.00	0.00	0.00	0.00	0.00	0.00	2.65	1.18
Sikkim	0.00	0.00	7.59	1.88	0.00	0.00	0.00	0.00	0.00	0.00	2.34	0.23
Tripura	0.00	0.00	17.99	5.56	9.37	1.04	27.79	0.00	0.00	0.00	11.61	2.06
Northern Region												
Haryana	18.83	0.00	79.53	0.00	14.15	0.00	6.06	0.00	0.00	0.00	27.13	0.00
Himachal Pradesh	14.45	0.00	1.75	0.00	0.49	0.00	11.29	0.00	0.00	0.00	2.32	0.00
Jammu & Kashmir	0.00	0.00	42.06	0.00	2.20	0.00	2.12	0.00	0.00	0.00	7.96	0.00
Punjab	63.90	0.00	77.08	1.85	7.35	0.00	4.57	0.00	3.22	0.00	37.99	0.81
Uttar Pradesh	70.20	1.59	31.15	0.56	4.43	0.00	4.00	0.00	0.00	0.00	10.64	0.16
Delhi	0.00	0.00	81.19	0.00	20.52	0.00	0.00	0.00	0.00	0.00	55.39	0.00
Chandigarh	0.00	0.00	44.79	0.00	10.33	0.00	0.00	0.00	0.00	0.00	28.14	0.00

Table 2.11: Percentage Distribution of Operational Holdings by Main Use of the Holding for Broad Size-Class of Operational Holdings for Kharif and Rabi Season (Contd.)

States/ Region	Less than 0.002		0.002-0.20		0.21-0.50		4.01- 10.00		10.01 & above		All sizes	
	(a) Livestock keeping	(b) Poultry raising	(a) Livestock keeping	(b) Poultry raising	(a) Livestock keeping	(b) Poultry raising	(a) Livestock keeping	(b) Poultry raising	(a) Livestock keeping	(b) Poultry raising	(a) Livestock keeping	(b) Poultry raising
(1)	(2)	(3)	(4)	(5)	(6)	(7)	(8)	(9)	(10)	(11)	(12)	(13)
Southern Region												
Andhra Pradesh	22.37	43.64	24.79	12.45	3.34	0.00	1.87	0.00	3.70	0.00	7.08	2.83
Karnataka	50.41	12.97	41.76	8.35	10.65	0.00	3.60	0.00	3.44	0.00	13.46	1.87
Kerala	0.00	57.97	5.56	6.41	4.25	0.70	0.00	0.00	0.00	0.00	4.60	4.20
Tamil Nadu	18.48	18.70	33.27	9.19	2.79	0.33	0.76	0.00	0.00	0.00	16.09	4.34
Andaman & Nicobar Islands	0.00	10.00	5.25	9.15	0.00	6.47	0.00	0.00	0.00	0.00	3.05	7.26
Lakshadweep	0.00	0.00	0.00	0.00	0.00	0.00	0.00	0.00	0.00	0.00	0.00	0.00
Pondicherry	0.00	36.62	5.75	18.54	0.00	0.00	0.00	0.00	42.77	0.00	6.19	13.58
Western region												
Gujarat	66.17	13.88	47.36	1.20	10.42	0.00	1.04	0.00	4.53	0.00	14.32	0.91
Madhya Pradesh	33.69	39.76	37.06	11.07	6.62	0.00	6.50	0.00	3.71	0.00	11.52	3.18
Maharashtra	71.64	20.60	51.75	11.17	0.00	0.00	0.00	0.00	0.38	0.00	11.53	2.67
Rajasthan	95.77	0.00	63.34	0.00	9.83	0.00	3.64	0.00	2.65	0.00	10.63	0.00
Goa	86.4	13.59	45.44	0.00	4.75	0.00	0.00	0.00	0.00	0.00	17.60	2.38
Dadra & Nagar Haveli	0.00	10.00	18.75	48.90	0.00	0.00	0.00	0.00	0.00	0.00	3.03	7.96
Daman & Diu	0.00	10.00	0.00	27.82	0.00	0.00	0.00	0.00	0.00	0.00	1.31	35.15
India	47.52	17.34	28.37	6.30	4.41	0.22	3.50	0.00	2.38	0.00	10.76	2.07

Table 2.11: Perentage Distribution of Operational Holdings by Main Use of the Holding for Broad Size-Class of Operational Holdings for Kharif and Rabi Season (Contd.)

States/ Region	Less than 0.002		0.002-0.20		0.21-0.50		4.01- 10.00		10.01 & above		All sizes	
	(a) Livestock keeping	(b) Poultry raising	(a) Livestock keeping	(b) Poultry raising	(a) Livestock keeping	(b) Poultry raising	(a) Livestock keeping	(b) Poultry raising	(a) Livestock keeping	(b) Poultry raising	(a) Livestock keeping	(b) Poultry raising
(1)	(2)	(3)	(4)	(5)	(6)	(7)	(8)	(9)	(10)	(11)	(12)	(13)
					RABI							
Eastern Region												
Assam	2.02	6.22	5.04	2.08	0.00	0.00	0.00	0.00	0.00	0.00	1.49	0.63
Bihar	25.75	0.00	14.81	0.97	2.30	0.00	0.48	0.00	0.00	0.00	14.06	0.44
Orissa	0.00	12.95	35.68	9.15	2.02	0.25	15.44	0.00	0.00	0.00	12.19	3.39
West Bengal	36.54	19.14	19.96	11.23	3.15	0.87	2.70	0.00	0.00	0.00	0.00	5.82
Arunachal Pradesh	0.00	0.00	0.00	0.00	0.00	0.00	0.00	0.00	0.00	0.00	0.00	0.00
Manipur	0.00	0.00	6.38	2.72	0.00	0.00	0.00	0.00	0.00	0.00	4.39	1.87
Meghalaya	5.47	0.00	7.66	5.08	1.75	2.07	0.00	0.00	0.00	0.00	4.11	1.79
Mizoram	0.00	0.00	0.00	9.13	6.93	1.73	0.00	0.00	0.00	0.00	2.45	2.52
Nagaland	0.00	0.00	19.98	0.00	1.62	0.00	0.00	0.00	0.00	0.00	6.06	0.00
Sikkim	0.00	0.00	15.41	5.95	0.00	0.00	0.00	0.00	0.00	0.00	1.95	0.75
Tripura	0.00	0.00	1.59	1.82	0.00	0.00	0.00	0.00	0.00	0.00	0.96	0.97
Northern Region												
Haryana	18.83	0.00	79.53	0.00	14.15	0.00	0.00	0.00	0.00	0.00	23.58	0.00
Himachal Pradesh	1.45	0.00	1.50	0.00	0.00	0.00	0.00	0.00	0.00	0.00	0.38	0.00
Jammu & Kashmir	0.00	0.00	43.21	0.00	6.79	0.00	11.21	0.00	0.00	0.00	13.09	0.00
Punjab	10.00	0.00	84.85	0.54	6.88	0.00	0.13	0.00	0.00	0.00	42.33	0.26
Uttar Pradesh	46.96	1.11	25.62	0.62	0.84	0.00	0.59	0.00	0.00	0.00	7.44	0.16
Delhi	0.00	0.00	97.72	0.00	0.00	0.00	0.00	0.00	0.00	0.00	58.20	0.00
Chandigarh	0.00	0.00	32.94	0.00	7.46	0.00	0.00	0.00	0.00	0.00	22.41	0.00

Table 2.11: *Percentage Distribution of Operational Holdings by Main Use of the Holding for Broad Size-Class of Operational Holdings for Kharif and Rabi Season (Contd.)*

States/ Region	Less than 0.002		0.002-0.20		0.21-0.50		4.01- 10.00		10.01 & above		All sizes	
	(a) Livestock keeping	(b) Poultry raising	(a) Livestock keeping	(b) Poultry raising	(a) Livestock keeping	(b) Poultry raising	(a) Livestock keeping	(b) Poultry raising	(a) Livestock keeping	(b) Poultry raising	(a) Livestock keeping	(b) Poultry raising
(1)	(2)	(3)	(4)	(5)	(6)	(7)	(8)	(9)	(10)	(11)	(12)	(13)
Southern Region												
Andhra Pradesh	26.48	41.38	37.71	10.35	15.73	3.61	2.71	0.47	0.00	0.00	17.49	4.94
Karnataka	46.03	12.92	54.99	4.15	13.43	0.00	8.31	0.00	1.67	0.00	30.57	2.22
Kerala	0.00	9.76	2.67	3.51	0.40	0.30	0.00	0.00	0.00	0.00	1.84	2.30
Tamil Nadu	18.29	9.28	40.43	9.60	12.13	5.97	13.03	0.00	0.00	0.00	26.45	6.01
Andaman & Nicobar Islands	0.00	10.00	9.67	14.47	0.00	0.00	0.00	0.00	0.00	0.00	7.58	9.95
Lakshadweep	0.00	0.00	0.00	0.00	0.00	0.00	0.00	0.00	0.00	0.00	0.00	0.00
Pondicherry	47.75	0.00	20.35	8.65	1.86	0.00	4.34	0.00	0.00	0.00	15.52	6.09
Western Region												
Gujarat	72.97	10.65	55.37	0.03	0.67	0.00	14.17	0.00	23.49	0.00	27.75	0.91
Madhya Pradesh	37.94	3.25	30.21	0.79	3.45	0.00	11.98	0.58	8.25	0.00	14.50	0.45
Maharashtra	76.19	13.95	72.52	9.15	0.67	0.00	6.26	0.00	2.43	0.00	38.04	4.99
Rajasthan	68.67	0.00	66.97	0.00	3.42	0.00	24.39	0.00	25.19	0.00	27.11	0.00
Goa	0.00	22.38	41.48	0.00	0.00	0.00	0.00	0.00	0.00	0.00	20.95	0.24
Dadra & Nagar Haveli	0.00	0.00	0.00	0.00	0.00	0.00	0.00	0.00	0.00	0.00	0.00	0.00
Daman & Diu	0.00	0.00	0.00	0.00	0.00	0.00	0.00	0.00	0.00	0.00	0.00	0.00
India	**49.68**	**8.41**	**33.49**	**4.48**	**3.50**	**0.70**	**8.67**	**0.14**	**11.94**	**0.00**	**16.04**	**0.00**

Source: Livestock Census, 1992

Table 2..12: Families with Milch Animals According to Holding Size

Category	Landless	Marginal	Small	Medium	Large	All
(1)	*(2)*	*(3)*	*(4)*	*(5)*	*(6)*	*(7)*
Families	2.131	1.690	1.025	0.675	0.508	6.029
(million)	(35)	(28)	(17)	(11)	(9)	(100)
Families owning	0.770	1.052	0.799	0.559	0.445	3.625
milch animals	(21)	(29)	(22)	(16)	(12)	(100)
(million)						
Animals (million)	1.390	1.390	1.932	1.651	1.377	8.941
	(16)	(23)	(22)	(18)	(21)	(100)
Animals*Per	1.8	2.0	2.4	2.9	4.2	2.5
Owner (No.)						

Source: NDDB village enumeration, 1984. A census of six million households in 20,386 dairy co-operative villages spread over 108 milksheds (2).

Definition of farmers according to holding size of irrigated land: Landless: No land; marginal farmer: Upto 1 ha;

Small farmer: 1 to 2 ha; Medium farmer: 2 to 4 ha; Large farmer: 4 ha. Or more.

*Buffaloes and cattle; male and female of all age groups figures in parentheses are percentages of the total.

rest produces coarse, hairy and coloured fleeces. The breeds identified are Deccani/Bellary, Nallore, Mandya, Mecheri, Ramnad, Madras Red, Nilgiri, Coimbatore, Hassan and Trichi Black. Of these Deccani/Bellary, Mandya and Coimbatore produce extremely coarse and hairy fleece. Other breeds except Nilgiri do not produce any wool and primarily used for meat production. The Nilgiri which has been evolved by crossing indigenous hairy breeds with exotic breeds (Cape Merino, South Down, Chevoit etc.) produces fine wool.

(iv) The eastern region comprising Bihar, West Bengal, Orissa, Sikkim, Assam, Meghalaya, Manipur, Tripura, Mizoram, Nagaland and Arunachal Pradesh possess 5 million sheep mostly reared for meat. The region carries 10 per cent of the total sheep population. The region has no distinct breed of its own except in case of Bihar where Shabhadi and Chotta Nagpuri breeds are found.

Goats

With more than 102 million (1997 census) goats, India ranks second among the countries of the world in goat population. The census carried out quinquennially during the period 1951 to 1997 showed the goat population maintained a continuous rising trend but for the last quinquinium. Between 1951 and 1992, the goat population in the country increased almost by 3 times but declined slightly by 1997. This increase in the number of goats has occurred despite the fact that no special goat development programmes are in operation and almost 40 per cent of the total population of goats is

Table 2.13: Distribution of Holdings According to Operational area and Posession of Livestocks —1995-96*

	No. and area operated		No. and share in GDP		Irrigated/ Unirrigated area 000' (hect.) All Crops	
	Number (million)	Area operated Holding size(000 hectares)	In Millions	Share of GDP from Livestock Rs. Crore	Irrigated	Unirrigated
(1)	*(2)*	*(3)*	*(4)*	*(5)*	*(6)*	*(7)*
Marginal Cultivators	71.2	28121	161.56	46236	13282	17432
(Less than I hectares)	(61.6)	(17.2)	(36.8)			
Small Cultivators	21.6	30722	102.85	29526	12174	20857
(1.0 to 2.0 hectare)	(18.7)	(18.8)	(23.5)			
Semi-Medium	14.3	38953	88.48	25379	14627	28001
(2.0 to 4.0 hectares)	(12.4)	(23.8)	(20.2)			
Medium	7.1	41398	64.44	18469	14961	32021
(4.0 to 10.0 hectares)	(6.1)	(25.3)	(14.7)			
Large	1.4	24163	20.98	6031	6615	19328
	(1.2)	(14.8)	(4.8)			
Total	115.6	163357	438.31	125641	61659	117639
	(100.0)	(100.0)	(100.0)			

Note: Figures in brackets are the percentages of the total
* -Data for column Nos. 4-7 relates to 1991-92

being slaughtered every year. The reason is that very nominal expenditure on their upkeep has to be borne by the goat owners since goats can thrive on shrubs, bushes, thorny vegetation and top feeds of a variety of trees. The number also multiplies due to the high incidence of twinning. In the north-western region, Barbari, Beetal, Jamnapari, Kutchi, Marwari, Mehsana, Sirohi and Zalwadi are the important breeds while in the Peninsular region, Osmanabadi, Malabari/Tellicherry are found. In the eastern region, black, brown and white Bengal and Ganjam are the important breeds. Of these, the Bengal, Sirohi and Barbari are small size breeds while the others are either of medium size or tall, the tallest being Jamnapari.

Pig

Pig is one of the most efficient feed converting animals among domesticated stock. It is revealed from the livestock census data that the pig population remained more or less stationary from 1951 to 1966. But during

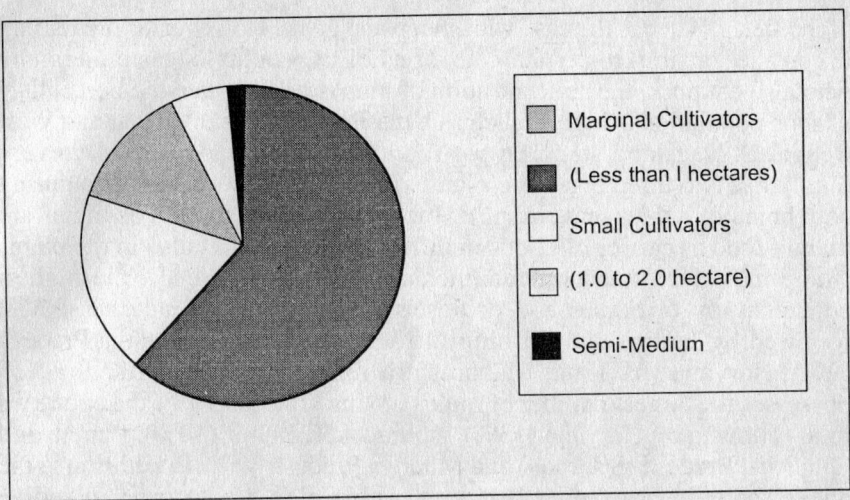

Graph 2.3: Distribution of Holdings According to Operational area and Posession of Livestocks

quinquennial ending 1972 there was a conspicuous rise in recording an annual growth rate of 6.65 per cent. Though during the next 5 years the annual growth rate in pig population was moderate being only about 2 per cent, there was a spurt in the growth rate by 5.79 per cent during 1977-82. The pig population thereafter remained more or less steady at around 10 million. However, during 1987-92, the growth rate was significantly high being almost 4 per cent per annum. During this period pig population increased in almost all the states and union territories except in Andhra Pradesh, Arunachal Pradesh, Himachal Pradesh, and Delhi. The period 1992-97 has, however, shown a slight decline for the first time.

Both indigenous and crossbred pigs are reared in the country. However, the number of crossbred pigs is still very small. As per 1992 census, the proportion of crossbred pigs in the total number of pigs was only 14.5 per cent. The number however showed an increasing trend as the proportion of crossbred pigs was only 10.5 per cent in 1987. A major constraint in piggery development is the lack of adequate high quality breeding stock. Exotic breeds like Largewhite, Yorkshire, Hampshire, Berkshire, Saddleback, etc. are maintained in the 200 pig breeding farms of state governments, Agricultural Universities and Krishi Vigyan Kendras. To overcome the shortage of high quality breeding stock, exotic breeds of 280 pigs of Largewhite, Landrace and Hampshire were imported from USA during 1999-2000 by the Department of Animal Husbandry, Government of India which would significantly assist in the development of piggery in the country. These pigs have already started producing piglets.

It has already been stated that bovine population is most predominant in most of the states. However, the size of bovine population, as already mentioned, depended on the geographical area and socio-economic milieu of the states. Same is the case with sheep and goats. However, as pig rearing is confined mainly to certain categories of the country's caste hierarchy who also eat pork, the concentration of pigs is more where the percentage of such population is higher, such as Uttar Pradesh, Assam, Bihar and West Bengal. A Nagaland study on pig rearing showed that practically every family has two three pigs. These animals are left loose in the open during cool hours of a day (scavenging). Horses and Ponies as well as mules are mainly used as carrier of goods in difficult hilly areas as also in the plains where motorized transport facilities are inadequate. Hence, the highest concentration of horses and ponies is found in Uttar Pradesh (30.5%) followed by Jammu and Kashmir (15%), Bihar (14%), Madhya Pradesh (9%), Haryana (6%) and Maharashtra (5%). Similarly Uttar Pradesh possesses the largest number of mules having almost 53% of the country's total followed by Haryana (13%), Jammu & Kashmir (10%), Punjab and Himachal Pradesh (8% each) and Madhya Pradesh (4%). In addition to the above there are few other livestock which play a great role in Indian economy. However, there is a need for special mention about mithun and yak which are available only in the Himalayan states of the country.

Uttar Pradesh Study

The successful production of pigs depends entirely upon good management for the organized operation of a swine enterprise. According to a study in Uttar Pradesh[3], existing managemental practices in pig rearing are based on management of breeding, housing, piglets, feeding and marketing. The majority (54.57%) of the pig owners reared upgraded pigs with superior quality of meat (Table 2.14), 30% farmers reared *desi* pigs and 12.08% farmers reared both *desi* and upgraded pigs. Only a few respondents (3.75%) reared exotic breeds (large white yorkshire) which had good pork quality, high conversion efficiency and large litter size. The respondents for the study area reported that the average age of gilt when it first came in heat was 9.65 months (SD = 2.34). the average number of piglets born per sow was 7.62 (SD=1.98) in the study area. Majority (53.34%) of the pig owners inseminated their gilts with the boar of other villagers due to their

Table 2.14: Breeds of Pigs Reared by the Farmers

Breeds	Frequency	Percentage
Desi pigs	72	30.00
Upgraded pigs	130	54.71
Desi and upgraded both	29	12.08
Exotic breeds	9	3.75
Total	240	100.00

[3]Rahul Tiwari, et al, Pig Husbandry in Uttar Pradesh, Indian Farming, January 2002.

inaccessibility to reach the veterinary hospitals, which are situated it far off places. The average age at first farrowing of sow was 7.62 (SD=1.98) in the study area. Majority (53.34%) of the pig owners inseminated their gifts with the boar of other villagers due to their inaccessibility to reach the veterinary hospitals, which were situated at far off places. The average age at first farrowing of sow was 12.38 months and the average farrowing intervals was 6.69 months in the study area. According to most of the pig owners the sow farrowed twice in a year.

Majority (88.75%) of the pig owners reported that when the animals retained the placenta they fed the sow a mixture of jaggery and dried ginger after which the placenta dropped successfully, a few respondents (11.25%) said that they called the veterinary doctor, in case the animals retained the placenta after birth. Almost all the respondents reported that they buried the placenta in a pit away from the home immediately after its expulsion. The majority (96.25%) of the pig owners constructed separate houses for pigs (Table 2.15). Only 3.75 percent farmers reported that the pigs shared the same houses with the owners. The majority (78.33%) of the pig owners cleaned the pigsty daily, since they had included it in their routine work. Approximately 15% respondents cleaned the pigsty weekly. Only 5.84% pig owners reported that they cleaned the pigsty when they got free time from the routine schedule.

Majority (92.91%) of the pig owners bathe their pigs themselves. Only a few respondents (7.09%) did not bathe their animals. The pigs wallowed in the pond, canal or river on their own to keep their body cool. The majority of the pig owners (98.58%) did not use any soap or detergent for bathing their pigs. Only 9.42% respondents used soap/detergent for bathing their pigs. Almost all the pig owners reported that they disposed the dung in garbage dumps away from the house. Nobody used the pig dung as manure for their fields.

Majority (67.50%) of the pig owners did not clean the mucous and nostrils of newborn pigelet presumably due to their illiteracy and lack of required knowledge. Only 32.50% exercised this practice. The female members in the family generally attended the farrowing and cleaned mucous from mouth, nostrils and various body part of piglets with the help of cloth or soft dry grass after brith. Only 17.50% of the pig owners clipped the needle teeth of young piglets. Among the pig owners who clipped the needle teeth, majority (50%) of the respondents clipped the needle teeth, when the piglets were 2-3 days old, while 28.57% respondents clipped the needle teeth within

Table 2.15: Night Shelter of Pigs

Items	Frequency	Percentage
Constructed separate houses	231	96.25
Share same house with owners	19	3.75
Total	240	100.00

24 hr after the birth of the piglets. Remaining 21.43% farmers clipped the needle teeth after 3 days of the birth.

Majority (65.42%) of the pig owners provided bedding materials for their piglets. Only a few respondents (34.58%) did not provide any bedding materials. Among the pig owners who provided bedding materials for their piglets, majority (47.13%) of the farmers used gunny bags, followed by 21.66% pig owners who used wheat straw. About 18.47% pig owners used dry leaves as bedding material for their piglets. The study showed that 65% of the respondents castrated their male piglets for maintaining the meat quality. Only 35% pig owners did not exercise this practice, since they were maintaining pigs for breeding purpose. All the pig owners who castrated their piglets used a new blade or knife for castration. They did not apply any antiseptic lotion or cream at the site of the operation. Further the respondents reported that they castrated their pigs within 2 months after birth.

Feeding Management

Almost all the respondents reported that they fed the undermentioned materials to the pigs as per their availability during the time of breeding. They were fed on molasses, wheat bran, rice polish, broken wheat, waste from sweet shop, kitchen waste, hotel waste, wheat flour, ground rice husk, grams (unfit for consumption), etc.

Besides stall feeding, almost all the pig owners left their pigs for grazing but the time of grazing differed. Majority (57%) of the respondents reported that the grazing period of pigs was more than 5 hr/day. Approximately 34% pig owners mentioned that they left their pigs for 3-5 hr/day for grazing. Rest 8.33% pig owners said that their pigs grazed for only 1-3 hr/day. Pigs went for grazing in the surrounding of the house, and even sometimes to the farmers' fields. Among the 240 respondents, 66.25% pig owners reported that during grazing, pigs had grasses, kitchen waste, standing crops, green leafy vegetable and sugarcane. Approximately 22.50% farmers said that their pigs consumed kitchen waste, grasses, leafy vegetables and roots of different plants during grazing. Only a few respondents (11.25%) mentioned that the pigs had grasses, kitchen waste, potato, barseem and bajara during the grazing.

The majority of the respondents (59.80%) left their pigs alone during grazing, whereas 40.20% mentioned that they accompanied the pigs for grazing, since they felt that the pigs might cross the roads or get injured while grazing alone. Also, they kept an eye on the pigs so that the pigs did not eat any dirty materials and destroy the crops of others during grazing. One more reason for accompanying the pigs was the fear of theft of piglets while grazing.

Marketing Management

Nearly 51.67% pig owners sold their pigs to the middleman due to lack of easily accessible markets for sale of pigs. Most of them (80.42%) sold the pork, while a few (19.58%) sold the live animals as such. The average selling price/kg live weight of *desi* pigs was Rs. 41.25, as reported by the pig owners. Majority (71.67%) of the pig owners did not sell the bristles of the pigs. They either sold the pigs as such or when selling as pork, they removed the bristles and threw them. Only 28.33% respondents reported that they cut the bristles of pigs for selling. The average age of slaughtering the pigs in the study area was 7.52 months (SD=2.61). Since at this age the pigs obtained a body weight of 80-100 kg and according to pig owners the pork quality is best when the pig is between 7 and 8 months. The meat quality deteriorated, as the pigs grew old, due to the deposition of fat under their skin.

Majority (72.90%) of the pig owners did not slaughter their pigs themselves. They took their pigs for slaughtering to the market meat shops. Only 27.10% pig owners killed their pigs themselves by poking a speer underneath the front leg of the animal a number of times till the animal died. They then removed the hairs of the animal and cut the body into a number of pieces for selling.

Mithun

Of the domestic animals, mithun is the most important in the sub-Himalayan region. west of the Buddhist areas in Kameng district of Arunachal Pradesh. The state is the habitat of nearly 70% of the total in the country. Remaining 30% are in Nagaland and Manipur states. This animal plays a very important role in the socio-economic life of the people. As in the biblical days, a man's wealth is estimated by the heads of mithun he possesses. As indicative of social status an essential item of requirement in most of their feasts and festivals and religious rites, they are also in great demand, and so are useful as means of payment. But as the mithun is the highest 'denomination coin' which has to be taken and paid in full, it is used in big transaction only. The bride-price is also determined by the number of mithuns to be paid. Earlier, it was the ransom to be paid for captives. Even at present compensation for crime is paid in terms of mithun.

Sachin Ray[4], then Cultural Research Officer, North-East Frontier Agency (now Arunachal Pradesh) stated that from January to July, the Tibetans used to come down through the Kepung La Pass with rock salt, iron, warm durable, aesthetically pleasing hand-woven cloth, swords, mask, imitation tarquoise necklaces, blue porcelain beads, yarn of different colours, snuff, small quantities of china, silver and wooden bowls and metal pots and exchanged these commodities with mithuns, raw hides, deer horns, white and red rice.

Mithuns are mainly used as means of appeasing deities and spirits, for bringing good luck to, and averting bad luck from, the sacrificer, they are considered good or bad according to the good or bad luck they are supposed

---

[4]Sachin Ray: Aspects of Padm-Minfang Culture, North-East Frontier Agency

to bring. The quality of individual animals is judged from special marks they bear, certain peculiar formations or particular features of appearance to which is ascribed ominous significance. A mithun is invariably considered unlucky if it has only a little hair on its breast, or if its colour is entirely white, or it is lean and thin. The price of the animal consequently goes down in such cases. On the other hand the animal is considered lucky if the colour of the forehead is partly red and partly black or if it has moist lips. Animals are considered moderately good if they are shaggy even if the body is smaller than average, or, if they are entirely black and lastly if they have white spots on two sides and one or two on the forehead.

Yak

The Yak, also called the grunting ox, is an animal adapted to high altitude. Yak is a native of the Tibetan Plateau and the surrounding countries of Central Asia. They are found in altitudes of about 4,300 to 6,100 metres above sea level. Wild yaks live in large herds in cold, high altitude, desolate regions where other livestock would not survive. Agile, sure climbers, and good swimmers, yaks roam icy mountainsides and valleys, grazing on coarse grasses. A wild bull may be 2.4 to 2.7 m (8 to 9 ft.) long, stand 1.8 m (6 ft.) tall at the shoulder hump and weigh approximately 545 kgs. Yaks have long hair that hangs nearly to the ground like a fringe. Wild Yaks are blackish brown but smaller domesticated forms may be red or brown mottled with white. All males have large horns. Domisticated Yaks are used for transportation, as pack animals, and as a source of milk, meat, leather and cloth.

In India Yaks are found mainly in Ladakh valley of Jammu & Kashmir (56.9%), Sikkim (17%), Arunachal Pradesh (15.5%), Lahaul & Spiti valleys of Himachal Pradesh (8.6%) and a small number in Meghalaya (1.8%). These animals generally live along the snow line moving up on grasslands at high altitudes which other species of livestock are unable to utilize.

Poultry

In respect of poultry, which of late, has assumed increasing importance in the livestock economy of the country, it may be pointed out that its existence is more dispersed among the states.

However, highest number of poultry is found in Andhra Pradesh (16%), closely followed by West Bengal (12%), Maharashtra (10.5%), Tamil Nadu (8%) and Madhya Pradesh (7%). Other states which have cognizable percentages of poultry population are Bihar and Punjab (6% each), Assam and Kerala (5 % each), Orissa and Madhya Pradesh (4% each) and Uttar Pradesh (3.5%). The rest of the states and Union Territories possess the remaining 13 per cent of the poultry population of the country.

Appendix I

Table 2AI.1: Total Number of Livestock and Poultry in India-1997- Statewise

(in '000 nos.)

States	Total Crossbred Cattle	Total Indigenous Cattle	Total Cattle	Total Buffaloes	Total Yaks	Total Mithuns	Total Sheep	Total Goats	Total Horses & Ponies	Total Mules	Total Donkeys	Total Camels	Total Pigs	Total Livestock	Total Poultry
1. Andhra Pradesh	751	9851	10602	9658	0	0	9743	5213	7	1	37	0	748	36009	63396
2. Arunachal Pradesh	11	441	451	12	14	124	27	154	6	0	0	0	249	1037	1292
3. Assam	369	7727	8097	728	0	0	84	2717	12	0	0	0	1082	12720	18210
4. Bihar	232	24366	24598	5879	0	0	1956	20229	120	8	28	0	924	53742	19890
5. Chhatisgarh	105	8680	8786	1941	0	0	196	2154	9	0	1	0	456	13543	6771
6. Goa	7	81	88	40	0	0	0	13	0	0	0	0	105	247	790
7. Gujarat	342	6406	6749	6285	0	0	2158	4386	14	0	74	0	198	19930	7236
8. Haryana	848	1552	2401	4823	7	0	1275	968	49	34	63	65	700	10413	9225
9. Himachal Pradesh	368	1805	2174	748	0	0	1080	1168	13	18	8	99	7	5224	865
10. Jammu & Kashmir	1083	2092	3175	787	33	0	3170	1864	141	21	23	0	12	9228	5557
11. Karnataka	1293	9539	10831	4367	0	0	8003	4875	16	0	28	4	405	28526	21399
12. Kerala	1957	533	2491	111	0	0	3	1598	0	0	0	0	88	4292	18397
13. Madhya Pradesh	177	19320	19497	6648	0	0	657	6470	55	7	49	0	375	33768	7261
14. Maharashtra	2457	15615	18072	6073	0	0	3368	11434	42	1	71	10	567	39630	35392
15. Manipur	69	439	508	95	17	17	8	33	2	0	0	3	388	1051	3055
16. Meghalaya	17	738	756	17	0	0	17	280	2	0	1	0	351	1424	2152

Table 2AI.1: Total Number of Livestock and Poultry in India-1997- Statewise (Contd.)

(in '000 nos.)

States	Total Crossbred Cattle	Total Indigenous Cattle	Total Cattle	Total Buffaloes	Total Yaks	Total Mithuns	Total Sheep	Total Goats	Total Horses & Ponies	Total Mules	Total Donkeys	Total Camels	Total Pigs	Total Livestock	Total Poultry
17. Mizoram	8	26	33	5	0	0	0	15	2	0	0	0	163	222	1307
18. Nagaland	154	230	383	36	0	3	2	161	1	0	0	0	571	1188	2444
19. Orrisa	912	12898	13810	1388	0	33	1765	5772	0	0	0	0	602	23338	18435
20. Punjab	1828	810	2638	6171	0	0	436	414	34	17	22	0	96	9858	11022
21. Rajasthan	211	11931	12141	9770	0	0	14585	16971	24	3	186	30	305	54655	4406
22. Sikkim	52	91	143	2	5	0	5	86	5	0	0	669	27	273	221
23. Tamil Nadu	3506	5541	9046	2741	0	0	5259	6416	11	0	43	0	609	24126	36511
24. Tripura	73	1155	1228	18	0	0	6	639	2	0	0	0	211	2105	3595
25. Uttar Pradesh	2105	17911	20016	18996	0	0	1905	11784	216	84	245	0	3135	56414	12116
26. Uttaranchal	103	1927	2031	1094	0	0	311	1070	23	24	1	31	32	4586	971
27. West Bengal	936	16895	17832	1233	0	0	1462	15648	18	0	0	0	805	36998	33309
28. Nicobar	6	54	60	14	0	0	0	71	0	0	0	0	43	188	801
29. Chandigarh	6	1	7	23	0	0	0	1	0	0	0	0	3	35	304
30. Haveli	1	59	60	4	0	0	0	20	0	0	0	0	0	86	411
31. Daman & Diu	0	5	5	1	0	0	0	5	0	0	0	0	0	11	24
32. Delhi	60	36	96	203	0	0	11	25	1	1	1	0	31	369	647
33. Lakshadweep	1	3	3	0	0	0	0	26	0	0	0	0	0	29	79
34. Pondicherry	50	23	73	4	0	0	2	41	0	0	0	0	1	121	121
Total	20099	178782	198882	89918	59	177	57494	122721	826	220	881	911	13291	485385	347611

Note: The census work was not conducted in Bihar, Himachal Pradesh, West Bengal and Dadra& Nagar Haveli. In

3

Role of Livestock in the Economy

Livestock is an important component of the agricultural sector in countries all over the world. Animal husbandry plays an equally important role in the national economy and in the socioeconomic development of India. It forms one of the important sub-sectors of the Indian agriculture. For a country like India, which derives over 23 percent of its Gross Domestic Product (GDP) from agriculture (Table 3.1), the sector plays a crucial role in its rural economy. Livestock is an important source of supplementary income for some 70%, of rural households who derive 15-40 percent of their farm income from livestock. Although at current prices the share of GDP from agriculture as a whole has been declining over the years, the contribution of livestock to the GDP increased from less than 5 per cent in 1980-81 6 per cent in 2000-01. It is a most important productive asset in rural areas serving as a critical store of wealth for farm facilities and an insurance mechanism to cope with household related crisis.

According to provisional estimates of the Central Statistical Organization (CSO), the gross value of output from the livestock sector at current prices was about Rs. 1502 billion during 2001-02, (Table 3.2). Among livestock products, milk group contributes 67 per cent of the total livestock sector output value, meat group is the second most important with 18 per cent (static though during the last five decades), while the share of poultry and eggs increased substantially to 9 per cent. Export earnings from livestock and related products was Rs. 2073 crore in 1998-99, leather and leather products accounting for 54 per cent of it, meat and meat products some 37 per cent. Interestingly, however, total plan investment for the sector is less than 1% and hardly 5% of the outlay in agriculture (Table 3.3). Revenue from exports of live animals and livestock products constituted about 8 percent of the total value of Indian exports.

ROLE OF BULLOCKS

Bullocks are being used for a variety of purposes, including ploughing, transportation of goods and passengers and drawing water from Persian wheels. There are a number of reasons why bullocks continue to hold an important place in rural life. However, two of these are the most important.

Table 3.1: Share of Livestock in GDP

(Rs. crores)

Year	GDP at current prices				Share in GDP (%)		Live-stock's share in Agri. (%)	GDP at constant (1993-94) prices				Share in GDP (%)		Livestock share in Agriculture (%)
	Total	Agri-culture	Live-stock	Agri-culture and allied	Agri-culture	Live-stock		Total	Agri-culture	Live-stock	Agriculture & allied	Agri-culture	Live-stock	
1993-94	781345	221834	50724	241967	28.39	6.49	20.96	781345	221834	50724	241967	28.39	6.49	20.96
1994-95	917058	255193	57718	278773	27.83	6.29	20.70	838031	233099	53511	254090	27.82	6.38	21.06
1995-96	1073271	277846	64970	303102	25.89	6.05	21.44	899563	230469	55827	251892	25.62	6.21	22.16
1996-97	1243546	334029	74710	362605	26.86	6.01	20.60	970083	253750	58168	276091	26.16	6.00	21.07
1997-98	1390148	353490	81927	387008	25.43	5.89	21.17	1016594	246598	59336	269383	24.26	5.84	22.03
1998-99	1598127	408498	91107	442494	25.44	5.70	20.59	1082748	263540	62074	286094	24.34	5.73	21.70
1999-00	1761932	422392	99209	461964	23.97	5.63	21.48	1148442	263258	64199	286094	22.92	5.59	22.70
2000-01	1917724	435135	112059	478468	22.69	5.84	23.42	1198385	261587	67780	285877	21.82	5.65	23.71

Source: National Accounts Statistics, various issues, Central Statistical Organisation, Govt. of India

Table 3.2: Value of Livestock Output at Current Price and its Share in GDP

(*Rs. crores*)

Item	1970-71	1990-91	1993-94	1994-95	1995-96	1996-97	1997-98	1998-99	1999-00	2000-01	2001-02
1. Milk	2167	27508	43408	50448	57231	64334	70729	79876	87608	98146	103804
2. Meat	294	7208	10860	11632	13255	15100	16940	17694	19646	20773	21607
2.1 Beef	41	686	1460	1338	1509	1748	1970	2160	2377	2579	2949
3. By-products		696	1249	1354	1687	2138	2247	2488	2532	2355	2545
3.1 Hides	47	270	541	591	697	889	882	934	1010	944	960
3.2 Skins	26	306	515	575	779	1004	1052	1189	1122	1037	1179
3.3 Others		120	193	188	211	245	313	366	400	374	406
4. Dung	320	4307	6214	6741	7379	8242	9047	9804	10937	11475	11835
4.1 Dung fuel	153	2161	2875	3175	3356	3701	3957	4076	4619	4823	4974
4.2 Other Dung	167	2146	3339	3566	4023	4541	5090	5728	6318	6653	6861
5. Value of Live-stock Product	3197	42040	66965	76043	85837	97158	107206	118367	129952	142487	150241
6. Value of Agri-culture Output	17531	128657	204874	236607	256698	302744	319586	370365	384766	391537	429410
7. Total Value (5 + 6)	20728	170698	271839	312650	342535	399902	426792	488732	514718	534024	579651
8. Total GDP	36736	477800	781345	917058	1073271	1243546	1390042	1598127	1761932	1917724	2094013
9. Share of Livestock (in GDP percent)	8.70	6.45	8.57	8.29	8.00	7.81	7.71	7.41	7.38	7.43	7.17
10. Share of Livestock (in Agriculture)	15.42	24.63	24.63	24.32	25.06	24.30	25.12	24.22	25.25	26.68	25.92
11. Share of Agriculture (in GDPPercent)	47.72	28.30	26.22	25.80	23.92	24.35	22.99	23.17	21.84	20.42	20.51

Source: National Accounts Statistics, 2002, Central Statistical Organisation, Govt. of India

Table 3.3: *Investment in Animal Husbandry in various Five Year Plans*

(Rs. crores)

Plan	Total Outlay*	Plan allocations on Agriculture & Allied (figure in parenthesis is % of total plan outlay)[1]	A.H. &Dairying (figure in parenthesis is % of outlay in agriculture)[2]	Animal Husbandry as % of total outlay
1st Plan (1951-56)	1960.0	289.9 (14.8)	22.00 (7.6)	1.1
2nd Plan (1956-61)	4671.8	549.0 (11.8)	55.94 (10.2)	1.2
3rd Plan (1961-66)	8576.5	1088.9 (12.7)	90.92 (8.3)	1.1
Annual Plans (1966 to 1969)	6625.4	1107.1 (16.7)	67.47 (6.1)	1.0
4th Plan (1969-74)	15778.8	2320.4 (13.4)	233.10 (11.0)	1.5
5th Plan (1974-79)	39426.2	4864.9 (12.3)	437.54 (9.0)	1.1
Annual Plans (1979 – 1980)	12176.5	1996.5 (16.4)	N.A.	—
6th Plan (1980-85)	97500.0	5695.1 (5.8)	396.56 (7.0)	0:4
7th Plan (1985-90)	18000.0	10523.6 (5.8)	467.94 (4.4)	0.3
Annual Plan (1990 to 1992)	123120.5	7255.9 (5.9)	278.84 (3.8)	0.2
8th Plan (1992-1997)	434100.0	22467.2 (5.2)	1300.00 (5.8)	0.3
9th Plan (1997-2002)	859200.0	42462.0 (4.9)	1545.64 (3.6)	0.2
10th Plan (2002-2007	1525639.0	58933.0 (3.9)	2500.00 (4.2)[3]	0.2

Source: [1] Economic Survey, Government of India.

[2] Basic Animal Husbandry Statistics 2002, Department of Animal Husbandry and Dairying, Government of India.

[3] Government of India, Planning Commission:Tenth Five Year Plan,Vol.II.

The first is tradition. Cows being revered in the Indian society, their male calves are traditionally reared lovingly by farmers and then used as bullocks in farming. This emotional bond between the farmer and his bullocks is still strong. Secondly, bullocks still make economic sense for medium and small farmers. A tractor-trailer for these farmers is a liability. The initial expenditure and later operational costs and maintenance are too high for farmers with smaller holdings. Most such farmers have already burnt tractors on loan and then selling land to repay it. They have reverted to bullocks. A young pair of bullocks costs around Rs 10,000, which is negligible as compared to tractors. Likewise, a bullock cart costs just Rs 12,000 to 15,000. The trailer for tractor costs significantly higher. Rural economy has a self-contained production system in which small farmers keep livestock in proportion to the crop residues available to sustain the cattle virtually free of cost. Largely, family labour is used to look after the cattle. This explains why bullocks fit in so well despite the changing agricultural scenario.

The role of livestock within agriculture sector is also increasing fast though it does not include the contribution of draught power and value of dung which is highly underestimated. Draught Animal Power (DAP) of bullocks (60 million) and buffaloes (7 million) as well as equines (1 million) horses and donkeys and camels (1 million), make available 50,000 million units of energy per year, worth Rs. 10,000 crores. Draught Animals (DAs) plough 100 million hectares of farm land, forming 60% of the area cultivated. They transport 25,000 million tonnes kms. of freight per year in 15 million carts, of which one million are improved type. DAP saves 6 million tonnes of petroleum per year, worth Rs. 4,000 crores, in foreign exchange. DAP is an appropriate technology, inevitable for 60 million small farms and for small scale transportation. Asset value of DAP is Rs. 20,000 crores and replacement by mechanized system would need Rs. 100,000 crores. The Institute of Economic Growth, Delhi University made a study and found that to replace draught animals, India would require about twenty million tractors and the petroleum products worth $20 billion. Another study by Dr Jugner Lansh, who stayed in Indian villages for three months found that if the cattle were to be eliminated then 100-200 million people would migrate to cities. In spite of its magnificent contribution, DAP is neglected, and therefore, is in a low level of productivity, resulting in enormous loss to farmers and huge wastage to the economy.[1]

Bovine animals, viz. cattle and buffaloes occupy a pivotal position in the national life. In fact, the cultural life in India, particularly in the rural areas, is intimately connected with these animals in several ways. This is more so with the cattle. The contribution of cattle and buffalo to the national economy is indeed vast. Briefly, they are the main source of draught power in agricultural operations and rural transportation. They provide essential foods of animal origin like milk and meat. Large quantities of animal byproducts such as hides, bones, blood, guts, etc. and organic manure valued at around Rs. 21,019 crore is also provided by these animals. Distribution of livestock and their contributions are indicated in annexure I-V. Sheep farming provides employment opportunities to a large section of the population, particularly to the weaker sections of the community in hilly, drought prone and desert areas. Sheep droppings improve the fertility of soil considerably and penning of sheep in harvested fields brings in

---

[1]First Conference and Photo Exhibition on Modernization of the Draught Power Systems (Sponsored by the Ministry of Non-Conventional Energy Sources & organized by the CARTMAN, the Centre for Action, Research & Technology for Man, Animal and Nature, Bangalore), March 4-5, 1994.

additional income to the flock owners. Since sheep rearing does not require any large investment in buildings and equipment, it offers good scope for exploitation by the small and marginal farmers and agricultural labourers. In fact, sheep rearing is extremely important in the rural economy of a number of states. Wool and mutton, the two main products from sheep, provide livelihood to a large number of people in many states.

India ranks first in respect of cattle and buffaloes, second in goats, third in sheep and sixth in poultry population in the world. About 19 million people working in livestock sector

Goat contributes about 16 per cent of the total meat and about 4 per cent to the total milk produced in the country. Besides, by export of goat skins, casings and hair, valuable foreign exchange is earned. The manure produced from droppings enriches the soil. However, because of its habit of nibbling at young plants and grasses, it can cause extensive damage to forest areas. Thus, if the economic value of the goat is to be fully exploited, suitable forest management systems will have to be devised to exercise greater control over their movement and feeding habits. It is also necessary to reduce their number in areas where afforestation, soil conservation and pasture development programmes have been introduced.

According to estimates of the Central Statistical Organization (CSO), the value of output from livestock and fisheries sectors together at current prices was about Rs. 1,70,205 crores during 2000-01; (Rs.1,44,088 crores for livestock and Rs. 26,117 crores for fisheries) which was about 30.3 per cent of the value of the output of Rs.5,61,717 crores from total agriculture and allied sector. The contribution of these sectors in the total GDP during 2000-01 was 7.35%

Poultry farming has become a popular avocation within rural and semi-urban areas, as it provides an excellent opportunity for gainful employment to idle or underemployed families since the poultry can be reared with ease even by women and children. Further, poultry farming is possible in varied agroclimatic environment as the fowl possesses marked physiological adaptability. Poultry farming is also remunerative following its small space requirements, low capital investment, with good returns from outlay and well distributed turnover throughout the year. Amongst farm animals, poultry is one of the quickest and most efficient converters of plant products into food of high biological value. About 14 per cent of the total meat and almost 95 per cent of the eggs are available from poultry farming. Poultry litter, if properly collected, as in the deep litter system, has a high manural value.

Pig is one of the most efficient feed converting animals among domesticated stock. It is the only litter bearing animals among meat producing livestock having the shortest generation interval and high feed conversion efficiency. Pork constitutes about 10 per cent of total meat production in the country. Processed pork products are becoming more and more popular in the country and thereby increasing employment opportunity. It may be mentioned that while the slaughter rates for cattle, buffaloes, sheep and goat are 6,10,30 and 40 per cent respectively, it is 99 per cent for pigs.

Sale of milk accounts for 30 to 50 percent of the rural household income with wide variations between regions and households. An extensive nationwide study carried out by the NCAER in 1990 reported that revenue from the sale of milk alone accounted for 22% of the family income. By the end of Year 2000 milk production shot up to almost 75 million tonnes as against only about 17 million tonnes in 1950-51.

The major contribution of animal husbandry to national economy is its support to self sufficiency in food production popularly known as the "green revolution", by providing the animal power valued at 37,000 MW. Such stable draught power was achieved through the reduction and control of animal diseases. If the green revolution has made the country self-reliant in grain production, the technologies developed in the areas of animal production and health have made White Revolution possible as an alternative model of rural change with little public investment and incentives. In contrast to the Green Revolution, White Revolution narrowed the gap between the rich and the poor. For instance 80 percent of milk produced in the country comes from small and marginal farmers and landless labourers.

About three-fourths of India's population in India live in rural areas, and over 70 percent of rural households own livestock. Dairy products are a major source of nutritious food to millions of people in India and the only acceptable source of animal protein for the large vegetarian segment of the population. However in triennium ending 1993, per capita availability of protein from milk was insignificant, being only about 6 gm, which constituted only 10 per cent of the total protein availability from different sources. The organic fertilizer produced in the livestock sector is a key factor of agricultural production and dung from livestock is a major source of cooking energy in rural areas especially among low-income households. Not only it is one of the most important productive assets in the rural areas, it also serves as a critical store of wealth for farm families and an insurance mechanism to cope with household related crisis.

NUTRITION

Whey: A protein source

Whey protein, with a biological value of 104, is by far the best naturally-available protein source. Whey proteins are present in soluble form in milk (a fraction of 0.62 per cent). Separating these proteins from milk requires high technology ultrafiltration process. This process subjects the whey to gentle processing, ensuring that the whey proteins are recovered and retained. Whey proteins contain essential amino acids in amounts proportion to the needs of the body and are easily digestible. A study by scientists at the National Institute of Nutrition, Hyderabad, has shown that whey proteins have the highest amount of almost every category of essential amino acids like leucine, isoleucine, lysine than any other protein source. These proteins have both nutraceutical and dietetic applications. In clinical foods, whey proteins are much in demand for their twin properties: a rich source of protein, so essential for repair of body cells and growth; and easy digestibility.

Whey proteins provide the nutritive value of milk minus the fat, lactose and other constituents of milk, that are difficult to digest. Whey proteins are deemed essential for infant food formulations, especially for infants with a low birth weight problem. Mother's milk has whey protein: casein ratio of 60:40. The only way in which this can be achieved in milk product formulations is fortification by whey protein powder. The area of greatest interest as far the application of whey proteins go are sports food. These proteins supply the much-needed quality amino acids to 'hungry muscles'. A cursory glance at various sports food websites on the Internet would convince one how seriously sports food manufactures take whey protein. Scientists have recently discovered that whey proteins, besides building muscle mass so critical for athletes and bodybuilders also offer numerous other benefits like immune-system reinforcement, antioxidant protection and support to muscle tissue repair and regeneration.

Whey proteins have been around for a decade in the developed world. In India, though, whey proteins have only recently entered the market. Mahaan Proteins Limited have set up a plant in Kosi Kalan (Mathura) for processing whey proteins, apart from a range of other milk products. Apart from nutraceutical and dietetic applications, whey proteins have applications in the bakery industry as well. "Mongini's have just launched an egg-less cake, using whey proteins. The cake has all the qualities of an egg cake.

Separating Milk and Water

The dairy revolution launched under Operation Flood in 1970 has raised the availability of milk in India from 112 grams per-person per-day in 1970-71 to 211 grams in 1998-99. While this is an impressive performance, milk availability remains inadequate for the predominantly vegetarian India. Most diet specialists would advice the vegetarians in India to drink at least 500 grams of milk per day. Add to that the milk needed for making ghee, curd, butter, khoya, milk powder and cheese, which currently account for a little more than half of the milk consumption in India. Even adjusting for the population that eats meat, fish and poultry and therefore, require less milk, these facts imply the need for a much larger quantity of milk than is currently available. Furthermore, given that millions of children still go without any milk because their parents are unable to afford it, the case for bringing milk processing costs down seems irrefutable.

Livestock Sector not only provides essential protein and nutritious human diet through milk, eggs, meat etc., but also plays an important role in utilization of non-edible agricultural byproducts. Livestock also provides raw material/by products such as hides and skins, blood, fat etc., The value of output from meat at current prices was Rs. 22,513 crores during 2000-01 as compared to Rs. 15,422 crores during 1995-96. Total export-earnings from livestock, poultry and related products was Rs. 3841 crores in 2001-02. Out of the total exports, leather sector accounted for Rs. 2198 crores in value terms.

Unfortunately, the issue is more complex. Unlike developed countries where milk is produced in big farms of 100 or more cattle on farm, the average farmer in India has just one or two cattle. Most of such cattle owners are small or marginal farmers or landless labourers. In all, nine million of them, spread over 100,000 villages, sell 12 million litres of milk every day to urban consumers. In all likelihood, production costs of these farmers are higher than the current world prices so that larger quantities of imports would displace many of them. Even though some poor people will benefit from lower milk prices, the net impact of imports on poverty is likely to be negative. There is also a politico-economic factor that suggests policy against free imports. Milk production and exports are subsidized in developed countries. Good economics says that we should enjoy the benefits of such subsidy: if these countries want to give us milk for free (or at throwaway prices), we should gladly take it, providing our children an adequate source of protein and calcium. Yet, politicians are likely to find it difficult to convince domestic industry to accept free flow of subsidized imports.

Thus, to ensure that the adverse impact of liberalization on poverty does not block other, more urgent reforms, pragmatism dictates a compromise solution whereby a modest protection to the domestic dairy industry is provided against milk imports. Contrary to some claims, the government has not tied its hand entirely under the WTO agreement. According to World Bank's Garry Pursell, a leading trade-policy expert on India, our current WTO obligations require us to import only 10,000 tonnes of powered milk at a tariff rate of 15 per cent. Beyond this quantity, the tariff rate can rise up to 60 per cent. Taking the interests of consumers and long-term efficiency into account, the tariff rate on out-of-quota imports should be set at approximately 30 per cent.

Of course, we should not lose sight of the fact the ultimate goal of the policy should be to lift the small farmers and landless labourers out of their marginal existence. Rather than freeze these individuals in their current employment, which condemns them to living on sales of a few litres of milk every day, we must create better opportunities for them. This means treating the protection to dairy industry as a transition measure. The ultimate cure for poverty lies in outward-oriented rapid growth that generates high-paying jobs- a prescription that the current president of the World Bank, James Wolfensohn, has chosen to ignore. On the one hand, we must continue with our broad liberalization programme and on the other, we must support the launch of a new WTO round that brings an end to agricultural subsidies in the rich countries.

POVERTY ALLEVIATION

Livestock Production Systems are based on low cost agro byproducts as nutritional inputs, using traditional technologies. Gender equity is more pronounced here as women participation is 71% of the labour force while it is only 33% in crop farming. About 10 million families in India are engaged in sheep, goat, rabbit and pack animal rearing, fur/skin processing, fibre/wool handling and meat production. Livestock indeed is considered as an important economic activity that can help to alleviate poverty. The spectacular growth of livestock products especially milk, meat, eggs and poultry meat is, however, attributed to the initiatives taken by the Government through its schemes and organized sector and the rising demand for these products in response to rising incomes in urban and rural areas. It has been observed that with increasing income, demand for cereals is decreasing. While Green Revolution was supply driven, Livestock Revolution is demand driven. With ever increasing demand for livestock products, its impact on agricultural economy becomes immensely important.

Far from being a drain on the food available to the poor, increased consumption of animal products can help augment the food purchasing power of the poor. Considerable evidence exists that the rural poor and landless, especially women, get a higher share of their income from livestock than better-off rural people. Furthermore, livestock provide the poor with fertilizer and draught power, along with the opportunity to exploit common grazing areas, build collateral savings, and diversify income. The Livestock Revolution could well become a key means of alleviating poverty in the next 20 years. But rapid industrialization of production abetted by widespread current subsidies for large-scale credit and land use could harm their major mechanism of income and asset generation for the poor. Policy makers need to make sure that policy distortions do not drive the poor out of the one growing sector in which they are presently competitive.

Livestock products also benefit the poor by alleviating the protein and micronutrient deficiencies prevalent in the country. Increased consumption of even a small additional amount of meat and milk can provide the same level of nutrients, protein, and calories to the poor that a large and diverse amount of vegetables and cereals could provide.

Some 80% of the main agricultural work force of 185 million were involved in livestock production either as producers or hired labour in 1991. Total employment potential in the livestock sector in terms of man –years had been variously estimated

> The rural women play a significant role in animal husbandry and are involved in operations like feeding, breeding, management and health care. The actual farm operations and participation of women vary from place to place with the system of production and socio-economic status. Women constitute 71% of the labour force in livestock farming. In dairying, 75 million women are engaged as against 15 million men. About 0.5 million women are employed in pre and post harvest operations in marine sector.

by different groups—the National Commission on Agriculture's estimate was 32.8 million man-years in 1970. Another estimate puts down to 36.07 million man years for the care and management of milch animals alone in 1987. According to an estimate of authors, nearly 35 million people were employed in livestock sector, of which nearly 80 per cent was in bovine animal sub-sector. The employment potential in livestock sector has been discussed in a separate chapter.

As the ownership of livestock is more evenly distributed with landless labourers, small and marginal farmers, the progress in this sector will result in a more balanced development of the rural economy. In India food consumption basket is also diversified in favour of non-food grain items like milk, meat, egg and fish. Women will be playing a larger role in value addition and marketing of these items.

Recently the processing industry for milk, poultry and leather has also become quite important with urbanization and improved living standards and demand for processed products is also increasing substantially. However reliable information is not available about the employment potential of such an important sector of the economy. While a large number of small/ marginal farmers and landless labour (particularly women folk) are getting part time employment throughout the year, a proper methodology, with an empirical data base, to tackle this problem has yet to be evolved. A study conducted by NDRI, Karnal provides useful data on labour employment in the dairy industry (Table 3.4). There is no justification for a large variation in various estimates with regards to the number of persons employed in the sector. NSSO data also shows wide changes from year to year (Table 3.5). Leather industry alone is estimated to employ over 16.65 million mostly women and other weaker sections of the society.

It may be stressed that livestock employment, particularly under Indian conditions has its own peculiarities. There is perhaps an urgent need to look into this aspect by a multi-disciplinary team to evolve an appropriate

Table 3.4: *Labour Employment in Dairy Enterprise on Different Categories of Progressive Farmers (Mandays/Household/Year)*

S. No.	Particulars	Small	Medium	Large	Overall
1.	Male	83.06	112.82	200.56	120.49 (39.84)
2.	Female	72.05	112.11	135.63	115.31 (38.13)
3.	Child	47.81	64.90	104.21	66.64 (22.03)
4.	Total Labour Employment per:				
	Household	202.94	289.83	40.40	302.44 (100.00)
	Dairy animal	98.60	83.80	70.32	86.22

Note: Figures in parenthesis indicate percentage to total employment per household.
Source: V.P. Sharma and Raj Vir Singh (1994) NDRI, Karnal.

Table 3.5: Sectoral Growth of Employment in Rural Area (1972-86) All India

Sl. No.	Sector	Employment (million)				Average annual growth rate			
		'72-'73	'77-'78	'82-'83	'87-'88	'72-'73	'77-'78	'82-'83'	87-'88
1	Agriculture*	167.30	183.40	196.60	196.77	1.96	1.27	0.39	1.10
		(85.62)	(83.35)	(81.50)	(78.01)				
	Livestock	9.03	10.60	29.43	16.65	7.41	10.06	18.31	4.15
		(4.62)	(4.82)	(8.47)	(6.6)				
2	Mining & Quarrying	0.68	0.89	1.16	1.48	5.83	4.94	5.56	5.41
		(0.35)	(0.40)	(0.48)	(0.59)				
3	Manufg.	10.46	13.73	16.32	18.51	5.89	3.19	2.84	3.95
		(5.35)	(6.24)	(6.77)	(7.34)				
4	Electricity, Gas & Water	0.14	0.28	0.34	0.43	15.71	3.59	5.36	7.90
		(0.07)	(0.13)	(0.14)	(0.17)				
5	Construction	2.70	2.90	4.05	8.50	1.52	6.26	17.91	8.09
		(1.38)	(1.39)	(1.68)	(3.37)				
6	Trade	4.80	7.24	8.37	10.31	8.75	2.67	4.74	5.25
		(2.49)	(3.29)	(3.47)	(4.09)				
7	Transport	1.29	1.79	2.61	3.33	7.14	7.10	5.56	6.64
		(0.66)	(0.81)	(1.08)	(1.32)				
8	Services	7.97	9.80	11.77	12.90	4.45	3.39	2.06	3.82
		(4.08)	(4.45)	(4.88)	(5.11)				
	Total	195.40	220.06	241.22	252.22	2.53	1.68	1.00	1.75
		(100)	(100)	(100)	(100)				

Note: Agriculture includes employment in livestock sector.
Source: Sarvekshana, various issues, National Sample Survey Organisation, New Delhi.

methodology which should take note of the ground situation in the country and develop required norms. Converting the total employment into man years is not much of relevance and depicts, if at all, a completely distorted picture.

In the Indian context of poverty and malnutrition, animal husbandry especially the dairy sector has a special role to play for providing supplementary income to some 70 million farmers and landless labour in over 500,000 remote villages as well as for much nutritional advantage of milk and milk products. In the rural areas around 70 percent of the households own livestock. Income from livestock production accounts for 15-40 percent of total farm households incomes. More importantly, small and marginal farmers account for three-quarters of those households, raising 56 percent of bovine (cattle and buffalo). Dairy industry plays a vital role in the agro-based economy of India. India's programme of reform and economic liberalization opens significant market-led opportunities for the livestock sector. Sustained economic growth and rising incomes are driving the rapid growth in livestock product demand. This has fostered the rapid expansion of the livestock output during the last two decades.

Social Dimensions and Gender Issues

With increasing integration of farm households with output markets, livestock has started exerting considerable influence on household behaviour: enhancing viability of both households as well as the farming system. There are however social problems impeding progress, undermining livelihoods.

Government policies based on religious compulsions inhibit alternate use of large ruminants, limiting the scope and viability of smallholder dairy enterprise, denying them over 40 per cent of their potential income.

There are equity concerns in livestock ownership, as the succession laws of the country preclude women from inheriting land; and so deny them access to credit for owning livestock.

Patriarchal rural societies discourage women from acquiring livelihood skills, as training for such skills require them to be away from homes for days together. Worse still is the patriarchal ambience of the institutional set up in the livestock sector and the absence of women employees in large enough numbers in these institutions.

As mentioned earlier, bulk of the chores related to care and management of livestock in households however, fall on the shoulders of the family women folk. There is increasing evidence to show that women are influential in shaping family decisions related to livestock, even though such decisions are publicly articulated or acted upon by the male members of the family. It is also becoming clear that targeting women as development partners in animal husbandry development projects will be the key to successful project implementation.

LIVESTOCK AND DIVERSIFICATION

Of all the existing technologies, livestock offers a good scope for diversification as it assures regular income. Such a diversification in today's scenario is deemed essential not only for uplifting rural masses but also meeting the rising demand for milk and other livestock products. Today India is a global leader in milk production. About 70 million farmers maintain a milch herd of 100 million cattle. Indian dairy, therefore, becomes a unique case where its marginal farmers contribute their share of milk resources through cooperative unions, notwithstanding several handicaps. Nearly seven million rural milk producers are direct beneficiaries of the biggest economic development programme anywhere in the world. During the post-independence period, milk production registered a persistent increase from 17.4 million tonnes in 1948-52 to an estimated 74 million tonnes in 1998 and 81 million tonnes in 2001 with per capita consumption of milk of 204 gm per day. However, milk production is characterised by the presence of poor breeds of milch maintained on inadequate feeding, management and health care. About 85 per cent of Indian cows give less milk than 1 kg per day and cows giving more than 2 kg of milk per day are only about 5 per cent. An average Indian cow milk yield ranges from 200 to 500 kg per lactation of 300 days compared to 4, 154 kg in the USA, 3,950 kg in Denmark. A major proportion of indigenous stock is also plagued with longer age at first calving i.e. 36 to 50 months and an inter-calving period of 14 to 22 months.

The situation with buffaloes is little better as 10 per cent of the buffalo population yield little less than 1 kg milk per day and about 25 per cent yield more than 2 kg of milk per day. On an average an Indian buffalo gives about 650 kg milk per lactation. In nutshell, poor yields are direct reflections of poor breed, feed and management. Upgrading and selective breeding indigenous breeds would not be effective in bridging the gap between requirement and availability in reasonable period of time.

Crossbreeding Option

During the past two decades, crossbreeding has been prevalent countrywide. To boost productivity cross with European breeds have provided a good combination of heat tolerance and disease resistance, besides improving milk production. Crossbreeding experiences have clearly shown that 50 per cent exotic inheritance is most ideal for growth, production and reproduction performances. Exotic genes should be stabilized at this level through crossbreeding. In areas where green fodder is available in plenty and cool climate prevails Holsteins are recommended. Jerseys have been recommended for plains and other areas.

Buffalo Breeding

Buffaloes are considered to be the base of Indian dairy industry. More than 50 per cent of milk production of our country is produced by buffaloes. The Indian subcontinent is endowed with varieties of genetically potential breeds like murrah, nili, jaffrabadi, surti, nagpuri and bhadawari. Nili and murrah are heavy and they are the best milk producers giving 1650-2160 kg. of milk per lactation. They are very much resistant to deadly diseases and drought conditions. Apart from this, they are efficient in utilising course fodder and converting it into milk.

Improving of nondescript buffaloes, grading up may be done with murrah or surti according to agroclimatic regions. Surti is preferred in coastal areas because of its compact size and better heat tolerance. Murrah may be used for grading up of nondescript animals in dry plains, all over India for improving milch production.

Thus, Diversification with dairying requires an appraisal by the farmer of his own resources. Choice of breed has to be made depending on available feed resources. An exotic cross requires more available feed, while the indigenous could subsist even in fecal deficit. It is the small farmers who can entirely change the picture of milk production in the 21st century since 85 per cent of Indian cows yield less than 1 kg milk per day Even a marginal increase by such low yielders can bring about a big revolution. Therefore, dairy of these types has vast scope for which technology dissemination aimed at small farmers is needed.

LIVESTOCK – A SOURCE OF ORGANIC MANURE

According to the livestock census (1992), total manurial potential of this source was over 45 million tonnes of NPK (Table 3.6). Assuming that 50 per cent of this is burnt/wasted, value of only manure at current prices would calculate to say Rs. 21019 crores (Table 3.7). The CSO estimate as against this calculates at hardly Rs. 5700 crores which is less than 27 per cent of the estimated manurial value. In addition, organic manure adds humus to the soil and improves its quality, while absorptive capacity of chemical fertilizers is low and some chemicals are not only waste, but create additional problems. Organic manures are thus contributing much more towards the supply of basic nutrients to the soil. Part of the dung which is being consumed as fuel is being diverted to Gobar-gas plants numbering around 3.2 million which in addition to supplying of necessary energy, also provides better quality of manure.

Gobar Gas Plants

Oil crisis and the consequent steep rise in prices of imported crude and chemical fertilisers created an urgent need for finding alternative sources

Table 3.6: Manurial Potential of Livestock In 1992

Source	Number	Quantity per unit	Total annual	Percentage constituents			Total constituents per year (million tonnes)		
	(Million)	Per day (kg.)	Quantity (million tonnes)	N	P_2O_5	K_2O	N	P_2O_5	K_2O
Cattle	204.53	15.2	1135.3	0.3	0.15	0.2	3.41	1.70	2.27
Adult	138.78	18.1	916.9	0.3	0.15	0.2	2.75	1.37	1.83
Young Stock	65.75	9.1	218.4	0.3	0.15	0.2	0.66	0.33	0.44
Buffaloes	83.5	17.7	531.5	0.3	0.15	0.2	1.59	0.80	1.06
Adult	51.18	22.7	424.1	0.3	0.15	0.2	1.27	0.64	0.85
Young Stock	32.32	9.1	107.4	0.3	0.15	0.2	0.32	0.16	0.21
Total Cattle &	**288.03**	**15.8**	**1666.8**	**0.3**	**0.15**	**0.2**	**5.00**	**2.50**	**3.33**
Buffaloes									
Sheep & goats	166.08	6.8	412.2	0.8	0.6	0.3	3.30	2.47	1.24
Horses & Ponies	0.82	18.1	5.4	0.5	0.4	0.3	0.03	0.02	0.02
Other Livestock	15.00	11.3	61.9	0.6	0.5	0.5	0.37	0.31	0.31
Total Livestock	**469.93**	**12.5**	**2146.3**	—	—	—	**8.70**	**5.30**	**4.90**
Poultry	407.00	0.4	5.9	1.6	1.5	0.9	0.10	0.09	0.05
Total	**876.93**	**6.7**	**2142.0**	—	—	—	**8.80**	**5.39**	**4.95**
Livestock urine	470.14	6.8(a)	1166.9	0.8	0.01	1.4	9.34	0.12	16.34
Cattle bones	43.24(b)	13.6(c)	0.6	3.0	23.5	—	0.02	0.14	—
Grand total	**1347.07**		**3309.5**				**18.16**	**5.65**	**21.29**

Note: (a) Quantity of urine per cattle per day, (b) This has been calculated at 15 per cent cattle mortality, (c) Quantity of bones per cattle.

Table 3.7: Value of Animal Dung and Urine for Manurial Use

Item	Quantity/ year (Million tonnes)	Million tonnes			Value Rs. Crores			Total Rs. crores
		N	P	K	N (Rs. 10/kg.)	P (Rs. 15/kg)	K (Rs.7/ kg)	
Dung.	1073.1	4.35	2.65	2.45	4350	3975	1715	10040
Poultry	5.9	0.10	0.09	0.05	100	135	35	270
Urine	583.4	4.67	0.06	8.17	4670	90	5719	10479
Bones	0.6	0.02	0.14	—	20	210	) —	230
TOTAL	1663.0	9.14	2.94	10.67	9140	4410	7469	21019

Notes: 1. Based on 1992 Livestock Census, 2. Only half dung and urine is assumed to be available for manurial use. Value of N.P.K. is calculated on the basis of current sale price.

of fuel and fertilisers by utilising the locally available materials. This has resulted in the commissioning of 'gobar gas plants' which are economically operated, with raw materials available in the country.

A foreign company has taken a step forward in the commercial application of gobar gas. A new development has taken place in the US. It is a million dollar business project in the US; where a corporation, *Calorific Recovery Anaerobic Process Inc.* has been formed to produce methane from cattle ranches in Oklahoma. The gas so produced would be supplied to the neighbouring states through interstate pipelines, the construction of which has already been authorised by the authorities concerned. This can be sufficient evidence for us to apply the gobar gas technology on a mass scale for preserving, 'both environmental and resources', disposing of the sewage in a scientific and useful manner. In the ultimate analysis, the application of this technology in our rural areas will have a far reaching effect and help rural reconstruction. The gobar gas as an alternative, yet cheap source of energy has been endorsed by an international workshop on 'biogas technology and utilisation' under the auspicious of the Economic and Social Council for Asia and Pacific. We should, therefore, view the implication of this technology in the light of our heavy dependence on oil as a source of energy.

Biogas — An Energy Alternative

Biogas is a clean, nonpolluting, smoke and soot free fuel for cooking, lighting and running of engines*. It contains 50 to 65% methane which is inflammable. Biogas is produced from cattle dung, human excreta and other organic matter in a "Biogas Plant" commonly known as "Gobar Gas Plant" through a process called digestion. One cubic meter biogas can keep one

---

*For more details on Rural Energy, please refer to Annual Reports of the Ministry of Non-Conventional Energy Sources.

biogas lamp of luminosity equivalent to 60 watt electric lighting for 6-7 hr. Biogas is also a superior fuel for producing power. One cubic meter can keep one h.p. engine working for two hours roughly equivalent to 0.6 lt of diesel. The use of energy of one cubic meter biogas can save 3.5 kg of wood or 1.6 kg of coal or 4.7 kW of electricity. Biogas can be used for following purposes:

Domestic Fuel and Motive Power

Biogas provides a clean and efficient fuel for domestic purposes. Conventionally, agriculture residues and dung cakes are used as cooking fuel. It is a wasteful practice as hardly 9-12% of their fuel value is utilised. However, a biogas plant eliminates the age-old practice of burning cow dung for fuel purposes. It saves consumption of wood, charcoal, kerosene and diesel. Thus, it saves the labour of women and children in rural areas who normally spend considerable time and energy to cover long distances daily to collect fuel wood. It would eliminate the practice of indiscriminate felling of trees and consequently soil erosion. The biogas is a smokeless fuel, so the utensils and kitchen remains clean. Biogas is also used for lighting purposes in the villages.

Biomass, such as firewood, agricultural residues and dung cakes, is still the dominant source of fuel in our rural areas; and women and girl children are the key players in producing, collecting and using these fuels. However, inefficient burning of such fuels in traditional chulhas is causing not only an economic loss to the nation but also a serious problem of indoor air pollution and consequent health hazards. An additional cause for concern in recent years has been the unsustainable level of consumption of fuel wood, which leads to deforestation and desertification. In this context, technological solutions, institutional arrangements, financial support and training schemes for ensuring adequate and affordable clean energy systems and services assume great significance in the rural energy policy and programmes. Therefore, the Ministry of Non-Conventional Energy Sources (MNES) has been promoting indigenously developed technologies for efficient utilisations of biomass fuels with a focus on extraction of more energy, reduction of household consumption of firewood, generation of employment and improvement in the living standard of rural people.

Delhi might soon have its first power plant fuelled by cow dung. The Municipal Corporation of Delhi (MCD) is planning to set up one such plant and use the dung, which otherwise pollutes the Yamuna, in a productive manner. The corporation has asked the ministries to consider it a part of the Yamuna Action Plan (Phase II). The plant is estimated to cost Rs. 12 crore approximately. A large number of clusters of dairy farms located in the city and along the river are now directly discharging the cattle dung into the river. There are nine authorized clusters of dairy farms in the outskirts of Delhi. These farms were developed by the DDA and MCD about 20 years ago for relocation of dairies which were earlier operating from within the city.

The most important and popular technology developed indigenously is the "biogas plant" for processing of cattle dung. It serves the purpose of meeting fuel as well as the manure requirement from the same quality of cattle dung available in the rural households and institutions. Another important technology is improved smokeless chulhas, which help in reducing the consumption of firewood per unit of heat energy used and in simultaneously reducing air pollutants in rural kitchens. These two technologies have the potential of meeting the cooking fuel requirement of all our rural households on a sustainable basis in an environmentally benign manner. Besides promoting these technologies through publicity, training, financial and other incentive package, the felt need is to develop and strengthen local institutions, participation of the people, particularly women, and village based energy service entrepreneurs.

The rural energy programmes, implemented by the MNES during 2001-02, comprised of (i) National Project on Biogas Development (NPBD) catering to family type biogas plants, (ii) Community, Institutional and Night-soil based Biogas Plants (CBP/IBP/NBP) Programme, (iii) Research and Development on Biogas, and (iv) National Programme on Improved Chulhas (NPIC). Besides these, pilot schemes on Rural Energy Entrepreneurship and Institutional Development (REEID) and Women and Renewable Energy Development (WRED), which were continued in 2000-01.

NATIONAL PROJECT ON BIOGAS DEVELOPMENT

Biogas, which contains about 55% to 70% inflammable methane gas, is a clean and efficient fuel for rural areas. It is produced when organic materials such as, cattle dung, leafy biomass, etc. are decomposed in absence of air (oxygen). It is piped for use as cooking and lighting fuel in specially designed stoves and lamps respectively. It can also be used for replacing diesel oil in fuel engines for generation of motive power and electricity. The leftover digested slurry serves as an enriched manure for use in agricultural fields, for growing mushroom and preparing vermi-compost or as feed in pisciculture.

The National Project on Biogas Development (NPBD), which was started in 1981-82, seeks to provide clean and convenient fuel for cooking and lighting purposes in rural areas; produce enriched organic manure for use in conjunction with chemical fertilisers in agricultural fields, improve sanitation and hygiene by way of linking household biogas plants with toilets and reduce the drudgery of woman. So far, about 32.75 lakh rural families have been benefited, representing coverage of 27 per cent of the estimated potential of 12 million plants.

Target and Achievement

A target of setting up of 1.80 lakh family type biogas plants was fixed for the year 2001-02 with a Budget Estimate of Rs. 59.50 crore. Against this over 75,000 plants had been installed during the period April to December 2001. Information on statewise coverage of estimated potential, achievements up to 2000-01 is given in (Table 3.8).

Table 3.8: National Project on Biogas Development

State/UT	Estimated Potential	State-wise Coverage of Estimated Potential Achievements in 2000-01	
		Number of Plants Plants Installed	Annual Target Percentage
Andhra Pradesh	1065600	308519	29
Arunachal Pradesh	7500	1142	15
Assam	307700	48059	16
Bihar	939900	119110	13
Goa	8000	3283	41
Gujarat	554000	343686	62
Haryana	300000	42120	14
Himachal Pradesh	125600	43354	35
Jammu & Kashmir	128500	1932	15
Karnataka	680000	306845	45
Kerala	150500	72339	48
Madhya Pradesh	1491200	192951	13
Maharashtra	897000	662120	74
Manipur	38700	1939	5
Meghalaya	24000	1859	6
Mizoram	2500	2376	95
Nagaland	6700	1477	21
Orissa	605500	171761	28
Punjab	411600	62708	15
Rajasthan	915300	66026	7
Sikkim	7300	2971	39
Tamil Nadu	615800	198838	34
Tripura	28500	1438	5
Uttar Pradesh	2021000	356311	18
West Bengal	695000	187266	27
A& N Island	2200	137	6
Chandigarh	1400	97	7
Dadra & Nagar Haveli	2000	169	8
Delhi	12900	675	5
Pondicherry	4300	675	5
Total	**12049900**	**3202047**	**26.57**

Manure for Agriculture

A biogas plant is an asset to a farming family. It provides larger quantities of better quality manure. A biogas plant, in many situations doubles the availability of organic manure. Traditionally one third to half of all cattle dung is burnt as fuel and is thus lost to the soil. The manure produced through a biogas plant has a comparative advantage over ordinary in terms of both quantity and quality. About 70-75% of the original weight of cattle dung is conserved in a biogas plant whereas in open compost pits 50% or more is lost. Similarly a substantial part of plant nutrients is lost during composting. Besides, digested slurry is a good source of micronutrients. It kills the weeds and disease causing organisms and hence increases the yield. The applications of digested slurry to crop serves dual purpose; as source of plant nutrients as well as a soil conditioner. The digested slurry, besides furnishing plant food, is beneficial to the soil as it increases the water holding capacity and improves its structure.

Biogas is a new source of fuel for mechanisation of agriculture. It can be used for running both SI (petrol) and CI (diesel) engines. Biogas in diesel engines is used in combination with diesel whereas petrol engines can be run on 100% biogas. Use of biogas as an engine fuel offers several advantages. Biogas being a clean fuel causes clean combustion and reduce contamination of engine oil. It also reduce deposits on piston and combustion chamber. Biogas engines are now available in the market.

Sanitation

Biogas plants are effective means for the sanitary disposal of human excreta. By putting all human and animal excreta into a biogas plant, the problem of waste disposal is solved at the family level itself. During decomposition in biogas plant, most of the disease causing organisms are killed. This can serve as an effective control of parasitic diseases. Digested slurry remains free of foul smell and most of the pathogens. Mosquitoes and flies do not breed in digested slurry. Thus biogas plants improve sanitation.

Health

The incidence of eye diseases and respiratory diseases among women and children is also reduced as burning of biogas does not cause any smoke in the kitchen. It does not cause air pollution and is free of sulphur dioxide when burnt. The danger of explosion is very less as it contains carbon dioxide which acts as fire extinguisher.

Implementation

A multi-agency approach has been in vogue. Besides the State nodal departments and corporate bodies and registered societies, the KVIC and nongovernmental organisations (NGOs)—both national-level and regional-level—are implementing the project. The KVIC is implementing in almost all the States and Union Territories, except Orissa. The All India Women's Conference (AIWC), New Delhi and the Sustainable Development Agency (SDA), Kanjirapally (Kerala) are implementing in seven northern States and five Southern States respectively. Recently, an NGO named BIOTECH, Thiruvananthapuram has been assigned on a trial basis a target of 500 biogas plants for promoting biogas in Kerala and Tamil Nadu.

The State nodal departments and implementing agencies are involving a large number of entrepreneurs on a turnkey basis with free-maintenance warranty for the first three years. Efforts have made to select a cluster of villages for implementing project on a 'saturation area' basis. Some State Governments have dovetailed the NPBD with other programmes, such as "Anila Yojana" in Karnataka "Janmabhoomi" in Andhra Pradesh. Many State Governments have linked the implementation of the NPBD earlier plant, as the SKD College, Gurdaspur has installed a 60 cubic metres capacity plant. The biogas is used in the hostel to save daily about 4 LPG cylinders. The Government of Rajasthan has installed two NBPs of 35 cubic metres capacity in the Central Prison, Jaipur and is using the biogas for cooking and water heating purposes, thereby saving daily about five LPG cylinders. A 3 kVA genset has also been installed to generate electricity for lighting the jail boundary and for powering emergency lights. A 35 cubic metres capacity NBP has been installed at Idgaah, Ajmer where a 5 kVA generator set is lighting the complex and pumping water. The Non-Conventional Energy Development Agency (NEDA), Lucknow (Uttar Pradesh) is promoting NBPs to benefit 'malin bastis' by providing not only sanitation facility but also drinking water, besides lighting. The NBPs have also been set up at bus stands, hospitals, schools, Police Lines, Collectorate compound and other public places. Women have found such facilities very useful. The NEDA has assigned the task of operation and maintenance of NBPs to entrepreneurs through lease agreements for a period of 30 years. The entrepreneurs manage the complexes on a "pay and use" basis. Recently, the NEDA has taken up the installation of NBPs in association with the State Urban Development Agency (SUDA). The West Bengal Renewable Energy Development Agency, Kolkata has installed NBPs in public places with the involvement of NGOs. The NBPs have been set up at Durgapur Children's Academy of Culture; Millennium Park, 24-Parganas; and Fishermen and Fish Traders Association, Midnapur.

Community and Institutional Biogas Plants Programme

The Community and Institutional Biogas Plants (CBP/IBP) Programme was initiated in 1982-83 with objective of recycling the large quantity of cattle dung available in the villages and institutions for the best of the weaker section as well. Under this programme the biogas is generally used for motive power generation of electricity, besides meeting the cooking fuel requirements. A component on biogas plants with community toilet complexes was added in the industrial establishments. At such sites, the biogas is used as fuel for cooking in canteens and boiling water for patients, besides generating electricity. Maharashtra Energy Development Agency (MEDA), Pune is promoting NBP in close cooperation with the community, local bodies and NGOs right from initial stages of determining the site feasibility. This had helped in improving social acceptance of NBP and encouraging urban local bodies as well as Members of Parliament to provide funds to meet the balance cost. The Solapur Municipal Corporation has installed 11 NBPs to supply biogas to about 132 families in slum areas. The Sangli-Miraj Kupwapal Corporation has used treated slurry for gardens and parks. Further, two more NBPs taken up in Amravati and Solapur each by Municipal Corporations with additional finance maintenance under Member of Parliament Local Arrangement Scheme and Member of Legislative Assets Area Development Scheme respectively. In Punjab, these have been installed in Gurudwaras and institutions where biogas is used for generating electricity.

A biogas plant of 85 cubic metres capacity based on kitchen wastes has been commissioned at Bharat Petroleum Corporation Ltd, Mumbai. It treats about 975 kg of kitchen wastes per day. The wastes, after segregation, are predigested for three days before being fed into the plant. The gas is used in the canteen to save about 40 kg of LPG per day. The digested slurry is used as organic fertiliser. The Department of Rural Development, Government of Rajasthan has set up two IBPs of 60 cubic metres capacity each at Sant Asharamji Goshala, Newai in Tonk district. The biogas is used not only for cooking but also for generation of electricity in a KVA generator and for distillation of cow urine for medicines. The digested slurry is used for the preparation of vermi-compost. One IBP of 45 cubic metres capacity has been set up at the Leprosy Rehabilitation Centre and Hospital, Missionary of Charity, Santinagar in Burdwan district of West Bengal. Besides these, the Animal Welfare Board of India, which was first associated with the implementation of IBPs in 2000-01, has taken up construction of plants in several gaushalas in Gujarat, Karnataka, Rajasthan, Tamil Nadu and Uttar Pradesh. A total of 32.75 lakh family type and 3,600 large-sized plants have been installed so far. These are estimated to have resulted in a saving of about 42 lakh tonnes of fuel wood equivalent per year and in producing 430 lakh tonnes manure containing nitrogen equivalent to 9.50 lakh tonnes of urea per year.

Chicken Droppings as a Fuel for Boilers

A 12.6 MW power station, the first in the world, to use chicken droppings as fuel has now been operating successfully at Eye in Suffolk, Eastern England, for the last 10 years. This has new breed of electricity plants, developed to use a truly renewable energy source, offers advantages both in terms of electricity generation and in terms of environmental protection, for developing and developed countries of the world. Chicken dropping is a mixture of wood shavings, or straw, and droppings cleared from poultry farms, where birds are raised for the table or for laying eggs. The droppings are collected in bulk and transported in covered lorries to the power stations where they are stored in closed warehouses to reduce both odour and dust emissions. The handling cranes feed the droppings into the specially designed furnaces, which heat the boiler to produce the steam driving a turbine, which in turn drives an electricity generator. Power stations fuelled by chicken droppings could be particularly attractive to rural communities in developing countries like India as they could provide local power production on a small scale, while providing a profitable outlet for potentially polluting waste products.

Such facilities are best sited close to chicken farming areas and a network of small power stations offers the potential for local, stable power sources. These would stimulate local power production and reduce the problems associated with distant, centralised and frequently unreliable power supplies. In terms of cost, such powerhouses would provide electricity that is comparable with that from coal or gas fired power stations. Another advantage of chicken droppings as a fuel is that it is far cleaner than coal-fired generation. The chemical composition of dropping, which is low in sulphur, chlorine and heavy metals means that the levels of noxious gases released, such as sulphur dioxide and various oxides of nitrogen, are very low 11 percent and 2 percent, respectively, of the levels released by comparable coal-fired stations. The plant is virtually smoke-free, and careful design can minimise the levels of noise near the power station. This constructive use of chicken droppings will also help to solve the problem of their disposal, which may cause concern in areas of intensive poultry farming. Chicken droppings are traditionally used locally as fertiliser, but intensive farming may lead to oversupply, and a subsequent tendency to apply too much. This may lead to certain areas becoming saturated with phosphates and potash.

In spite of such heavy use, in some instances there is a surplus, which must be sent for landfill. Its nitrogen content may cause contamination of ground water, not only following fertiliser application, but because seasonal application means that droppings are stored for several months, usually on open sites. This also allows generation of significant quantities of methane, a greenhouse gas 25 to 30 times more damaging to the atmosphere than carbon dioxide, to be released into the atmosphere. In cases when the droppings are used as a fertiliser, there is also a risk of salmonella entering the food chain. The smell from storage sites and from open farm vehicles used traditionally for transportation may also cause considerable local nuisance. Burning, however, does not only generate electricity and solve the environmental problems associated with storage and use as manure; the resultant concentrate ash is still available as fertiliser and is in fact improved in the process. It retains the important phosphate and potash content, but is nitrogen-free and sterile. Since, it is lighter and easier to handle, it can easily be transported over a far wider area.

Table 3AI.1: Population of Draught Animals for Field Operations

(Million)

Livestock	1971-72	1976-77	1981-82	1986-87	1990-91	1991-92	1996-97
Cattle							
Male	72.56	73.23	61.05	63.78	61.62	61.10	58.53
Female	2.07	2.05	2.04	1.95	1.92	1.91	1.87
Buffalo							
Male	7.61	7.93	7.32	6.56	6.31	6.25	5.94
Female	0.37	0.34	0.33	0.68	0.81	0.84	1.03
Camels**							
(Male & Female)	0.49	0.47	0.41	0.36	0.33	0.32	0.29
Total animal pairs*	**41.80**	**41.25**	**35.79**	**36.86**	**35.66**	**35.77**	**33.98**

Note: 1. * Bovine in Pair and Camels in single
2. ** Camels are mainly used in Rajasthan & Haryana for field operation and thus, 60% of its total camel population assumed for field operations.

Source: "Data Book on Mechanization and Agro-Processing Since Independence" by Dr. G. Singh, Director, CIAE, Bhopal 462038, December 1997.

Authors' Source: Agricultural Research Data Book 2001, Indian Council of Agricultural Research, New Delhi 110 001.

Table 3AII.1: *Acreage Per Draught Animal Pair in India*

States	DAP intensity (ha/animal-pair)			
	Net sown area basis	Gross cropped area basis		% change
	1986-87	1976-77	1986-87	1976-87
A. High DAP Intensity States				
1. Himachal Pradesh	1.29	2.24	2.21	-1.34
2. Manipur	1.65	3.18	1.17	-63.21
3. Bihar	1.79	2.84	2.50	-11.97
4. Uttar Pradesh	2.50	3.12	3.68	17.95
5. Orissa	2.51	2.68	3.91	45.90
B. Medium DAP Intensity States				
1. West Bengal	2.70	3.02	4.12	36.42
2. Assam	3.06	2.48	4.11	65.73
3. Jammu & Kashmir	3.16	2.09	4.46	113.40
4. Tamil Nadu	3.36	3.22	3.76	16.77
5. Madhya Pradesh	3.96	3.90	4.56	16.92
6. Sikkim	4.68	2.95	9.24	213.22
7. Andhra Pradesh	4.87	3.76	5.46	45.21
C. Low DAP Intensity States				
1. Maharashtra	5.35	6.05	5.86	-3.14
2. Rajasthan	5.60	8.21	13.30	62.00
3. Punjab	6.07	8.13	10.54	29.64
4. Karnataka	6.79	5.00	7.48	49.60
5. Gujarat	7.17	7.20	8.37	16.25
6. Haryana	8.62	10.30	15.10	46.60
7. Kerala	14.00	10.13	18.60	83.61
All India	**3.87**	**4.12**	**5.03**	**22.09**

Source: "Data Book on Mechanization and Agro-Processing Since Independence" by Dr. G. Singh, Director, CIAE, Bhopal 462038, December 1997.

Authors' Source: Agricultural Research Data Book 2001, Indian Council of Agricultural Research, New Delhi 110 001.

Annexure III

Table 3AIII.1: Distribution and Growth of Bullocks

(Million)

Zones/States	1972	1977	1982	1987	Growth, % 1972-87
Northern	**21.42**	**20.90**	**17.56**	**17.43**	**-1.36**
Madhya Pradesh	0.89	0.82	0.73	0.86	-0.24
Uttar Pradesh	13.58	13.02	11.40	11.67	-1.00
Jammu & Kashmir	0.76	0.86	0.46	0.42	-3.87
Rajasthan	3.86	3.94	3.12	2.55	-2.73
Punjab	1.39	1.32	1.11	1.30	-0.45
Haryana	0.94	0.94	0.73	0.63	-2.61
Southern	**13.49**	**13.54**	**9.49**	**9.86**	**-2.07**
Tamil Nadu	4.38	4.37	3.25	3.00	-2.50
Andhra Pradesh	5.25	5.13	3.84	3.63	-2.43
Karnataka	3.48	3.67	2.17	2.96	-1.07
Kerala	0.38	0.36	0.23	0.27	-2.26
Eastern	**14.56**	**15.13**	**14.03**	**14.44**	**-0.06**
Manipur	0.12	0.12	0.22	0.29	6.29
Bihar	7.22	7.21	7.18	7.64	0.38
Orissa	4.54	4.80	4.45	4.41	-0.19
West Bengal	0.50	0.50	0.53	0.46	-0.54
Assam	2.19	2.46	1.64	1.60	-2.06
Sikkim		0.04	0.02	0.03	-4.08
Western	**18.61**	**18.66**	**16.89**	**17.75**	**-0.32**
Madhya Pradesh	9.47	9.57	8.59	8.68	-0.58
Gujarat	3.04	2.85	2.74	2.60	-1.04
Maharashtra	6.10	6.24	5.55	6.47	0.39
All India	**72.56**	**73.23**	**61.05**	**63.78**	**-0.86**

Source: "Data Book on Mechanization and Agro-Processing Since Independence" by
   Dr. G. Singh, Director, CIAE, Bhopal 462038, December 1997.
   Authors' Source: Agricultural Research Data Book 2001, Indian Council of Agricultural
Research, New Delhi 110 001.

Annexure IV

Table 3AIV.1: Average Quantity of Dung and Urine Excreted by Different Animals
(Kg)

Type of animal	Quantity excreted per day*		Type of animal	Average Weight	Quantity Excreted at night (15 hr)	
	Dung	Urine			Dung	Urine
Horse	16.10	3.6	Cow (cultivators)	172	2.8	1.31
Cattle	23.50	9.0	Bullock (Govt. Farm)	279	3.8	1.40
Sheep	1.13	0.6	Breeding Bull (Govt. Farm)	530	7.7	4.50
Pig	2.70	1.5	She-buffalo	374	5.3	2.20
Poultry	0.04	-	He-buffalo	617	7.7	4.40

Note: * American data
Source: Handbook of Manures and Fertilizers (Revised Edition) 1971, Indian Council of
Agricultural Research, New Delhi.
Authors' Source: Agricultural Research Data Book 2001, Indian Council of Agricultural
Research, New Delhi 110 001.

Annexure V

Table 3AV.1: Average Nutrient Content of Animal Urine
(Per cent on original matter)

Content	Horse	Cattle	Buffalo	Sheep	Pig
Water	89.60	92.60	81.00	86.30	96.60
Organic matter	8.00	4.80	-	9.30	1.50
Mineral matter	8.00	2.10	-	4.60	1.00
Nitrogen	1.29	1.21	0.62	1.47	0.38
Phosphoric acid (P_2O_5)	0.01	0.01	Trace	0.05	0.10
Potash (K_2O)	1.39	1.35	1.61	1.96	0.99
Lime (C_aO)	0.45	0.01	Trace	0.16	0.00

Source: Handbook of Manures and Fertilizers (Revised Edition) 1971, Indian Council of
Agricultural Research, New Delhi.
Authors' Source: Agricultural Research Data Book 2001, Indian Council of Agricultural
Research, New Delhi 110 001.

4

Production Performance

Livestock production in India takes place in millions of holdings scattered across the country, over 75 per cent of them in small and marginal holdings. Traditional mixed crop-livestock farming is the most preponderant farming system in the country, accounting for over 90 per cent of all operational holdings, with wide variations in practices and farming culture between the irrigated and rain fed areas.

Livestock are farmed predominantly in mixed crop-livestock farming systems (over 90 per cent) and to a much lesser extent in landless livestock farming systems, pig farming systems in marginal areas restricted to special categories among the socially weaker sections, back yard pig farming systems as part of the mainstream farming in Kerala, Goa and the North-Eastern states; and backyard poultry system made up entirely of *desi* birds (over 90 per cent) across the entire country.

There is then the large industrial livestock farming, systems mainly for commercial poultry production, and some large institutional dairy farms. There are also the large migratory herds of cattle, buffalo, sheep and goat owned by the transhumant tribes in Gujarat, Rajastan, Punjab, Haryana, Jammu & Kashmir, Himachal and Uttaranchal (Ahirs, Bharwads, Rabaris, Gujjars and Gaddis). Other classifications of livestock farming systems do exist, but most of them are armchair exercises without any empirical basis. Draught animal group in India is made up of the work bullock and male buffalo predominantly, along with camel, horse, pony, mule, donkey and yak. Among all work animals the work bullock occupy the pride of place, as the crop production system in Indian agriculture is overwhelmingly dependent on them as the prime source of farm power. On the whole however, dependent on them as the prime source of farm power. On the whole however, dependence on animal power for farm operations as well as transport and haulage has considerably diminished over the years and is fast being replaced by electrical and mechanical sources of power.

According to FAO estimates, India possesses cattle population of 220 million and 94 million buffaloes, which is about 16.3% and 56.6% of the total world population, respectively. India is currently the largest producer of milk in the world. The Indian share of cow milk production to world is about 6.4% in comparison to 63.06% from buffaloes. There are significant differences in productivity of cows and buffaloes in different region/states of the country. Milk production is highest in Uttar Pradesh followed by Punjab and Rajasthan. The productivity of India's milch breeds is far below the world average (2,026 kg per year). The reasons for low productivity are multifactorial. Indigenous cattle are unique in its qualities like heat tolerance, disease resistance, ability to withstand stress, but are low producers due to their genetic endowment and low grade nutrition. Conservation and management of animal genetic resources and dovetailing of breeding programmes with conservation are being attempted.

Milk and milk products, meat and meat products, eggs and poultry meat, animal draft power, dung, hides and skins, wool & hair etc. are the major components of output from the livestock sector. The total value of output from livestock sector at current prices increased from about Rs.106 billion in l980/81 to Rs. 1,230.8 billion in 1998/99 and further to 1302.3 billion in 1999-00. Gross domestic product from the livestock sector rose from Rs. 59 billion to Rs. 923 billion during this period. The share of livestock sector in total value of agricultural output increased from 22 percent in 1980/81 to 32 percent in 1999-00.

Milk products continue to account for about two-thirds of the total value of livestock output. Meat and meat products account for around l7 percent of total output, eggs about 4 percent, wool only 0.3 percent, dung almost 11 percent and other products accounted for the remainder (Table 4.1). As livestock population expanded, output from most livestock categories also grew. Milk and broiler production displayed the highest annual growth rates. Growth rates in the value of output of agriculture and livestock sectors and the livestock major sub-sector, during each decade from 1950/51 to 1998/99 are discussed below. Overall performance of the livestock sector has been slightly better than the agriculture sector during the past 45 years. Annual rates of growth were 2.9 percent and 2.8 percent respectively (Table 4.2 and Graph 4.1). However, during the last two decades livestock registered higher rate of growth, annual increase being 4.6 percent against 3.l percent for the agriculture sector. Performance has been varying among

Table 4.1: Share of Major Sub-Groups in Total Value of Livestock Output: All India

(Percentage)

Period *	Milk group	Meat group	Poultry meat	Eggs
1951/52	55.3	20.9	4.5	1.3
1961/62	54.5	21.3	5.7	1.6
1971/72	57.4	18.7	4.1	2.1
1981/82	62.2	16.3	5.2	2.7
1991/92	65.3	17.9	6.5	3.3
1997/98	66.3	17.3	6.7	3.4

* Three years average centred on the year shown.

Source: Central Statistical Organisation: Nations Accounts Statistics: 2000

Table 4.2: Value of Output of Agriculture and Livestock Sectors and Major Livestock Sub-sectors: 1950-51 to 1997/98: (at 1993/94 prices)

(Rs.billion)

Period *	Agriculture	Livestock	Livestock sub-sectors			
			Milk group	Meat group	Poultry meat	Eggs
1951/52	660.5	205.9	114.0	42.9	9.3	2.7
1961/62	889.2 (3.0)	235.8 (1.4)	128.5 (1.2)	50.2 (3.1)	13.5 (3.8)	3.9 (3.8)
1971/72	1,119.6 (2.3)	261.7 (1.0)	150.1 (1.5)	49.0 (-0.3)	10.7 (1.1)	5.4 (3.1)
1981/82	1,466.4 (2.8)	387.9 (4.0)	241.2 (4.9)	63.3 (2.6)	20.2 (6.6)	10.3 (6.7)
1991/92	1,930.5 (2.8)	612.3 (4.7)	399.7 (5.2)	109.9 (5.6)	40.0 (7.0)	20.4 (7.1)
1997/98	2,340.9 (3.9)	771.1 (4.6)	512.8 (5.1)	133.6 (3.8)	52.0 (5.4)	26.5 (5.3)
Overall annual growth during 45 years	(2.8)	(2.9)	(3.4)	(2.6)	(3.9)	(5.2)

* Three years average centered on the year shown.

N.B. Figures in brackets are annual growth rate in percentage over the previous decade.

Source: Computed from Central Statistical Organization: National Accounts Statistics 2001: Back Series 1950-51–1992-93, and National Accounts Statistics 2000.

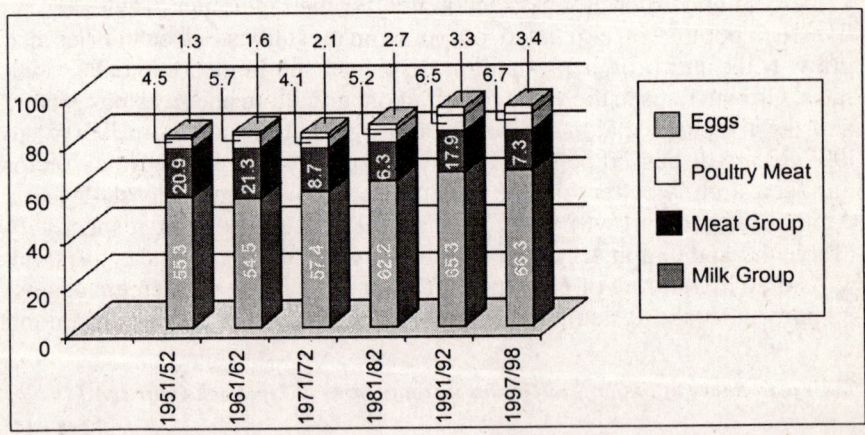

Graph 4.1: Share of major subgroups in total value of livestock output: 1993/94 prices

the various livestock sub-sectors. Whereas milk group has registered a continuous growth rate, performance of meat group is a mixed one, despite an impressive growth in the poultry and eggs over the past two decades.

A study by the National Centre for Agricultural Economics & Policy Research (NCAP), New Delhi has revealed that the livestock output grew at 2.59 per cent per annum over 1950-51 to 1995-96. The input index increased by 1.79 per cent per annum and Total Factor Productivity (TFP) grew at about 0.8 per cent, implying that technical change contributed about 30 per cent to overall output growth over the last 45 years. Period-wise results are more revealing. There was no TFP growth in the first period (1950-51 to 1970-71) implying no technical change. Output growth proceeded along the traditional production function and was entirely driven by growth in measured inputs, Not surprisingly, the resulting growth in output was a modest 1.3 per cent per annum. There was a sharp up trend since then. Output as well as TFP growth picked up. The results show that the real upswing started in the eighties when sector's output growth touched nearly 4 per cent per annum and TFP growth jumped to nearly 1.8 per cent, contributing about 45 per cent to total output growth. Backed by an improved market and institutional environment, investments in livestock research have begun to pay off. The above-mentioned results are confirmed by the analysis of the data on the growth rate in the value of livestock output based on three years averages and the 1993/94 prices. The total value of livestock output rose by almost four times during the period 1950/51 to 1998/99. Poultry meat and eggs displayed impressive growth; their value having increased by almost 7 times. Milk products followed this, with their value having risen by four and half times. The value of meat and meat products increased 3 times, hides & skins 1.74 times, dung 1.5 times and the value of output of draft power and wool hair remained almost constant during the period under review.

Milk and milk products constitute the lion's share in the value of output from livestock sector. Its share in the total value (in terms of 1993/94 prices) rose from 55 percent in 1951/52 to almost 67 percent in 1997/98 (Graph 4.2). The share of draught power was around 16 percent in 1951/52 and declined to a mere 6 percent in 1997/98[1]. Eggs and poultry meat have emerged next to milk as a contributor to the output from livestock sector in recent years. The share of eggs and poultry meat was 5.8 percent in 1951/52, which rose to a little over 10 percent in 1997/98. Meat and meat products (excluding poultry) are also major contributors to the output of livestock. However, their contribution has declined slightly from 20.9 percent to 17.3 percent. Hides and skins and wool & hair are relatively less important and have registered consistent decline. The share of wool and hair has gone down from 1.04 percent to 0.34 percent, while that of hides and skins has declined from 3.1 percent to 1.4 percent. Similar has been the case with dung, its share having declined from 21.8 percent in 1951/52 to 8.6 percent in the terminal year

MILK AND DAIRY PRODUCTS

The importance of milk and milk products for physical development and well-being of people can hardly be over emphasized. Since time

---

[1] There is hardly any reliable information available about draught power. These are all rough estimates.

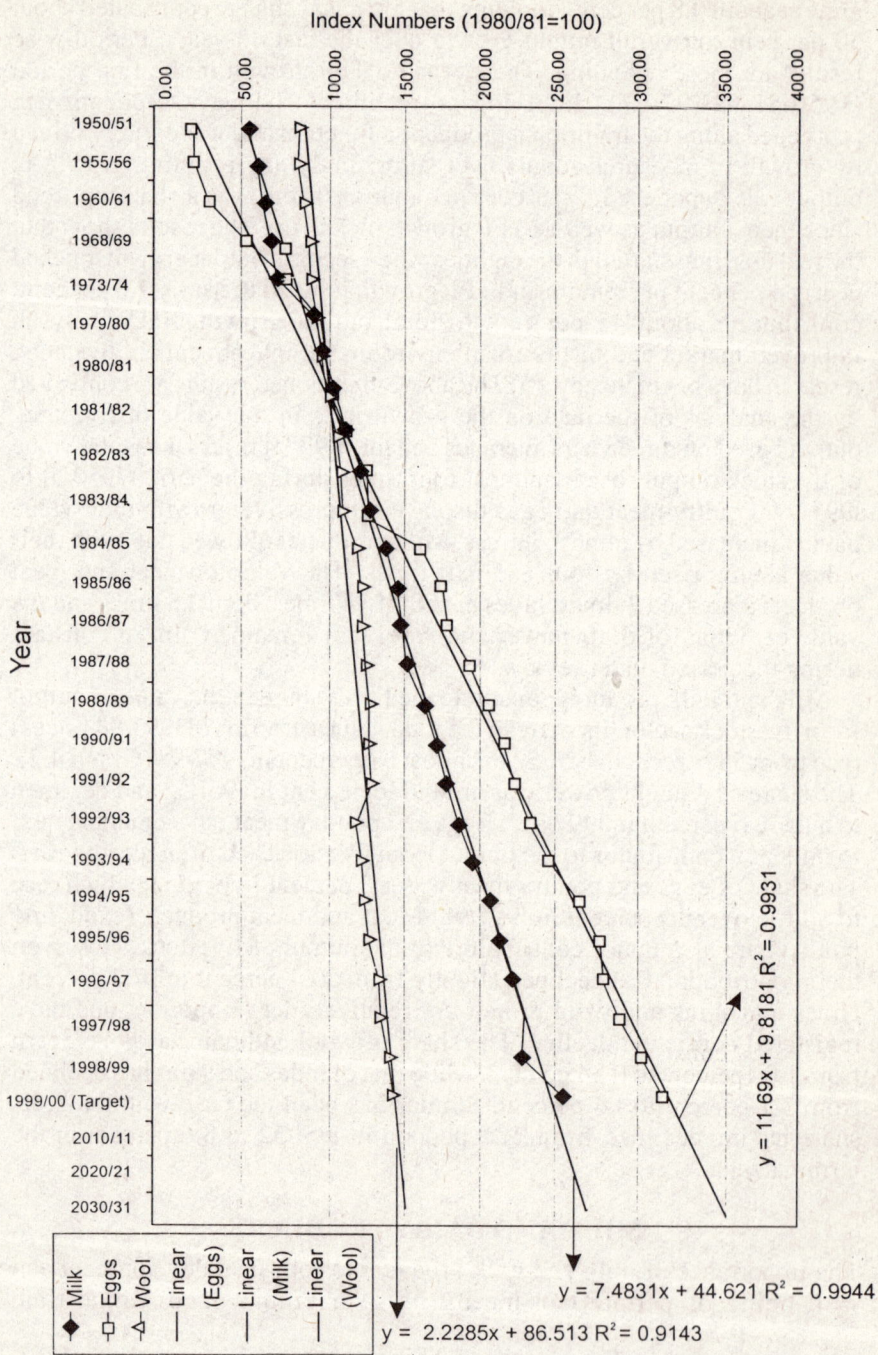

Graph 4.2: Production Index of milk, eggs and wool

immemorial, milk and milk products have been accepted as a must in the dietary of Indian people. In good olden days the population was small and life was simple and confined almost exclusively in rural areas. Cows were maintained in many homes in self-sufficient villages; there was no dearth of milk. The liking that people had developed for milk and its products continues and these items of food are equally acceptable to all communities in the country. Fluid milk and its products were generally not saleable commodities and there was no long distance movements of these products from one place to another.

With growth of population and change in the pattern of life with urbanization, there was rapid increase in demand for milk and its products particularly in urban areas where these items could not be and were not produced in any large quantity. And at the same time the increasing pressure on land, fragmentation of land holdings and decrease in pasture made it difficult for rural milk production to keep pace with the demands in the growing towns and cities. As a result, there was an upsetting in the ancient system of production and consumption of milk and milk products and there developed an imbalance between production in the villages and supply to fast growing demand centers in congested urban areas. Due to lack of attention to organize a system of dairying based on commercial rural milk production, bulk collection, transportation, processing and supply of milk and milk products as required for the altered situation, it became increasingly difficult to meet the demands in cities and towns.

The gap between supply and demand of milk in cities continued to grow and acute shortages became patent in more and more areas. Widespread adulteration of milk with water and undesirable practice of urban milk production came into existence and became a part of the general system of dairying in the country. Because of shortages, prices of milk and milk products continued to soar higher and higher taking these out of reach of the poorer sections of the community. Impoverishment of the villages and tempting price in urban areas funneled out milk and milk products from many rural areas leaving little to meet the village needs. Due to low per capita income of people in rural areas, milk consumption is at a low level even in those villages where milk does not flow out to the urban areas.

Milk production, which stagnated during the fifties and sixties, increased significantly during the next three decades. During the nineties the livestock sector as a whole, and milk production in particular, registered a higher growth rate as compared to the agricultural sector. Milk output grew by about 5.5 percent during the eighties and about 4 percent in the nineties, compared to 3.2 percent and 2.7 percent respectively for agriculture during the same period. A significant portion of milk production in India's countryside is consumed as liquid milk within the household itself. Only ad-hoc data are available on the quantities of milk and dairy products sold on the market. In the absence of the time series data on commercial sale of milk and dairy products, total production and availability of these commodities can serve as a proxy for the domestic market.

After Independence, with the initiation of Five Year Plan programmes, dairying has progressively been receiving more and more emphasis and getting greater allocation of funds. There is a growing realization that promotion of dairying not only contributes towards national health building but also creates substantial employment opportunities. Properly organized and developed, dairying could be effectively used as an instrument of social justice. With the launching of the Operation Flood and the livestock development programmes, milk production in India got a remarkable boost, especially since the mid-seventies. Major milk supply in India comes from buffalo and cows. However, the role of buffalo as a major milk producing species is well recognized in the country - percentage of cattle yielding more than 1.5 kg. milk per day is less than 2 per cent, whereas the percentage of such buffaloes is over 40 percent. With 53 per cent of the world buffalo population, India produces 64 per cent of the world buffalo milk. By contrast, 15 per cent of the world cattle population in India yields only 7 per cent of total world milk output. Following the launching of the Operation Flood and the livestock development programme, milk production in India got a remarkable boost, especially since the mid-seventies. The annual growth rate of total milk production from 1950/51 to 1998/99 is shown in Table 4.3. State-wise and Region-wise milk production from 1973-74 to 1998-99 is shown in Table 4AI.1 at Annexure I.

Table 4.3: Growth in milk production All India: 1950/51 – 2000-01

Period	Percent per year
1950/51 to 1960/61	1.64
1960/61 to 1973/74	1.15
1973/74 to 1980/81	4.51
1980/81 to 1990/91	5.50
1990/91 to 2000/01	5.10

Source: Ministry of Agriculture: Department of Animal Husbandry & Dairying: Basic Animal Husbandry Statistics: 2002

Milk from Barren Cows

Sterility and infertility in cattle account for major economic losses to dairy farmers in India. In almost all other countries, such animals find their way to the slaughterhouse, leaving room for new animals in the herd. However, the slaughtering of such unproductive cows in India is prohibited. At the same time, maintaining such animals is an economic burden on farmers. In case such cattle are turned out, it leads to the problem of stray cattle, which is already a menace. A high percentage of heavy milk-yielding cows suffer from or are prone to reproductive problems resulting in infertility. It is thus imperative to find acceptable yet productive ways of using them. Studies have led to development of methods to artificially induce lactation in otherwise infertile cows but having a viable healthy udder. Keeping in view the losses incurred due to sterility and infertility, artificial induction of lactation using hormones is an option worth adopting. The artificial induction of lactation at present is quite successful in cows, although the results in buffaloes are debatable.

It could be undertaken in cows with problems like chronic repeat breeder, anoestrus, infantile genitalia or having congenital abnormalities like free martin, undeveloped ovaries or genitalia. Animals that have calved earlier give better results and have good milk production potential.

Artificial induction of lactation, however, should be undertaken as a last resort and not as a substitute or supplement to pregnancy. All other recommended procedures and measures must be exhausted before instituting this therapy for induction of milk. The main aim of artificial induction of lactation is to improve utilization of unproductive cows through cost effective milk production in the absence of normal and physiological breeding. An additional advantage is that some of the animals might regain fertility during the course of lactation. Infertile/sterile cows that have attained the age of sexual maturity, good general body condition and a well-developed healthy udder qualify for artificial induction of lactation. The udder and all the teats should be healthy without any abnormality, either congenital or acquired. The treatment involves the use of sex hormones in a prescribed proportion and a systematic schedule, which should be strictly adhered to. Treatment should be started preferably 7 to 10 days after the animal is detected in heat. While the hormones are being injected for about 15 days, the udder should be massaged simultaneously twice daily until secretions from teats start. The milk secretions normally start within 5–15 days.

Hormones are excreted in milky secretions after the start of treatment and the milk produced during this period is unfit for human consumption for the first 3-4 weeks. The milk can be consumed only after about 30 days from the first injection of the hormone and this regime should be strictly complied with. Such animals may continue to give milk for a complete lactation period (300 days).

After the completion of one lactation period there should be a gap/rest for 50 days as dry period during which no milk is to be taken from the animals as is done normally. The next artificial induction of lactation can be done after this period. The quantity of milk produced by the animal is approximately 60-70 per cent of normal milk yield that the animal had yielded earlier after parturition. The decision of artificial induction of lactation, thus, should be made after weighing the costs involved and the benefits expected.

Special housing care is needed for the animal undergoing artificial induction of lactation, as the treated animal will exhibit increased estrus/heat behaviour due to hormones and precautions should be taken to avoid possible injury to the treated animal as well as to her herd mates. In some cases there can be decreased feed intake, constipation and ataxia, which subsides by itself and there is no need to treat the animal.

Precautions

- This therapy should be instituted strictly under the guidance of a registered veterinary practitioner.
- Correct selection of the animal is very important, as all animals are not fit for artificial lactogenesis.
- Proper feeding and deworming needs to be taken care of.
- Adequate housing and management is mandatory for the treated animals.
- Milk is fit for human consumption only after discarding it for the first 30 days.

Buffalo and Buffalo Milk

In milk production India has made impressive progress in the past 30 years, producing 75 million tones per year. Punjab contributes 10 per cent of the national produce. Buffaloes are the mainstay of this production in Punjab, as well as the rest of the country. While extensive genetic improvement in indigenous cows has been achieved through crossbreeding with exotic breeds, very little has been done in the case of buffaloes. That notwithstanding, buffaloes as dairy animals can be more efficient than crossbred cows in view of the following factors:

- Buffalo is an indigenous animal of the region, so it can adopt easily to the hot, humid and cold climates.
- Buffalo milk is preferred – as fluid milk, for *ghee* and *paneer* etc., The organized dairy sector prefers buffalo milk and the market prices also are favourable.
- Buffalo is better adapted to the Indian conditions in respect of poor feed quality and tropical diseases as compared to crossbred cows.
- The Punjab buffalo compares well with the best of the buffaloes from any other region and is known for its performance.
- There is no problem of stray buffaloes, as opposed to cows.
- No special care is required for the buffalo as for crossbred cows.
- With special care, we can achieve the following in the case of the buffalo too: early maturity and puberty; short calving during their life span of about 20 years; high fat percentage – almost 1.5 or 2 per cent more than a good cow's milk.
- That buffalo is a seasonal breeder is a wrong perception. Provided the required atmospheric temperature and nutrition, it can breed regularly.
- Buffalo breeding, housing and progeny testing, along with herd book registration, are must to make buffalo the main milk producing animal and make livestock owners prosperous.
- Buffalo calves suffer high mortality due to neglect. There is delayed maturity in both the sexes. Heat detection in buffaloes is considered a problem, which can be improved by proper management.

Improving Buffalo Milk Production

Buffalo Husbandry is an important source of income and means of employment for more than 70 million farmers in India. Buffaloes contribute more than half of the total milk produced in the country although buffalo population is 1/3rd of total cattle population. In spite of its large contribution to total milk production of the country, little efforts have been made to improve their genetic potentiality for milk production. Selective breeding among them is an important tool to enhance their genetic potential for milk productivity. A sire is more than half the herd as it contributes more than 60 per cent of the genetic improvement of the herd for milk production. The remaining improvement comes through dam selection. Therefore, availability of best sires or its service through artificial insemination to commercial breeders/ farmers is the primary key to increase milk production status of buffaloes. Moreover, selective breeding through progeny testing could not be initiated at the National Level to improve milk production status of buffaloes due to the following operational constraints:

Small sized herds (2-3 animals) in the country, lack of performance data recording facilities, lack of effective artificial insemination services, lack of education among the farmers, and lack of breed association/agency responsible for taking up the Improvement Programmes. The cooperative group breeding scheme is now being considered as an alternative to conventional breeding schemes. In this scheme, a sire breeding nucleus herd is established to breed replacement sires for itself and the associated herds.

Female replacements are reared in both the nucleus and the base herd (associated herds) and there is transfer of females in both directions between nucleus and base herds. The nucleus remains open to introduction of new genes from outside and hence; the system is termed as "Open Nucleus Breeding System" (ONBS). A group of interested breeders get together to discuss the concept and the business, legal and genetic aspects of the scheme. Each breeder contributes the top performing females in his herd to a central Unit (Nucleus). The group then decides where the nucleus is to be located and how it is going to be managed. They then decide on an exchange rate of top females between the nucleus and the base.

Selected females must be mated to top sires within the nucleus schemes to breed sires for use within the nucleus. Only the nucleus born males should be used in the base herds/breeding tract. With increased interest in the performance data, the progeny testing of the nucleus born males may further augment the mil productivity of buffaloes. However, to make the people understand the concept and to involve them in breeding programmes at grass root level, the existing farms of State Governments/Central Government should take lead in this direction. These farms have excellent infrastructural facilities and trained manpower to operate the nucleus schemes involving the commercial breeders and progressive farmers. Moreover, the nucleus schemes when implemented may be the vehicle for introduction of newer and latest molecular breeding technologies. The use of DNA/gene markers in the nucleus may assist in selection of the superior germplasm to produce the next generation. Therefore the nucleus schemes hold the promises to enhance and to sustain the milk productivity of buffaloes and thereby help to enhance the socioeconomic status of its stakeholders.

Gene Pool

Punjab is fortune to have some of the world's best dairy buffalo breeds. But there is a need for better understanding of these breeds and steps to be taken for proper conservation. A policy on organized breeding for genetic improvement is needed for good progeny from tested bulls. Good milking buffaloes should not be allowed to be crossed with inferior quality bulls.

Progeny testing of buffalo bulls for milk production should be done on a large scale. The involvement of farmers in animal-performance recording would be helpful. Open-nucleus breeding of animals with elite females and making use of multiple-ovulation embryo transfer can be a feasible alternative to the lack of a large population of pedigree performance-recorded females. Embryo transfer technology (ETT) should be for buffaloes, too. In Punjab, which has the highest per-capita availability of milk in the country, buffaloes contribute 75 per cent, but are underfed. Against the recommended 40 kg of fodder per day, buffaloes in Punjab barely get 12 kg. The area under fodder has decreased from 7.2 lakh hectare to 6.9 lakh, which constitutes about 9 per cent of the cropped area. This has happened while the buffalo population has doubled during the past 25 years. Punjab, thus, has a 'black revolution' in spite of the lack of any support or incentive base.

Health

Buffaloes also need adequate attention to their health problems. Surveillance and monitoring of important buffalo diseases have to be strengthened along with disease-investigation facilities. Calf diseases also need more attention as the loss due to calf mortality is relatively higher in buffaloes as compared to cows.

Meat Potential

Buffaloes are also potential animals for meat production. While the slaughter of cows is restricted, buffaloes can be slaughtered for meat any where in the country. Moreover, buffalo meat has low fat and is tender, especially if male Murrah buffaloes are properly managed for the purpose. Some of the developed countries are exploring the potential of buffalo as a meat animal. According to an estimate, about 10 million male buffalo calves are born annually. Rearing of these calves for meat can have good potential. Buffalo meat can be exported as it has high content of lean meat and has 25 per cent higher protein than beef and is 50 per cent lower in cholesterol, and is considered quality meat for human consumption. Even though there is no ban on the slaughter of buffaloes, much of the buffalo meat available at present is from old animals. Neglected male calves are also slaughtered at an early age to yield poor-quality meat. In the international market it is sold at a very low price. This area needs more attention. There is an urgent need to boost the breeding and maintenance of buffalo herds.

Milk Quality

The quality of the milk produced needs improvement. The main reason for the poor quality is the time lag between milking and reaching the chilling centre. The more the time lag the poorer the quality. Milk chiller should be installed at collection centres in the villages. The Animal Husbandry Department mainly provides health services, whereas extension services to educate farmers in animal husbandry are nonexistent. Strong and efficient extension, health and insemination services are required. Efforts are being made to organise dairy farmers' cooperatives, yet it is an unorganised sector. Most of the farms operate at a small level, unable to make use of machines and modern management practices.

Milk is regarded as a remarkable combination of food elements. It represents the perfect single food more than most other natural foods. However, it becomes harmful if it is not produced and handled under strict sanitary conditions. Due to the callousness or ignorance of dairymen, germs, drug-residues, dyes and pesticides in milk render it a health hazard. If certain practices are followed strictly and lapses looked into, most problems can be avoided.

Diseased Animals and Handlers

Milk can also be contaminated with germs of the diseases from which the animals may be suffering, like tuberculosis, foot and mouth, mastitis, brucellosis, etc., Similarly, persons suffering from infectious diseases handling the milk may also give germs to the milk.

Drug and Dye Residue

Drugs are at times used indiscriminately by dairymen as well as veterinary staff for the treatment of sick animals. Milk containing residues of most commonly used antibiotics, steroids hormones and deworming medicines is not fit for consumption. It is fit for consumption only after the "milk discarding time" specified for each drug. Toxic dyes contained in polythene bags lying on garbage when ingested by cows can also contaminate the milk. It is also reported that pesticide contamination of milk is not only excessive but widely spread all over the country.

Milking Operation

During the operation of milking, dung sticking to the udders and flanks may get detached and fall into the milk. This is most undesirable as dung carries a large number of bacteria with it. Due to lack of proper space for each animal in a shed, the skin of the udder and hindquarters is liable to be soiled when the animals lie down. The laxity in keeping the sheds free from dung is the reason for this avoidable contamination. If milking is done immediately after the cleaning of the sheds and the animals, the germs present in the atmosphere can find way to the milk. Also, the hands of the milkers and udders of the cows are usually not dry at milking, again resulting in contamination of milk. Veterinarians should give demonstration on how to clean, dry and disinfect the udder and hindquarters before and after milking. Milkers have also to keep themselves and their clothes clean. Sheds should be kept free of flies using suitable sprays.

Unhygienic Utensils

Cleaning, and sterilization of dairy utensils to render them germ free is often left to low paid and uneducated workers unaware of the concept of hygiene. As such, small quantities, of milky water left in the cans are sufficient for germ growth. The standard procedure for cleaning utensils should be demonstrated to dairymen by competent persons of the dairy development departments.

> It is essential that those engaged in the profession of dairy have a keen sense of the responsibilities of their job.

Milk in Transit

The faulty construction of containers for carrying milk to the doorsteps of the consumers also contributes to the contamination of milk. Containers with fixed lids should be used rather than containers with removable lids as at every point of delivery the lid comes in contact with dirty surfaces. During transit, if milk is not kept at the required low temperatures and is exposed to high temperatures as in summer, multiplication of the already present germs occurs. Dairymen need to be educated on the ideal temperatures for milk. Flies, dust and other atmospheric contamination at every stage of milk handling contribute to the degradation of milk. Flies are the worst offenders because they leave germs and filth on every thing they touch.

No matter how many norms and practices are demonstrated to dairymen, these cannot cover all the exigencies that may arise. It is essential that those engaged in the profession of dairy have a keen sense of the responsibilities of their job. In the joint camps held by the Dairy Development and Animal Husbandry Departments dairymen need to be told in simple language through lectures films about the need for adopting the approved dairy practices.

Milk Production

A time series data for buffalo and cow milk separately are not readily available from national sources. The total milk production in India almost doubled from 38.8 million tonnes in 1983-84 to 75 million tonnes in

1998-99. It is interesting to note that though there has been a higher rate of increase in cow milk production, buffalo milk still accounts for almost 52 per cent of the total milk output. In 1992/93, the latest year for which data is available, the milk yield per day per animal in milk for India was 3.46 kg. per buffalo compared to 2.1 kg. for cow. There is, however wide variation in milk production per animal among different states due to differences in species, feeding pattern, health and hygiene of animals. The milk production in India ranges from 5 kg. to 336 kg. per head of cattle per annum. This corresponds to 1260 kg. per lactating buffalo and 770 kg. per lactating cow. In 1992-93, the shares of lactating buffaloes and cows in milk production among total buffaloes and cattle were 31 per cent and 15 per cent respectively.

Out of the total production of milk, around 45 percent is consumed as fluid milk. About 35 percent is processed into butter or ghee, 7 percent into paneer (cottage cheese) and other cheese, 4 percent converted into milk powder and the rest is used for other dairy products such as yoghurt (*dahi*) and sweet meats. In recent years, ice cream production has been increasing. Annual production of butter and ghee totals about 1.2 million tons, most of which is produced by small businesses and households.[*] Annual production of milk powder and infant food is estimated at 160, 000 tons, malted milk food at 45,000 tons, cheese at 3,000 tons and condensed milk at 8,500 tons. The production increased impressively in per cent terms. In the coming decade the products that are likely to enter the market in a big way will be the fermented products like dahi/yoghurt and acidophilus health drink, health foods like milk with fruits, calcium rich and low fat dairy products. Lastly there is also immense potential for the Indian milk sweets like the traditional rasogollas, pedhas, halwas, payasam in ready to consume form. The combined market of these products exceeds Rs. 100 billion and organized dairy sector perhaps today accounts for less than 10 percent of market share. The Government is attaching great importance to the processing industry. During 1991-2000 investment in the livestock processing industry totalled Rs. 166 billion (Table 4.4).

As regards regional distribution of milk production in India, the Central region consisting of UP and MP accounts for around 26% of the total output. This is followed by Western region (22%), Southern region (21%), Northern region (18%) and Eastern region (11%) (Table 4AI.1 at annexure -I).

The rise in international prices in late 2002 was mainly attributable to limited production growth, and in some cases declining production, in Oceania and South America leading to a reduction in export supplies. As world prices rose, export subsidies paid by some high-cost producing countries in the northern hemisphere also fell. For example, average United States monthly export subsidies for skimmed milk powder were US\$ 329 per tonne in November 2002 compared to US\$ 864 per tonne in March of

---

[*]USDA: Indian Agricultural Situation: 1994: AGR No. IN 4084 and Department of Animal Husbandry Basic Animal Husbandry Statistics: 1997, p.101.

Table 4.4: Investment in the Processed Food Sector
(From July 1991 to December 2001)

(Rs. in million)

S. No.	Sector	Industrial Entrepreneur Memorandum		Industrial Approvals (100% Export Oriented Units/ Industrial License)		Total		Foreign Investment out of total Investment
		No.	Invest.	No.	Invest.	No.	Invest	
1.	Meat & Poultry Products	89	3840	59	13940	148	17780	2670
2.	Milk & Milk Products	1104	137510	26	10820	1130	148330	10040

Source: Ministry of Food Processing Industries, Annual Report 2001-2002.

the EU, skimmed milk powder export subsidies fell from 850 per tonne in mid 2002 to 540 per tonne in early December. Over the same period, EU export subsidies for whole milk powder also decreased. Should world prices continue to rise, further cuts in export subsidies are anticipated. However, even at the lower rates, for a number of high-cost dairy producing countries in the northern hemisphere, the amount of subsidy required to export dairy commodities at prevailing international prices is substantial. Table 4.5 shows indicative dairy products export prices.

Table 4.5: Indicative Dairy Export Prices

	2002		2003	
	Oct.	Aug.	Sept.	Oct.
Skimmed milk Powder	1361	1727	1765	1829
Whole milk powder	1352	1748	1789	1853
Acid Casein	3539	3926	4012	4156
Cheddar cheese	1501	1848	1916	1995
Butter	1067	1393	1432	1542

Source: Midpoint of price ranges reported by Farmnet (NZ) and USDA.

Soya Milk a Variable Alternative

According to a new study by the Physician Committee for Responsible Medicine (PCRM). Milk proteins, which are difficult for babies to digest, are passed through the breast milk. Infants who are sensitive to milk proteins often suffer from colic, skin reactions and asthma. Consumption of milk has also been associated with more serious conditions, including Type (T) juvenile diabetes and symptoms similar to autism.

These health threats have also prompted the Indian medical community to follow the example of the American Academy of Pediatrics by recommending against feeding milk to infants less than a year old. Many physicians believe there is no safe age to begin drinking cow and buffalo milk. This is one view based on American experience. It may not be of general acceptance for the people at large. One would surely welcome soya milk as a superior nutritional and healthy product to replace milk for everyone. An estimated 50 to 90 percent of Indians are having lactose intolerant symptoms, and gastrointestinal distress, diarrhoea and flatulence, occur because these individuals do not have the enzymes to digest the milk sugar lactose.

Additionally along with unwanted symptoms, milk-drinkers are also putting themselves at risk for the development of other chronic diseases and ailments. Dairy products — including milk, cheese, ice-creams, ghee and curd – contribute significant amounts to cholesterol and fat to the diet. Diets high in fat and saturated fat can increase the risk of cardiovascular disease. Heart disease and several cancers, including ovarian, breast and prostate, have been linked to the consumption of the dairy products. Soya milk, which lacks the dangerous fat and cholesterol of dairy, may help ward off these life-threatening ailments. The World Health Organisation predicts that heart disease will double and cancer rates will treble in India by 2015, The time to find healthy alternatives to dairy is right now.

The health benefits of soya have spurred a growth in soya beverage sales overseas. Sales in Canada reached $33 million in 1998, and they were a staggering $300 million in the United States. Chemical contamination of cow and buffalo milk poses yet another health threat. Studies by the Indian Agricultural Research Institute in New Delhi reveal that pesticide residue in milk and dairy products often exceeds the limits recommended by the World Health Organisation. A 1995 study by the Food and Drug Toxicology Research Centre, National Institute of Nutrition in Hyderabad found that some pharmaceutical drugs, including oxytocin and oxytetracycline (used by veterinarians in treating cows), has contaminated as much as 73 percent of individual milk samples tested. Adulteration of milk which toxins and detergents, the so-called "chemical milk", is also common. Parents who knowingly purchase chemical milk may be poisoning their children.

Soya milk reduces these hazards and is highly nutritional. It is also much less expensive. The cost is of particular concern. Ours is a poor country, overwhelmed by people below the poverty line. It is here the soya been offers a relief in disguise for this majority. More than half of all Indians suffer from malnutrition. For the poor, soya milk is a high protein, affordable drink. For more affluent Indians, who increasingly suffer from diet-related diseases of the West (such as heart disease and cancer), soya milk is a healthy alternative to dairy.

WORLD MILK SCENARIO

International dairy product prices strengthened during the second half of 2003 as a result of limited export supplies and sustained import demand.

The FAO price index for dairy products stood at 123 in October 2003, compared to an average of 114 during the first six months of the year; in October 2002, a year earlier, the index value was 90. To date this year, butter and cheese prices have increased more strongly than those of milk powder (powder had risen strongly in the second half of 2002). Compared to mid-2003 prices (June-July average), October prices increased as follows: butter by 18 percent, cheese by 11 percent, skimmed milk powder by 6 percent and whole milk powder by 5 percent. International prices were higher in terms of US dollars; this rise was tempered, however, by an increase in the value of several important exporters' national currencies (European euro, New Zealand and Australian dollars and Argentine peso) against the US dollar. As a result of rising international prices, the domestic industries in developing countries with relatively open markets have been less subject to competition from low- priced imports.

The increase in international prices is attributable mainly to marginal production growth and, in some cases, to declining production in exporting countries in Oceania, South America and some parts of Europe, leading to limited export supplies. As world prices rose, export subsidies paid by some high –cost producing countries in the Northern Hemisphere fell. In the case of the United States, average monthly export subsidies for skimmed milk powder declined from US $ 142 per tonne in March 2003 to US $ 121 per tonne in August 2003. In the EU, export subsidies for dairy products also fell, particularly for cheese – reflecting relatively stronger international prices for this product. In the EU at the end of August, subsidies for Gouda cheese were reduced from Euro – 1 108 per tonne to Euro 1 000 per tonne – a 10 percent decline. At the same time, EU export subsidies on milk powder and butter were reduced by around 4 percent. Despite declines in export subsidies, the amount of subsidy required to bring domestic prices for dairy products in high –cost producing countries down to world market levels remains substantial. As an illustration, recent levels of subsidy needed to export butter were US $ 1 973 per tonne in the United States and Euro 1 780 per tonne in the EU.

World Milk Production

Global milk output is expected to rise by approximately 1 per cent during 2003, mainly as a result of increased production in Asia, Central America and New Zealand (Table 4.6). In Oceania, milk production for the 2003/04 dairy year in New Zealand is anticipated to be 5 percent higher than for last year. Most areas of the country received plentiful rainfall during the spring, and prospects for pasture growth are good, although in some sections of North Island pastures were waterlogged. In Australia, continued reduced rainfall in some areas of the country is expected hinder recovery form last year's drought. Consequently, milk production could rise only marginally, perhaps by 1-2 percent, in the coming 2003/04 season. In the light of these factors, milk production for the end of the current dairy year for New Zealand is forecast at 15 million tonnes and for Australia at 10.6 million

Table 4.6: Milk Production

(*in million tonnes*)

	2001	*2002 Prov.*	*2003*
World	**579.9**	**594.0**	**599.1**
EU	126.1	126.7	126.8
India [1]	82.0	84.6	88.0
United States	75.0	77.3	77.5
Russian Fed.	33.0	33.5	33.2
Pakistan	27.0	27.7	28.4
Brazil	22.4	22.8	23.5
Ukraine	13.4	14.1	14.3
New Zealand [2]	13.2	13.9	14.2
Poland	11.9	12.0	11.8
Australia[3]	10.5	11.3	10.3
Mexico	9.5	9.6	9.8
Argentina	9.6	8.2	7.7

Source: FAO

[1]Dairy years ending March of the year shown.
[2]Dairy years ending May of the year shown.
[3]Dairy years ending June of the year shown.

tonnes. In both countries, the national dairy herd is in a phase of expansion, in contrast to most other developed countries; however, in the case of Australia, culling linked to the last season's drought could lead to a temporary reversal in herd growth. Since the beginning of 2003, the currencies of Australia and New Zealand have strengthened by 19 percent and 13 percent respectively against the US dollar, computing the strong growth seen in 2002. As international prices for dairy products are quoted in US dollars, the appreciation has had the effect of diluting the rise in international prices during 2003, in terms of local currencies. For example, in Australia, despite a fall in production, farmgate prices for milk for the 2002/03 season were 9 percent below last year's Australia exports more than 50 percent of its milk production as milk and milk products, thus domestic returns are highly sensitive to changes in international prices and exchange rate fluctuations.

In the United States, 2003 milk production is expected to be slightly higher than for last year to reach 77.5 million tonnes. Growth should stem from increased yields and cyclical herd rebuilding. During the second half of 2003, US producers introduced a scheme intended to reduce milk production and increase milk prices: " Cooperatives Working Together" (CWT), which may have some impact on national milk production in 2004. Milk production in a number of other developed countries (Canada, EU and Japan) is subject to policies that restrict output and consequently changes little from year to year.

In eastern Europe, milk production is not expected to increase in most countries in 2003, as a result of dry summer conditions. In most countries, yield per cow is increasing while the size of the national herd is decreasing. Also in eastern Europe, for example in Poland and Hungary, the impetus of imminent membership to the EU has resulted in dairies raising quality standards for milk and milk products – one result of which has been a reduction in the number of small-scale dairy producers, some of whom were not able to meet the required standards. In Hungary, it is estimated that 10 000 such producers may cease production. Other countries in the region, such as Bulgaria and Romania, have introduced government funded incentives to raise milk quality standards. For example, Bulgaria has announced that in 2004 it will begin closing dairy farms and dairies that do not conform to EU standards; moreover, along with this process, domestic quality standards for milk will be raised.

Milk production in the Russian Federation, after a decade of decline, has stabilized in recent years, although an expected phase of growth has yet to materialize. In general within the Federation, the size of the milking herd has continued to decrease, but feed availability has improved, raising yields per cow. Russian production is moving away from the large former state-run farms to small-scale ownership and production. Similarly, in a number of other member states of the CIS, where milk production also declined markedly throughout the 1990s, milk output in 2003 is expected to be stable compared with last year.

In the developing countries overall, growth in milk production is expected to continue; however, a number of countries in Latin America could see a decline in output. In Asia, India's milk production during the 2003/04 (April/March) marketing year could rise to above 90 million tones. This year, heavy rainfall during the monsoon season points to greater availability of fodder in India. Increased milk output in India is based more on improved feeding and genetics than on herd expansion. In China, milk output is also projected to rise as a result of strong consumer demand and the profitability of dairying compared with other types of agricultural production. As a result of rising international prices, dairy companies turned to expanding domestic supplies of milk during 2003 – principally by increasing herd size. In Thailand and the Philippines, milk output will probably increase further in 2003 as a result of the rest of South East Asia, demand for dairy products in these countries continues to grow as people's diet becomes more diversified.

In Latin America, milk production was affected in many areas by low prices; consequently, it is anticipated that output in a number of countries will decline. In Argentina, milk output is set to decline further in 2003, following a sharp reduction in 2002, as a result of variable pasture quality and low milk prices. Most recently, improved international prices and some recovery in domestic demand led to growth in intake by processors and to higher farmgate prices: in October 2003 prices were between US $0.15 and US$0.17 per litre. For 2004, this price increase may be sufficient to halt, or at least stem, the sharp falls in Argentine milk output experienced over the past three years. Producers in Uruguay also suffered from low farmgate prices as result of decreased domestic and regional demand and low international prices. For the 2002/03 season, prices averaged US$0.10 per litre, the lowest price in 25 years. As a result, production has dropped despite a government support programme and favourable weather conditions for pasture growth. Since mid-2003, however, farmgate prices in Uruguay have risen significantly. Not only have higher international prices contributed to this rise, but there has also been increased competition for milk supplies as Argentine dairies have begun sourcing milk in Uruguay. It appears that the dairy industry in Uruguay has passed the most difficult period; however, it is doubtful if production growth will return to the levels seen in the 1990s, as other activities – such as meat and oilseed production – are yielding higher returns than milk. Following a fall of 1 percent in 2002, milk production is expected to decline further in Chile in 2003, perhaps by as much as 5 percent. Major factors in this drop are low prices and stagnant domestic demand.

Elsewhere in Latin America, milk production in Peru is expected to grow in 2003 in response to higher prices resulting from rising domestic demand, including purchases by the government for social assistance programmes. Output is also anticipated to increase in Honduras as a result of improved infrastructure stemming from the construction of milk collection centers around the country's main producing regions, where groups of 10 to 15 farmers cool their milk before selling and delivering it to processing plants, receiving a premium prices over their once-warm milk.

Some countries in West Africa suffered from a lack of rainfall during 2002. In 2003, while rainfall has been generally good, milk production has been slow to recover as the number of cows in calf was severely reduced in the afternath of the previous year's drought. In some areas, for example Senegal and Mauritania, farmers migrated with their cattle in search of better pastures. This caused a shortage of fresh milk supplies for dairies in urban areas, which found themselves obliged to turn to supplies of imported milk powder to meet their processing needs. In Senegal, a large private-sector dairy withdrew from processing domestic milk in September 2003 to concentrate on producing dairy products based on imported materials. While the company's processing capacity was taken over by a government agency, the development of a domestic industry in the face of competition from imports is expected to be a significant challenge. In Kenya, well-distributed rains I 2003 provided good fodder availability and a favourale production outlook. Production has also been encouraged by stronger retail prices for milk in the main market – Nairobi – which also led to milk being shipped in from outside the usual Nairobi milk shed. Many other countries in East Africa received abundant rain during the year, resulting in favourable conditions for fodder and pasture growth.

Import Demand

International demand for dairy products is expected to remain firm, particularly in certain Asian countries. Increased purchases of milk powder by countries in Southeast Asia and China, are anticipated to meet rising domestic demand. Elsewhere, imports by Central American countries and the important markets of Mexico and Algeria could increase. Imports of milk products by Brazil had fallen by 60 percent from January to September compared to the same period in the previous year. This drop reflected a fall in domestic demand caused by a lack of economic growth purchases of milk powder by Venezuela were also anticipated to be lower, in part as a result of difficulties faced by traders in obtaining import licenses. Imports of butter and cheese by the Russian Federation grew substantially in 2003, despite an increase in tariffs in the previous year. However, purchases of butter by some countries in the Near East and Africa, which are the most price-sensitive importing regions, could fall in the light of the higher international which may reduce imports are Egypt, Lebanon, Nigeria and Kenya.

Export Supplies

For the 2003/04 dairy year, export supplies of dairy products are anticipated to be moderately higher from New Zealand and slightly higher from Australia - reflecting different rates of milk production growth. Export availabilities from South America are expected to be similar to the previous year, while those form eastern Europe and the Baltic States could be lower as a result of reduced milk production. Following a WTO ruling at the end of 2002 against Canada's dual pricing system for milk, which allowed milk produced outside the country's quota system to be exported, Canadian dairy product exports are expected to fall in 2003. As a result by both the EU and the United States are anticipated to be higher in 2003. While exports of bulk dairy commodities from both countries are constrained by the Uruguay Round Agreement limits on the use of export subsidies, recent years have seen a growth in the export of higher value products, which do not such exports now account for a greater volume of exports than bulk items requiring subsidy.

POULTRY PRODUCTS

Before the advent of the plan era, commercial poultry production was practically nonexistence. Poultry farming was then however fairly extensive but limited to backyard poultry keeping with low productive desi fowls maintained under peasant husbandry practices. The benefits derived were, therefore, only a small fraction of what could be obtained from scientific poultry farming. No doubt, superior exotic poultry breeds with high egg productivity were introduced in the country from time to time for improving the indigenous stock but in the absence of a systematic large-scale development programme such efforts proved abortive. Poultry farming, however, over the past 25 years has developed as a healthy and forward looking industry, and the global market now takes it seriously. India ranks fifth in world egg production, with an annual production of about 28 billion. In broiler production, the country ranks among the first ten countries. About

450 million broilers are produced annually for domestic consumption. Nevertheless, the per capita consumption in India of eggs (33 eggs/ year) and broiler meat (1.0 kg. per year) is one of the lowest in the world.

Commercial poultry, mainly egg production, had its beginning in India in the sixties. Broilers became popular during the seventies. Eighties saw a boom in both egg and broiler production. During nineties the processing industry gained importance, Today, India is producing about 28 billion eggs and nearly 900,000 tonnes of broiler meat and nearly 88% eggs and 100% broilers are produced by commercial farmers. Egg production is concentrated in the South (40%), East (20%), North and West (each accounting for 13.5%). Uttar Pradesh and Madhya Pradesh contribute only 8% to egg production (Table 4AII.1 at Annexure II). Urban areas produce 75% eggs and per caput consumption is about 80 eggs per annum. The remaining 25% is from rural areas where per caput consumption is only 10 eggs per annum. Within rural areas also, relatively developed regions account for nearly half of the rural population, producing 66% of eggs. Broiler production in the rural areas is practically nil. Poultry industry in India plays a very important role in employment and wealth generation, and occupies a place of pride in the Indian economy. This will continue to be so during the 21st century also. Ironically, however, the per capita consumption of eggs in India is just around 33 eggs per person per year as compared to 120 in more developed countries. In 1970, the figure in India was 10 eggs per person per year.

The Public sector, as of today, plays quite an insignificant role in the growth of this industry. At present there are 3 clear-cut segments responsible for development and production of poultry:

   (i) Organizations with the State and Central Government (DAH&D),

  (ii) ICAR and other bodies, and

 (iii) Private sector.

An attempt has been made here to look at the industry as a whole, and present a composite picture of its development both in the public and the private sector. One very interesting feature of the industry in India is the development of both production and consumption of poultry in the rural areas. The organic egg as well as broiler has a large potential for export.

The process of transformation of this agro-based activity from the nascent stage to the present gigantic form started in 1960. The concept of backyard poultry keeping yielded place to poultry farming as a commercial enterprise. The development is not only in number but also in size, productivity, sophistication, image and versatility. Factors which contributed to this gigantic growth within a short span of period were planned research and development strategies adopted since the mid-sixties leading to the massive application of modern technology of intensive system of housing and management, availability of genetically superior hybrid layer and broiler chicks, nutritionally balanced feed, better health care, and sizeable investment in both public and private sectors. Initiation of an Intensive Egg and Poultry Production-Cum-Marketing Programme, popularly known as the Intensive Poultry Development Project (IPDP), with an area development and package approach, was also one of the most important factors for bringing about this favourable development. Introduction of deep litter system of management and further importation of high quality stock and mass preventive vaccination against common avian diseases, income tax exemption for the poultry sector in agriculture, progressive industrialization with resultant higher purchasing power of people, were among other major contributing factors.

While commercial poultry production was increasing rapidly following the measures taken so far, no systematic efforts were undertaken till the VIIIth Plan for developing backyard poultry for small farmers which still contributed about 30% of the total egg production in the country. Hence a new scheme was launched during 1999-2000 to encourage backyard poultry in the country.

In India poultry meat constitutes around 12 per cent of the total meat. Poultry meat, today, accounts for 27% of all meat consumed in the world. But considering the rate at which consumption is growing, the equations can change within the next 20 years or so and will account for 45% of meat consumption globally. India is not isolated from these developments and the poultry industry appears ready to take in the benefits.

Poultry Production in Villages

An essential requirement to meet village needs is to find a suitable marketing system by which eggs can be made readily available at affordable prices. This will call for a new approach. Village poultry production offers hope. By setting up a local unit to serve a cluster of villages, the birds will be scavenging in the backyard supplemented by kitchen waste and feed containing locally available ingredients. At night, the birds can be provided shelter through small low-height houses constructed with cheap wood or bricks utilizing some corner of the house. It is obvious that villages with small population cannot really sustain industrial approach to poultry production. The clue perhaps lies in developing egg production in villages not as an occupation but as a supplemental household activity. Using management methods which, even if they do not lead to high levels of production per bird, do enable eggs to be produced at least possible cost. One must remember that the cheapest egg is the backyard egg which is produced by a foraging hen, scavenging in the backyard and feeding on nothing specific. The output of these birds can be sold readily within the village or in its neighborhood. Such flocks certainly cannot be left at the mercy of nature altogether, as the traditional backyard flocks were.

The task is to induct an appropriate husbandry technology which will permit effective management of small flocks of say, 20-25 birds. For example, improved birds may be distributed to villages within the periphery of a breeding farm. Also free-range poultry products command a higher price than factory-farmed ones. Poultry farming has a very bright future both for home as well as external markets. The important thing is to strike a right balance between making poultry production profitable for the backyard producer and affordable to the rural consumer.

Latest production estimates indicate a phenomenal growth during the current decade. The industry is highly research driven and huge resources have been put into research activities, particularly by private sector. To ensure that Indian egg and poultry products are among the best in the world, research is concentrated on genetics, breeding of birds, vaccines and virology. The Venkateshwara group has impressive laboratories across the country, peopled by a highly qualified technical pool that provides support to the industry. Almost all major European and American commercial breeds are available in India today. More than 500 hatcheries supply day old chicks to farmers to raise layers and broilers. The egg production per hen increased from 270 eggs in 1980 to 310 in 2000. This increase in production provided an additional income of Rs. 5630 million to layer farmers in just one year. All basic equipment required for rearing and breeding poultry is available here in the country and with the growing size of breeder and commercial farms, automation is gaining strength.

The industry has been built with an investment of Rs. 100 billion. In a recent study of the Indian Food Industry, CII and Mckinsey & Co. have projected a very bright future for the Indian poultry industry: This sector in India has a potential to grow at over 20% a year over the next 10 years. This will enable it to at least quadruple in size, growing from the present Rs. 75,000 million to approximately Rs. 300,000 million. Unlike other sub sectors of agriculture, development of poultry is based on the role of private sector. In addition to various developmental activities, research programmes have also been pioneered by the private sector where investment has been increasing at a faster rate.

Much of the credit for the present status of the poultry industry goes to Dr. B. V. Rao, whose dream of providing total support to the small poultry farmers has today resulted in the mega Venkateshwara hatcheries group, indisputably forerunners in their field. In his lifetime he was able to establish a totally farmer-oriented Corporation with total backward and forward integration. Single handedly he provided impetus to a fledgling industry. The Group today continues to stress on quality in whatever it produces-whether chicks, vaccines, medicines, equipment or processed eggs/chicken. Their technical support to farmers has been impressive, resulting in increased productivity and a better lifestyle for a large number of farmers. With a market share of 85% in the layer business and 60-65% in the broiler business, the group plays a significant role in the poultry business today.

The cost of egg production is very low in India, as a result, a few joint ventures have come up for egg processing. There are about six large size units, each with a capacity of more than 5,00,000 eggs per day. Products such as albumin, whole egg powder, yolk powder, lysozyme and calcium are recovered from table eggs. The annual output of poultry feed exceeds 8 million tons. The bulk of this production, estimated at 85%, is accounted for by farms and custom manufacture units. The feed industry is increasingly relying on computers to work out low cost feed formulation with locally available ingredients. Though maize is an important ingredient in poultry feed, the production of this grain has not matched the growth of the poultry industry. The feed required per k.g. of body weight in broilers has been reduced from 2.5 kg. in 1980 to 1.8 kg. in 2000, resulting in savings of an estimated Rs. 3800 million.

Highly labour intensive, the poultry industry has a huge employment potential and is one of the few industries that can provide employment in the rural areas, preventing the need for migration to overcrowded cities. An increase of just one egg per capita per annum, or an increase of 50 gm. per capita per annum in broilers, can create 26,000 additional employment opportunities. The industry gives employment to 1.6 million people. In addition, many other ancillary industries provide employment and generate income.

Research Requirements

Layers

1. Evolve high-yielding strains/strain crosses capable of yielding 250 eggs with more than 50 g. egg weight during 500 days of age and without more than 1% layer-house mortality per month. This is to be done through testing the purebred and crossbred performance of a number of purelines/strains.
2. Estimate genetic and phenotypic parameters and components of genetic variability like GCA, SCA and reciprocal effects, using complete diallel crosses to facilitate decision on selection criterion and mating system.
3. Estimate genetic gains from selection in the principal and correlated traits.
4. Compare different breeding methods for improving the principal performance traits.

Broilers

1. Evolve pureline/crossbred broilers weighing at least 100 g at 6 weeks or efficiency better than 2.4 and mortality less than 5% up to 6 weeks of age. This is to be done through testing the purebred and crossbred performance of a number of strains/purelines.
2. Estimate genetic and phenotypic parameters of important performance traits in these lines, and estimate various components of genetic variability like GCA, SCA, reciprocal and maternal effects, using complete diallel crossing to allow decision on selection criteria and mating system(s).
3. Estimate genetic gains from selection in the principal and correlated traits.

4. Compare the different breeding methods for improving the principal performance traits and consider reducing the size of the broiler female through the introduction of dwarfing gene. Graph 4.3 gives an idea of investment in research.

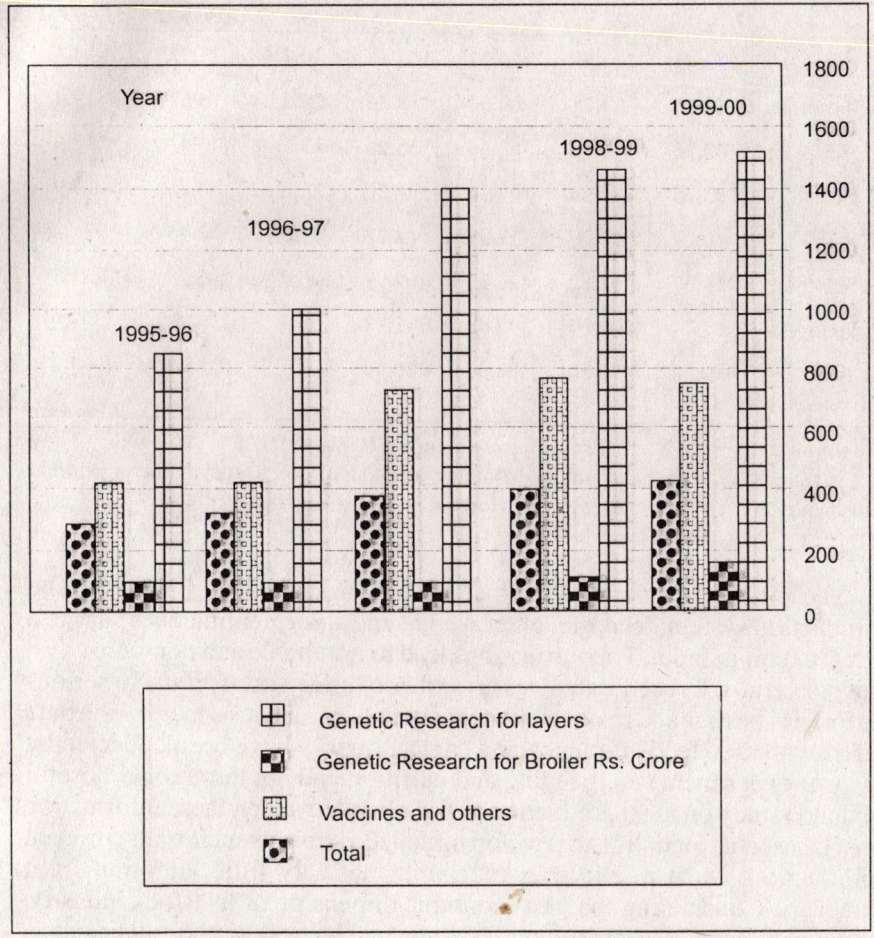

Graph 4.3: Investment in Research over last five years in Private sector

MEAT

The source of meat in India is from goats, sheep, buffaloes, cattle, pigs and poultry. The population of different animals in India is shown in Table 4.7. Total meat output (including poultry meat) accounts for 24 percent of the value of livestock production. No official time series data of production of meat in the country are available. The discussion on the performance of meat sector is based on the FAO time series. However, as discussed later in Chapter 7 this series suffers from several limitations.

Table 4.7: Population of Different Animals in India: Selected Years

(Million)

Category	1982	1992	1997	1999*	% share	Increase in 1999 over 1982	
						Numbers	Percent
1. Cattle	192.45	204.58	174.97	164.68	40.2	-27.77	-14.4
2. Buffaloes	69.78	84.21	84.02	83.35	20.3	13.57	19.4
3. Sheep	48.76	50.98	53.30	55.24	13.5	6.48	13.3
4. Goats	95.25	115.26	102.26	94.50	23.0	-0.75	-7.9
5. Pigs	10.07	12.79	12.37	12.22	3.0	2.75	21.35
6. Sub-total	416.37	467.82	426.92	409.99	100.0	-6.38	-1.5
7. Poultry	207.74	307.07	342.48	381.97	....	174.23	83.9
8. Total Livestock	419.50	470.86	452.45	416.48	....	3.02	-7.2

• Projected on the basis of rate of growth during 1992 to 1997.

Source: Government of India, Ministry of Agriculture, Department of Animal Husbandry & Dairying: Basic Animal Husbandry Statistics: 2002.

The production of meat animals is not an organized business. The production system, feed, slaughter weight and slaughter practices vary to a great extent in India. These situations lead to unreliable and non-consistent raw materials. Usually carcasses are either overlean or overfat. No serious effort has been made to develop meat animals of various species. The data of growth rate, feed efficiency and carcass quality have been collected by way of experiments on breeding and nutrition and not through purposeful planned study on meat production and quality. However, these information can be used as guideline to develop organized experimental trials for meat production. Meat quality has received relatively little attention from breeders. Considering the vast economic dimension of livestock industry, there has recently been some awakening of interest in the quality. It is hoped that the availability of improved meat animals will increase, still in the years to come; major meat production will depend on presently available raw material.

Cattle population declined during the 1997 compared to the 1982. This welcome trend had partly been due to the replacement of bullock power by tractors and other agricultural machinery in Northern states especially in Punjab, Haryana and West Uttar Pradesh. Population of goats also declined compared to 1982. This trend is assumed to have since continued. By contrast population of other species increased with faster increase in pigs, followed by buffaloes and sheep. These trends were assumed to hold good thereafter too.

Meat production increased at a slower pace, around 3 percent during the period 1981 to 1999. This was partly due to the non-availability of cattle and breeds. Meat animals are, as mentioned above, not optimally utilized due to unorganized meat sector and social reasons in the country. Due to poor slaughterhouse conditions, meat cannot be produced under strict hygienic conditions; however, cooking and consumption practices limit the risks. Number of animals slaughtered and meat production from them are shown in Table 4.8. Total number of animal slaughtered in India rose from 67.95 million head in 1981 to 102.79 million head in 1999, representing 51 percent increase. This translated in total meat production increasing from 2.57 million tonnes in 1981 to about 4.55 million tonnes in 1999. Total cows and buffaloes slaughtered for meat increased from 15.6 million head in 1981 to 23.8 million head in 1999. Total production of beef and buffalo meat rose from 1.67 million tonnes to 2.83 million tonnes. The 53 percent rise in the number of animal slaughtered resulted in about 70 percent increase in meat output. This reflects improvement in the carcass weight per animal assumed in the FAO series.

Table 4.8: **Number of Animals Slaughtered and Meat Production: 1981 and 1999**

Category	No. slaughtered (in 000)		Increase over the years		Meat Production (000 tonnes)		Growth in output in 1999/ 1981(%
	1981	*1999*	*No. ('000)*	*Percent*	*1981*	*1999*	*per annum)*
1. Cattle	9,636	13,800	4,164	43.2	845	1,421	2.8
2. Buffalo	5,969	10,000	4,031	67.5	824	1,410	2.9
3. Sheep	12,750	19,000	6,250	49.0	153	228	2.1
4. Goats	30,250	46,600	16,350	54.0	302	466	2.3
5. Pigs	9,333	13,386	4,053	43.4	327	469	1.9
Sub-Total	67,948	102,786	34,838	51.3	2,451	3,994	2.6
Poultry meat	......	......	......	......	120	551	6.9
Total Meat	......	......	......	......	2,571	4,545	3.0

Source: FAO: Production Yearbook: various issues.

Graphs 4.4 and 4.5 indicate shares of different categories of meat in the total production in 1981 and 1999. In total meat output, beef accounted for 32 percent in 1999 almost the same as in 1981. Buffalo meat share was 31 percent. Lamb and goat meat together contributed over 15 percent, while the share of poultry meat increased from 5 percent in 1981 to 12 percent in 1999. Production of beef and buffalo meat in India is more than 4 times the mutton and goat meat. The per capita availability and consumption of beef and buffalo meat of 2.8 kg, is about half of fish, but more than twice the average intake of mutton, pork and poultry.

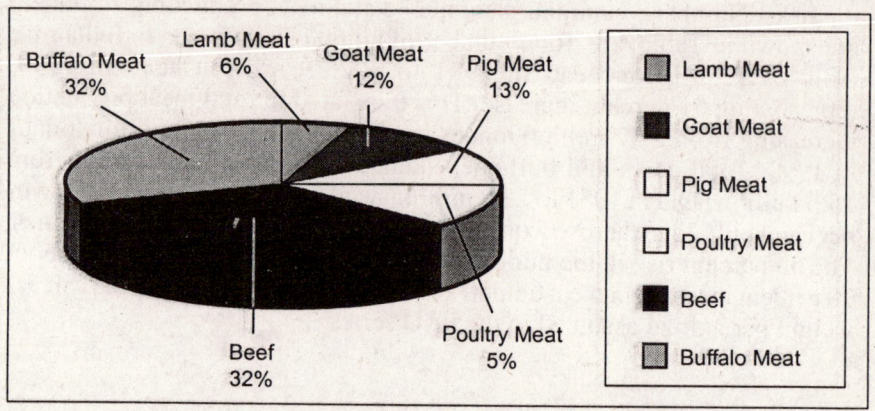

Graph 4.4: Share of different types in total meat in 1981(%)

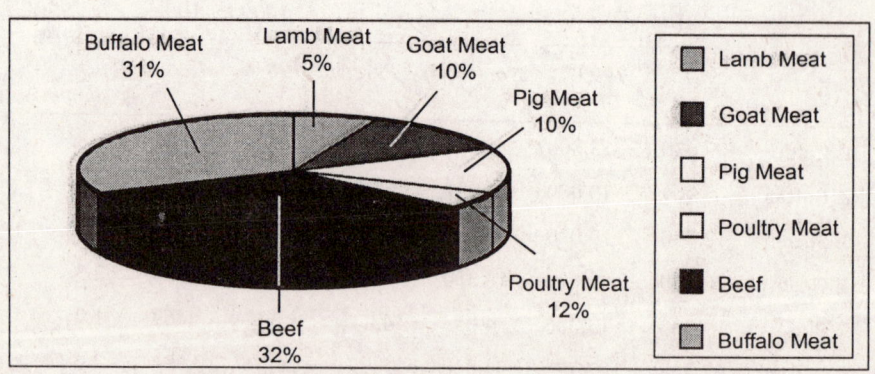

Graph 4.5: Share of different meats in total output in 1999

Production of different types of meat in India in 1981, 1991, 1997 and 1999 is shown in Table 4.9. In the total increase in meat output of 1, 974 thousand tonnes from 19981 to 1999, buffalo meat contributed around 30 percent, followed by beef (29 percent) and poultry meat (about 22 percent). Goat meat and pork contributed 8 and 7 percent respectively. Lamb meat share in the increase comes to only 3.8 percent. The rate of growth of meat production seems to have slowed down during the last decade. This reflects lower increase for most categories of meat, except lamb meat and pork.

Even for poultry meat the rate of increase was lower than during 1981-1991. The low rate of increase in red meat i.e. beef and buffalo meat, is due to the following reasons:

(i) High feed cost and poor feed conversion ratio compared to poultry where l: 8.8 conversion is being taken as compared to l:4 by goats and sheep.

(ii) The requirement of land for grazing is a limiting factor.

(iii) The turnover for broilers is much faster, i.e. within 6-8 weeks the broilers are ready for consumption whereas in the case of goats it takes much longer before they are ready for consumption.

(iv) The requirement of land to produce 1 kg. of red meat is far higher than for the production of poultry meat.

(v) Even on health grounds, doctors advice people to consume white meat.

Table 4.9: Meat Production in India

('000'tonnes)

Types of meat	1995	1996	1997	1998	1999	2000	2001	2002
Mutton & Goat Meat	647	669	670	675	800	825	850	870
Pork Meat	420	420	420	520	464	480	495	505
Buffalo Meat	1204	1204	1205	1210	1250	1270	1300	1365
Other Cattle Meat	1292	1292	1292	1295	1295	1300	1305	1330
Poultry Meat	578	480	600	675	725	775	875	975
Total	4141	4065	4187	4375	4534	4650	4825	5045

Note: Data shown relate to animals slaughtered within national boundaries irrespective of their origin

Source: FAO Production Yearbook: various issues.

Increases in livestock numbers and offtake rates have been the dominant sources of growth in meat output in the country. Much of the increased output in the future should come from intensive and semi-intensive commercial production with the use of supplementary feeds. The overall pattern is likely that most of the additional meat production will be derived from a higher number of animals. However, yields per animal are expected to increase faster than in the past twenty years as a consequence of improvements in health, feed and pasture carrying capacity.

In India, buffalo population increased proportionately higher than cattle population and contributed significantly to total milk output production (about 55 percent) though systematic improvement of buffaloes through breeding did not take place. The meat potential of the buffalo remains largely unexploited so far. The concept of fattening young buffaloes is largely unknown. Mostly infirm or diseased animals are brought to abattoirs. The buffalo keeper gives away the animal against a nominal charge or even free and thus feels relieved of the burden of the act of killing, for which he has to overcome his religious sensibilities. He does not seek to ameliorate his economic condition by such means. However, the buffalo meat processing has developed into a full-fledged business and relevant products are marketed at various stages to meet domestic as well as the export demand (canned meat). The Brooke Bond meat industry in Aurangabad illustrates the role of an efficient system of meat production. Buffaloes are bought directly from the individual farmers, thus avoiding the animal markets and middlemen. The Company guarantees the buffalo keepers who are willing to sell their animals, quite at a reasonable price. It also makes its own arrangements for transporting the animals to the slaughter facilities, where they are processed into canned meat. The processing capacity finds use of all edible and non-edible products.

Except in a few export-oriented units, unsophisticated slaughtering practices contribute to poor meat quality and low recovery of various byproducts such as hide and skins, tallow, blood, viscera and organs. Most meats are sold without the benefit of sanitary inspection. Butcher shops often lack chilling equipment, further contributing to product deterioration and increased marketing losses. Poor enforcement of hygienic standards constrains India's export competitiveness. Capital investment in existing slaughterhouses would contribute significantly to the collection of byproducts. For example, blood and other offals could be used as animal feed supplement. Political and social pressures, however, continue to impede efforts to modernize the slaughtering sector.

The prospects of buffaloes for meat production are excellent in view of their triple function, efficiency for converting roughages into valuable products and superior quality of buffalo milk and meat. An immense potential exists for an organized buffalo meat industry on scientific and modern lines. The following approaches are recommended for development of buffaloes for meat**:

(1) The recommendations made by the National Commission on Agriculture in 1976 on development of buffaloes in general and for meat production for domestic and export trade are appropriate even today and need to be implemented. These recommendations include: (i) A fresh review and a study in greater depth should be carried out for a more satisfactory breed classification of the Indian buffalostock; (ii) The buffalo should be developed not only for enhancement of milk, production but also for making it a source of production of quality meat; (iii) Attempts should be made to develop distinctly separate milk and meat breeds or types of buffaloes; (iv) A number of seed stock farms with at least 150 breeding she-buffaloes should be established; (v) In buffalo farms

---

**Kondaiah, N: Improvement of Buffaloes for Meat Production: Methods and Organization. In Indian Journal of Animal Production : NO.1-4: January-December 1998, pp.57-58.

and research institutes wide scale investigations and studies should be undertaken on early weaning of buffalo calves and their rearing on low cost calf starters; (vi) Research studies on the effect of feeding and husbandry on fattening buffalo calves should be undertaken. Promotional activity for consumption of buffalo meat in the country and consumer educational programme should be undertaken on a countrywide scale; and (vii) A deliberate and energetic drive should be made to develop export trade in buffalo meat.

(2) Salvaging male buffalo calves from early death both to conserve germplasm and increase meat production and availability of draught animals. Improved extension services should be adopted for salvaging buffalo calves.

(3) Entrepreneurial programmes for salving buffalo calves from early death. Meat exporters need to provide the required assistance before the activity is adopted.

(4) Simple breeding programme for increasing availability of large number of buffalo bulls for natural service. Based on dam's milk production and growth rate of male calf with better conformation could be considered for selection and distribution of buffalo bulls for improving large number of nondescript buffaloes.

(5) At least ten more integrated meat processing complexes should be established in the buffalo population rich states with backward integration of improved buffalo production programme by providing input services and marketing of animals to the farmers.

(6) Meat exporters should organize selection programme to identify superior buffaloes in the abattoir project area and provide necessary facilities for effective use of the superior animals in the overall improvement of buffaloes.

(7) The superiority of buffalo meat need to be demonstrated through continuous experimentation for promotion of buffalo meat for domestic and export market.

(8) Fattening buffaloes through economical feeding to exploit compensatory growth phenomenon and increase buffalo meat and hide production potential need to be actively adopted.

(9) Pragmatic approach in culling and utilization of spent buffaloes need to be adopted for better utilization of feed resources and sustainable buffalo production.

(10) Concerted efforts for defending and promoting meat exports by demonstrating the public interest involved are required in view of the demand raised for ban on meat exports.

(11) A review of the State Animal Preservation Acts for effective utilization of the buffalo resources in view of the changing agricultural practices and growing buffalo population.

(12) Quality assurance of buffalo meat for domestic and export market to promote buffalo meat.

ROLE OF LIVESTOCK BREEDS

Livestock productivity is directly related to the quality of animals/birds. While Livestock Census provides details of the distribution of the number of cattle as between improved breed and indigenous, such information is not available for buffalo. All the same, it would be useful to have some idea about the breeds and breeding programmes for livestock. At present there are 26 recognised breeds of cattle and 8 that of buffalo. A central Herd Registration Scheme is in operation. Under this scheme 4 Central Herd Registration Units have been established at Rohtak (Haryana), Ahmedabad (Gujarat), Ongole (Andhra Pradesh) and Ajmer (Rajasthan). Under these units Gir, Kankrej, Haryana and Ongole cows, and Suri, Jaffrabadi, Murrah and other buffalo breeds conforming to specific breed characteristics and prescribed level of milk production are identified in their breeding tracts and registered. The registration is done after recording the lactation yield of cows and buffaloes through field milk recording programme. Breeders possessing registered animals are awarded prizes depending on the level of production to encourage them to preserve and improve the indigenous milch breeds. Farmers are also educated on scientific management practices to improve production potential, and are advised to form associations for the scientific breeding of their animals by using outstanding bulls and their germ plasm. During 1998-99, Primary Registration of milch animals of various breeds was done against the target of registering 12000 animals.

For any increase in milk production, it is necessary to improve the quality of animals to be followed by proper feed and disease control. According to available information productivity levels of indigenous cows are quite low as compared with crossbred (Table 4.10). Of late, it has been felt to recognize a number of indigenous farm animal breeds which have been developed over the ages through natural selection in different agro-ecological zones. During the process of development such animals have developed remarkable tendency to withstand hot climatic stress and disease. Such well defined cattle breeds merely constitute one-fifth of the country's total cattle population. The rest is an admixture of desi cattle.

Indigenous or zebu cattle in the Indian subcontinent, Asia pacific region and other tropical countries are low producing except for some important

Table 4.10: All-India Average Milk Production of Cross-Bred and Non-Descript cows
(kg per day)

Year	Cross-Bred	Non-Descript
1993-94	5.65	1.66
1994-95	5.81	1.69
1997-98	6.36	1.83
1998-99	6.46	1.89

Source: Government of India, Ministry of Agriculture, Department of Animal Husbandry & Dairying: Basic Animal Husbandry statistics, 1999 and 2002, New Delhi.

cattle breeds of Sahiwal, Red Singhi, Hariana Gir and Kankrej of India and Pakistan. These cattle breeds have been exported to adjoining countries and have been used in upgrading the local cattle stock for hardness, heat and tick infestation quality as well as high butter fat content in milk. The spread of Indian zebu cattle in foreign countries has been in vogue since the 19th century to Africa, Asia, North America, South America and Australia where zebu cattle germplasm is utilised to upgrade cattle for draught purpose.

Although rampant crossbreeding has a desired result in improving the milk production scenario, yet unfortunately its consequences are being felt now. A number of indigenous farm animal breeds are gradually getting genetically degraded and diluted because of unplanned breeding and introduction of exotic germplasm. As a result indigenous breeds are getting endangered at an alarming rate, while others are in the process of replacement by certain high-yielding strains. If this trend continues, the invaluable native germplasm which is relatively better to withstand stress, disease, food conversion and adaptation to local environment, would grossly be depleted or even lost forever.

Collective efforts by all concerned organizations are needed to ensure the conservation of such threatened forms of farm diversity. Various techniques for cellular and genetic manipulation of mammalian eggs and embryos are now being employed in conserving genetic diversity. Such technology having wider application in the frontier of preservation are as follows:

Cryo preservation of semen: The technique of semen preservation is now in practice and has been routinely used for improvement and development of crossbreeds. However, the technique can only satisfy to conserve germplasm of male parent.

Ooctyle preservation: This technique provides opportunity for conservation of female oocyte in the same way as male semen. The oocyte can be recovered by surgery, laparotomy or even from slaughtered female. Hence individual genome of male or female can be cryo preserved.

Embryo preservation and transfer: This technique has been developed to preserve a complete genome of a species and has distinguished role in conserving them. Embryos can be obtained by flushing the oviduct or the uterus by surgical or nonsurgical methods. Such an embryo can be kept resurrected any time.

Preserving of ovaries: Preservation of slices of ovaries in liquid nitrogen is the new technology coming up for conservation. Ovaries sliced can be cryo-preserved for longer period of time and can be thawed when required to produce viable ooctyle.

Embryo splitting: This technique of manipulating embryos could be helpful in producing more number of animals from a few stored embryos or rare or endangered animals. This technique needs to be standardized, and the 21st century could see fruitful results in adopting technology for conservation of not only milch animals but also endangered wildlife species.

It may be reiterated that a number of indigenous milch breeds are gradually declining in population and are in the process of becoming extinct. A few of them are already on the verge of extinction. Immediate measures are needed to be taken to conserve these valuable genetic resources. As variation is a tool for genetic upgradation, such a tool should not be lost at any cost. Therefore, conservation is the key word in preserving the vast genetic diversity.

National Project for Cattle and Buffalo Breeding

National Project for Cattle and Buffalo Breeding is a 10-year programme and was launched in the year 2000 with an allocation of Rs. 402 crore for the first phase of five years. Under the programme, the genetic quality of cattle and buffaloes will be improved through extensive artificial insemination and increased availability of superior quality of indigenous breeds for natural insemination. Artificial insemination services will be made available at the farmers doorsteps. All breedable females among cattle and buffaloes will be progressively brought under artificial insemination or natural service by high quality bulls. Emphasis will be laid on conservation and improvement of indigenous cattle and buffalo breeds. Quality control and certification of bulls and services at sperm stations, semen banks and training institute will also be taken up under this programme.

During the next three years, 700 superior quality bulls will be acquired for natural insemination, 300 bulls will be acquired for artificial insemination, 20 new semen banks will be set up 1,300 artificial insemination centers will be converted into mobile centers besides setting up 700 new centers, and 2,520 fertility camps will be organized. Storage and distribution of liquid nitrogen used by sperm station and semen banks will be strengthened. Educated rural youth will be provided with training and equipment to work as private artificial insemination workers. These workers would also take up vaccination, primary health care and cattle insurance activities. These are in addition to various activities like field recording, training, computerization, animal identification and evaluation studies, etc.

LEATHER

Hides and Skins

India's leather industry has a rich legacy of 200 years. At present, it is predominantly export –oriented. It is the second largest employer and the fourth largest forex earner in the country. About 2.5 million people, mostly the poor, are engaged in the leather sector. About 200,000 women work in the industry. The industry's annual turnover is estimated at $4 billion. The total value of production is estimated to have crossed Rs. 302 billion in the year 2000. A large part (60 to 65 per cent) of leather production is in the small/cottage sector. The basic raw materials for leather industry, viz. raw hides and skins are derived from livestock. Cattle, buffaloes, goats and sheep are the four species which supply hides and skins to the Indian Leather Industry. Of the four, buffalo's contribution to leather industry is significant not only in quantum but also in quality in respect of calf skins.

From official sources, little information is available with regard to the production of hides and skins. Even though India is the largest producer of hides and leather, it is not able to reap the full potential. This is because a good part of the hides are damaged due to poor flaying especially in the small and unregistered slaughterhouses. There is, therefore, a considerable scope for improvement of hides and tanning and using entrails and offal etc. that generally goes waste. Though the quality leaves much to be desired, there is considerable demand for quality hides. The only source of information regarding hides and skins production in India and other countries is the FAO's Yearbook. Besides the Central Statistical Organization publishes the value of Indian hides and skins in their National Account Statistics, but does not give either the unit value or the physical output. Based on data available from these two sources, production of raw hides and skins and their value in the selected years are presented in Table 4.11.

Table 4.11: All India Production and Value of Raw Hides and Skins: Selected Years

Years	Hides	Sheep	Goat skin	Total skin	Value (1993/94 Rupees million)		
	.... 000 tonnes				Hides	Skin	Total
1979-81	736	37	75	848	5,027	2,560	7,587
1989-91	860	44	107	1,011	4,417	3,320	7,737
(Growth rate %)	(1.5)	(1.9)	(3.6)	(1.8)	(-1.3)	(2.6)	(0.2)
1991	841	38	108	987	4,460	3,470	7,930
1992	850	38	109	997	4,760	3,330	8,090
1993	915	39	119	1,073	5,060	5,030	10,090
1994	924	45	120	1,089	5,410	5,150	10,560
1995	933	49	122	1,103	5,240	5,010	10,250
1996	944	50	124	1,118	5,380	5,080	10,460
1997	953	51	126	1,130	5,670	5,160	10,830

Source: FAO: Production Yearbook various issues and World Statistical Compendium for Raw Hides and Skins, Leather and Leather Footwear: 1974-1992, Rome 1994.
Central Statistical Organization: National Accounts Statistics; 2000

Hides and skins are derived both from animals slaughtered for meat purpose and also from fallen animals (i.e. mortality due to natural reasons like old age, diseases, etc.). While availability of slaughtered hides and skins depends on meat (in other words slaughters rate), the fallen hides/skins depends on the rate of mortality as well as extent of recovery. Table 4.12 shows the availability of hides and skins in India.

Table 4.12: Production of Hides and Skins–1998*

S. No.	Specie	In million pieces	In million sq. ft.	% Share in total
1.	Cattle Hides	25.16	503.2	30.54
2.	Buffalo Hides	21.74	543.5	32.98
3.	Goat Skins	88.02	440.1	26.71
4.	Sheep Skins	32.17	160.9	9.77
	Total		1647.7	100.00

*Estimated by the authors

The data in Table 4.12 show that India annually produces about 1650 million sq. ft. of leather of which buffalo contribution accounts for one third share. India by holding 58% of global buffaloes annually produces 63% of global buffalo hides. Buffalo hides and calf skins are very valuable raw material for the leather industry both in terms of quality and quality. Hides and skins recovered from slaughtered animals are collected, cured with common salt and then sent to tanneries for processing. Hides and skins from fallen animals are wasted, though majority recovered, due to several reasons which are listed below:

   (i) Non-availability of flayers in time;
  (ii) Due to occasional availability of carcasses, coupled with social change among flayers community, many of them have migrated and settled in other professions;
 (iii) Younger generation not willing to work in this profession; and
 (iv) Flayers do not attend damaged carcasses since they yield poor quality of hides/skins which even if recovered would fetch meagre amount.

As a result of non-recovery, annually an estimated 2.5 million hides and calf skins are wasted and the value of this material would be Rs. 700 million.

To minimise the wastage, it is essential to establish Carcass Recovery Centres wherever possible. It would be possible not only to recover hides and skins from fallen animals but also other byproducts like flesh/bones etc. to manufacture value added products. However, the site selection for such carcass recovery centres should be preceded by feasibility report which should take into account the availability of carcasses in and around the centre, present practices of disposal etc. since the viability of a Carcass Recovery Centre (CRC) would solely depend on the availability of sufficient number of carcasses. In addition, to make the CRC viable, the capital investment on building and equipment should be low with cost effective technology.

Centre Leather Research Institute (CLRI) under Leather Technology Mission (LTM) has upgraded 25 Carcass Recovery Centres in the country with improved equipment and technology and it is planning to establish a few more in the near future. The above data show that meat and other edible offals account for nearly 78% in the total value realised while the hide accounts for about 17%. The meat is sold for edible purpose in fresh condition whereas the raw hide is processed·into finished leathers and converted into products like shoes, bags and garments and as a result the value realisation would enhance by almost 5 times. Of course, other inputs like chemicals, labour and accessories are added in the process of manufacturing. As a result of value addition the basic raw hide price of Rs. 650/- would enhance to Rs. 3250/- by the time leather products are made and sold in the market. It amounts that the value of leather products often exceeds the value of meat. In addition to added value, sizable number of people are being employed during the process. The raw hide, though a by-product for the butcher in terms of value, it is treated as a coproduct, because of these twin advantages (value addition and employment generation). Government has been encouraging the exports of final finished products like shoes and bags instead of intermediary products to earn more foreign exchange and to provide employment.

The flow chart given in Graph 4.6 shows the different end uses of raw hides and calf skins.

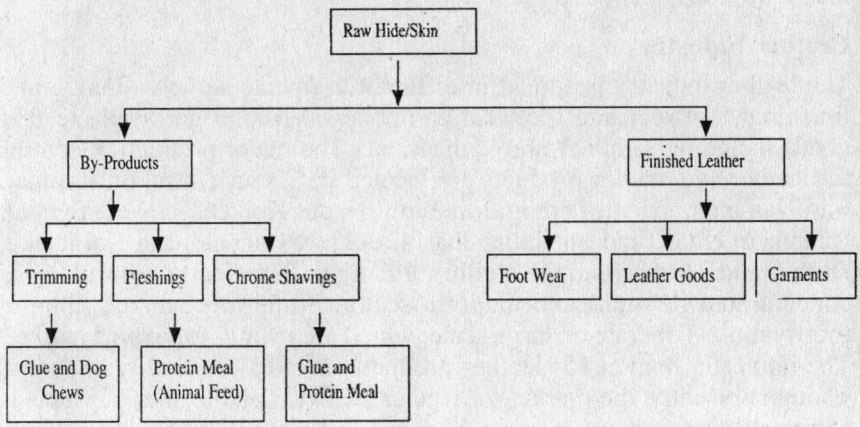

Graph 4.6: End uses of raw hides and calf skins

Production of cattle and buffalo hides increased from an average of 736 000 tonnes during 1979-81 to 953 000 tonnes, representing an increase of about 29 percent. Sheep and goatskin increased by 58 percent to 177 000 tonnes during this period. Goatskin contributed the bulk of this increase (about 80 percent). In term of value, the increase for raw hides was only 13 percent, while the value of sheep and goatskins more than doubled during this period.

At present nearly 35-40 percent of leather goes waste. The Committee set up by the Government had recommended the utilization of hides from fallen animals, upgradation of lower grade hides and skins, and commercial cattle farming to increase the quality. According to the forecasts prepared by the Indian Council of Leather Exports, by the year 2003, nearly 30 percent of the total demand for leather in India would have to be met through imports.

Types of Finished Leathers

Buffalo hides are best suited for the manufacture of sole leather because of their thickness. But the demand for sole leather is very limited. Today, because of the availability of splitting machines, the thicker hides can be split into two or more layers. In addition, technology to finish the spilt leather (inferior in quality) into high grade finished, softy uppers (Nubuck, oil pull up etc.) and garment leathers are produced. The buff calf finished leather are useful for manufacturing top quality women footwear. Calf skin based leathers and leather products are in great demand in developed countries, as they hardly get any calf skins because of regular fattening/farming, they mostly produce hides.

Hides and skins are converted into unfinished leathers, finished leathers and then utilised for manufacturing products like footwear, leather goods and garments. About 30-35% of the total buffalo hides and skins produced in the country are utilised for manufacturing footwear and other products meant for domestic market.

Leather Industry

The leather industry is spread in different segments namely tanning and finishing, footwear and footwear components, leather garments, leather goods including saddlery and harness, etc. The major production centres for leather and leather products are located in Chennai, Ambur, Ranipet, Vassiyambadi, Trichi, Dindigul in Tamil Nadu, Kolkata in West Bengal, Kanpur in Uttar Pradesh, Jallandhar in Punjab, Bangalore in Karnataka, Delhi, and Hyderabad in Andhra Pradesh. The leather industry is concentrated in small and medium sector. Some mechanized tanning footwear units operate on large scale, which are mainly for export market. The domestic market for leather products in India is steadily growing. Though presently, the market for leather footwear and leather products is extremely price sensitive, there is going to be a revolution in footwear consumption pattern within the country. As per the survey of the Leather Industry, the per capita consumption of footwear in the country is 0.5 pair. With the increase in middle class population, the consumption is likely to increase, the signs of which are clear during the last five years.

At present, India is producing 800 million pairs of leather footwear, 200 million pairs of leather shoe uppers, 20 million pieces of leather garments and a hundred million pieces of leather goods. Much of the credit for the expansion of leather industry goes to the Central Leather Research Institute at Chennai which has played a useful role in strengthening this industry. It may be mentioned here that in 1995, the Government of India announced the appointment of Leather Technology Mission with an outlay of $ 6.3 million for a period of four years to provide guidance in various fields, such as, improvement in the quality of raw hides and skins and cleaner production with reduced wastage. Since the quality of leather goods produced in our country is of the international class, the domestic market has also expanded. The industry has expanded its export without starving the domestic market. The country has now skilled, semiskilled and unskilled workmen whose relentless efforts are helping to win over new pastures.

The growth of the leather products industry was very encouraging in the last two years, namely, 1999-2000 and 2000-01. In both these years, production of leather goods recorded a double-digit rate of growth. Again, in the decade ending in 2000-01, the average rate of growth in production was more than six percent a year. Tanneries are the backbone of the leather sector. There are about 2500 tanneries, which are concentrated mainly in Tamil Nadu (60 per cent), Kolkata in West Bengal (15 per cent), Agra and Kanpur in Uttar Pradesh (12 per cent), and Jallandher in Punjab (7 per cent), producing more than 1.8 billion square feet of leather a year. More than 90 per cent of these are in the small-scale sector, but bulk of the production (more than 65 per cent) takes place in modern, medium and large-scale tanneries. Of course, the tanners urgently require modernization. The central government has launched a tannery modernization scheme.

Against the global annual import of $70 billion of leather and leather products, India's export of $1.93 billion in 2001-02 was only 2.76 per cent. The industry has drawn up plans to raise the share at least 7 per cent by the turn of the decade. The total shoe market in India in 2001 was estimated at Rs. 50 billion (organized and unorganized). Of this, the organized premium segment was approximately Rs. 12 billion,. The government has proposed to set up two integrated tannery projects on a pilot basis to attract foreign investment. It also intends to expand the scope of the Tannery Modernization Scheme to encourage industries to come forward and modernize the tanning industry in India. The industry is also paying attention to environment management. The industry has 17 common effluent treatment plants and over 180 individual effluent treatment plants set up all over the country. The tanning industry is able to treat more than 75 per cent of all effluent generated by it. Kolkata Leather Complex, when completed, would take care of more than 90 percent of all wastes generated by the industry.

The Tenth Plan allocation for leather sector had been hiked to Rs. 4 billion from just Rs. 120 million in the Ninth Plan. The enhanced allocation is expected to bring in at least Rs. 22 billion of investments into the sector by private players and create jobs for 300,000 hands. Apart from the anti-leather campaign of the People for Ethical Treatment of Animals (PETA), the environmental issues are proving to be an Achilles' heel to the exporters. The leather industry is caught between animal right activists and pollution watchdogs. Labour standards and work environment are receiving due

> Tamil Nadu accounts for 70 percent of the total installed capacity of 225 million pieces of hides and skins in the country. The state contributes about 45 percent to India's export of leather and leather related products such as shoe uppers, shoes, and garments. It is eyeing a share of nearly Rs. 50 billion in the target of $ 3.7 by 2005.

attention. Some of the importing countries, especially consumer organizations and green groups, are demanding environmental compliance by their suppliers.

Chrome tanning, the chemical procedure used to treat raw hides and skins in the manufacture of leather goods, caused enormous environmental pollution as the tannery effluents are discharged mostly untreated into local water bodies and even farmlands. In 2002, the Supreme Court ordered tanneries in Kolkata to close down immediately. It ordered the state government to evict those found violating the order. Earlier, in 1996 the apex court ordered the closure of tanning units in the city and their relocation to a modern leather complex with effluents treatment facilities. However, not a single unit had moved out. There are allegations of collusion between tannery owners and politicians.

As India enjoys a comparative advantage, the Tenth Plan (2002-07) aims at providing all the incentives and infrastructural facilities for accelerated development of the leather sector. The government has already de-reserved many leather products from the purview of the small-scale sector. This is expected to pave way for setting up of modern large production units to compete globally with economies of scale. In the coming years, there is bound to be a greater inflow of foreign direct investment and opportunities for joint ventures.

Annexure I

(In 000 tonnes)

Table 4AI.1: Milk Production Region and State-Wise

Region State/U.T	1973-74	1979-80	1980-81	1981-82	1982-83	1983-84	1984-85	1985-86	1986-87	1987-88	1988-89
NORTH											
Haryana	1344	1950	2187	2275	2262	2427	2441	2556	2624	2558	2785
Himachal Pradesh	64	304	315	339	358	376	404	431	459	478	500
Jammu & Kashmir	180	235	250	260	270	285	342	379	406	400	450
Punjab	2122	3059	3221	3494	3599	3758	3876	4093	4355	4365	4626
Chandigarh	15	N.E.	18.6	19.2	19	20	21	23	25	30	28
Delhi	136	N.E.	157	163	168	175	179	221	255	219	223
Sub-Total	3861	5548	6148.6	6550.2	6676	7041	7263	7703	8124	8050	8612
SOUTH											
Andhra Pradesh	1850	1802	2010	2127	2303	2375	2668	2783	2783	2807	2814
Karnataka	909	1375	1425	1590	1655	1758	1839	2013	2070	2189	2248
Kerala	414	854	908	982	1078	1150	1220	1282	1334	1426	1513
Tamil Nadu	1036	1860	1738	1886	1788	2562	2846	3118	3295	3109	3238
Lakshadweep	N.E.	N.E.	0.24	0.35	0.46	0.7	0.7	1	1	1	1
Pondicherry	13	N.E.	8.3	14.55	14.5	14.5	14.5	18	23	26	26
Sub-Total	4222	5891	6089.54	6599.9	6838.96	7860.2	8588	9215	9506	9558	9840
CENTRAL											
Madhya Pradesh	1679	2210	2282	2390	2510	2640	2784	2891	3530	4272	4382
Uttar Pradesh	4904	5665	5728	6461	6666	7004	7723	8015	8417	8595	8824
Sub-Total	6583	7875	8010	8851	9176	9644	10507	10906	11947	12867	13206

Table 4AI.1: Milk Production Region and State-Wise (Contd.)

(In 000 tonnes)

Region State/U.T	1973-74	1979-80	1980-81	1981-82	1982-83	1983-84	1984-85	1985-86	1986-87	1987-88	1988-89
WEST											
Maharashtra	1013	1506	1756	1909	2009	2228	2358	2466	2459	2657	2800
Gujarat	1746	2115	2153	2228	2529	3093	3239	3270	3246	2997	3041
Rajasthan	2394	3085	3250	3300	3400	3544	3884	4146	4168	3911	4036
Dadra & N. Haveli	1	N.E.	1	1	1	2	2	2	2	2	3
Goa, Daman & Diu	N.E.	N.E.	18.5	19	20	25	27	27	25	25	27
Sub-Total	5154	6706	7178.5	7457	7959	8891.8	9510	9911	9900	9592	9907
EAST											
Bihar	1744	1860	1942	2035	2133	2235	2330	2702	2814	2648	2826
Orissa	200	238	310	316	322	344	386	394	401	423	434
West Bengal	955	1231	1282	1782	2013	2107	2210	2400	2597	2664	2704
Andaman & Nicobar	2	N.E.	9.47	11.23	10.35	12	13	17	17	18	18
Sub-Total	2901	3329	3543.47	4144.23	4478.35	4698	4939	5513	5829	5753	5982
NORTH-EAST											
Assam	318	460	464	469	482	498	512	526	539	610	603
Arunachal Pradesh	20	30	31	32	33	34	35	36	37	37	38
Manipur	51	58	60	62	63	64	66	69	73	77	80
Meghalaya	42	54	56	58	60	40	44	46	47	41	47
Nagaland	2	3.25	3.05	3.04	4	4	4	5	5	30	33
Sikkim	—	14.2	17	18	19	19.6	20.2	22	22	22	25
Tripura	13	15.5	16.5	17.5	18	19	22	23	25	26	27
Mizoram	1	N.E.	2.7	2.85	2.95	4.28	5.5	7	7	8	8
Sub-Total	447	634.95	650.25	662.39	681.95	682.88	708.7	733	755	851	861
All-India	23168	29984	31619.36	34264.72	35810.3	38817.88	41516	43981	46061	46671	48408

Table 4AI.1: Milk Production Region and State-Wise (Contd.)

(In 000 tonnes)

Region State/U.T	1989-90	1990-91	1991-92	1992-93	1993-94	1994-95	1995-96	1996-97	1997-98	1998-99
NORTH										
Haryana	3151	3200	3565	3715	3850	4062	4055	4204	4373	4527
Himachal Pradesh	529	573	597	610	654	663	676	698	714	724
Jammu & Kashmir	487	557	581	937	780	641	869	992	1167	1232
Punjab	4972	5142	5395	5583	5970	6215	6424	6755	7165	7394
Chandigarh	31	33	34	37	38	39	43	42	43	43
Delhi	224	244	230	235	251	257	261	264	267	290
Sub Total	9394	9749	10402	11117	11543	11877	12328	12955	13729	14210
SOUTH										
Andhra Pradesh	3030	3010	3650	3103	3766	4221	4261	4471	4473	4842
Karnataka	2291	2389	2461	2590	2736	3003	3190	3460	3970	4231
Kerala	1600	1690	1780	1889	2001	2118	2192	2258	2343	2420
Tamil Nadu	3410	3375	3357	3468	3524	3695	3791	3976	4061	4273
Lakshadweep	1	1	1	1	1	1	1	1	1	2
Pondicherry	27	27	27	27	32	33	33	38	36	36
Sub-Total	10359	10492	11276	11078	12060	13071	13468	14204	14884	15804
CENTRAL										
Madhya Pradesh	4529	4700	4806	4879	4975	5047	5125	5224	5377	5442
Uttar Pradesh	9145	9692	10200	10649	10991	11321	11877	12387	12934	13618
Sub-Total	13674	14392	15006	15528	15966	16368	17002	17611	18311	19060
WEST										
Maharashtra	3266	3735	3955	4102	4250	4812	4991	5127	5193	5609
Gujarat	3351	3532	3386	3795	3935	4459	4608	4831	4913	5059

Table 4A1.1: Milk Production Region and State-Wise (Contd.)

(*In 000 tonnes*)

Region State/U.T	1989-90	1990-91	1991-92	1992-93	1993-94	1994-95	1995-96	1996-97	1997-98	1998-99
Rajasthan	1217	4339	4474	4586	4958	5103	5449	5874	6487	6923
Dadra & N. Haveli	3	3	8	10	7	1	1	1	1	1
Goa, Daman & Diu	25	25	25	31	34	44	40	41	42	49
Sub-Total	10862	11634	11843	12524	13184	14419	15089	15874	16636	17641
EAST										
Bihar	3000	3123	3240	3195	3227	3250	3321	3410	3420	3440
Orissa	455	470	505	542	565	584	648	687	672	733
West Bengal	2805	2912	3019	3023	3095	3250	3340	3376	3415	3441
Andaman & Nicobar	18	19	23	24	25	25	21	21	22	22
Sub-Total	6278	6524	6787	6784	6912	7109	7330	7494	7529	7636
NORTH-EAST										
Assam	617	653	704	658	676	698	699	714	719	725
Arunachal Pradesh	40	41	41	21	21	22	42	44	43	45
Manipur	82	82	95	83	84	64	57	61	62	65
Meghalaya	47	48	50	52	53	54	57	58	59	61
Nagaland	32	43	44	44	45	43	44	46	46	48
Sikkim	27	28	29	30	30	32	33	34	35	35
Tripura	27	29	32	34	35	38	39	44	57	76
Mizoram	9	8	10	9	9	9	9	9	17	20
Sub-Total	881	932	1005	931	952	960	980	1010	1038	1075
All-India	51448	53723	56319	57962	60607	63804	66197	69148	72127	75424

Source: Government of India, Ministry of Agriculture, Department of Animal Husbandry and Dairying, New Delhi. BasicAnimalHusbandryStatistics,1999and2002

Annexure II

Table 4AII.1: Egg Production Region and State-Wise

(In Million)

Region/State/U.T	1968-69	1973-74	1974-75	1978-79	1979-80	1980-81	1981-82	1982-83	1983-84	1984-85	1985-86	1986-87
NORTH												
Haryana	75	140	160	245	162	182	189	195	210	311	342	343
Himachal Pradesh	6	13	14	16	21	23	25	25	29	34	38	41
Jammu & Kashmir	116	165	176	200	220	200	200	230	229	215	228	243
Punjab	218	321	355	495	474	517	597	642	771	825	985	1247
Chandigarh	—	9	10	14	19	33	36	33	30	30	30	32
Delhi	47	37	41	60	53	61	62	67	68	61	63	64
Sub-Total	462	685	756	756	949	1016	1109	1192	1337	1476	1686	1970
SOUTH												
Andhra Pradesh	548	650	750	1200	1713	1741	2036	2168	2370	3072	3136	3145
Karnataka	700	1500	1800	3000	735	770	826	872	928	987	1072	1128
Kerala	658	800	880	1200	966	962	1018	1172	1260	1312	1360	1397
Tamil Nadu	650	500	625	630	853	835	917	898	996	1064	2067	2076
Pondicherry	—	0.1	0.12	0.2	1	1	1	1	1	1	2	2
Lakshadweep	—	2	3	10	4	4	5	4	5	8	11	9
Sub-Total	2556	3452	4058	6040	4272	4313	4803	5115	5560	6444	7648	7757
CENTRAL												
Madhya Pradesh	220	250	280	400	400	504	533	564	604	700	740	780
Uttar Pradesh	N.A.	241	275	372	318	326	328	329	341	374	375	386
Sub-Total	220	491	555	772	718	830	861	893	945	1074	1115	1166

Table 4AII.1: Egg Production Region and State-Wise (Contd.)

(In Million)

Region/State/U.T	1968-69	1973-74	1974-75	1978-79	1979-80	1980-81	1981-82	1982-83	1983-84	1984-85	1985-86	1986-87
WEST
Gujarat	88	134	150	215	201	191	205	211	237	261	251	253
Maharashtra	N.A.	720	755	900	1026	1153	1237	1286	1350	1428	1509	1589
Rajasthan	65	500	625	630	126	130	138	144	151	160	197	209
Dadra & N. Haveli	—	1.2	1.4	2.2	2	2	2	2	3	3	3	3
Goa, Daman & Diu	—	9	10	15	N.E.	67	69	71	73	76	78	78
Sub-Total	153	1364	1541	1762	1355	1543	1651	1714	1814	1928	2038	2132
EAST
Bihar	296	477	540	780	700	752	807	867	931	1000	1100	1175
Orissa	194	292	320	436	279	360	348	320	313	279	324	324
West Bengal	380	564	585	833	790	821	848	875	1381	1518	1656	2199
Andaman & Nikobar	—	3	4	6	13	13	18	23	24	23	23	23
Sub-Total	870	1336	1449	2055	1782	1946	2021	2085	2649	2820	3103	3721
NORTH EAST
Arunachal Pradesh	548	650	750	1200	24	23	23	24	24	25	26	27
Assam	115	234	250	300	271	280	291	298	315	328	347	351
Manipur	10	15	17	26	30	27	30	36	37	39	42	46
Meghalaya	13	19	21	28	30	32	34	40	51	55	58	60
Mizoram	—	4	5	7	10	10	11	12	13	14	14	19
Nagaland	6	9	10	13	14	14	15	16	17	18	19	20
Tripura	10	16	19	30	21	22	24	25	26	28	27	31
Sikkim					4	3	3	4	4	4	5	10
Sub-Total		947	1072	1604	404	411	431	455	487	949	538	564
All-India	4261	8275.3	9431.52	12989.4	9480	10059	10876	11454	12792	14691	16128	17310

(In million)

Table 4AII.1: Egg Production Region and State-Wise

Region/State/U.T	1987-88	1988-89	1989-90	1990-91	1991-92	1992-93	1993-94	1994-95	1995-96	1996-97	1997-98
NORTH											
Haryana	263	299	333	320	507	517	533	468	494	633	636.9
Himachal Pradesh	43	48	49	53	58	69	71	70	71	71	75
Jammu & Kashmir	201	258	267	283	294	288	348	360	381	396	412
Punjab	1328	1452	1619	1820	1900	2165	2330	2438	2510	2733	2910.3
Chandigarh	37	38	38	36	37	38	35	33	34	31	20
Delhi	67	53	53	53	58	60	64	65	66	67	68
Sub-Total	1939	2148	2359	2565	2854	3137	3381	3434	3556	3931	4121
SOUTH											
Andhra Pradesh	3210	3427	3710	3829	3700	3962	4475	5435	6001	5659	5751
Karnataka	1180	1230	1278	1285	1336	1359	1416	1469	1557	1630	1812
Kerala	1440	1468	1501	1540	1600	1774	1844	1916	1996	2069	2024
Tamil Nadu	2197	2287	2461	2551	3704	2844	2919	3050	3049	3042	3050
Pondichery	2	2	3	3	3	10	9	10	8	7	8
Lakshadweep	10	10	10	10	13	4	4	4	5	5	5
Sub-Total	8039	8424	8963	9218	10356	9953	10667	11884	12616	12412	12650
CENTRAL											
Madhya Pradesh	606	860	1006	1015	1040	1068	1098	1145	1195	1250	1347
Uttar Pradesh	398	411	494	519	536	566	602	626	671	699	722
Sub-Total	1004	1271	1500	1534	1576	1634	1700	1771	1866	1949	2069
WEST											
Gujarat	253	322	386	412	340	473	505	468	494	501	488
Maharashtra	1716	1799	1957	2098	2145	2290	2338	2501	2602	2687	2766

(In million)

Table 4AII.1: Egg Production Region and State-Wise *(Contd.)*

Region/State/U.T	1987-88	1988-89	1989-90	1990-91	1991-92	1992-93	1993-94	1994-95	1995-96	1996-97	1997-98
Rajasthan	214	226	230	280	317	349	395	417	450	475	500
Dadra & N. Haveli	4	4	5	5	6	7	4	6	4	5	3
Goa, Daman & Diu	87	92	92	92	92	99	101	102	104	110	111
Sub-Total	2274	2443	2670	2887	2900	3218	3343	3494	3654	3778	3868
EAST											
Bihar	1311	1280	1328	1335	1335	1380	1390	1398	1400	1410	1420
Orissa	343	405	418	420	480	526	568	560	586	599	825
West Bengal	2155	2197	2220	2219	2327	2330	2364	2500	2568	2603	2634
Andaman & Nikobar	27	31	33	39	43	45	51	51	52	52	41
Sub-Total	3836	3913	3999	4013	4185	4281	4373	4509	4606	4664	4920
NORTH EAST											
Arunachal Pradesh	28	29	30	31	31	22	23	22	33	33	34
Assam	438	440	461	500	532	434	449	460	604	487	499
Manipur	56	62	63	92	81	67	67	108	59	60	61
Meghalaya	62	63	64	66	67	70	72	75	77	79	81
Mizoram	18	18	19	2	2	13	18	19	20	20	3
Nagaland	29	35	32	40	43	39	43	42	39	45	46
Tripura	31	32	32	34	37	37	40	42	44	53	58
Sikkim	10	12	12	13	13	14	14	15	16	17	17
Sub-Total	672	691	713	778	806	696	726	783	892	794	799
All-India	17764	18890	20204	20995	22677	22919	24190	25875	27190	27528	28427

N.E.: Not Estimated

Source: Report of the Technical Committee of Direction for Improvements of Animal Husbandry and Dairying Statistics: Animal Husbandry Statistics 1997 and Agriculture Statistics at a Glance, 1999-2000. .

5

Dairy Industry in India

India's dairy industry generates an annual business worth Rs. 550 billion ($15.7 billion) and was expected to touch Rs. 880 billion ($25 billion) by the turn of the century. India's highly skilled manpower pool is another comparative advantage. The country has built up a strong base for education, research, extension and training in dairy and veterinary science and manpower resources available here are much cheaper than other countries. Since dairying in India is closely linked with agriculture, most milk production is based on utilisation of agricultural byproducts and crop residues. Because of this, the cost of milk production in India is much lower than many developed countries. Dairy infrastructure now comprises 23 state federations, 170 district unions and around 90,000 village cooperatives societies, through which the rural milk production and procurement system have been effectively linked to urban markets and consumption centres. Although India enjoyed several competitive advantages compared to other countries, it has failed to make a proper dent in the export market. The country has been adopting easier path by going in for occasional milk exports. Whenever we have seasonal surpluses resulting out of extra production, instead of maintaining a buffer stock, we have resorted to export. Similarly, advocating the prioritizing of branded product exports instead of occasional bulk exports, the government could provide all those who wanted to export branded products with incentive.

Other value-added products such as Indian sweetmeat and desserts are worth mentioning. With the Indian population migrating to various developing and developed countries, a good potential for export of such products is emerging and it should be fully exploited. The investment and achievements in research and modernising the Indian dairy industry have had a major impact on milk production. Presently, a large number of processing and allied facilities are available in India. There are 300 liquid milk plants, besides over 100 milk product manufacturing plants and more than 200 projects are in the pipeline. India is in advantageous position in terms of handling large quantity of milk and milk products, as some of the units have the latest technology. A serious impediment is the low milk productivity per animal. India's milk yield is the lowest compared to the developed countries. It is unfortunate that though India is the second largest milk producer, the density of milk production is low.

With the launching of the Operation Flood and the livestock development programmes, milk production in India got a remarkable boost, especially since the mid-seventies. With the rapid increase in its production India's share in world milk output had increased from about 9 percent in 1986 to almost 14 percent in 1999 (Table 5.1). Major milk supply in India comes

Table 5.1: *World Milk Production and India's share: 1985 – 2003*

(Million tonnes)

Year	Cow	Buffalo	Goat	Sheep	Total	Share of India
1985	462.2	34.2	7.6	0.0	504.0	44.0
	(91.7)	(6.8)	(1.5)	(0.0)	(100.0)	(8.7)
1986	463.5	36.0	7.9	0.0	507.4	46.1
	(91.3)	(7.1)	(1.6)	(0.0)	(100.0)	(9.1)
1987	460.6	38.4	8.2	0.0	507.2	46.7
	(90.8)	(7.6)	(1.6)	(0.0)	(100.0)	(9.2)
1988	466.2	39.0	8.5	8.6	522.3	48.4
	(89.3)	(7.5)	(1.6)	(1.6)	(100.0)	(9.3)
1989	470.6	40.1	9.5	8.9	529.1	51.4
	(88.9)	(7.6)	(1.8)	(1.7)	(100.0)	(9.7)
1990	482.4	41.4	9.9	8.2	541.9	5.0
	(89.0)	(7.7)	(1.8)	(1.5)	(100.0)	(10.1)
1991	472.8	43.9	9.8	8.0	534.5	58.4
	(88.5)	(8.2)	(1.8)	(1.5)	(100.0)	(10.9)
1992	462.8	45.8	10.2	7.9	526.7	62.6
	(87.9)	(8.7)	(1.9)	(1.5)	(100.0)	(11.9)
1993	463.6	46.0	9.9	7.7	527.2	61.0
	(87.9)	(8.7)	(1.9)	(1.5)	(100.0)	(11.6)
1994	464.4	48.3	9.9	7.9	530.5	63.0
	(87.5)	(9.1)	(1.9)	(1.5)	(10.0)	(11.9)
1995	464.4	48.3	9.9	7.9	530.5	66.0
	(87.5)	(9.1)	(1.9)	(1.5)	(100.0)	(12.4)
1996	467.0	53.6	10.4	8.1	539.1	69.5
	(86.6)	(9.9)	(1.9)	(1.5)	(100.0)	(12.9)
1997	466.4	59.7	12.2	8.1	546.4	71.1
	(85.4)	(10.9)	(2.2)	(1.5)	(100.0)	(13.0)
1998	478.1	58.1	12.2	7.9	556.3	74.5
	(85.9)	(10.5)	(2.2)	(1.4)	(100.0)	(13.4)
1999	480.7	60.3	12.1	8.0	561.1	78.2
	(85.7)	(10.7)	(2.2)	(1.4)	(100.0)	(13.9)
2000	490.8	67.6	11.6	8.0	579.2	81.0
	(84.7)	(11.7)	(2.0)	(1.4)	(100.0)	(13.9)
2001	495.6	68.7	11.7	8.1	585.4	82.0
	(84.7)	(11.7)	(2.2)	(1.4)	(100.0)	(14.0)
2002	506.5	70.5	11.8	8.0	598.0	84.0
	(84.7)	(11.8)	(2.1)	(1.4)	(100.0)	(14.1)
2003	504.7	72.6	11.8	7.9	601.0	87.0
	(84.4)	(12.1)	(2.1)	(1.4)	(100.0)	(14.5)

Note: Figures in brackets show percentage share of India

Source: FAO Production Year Book: various issues and FAOSTAT online

from buffalo and cows. However, the role of buffalo as a major milk producing species is well recognized in the country – percentage of cattle yielding more than 1.5 kg. milk per day is less than 2 percent, whereas the percentage of such buffaloes is over 40 percent. With 53 percent of the world buffalo population, India produces 63 percent of the world buffalo milk. By contrast, 15 percent of the world cattle population in India yields about 8 percent of total milk output (Tables 5.2A and 5.2B).

Table 5.2A: Production of Cow and Buffalo Milk by Major Producing Countries of the World: 1992-1999

('000 Tonnes)

Country	Cow milk production					Percentage share to world total				
	1992	1995	1996	1997	1998	1992	1995	1996	1997	1998
1. Canada	7633	7920	7890	8100	8200	1.6	1.7	1.7	1.7	1.7
2. Mexico	7204	7628	7822	8091	8574	1.6	1.6	1.6	1.7	1.8
3. Germany	27991	28621	28729	24917	24741	6.0	6.1	6.2	5.3	5.2
4. Italy	10898	11259	10746	11319	11236	2.4	2.4	2.3	2.4	2.3
5. Netherlands	10909	10900	11188	10922	11200	2.4	2.3	2.4	2.3	2.3
6. Brazil	15784	16985	18300	20600	21630	3.4	3.6	3.9	4.4	4.6
7. U.K.	14701	14844	14808	14848	14635	3.2	3.2	3.2	3.2	3.1
8. Poland	13153	11642	11696	12123	12596	2.8	2.5	2.5	2.6	2.6
9. India	29400	32000	33500	29576	35000	6.4	6.9	7.2	6.4	7.4
10. USA	68440	70527	70003	70801	71414	14.8	15.1	15.0	15.2	14.9
11. USSR*	47166	39098	35445	33835	32955	10.2	8.4	7.6	7.3	6.9
12. France	25738	25438	25065	24917	24741	5.6	5.5	5.4	5.4	5.1
13. Other countries	183763	189316	191818	196378	201159	39.7	40.6	41.1	42.1	42.1
14. World	462780	466171	467010	466427	478081	100.0	100.0	100.0	100.0	100.0

Country	Buffalo milk production					Percentage share to world total				
	1992	1995	1996	1997	1998	1992	1995	1996	1997	1998
1. Egypt	1421	1358	1365	1820	2022	3.1	2.7	2.5	3.0	3.5
2. China	2000	2200	2200	2450	2540	4.4	4.3	4.1	4.1	4.4
3. Pakistan	11884	13984	14800	15587	16456	25.9	27.5	27.6	26.1	28.3
4. India	29250	32020	33930	38392	35850	63.8	62.2	62.3	64.2	61.7
5. Other countries	1280	1272	1302	1478	1260	2.8	2.4	2.4	2.5	2.2
6. World	45835	50834	53597	59727	58128	100.0	100.0	100.0	100.0	100.0

Data from 1997 onwards relate to Russian Federation

Table 5.2B: Production of Cow and Buffalo Milk by Major Producing Countries: 1999-2003

Country	Cow milk production ('000 tonnes)					Percentage share to world total (%)				
	1999	2000	2001	2002	2003	1999	2000	2001	2002	2003
1. Canada	8,164	8,090	8,106	7,964	7,880	1.7	1.6	1.6	1.6	1.6
2. Mexico	8,877	9,311	9,472	9,658	9,871	1.7	1.6	1.6	1.6	1.6
3. Germany	28,334	28,331	28,191	28,012	28,012	5.9	5.8	5.7	5.5	5.5
4. Italy	11,895	12,309	11.275	11,335	11,000	2.5	2.5	2.3	2.2	2.2
5. Netherlands	11,174	11,155	11,291	10,842	10,842	2.3	2.3	2.3	2.1	2.1
6. Brazil	19,661	20,379	21,145	22,635	23,315	4.1	4.2	4.3	4.5	5.5
7. UK	15,014	14,488	14,709	14,899	15,045	3.1	3.0	3.0	2.9	2.2
8. Poland	12,284	11,889	11,884	11,872	11,845	2.5	2.4	2.4	2.3	2.3
9. India	32,800	34,000	34,400	35,300	36,500	6.8	6.9	6.9	7.0	7.2
10. USA	73,804	76,023	74,980	77,248	78,155	15.3	15.5	15.1	15.3	15.4
11. Russia Federation	32,001	32,000	32,600	33,100	32,800	6.6	6.5	6.6	6.5	6.5
12. France	24,892	24,998	24,903	25,197	24,800	5.2	5.1	5.0	5.0	4.9
13. Other countries	204,187	207,785	212,607	218,705	217,311	42.3	42.3	42.9	43.2	42.8
14. World	483,087	490,758	495,563	506,467	507,385	100.0	100.0	100.0	100.0	100.0

Country	Buffalo milk production ('000 tonnes)					Percentage share in world total (%)				
	1999	2000	2001	2002	2003	1999	2000	2001	2002	2003
1. Egypt	2,018	2,030	2,077	2,077	2,077	3.1	3.0	3.0	2.9	2.9
2. China	2,600	2,650	2,650	2,650	2,650	4.0	3.9	3.9	3.8	3.6
3. Pakistan	16,391	16,910	17,454	18,222	18,520	25.0	25.0	26.7	27.8	28.3
4. India	43,000	44,600	45,100	46,200	47,850	65.7	68.1	68.9	70.6	73.1
5. Other countries	1,443	1,454	1,483	1,319	1,518	2.2	2.2	2.3	2.0	2.3
6. World	65,452	67,644	68,737	70,468	72,615	100.0	100.0	100.0	100.0	100.0

Source: FAO Production Year Books – Various issues & FAOSTAT online information

DAIRY DEVELOPMENT

Growth Pattern

Dairying has become an important secondary source of income for millions of rural families and has assumed the most important role in providing employment and income. The per capita availability of milk has also increased to a level of about 221 g. per day, but is still very low as compared to developed nations or the world average of 285 g per day. Government of

India is making efforts to increase the productivity of milch animals and thus increase the per capita availability of milk. The efforts of the Department in the dairy sector are concentrated on promotion of dairy activities in non-operation flood areas with emphasis on building up cooperative infrastructure, revitalization of sick dairy cooperative federations and creation of infrastructure in the States for testing the quality of milk and milk products. Besides this, the National Dairy Development Board (NDDB) continues its activities for the overall development of Dairy Sector in Operation Flood areas.

India will create a new world record by crossing the 90 million tonnes mark in milk production by year 2005. The country which is already the world's largest milk producer with an output of 88 million tonnes, aims to increase its production by 2 million tonnes. In 2004, it produced 37.5 million tonnes cow milk and 50.5 million tonnes buffalo milk. This is expected to rise to 38.5 million tonnes and 53.5 million tonnes respectively. During 2004, the per capita milk consumption has risen to 227 gm/day, which is still below the WHO-recommended level of 283 gm/day.

National Dairy Development Board (NDDB), an institution of National importance was set up by the Government of India to promote, plan and organize programmes for development of dairy and other agriculture based and allied industries along cooperative lines on an intensive and nationwide basis. Operation Flood (OF), an integrated dairy development programme completed its third phase on April 30, 1996. The main thrust of the programme was to consolidate the gains already achieved, and to strengthen the dairy cooperative structure for sustainable development of the dairy industry in India. After the completion of Phase 3 of Operation Flood, a Programme implementation Agreement (PIA) was signed between the EEC and the NDDB to strengthen cooperatives at the grassroot level. The Agreement was endorsed by the Government of India on August 21, 1997. Consequently, measures were initiated from September 1997 and are continuing presently.

Perspective Plan, 2010

The National Diary Development Board (NDDB) has evolved a Perspective Plan 2010 to strengthen the country's cooperative dairy sector. During the year, NDDB continued to work in close partnership with the 126 identified district unions to help achieve their Perspective Plan goals. As on December 2002, under Phase-1, 79 district unions had submitted their Perspective Plans to NDDB with an outlay of Rs. 96000 million. NDDB has approved the Plans of 68 district unions with an investment outlay of Rs. 833 crores. Perspective Plans of 11 district unions are being appraised and Plans for the remaining 47 unions are being initiated. Majority of the Plans have taken off and NDDB has already released Rs. 760 million to these unions for activities such as productivity enhancement, quality assurance, cooperative business including milk marketing and building a national information network. It is expected that over Rs. 200 crores will stand disbursed under the Plans by the close of the financial year 2002-03.

Through institution building and women dairy cooperative leadership programmes organized during the year, NDDB supported dairy cooperative to become self reliant enterprises. The Cooperative Institution Building Programme seeks to strengthen dairy cooperatives on aspects like governance, management, economic viability and productivity. This is achieved through a multi-pronged initiative involving awareness building, education, extension and demonstration. The programme, being implemented in 48 district unions across the country, has enabled the management committees of village dairy cooperative societies (DCS) evolve business plans of their cooperatives.

NDDB's Business Orientation Programmes sensitizes board of directors of district unions about the need for a professional approach in conducting the business of the unions and helps evolve long term goals. So far, 60 board of directors have participated in these programmes. NDDB also organized eight training programmes for district union personnel to enable them to facilitate village level Institution Building programmes. In all, 135 district union personnel including 30 women participated. NDDB has also prepared audio visual aids and training manuals for use by union personnel. The Women Dairy Cooperative Leadership Programme (WDCLP) implemented in 50 district unions across the country, has greatly contributed in increasing women dairy farmer's participation in dairy cooperatives. The encouraging

> **WOMEN THRIFT STRENG-THENING THE COOPERATIVES COOPERATIVE PROJECT, SHAJAPUR (M.P.)**
>
> **Project started at Shajapur in 1999-2000 to finance dairying and to develop leadership skills among women.**
>
> 56 Women Thrift Cooperatives (WTC) have been recognized.
>
> More than 3000 women members.
>
> Total savings of these WTCs is Rs. 11.30 lakhs.
>
> Money saved is being provided to women are members as loan for productive purposes

response to the formation of thrift groups in district unions covered under WDCLP has encouraged NDDB to undertake women's thrift cooperative projects in Shajapur (Madhya Pradesh) and Tirupati (Andhra Pradesh). By the end of November 2002, 114 women thrift cooperatives with a membership of 8742 were organized.

Quality of Milk

Seventy per cent of the milk produced in the country has come into close watch in the wake of an udder disease prevalent among cattle. Mastitis, an intra mammary infection, spreads due to unhygienic conditions at cattlesheds. The disease among cattle is hampering the milk production in the country – an annual loss of over Rs. 6,000 crore due to reduced milk production, treatment cost, discarded milk and animal death. Though India is the largest milk producer in the world (86 million tonnes annually), only 15 percent of the milk is processed – which is safe to drink. Barring some Government owned and private firm dairies which together hold 30 percent of the share in the milk market, the rest of the 70 percent of the milk comes from the ordinary milkmen. It is this milk that is considered unsafe. The milk of animal suffering from mastitis should not enter the milk supply chain and be discarded immediately. As soon as an animal is infected with mastitis, it should be isolated. The infected milk can lead to tuberculosis, asthma, allergies and diarrhoea among human beings. Experts advise that only processed milk should be boiled before consuming. A few experts say that even after the milk is boiled several harmful substances like deformed proteins, deformed minerals and fats still remain in it.

Dabur Ayurved Limited was the first to come out with a diagnostic kit for identifying mastitis and its treatment at early stages. Its chairman said, "25 to 50 percent of the cow population may at any point of time suffer from clinical or sub clinical mastitis." It is this time that a paste should be plastered around the udder and the milk from the animal should not be used for at least five days. Though the Bureau of Indian Standard has laid down certain quality norms like total bacterial count and finding percentage of fat in milk, these measures are not mandatory.

The international dairy industry is passing through a critical phase. While farmers in the USA have recently won a legal battle, resulting in the continuance of subsidy to the dairy sector, the overall production of milk in the Commonwealth of Independent States (CIS) has registered a decline since 1990. However, the demand and production of milk are continuously increasing in India. The milk processing industry is, however, facing the challenge of demand constraints and changing consumer behaviour. Unhygienic milk collection practices, inefficient processing techniques and growing concern for environmental aspects regulations have posed a major challenge for the growth of the industry. It is estimated that more than 40 percent capacity of the milk processing plants had remained unutilised, resulting in higher production costs. The future of the Indian dairy industry lay in the organised sector. The industry would have to organise itself keeping in view the global demands. It would require strengthening of linkages among milk producers, animal health system, pricing and quality aspects.

Though the Indian dairy industry enjoyed locational advantage in the international market, it would have made milk products as per the specifications of the major market. The demand for milk products is also witnessing an increase in the South East Asian market. Since India is the lowest cost producer of per litre milk in the world, at 27 cents, compared with the US' 63 cents and Japan's $2.8, it should make efforts to tap the world market. India's dairy sector is expected to triple its production in the next 10 years in view of the expanding potential for export to European and other nations. Like the mineral water industry, the milk processing industry may also witness an exponential growth in the next few years. The advertising budget of the industry had already reached about Rs 15 crore annually against Rs 30 crore of mineral water. There is need for exploration of nontraditional milk channels to boost the domestic demand, such as the supply of flavoured milk to educational institutes, airlines and factories.

Modernisation

In Dairy Processing, emphasis has been given to the development of indigenous dairy products having longer shelf-life. Operation Flood III, like the previous phases, continued to modernise the manufacture of traditional milk products by developing or adapting appropriate technologies. Traditional dairy products have an established market and provide high operating margins, but as most of these are manufactured in the traditional sector, the quality of these products leaves much to be desired.

The development of process technologies and the manufacture of quality dairy products in the organised sector will benefit both milk producers and consumers. With this objective the technology for manufacturing *shrikhand, gulabjamun, peda, lassi, mishti doi, rasagulla, paneer, kalakand, khoa* and flavoured milks developed by the Applied Research and Development Group of the NDDB has been progressively transferred to the cooperative dairies to enable them diversify their marketing efforts. The advances already made in dairy technology will provide the means to explore and improve upon the quality and shelf-life of these products as well as more effective utilisation of raw material. Organised manufacture of *chhana* and *paneer*, for example, will help in utilising the whey produced as a by-product.

Work on improving animal productivity both in cattle and buffaloes has been essentially through application of embryo transfer (ET) technology and tissue culture for the development of the vaccines and biological products related to plant and animal biotechnology. Research facilities for embryo transfer, cloning and sexing of embryos has been strengthened. The programme also continues to support the animal disease diagnostic laboratory at Anand for continued research in the field of emerging animal diseases. Applied research on various aspects of animal productivity, husbandry practices, farm management etc. is being carried out in the two breeding farms — Animal Breeding Centre at Rae Bareli (Uttar Pradesh) and the Buffalo Breeding Centre at Nekarikallu (Andhra Pradesh), set up during the current phase.

Marketing Support

In 2003, NDDB further expanded its national campaign create an umbrella brand identify for associated cooperative milk brands. Campaign, initiated in 2002, has so far been launched in 16 states and include major cooperative brands in 72 district unions. It now covers more than 50% of the liquid milk sales by cooperatives. Growth in sales volume of liquid from cooperatives for April-November 2002 as compared to the same period last year, has shown a 4% growth. The unions/dairies participating cooperative brands required to conform to the quality guidelines worked out by NDDB to use the symbols.

The major highlight of the campaign is the standardized milk products design with the 'milk drop' and the use of colours on milk pouches to distinguish different milk types: blue for toned, green for standardized, orange for full cream, yellow for double toned and purple for skim milk. This enables consumers to identify the different milk types available under cooperative labels. To ensure a better recall for cooperative brands in the market place, the 'milk drop' is not only displayed on milk sachets, retail signs and distribution vehicles, but is also promoted through range of media activities – television commercials, outdoor and print advertisement, advertorials and point-of-purchase merchandise. Such media activities carried during 2002-03 in major cities of the country had been successful in creating a recall for the cooperative brands.

Apart from assisting district unions to prepare, implement and monitor market plans, NDDB also extended financial and technical support to unions during 2003, for retail and cold chain development as well as for undertaking sales promotion activities. NDDB has also been working towards the diversification of unions' product-basket and the 2003 year saw the launch of several new products.

As a part of its endeavour to sensitize consumers to qualify milk and milk products, NDDB has developed a documentary film for distribution to dairy cooperatives for use during their mass consumer contact programmes. With a view to making children understand the benefits of drinking quality milk, NDDB launched a website for children. During the year, NDDB continued to extend supply to a variety of consumer education programmes like dairy visits for consumers/children, milk-testing campaigns etc.,

Recognizing the need for more efficient marketing of cooperative brand milk and milk products in the face of increasing competition, NDDB has taken initiative to directly assist the cooperatives in the marketing of their milk and milk products. NDDB's wholly owned subsidiary company. Fruit and vegetables Company Limited has formed a marketing company. Mother Diary Food Limited which would offer to assist by forming JVS with various state cooperative federation if they so desire.

Milk production, which stagnated during the fifties and sixties, increased significantly during the next three decades. During the nineties the livestock sector as a whole and milk production in particular, registered a higher growth rate as compared to the agricultural sector. While milk production increased by only one percent during 1947 to 1970, its output grew by about 5.5 percent during the eighties and 5 percent in the nineties, compared to 3.2 percent and 2.7 percent respectively for agriculture during the same period.

The role of government in the sustainable growth of a sector such as that of dairy cannot be overemphasized. In India, the government's approach towards dairy has passed through three distinct phases. Though it is difficult to earmark the exact year for distinguishing these periods as a shift in policy action is often staggered over a couple of years. However, this may be roughly demarcated on the basis of plan periods, namely, first phase (Plan I-III), second phase (Plan IV-VII), third phase (since Plan VIII).

The first phase began immediately after independence when dairy produce like many other agricultural commodities was considered as an important item to be supplied to the urban consumers at the lowest possible price. Government monopolized the milk supply and distribution through the Milk Control Board. This has led to a proliferation of middlemen in the milk supply system, and finally, a decline in the share of producers in the consumer's price of milk. As a result of this set of policies, milk production observed a linear trend growth of less than 2 percent during the first two decades of planned development. This rate of growth was too low to match the growth in human population during the period and finally, the per capita availability of milk has declined during the period.

The per capita availability of milk in the country was already low; Government had therefore restored to import of milk powder to protect consumers' interest. Import of milk powders, which was highly subsidized, had further deteriorated the price incentive for domestic milk production in the country; this was apparent with an almost stagnant milk yield during the period. Increase in milk production during the period was primarily because of an increase in the breedable bovine population and the milk production system, which was subsistence in nature, remained so during the period. On account of this milk production in the country was in fact trapped in a vicious cycle of low price-production and yield of milk. This policy orientation continued, till the Third Five Year Plan.

The second phase of dairy development can be distinguished from the earlier plans with a high allocation for Operation Flood (OF) programme in the fourth Five Year Plan. The OF programme aimed at replicating Amul type milk cooperatives, which essentially provided a favourable price to milk producers. (A detailed discussion on OF has been made later.) The OF programme and similar other dairy development programmes to strengthen cooperative networks remained important throughout the planned development. The spread of the cooperative network is apparent with the growth in milk throughout. The role of Government in milk collection and processing was restricted during the period; import of low cost milk powder was also restricted.

As a result of these policies, the growth in milk production had experienced a structural break in its trend during the year 1973-74. The exponential trend in growth was visible during the later period. The per capita availability of milk, which started declining during the first two decades of the plan period, has shown an increasing tendency after the mid-70s. There has been an encouraging trend in the sources of milk production as well. The rate of growth in the breedable bovine population has slowed down after the 80s, suggesting that the increase in milk production is largely contributed to by an increase in the productivity of milch animals. This is further corroborated by an increase in crossbred cattle population, in the total bovine population. The average productivity of cattle, which was almost stagnant during the 1951-71 period increased especially during the 90s.

The third phase of shift in policy environment was more mandatory in a globalizing world. Following the Uruguay Round of Agreements, trade was liberalized; cost efficiency and quality was perceived as important for an economy. Many of the earlier laws and government policies underwent drastic changes in 1991s. As far as the dairy sector is concerned the manufacture of milk products was delicensed, that is, it was removed as a scheduled industry under the Industrial Development Regulation Act of 1951. Recognizing some anomalies in the pattern of investment in dairy processing, the Government of India has notified the Milk and Milk Product Order (MMPO) in June 1992, which reintroduced registration for milk processing units. The MMPO was however perceived as an entry barrier for private sector investments, and in March 2002, the government made some important amendments so that the MMPO would basically regulate food safety, quality, sanitary and hygiene conditions of all registered units. Thus most of the draconian rulings inhibiting private investments in dairy have been withdrawn. The cooperative processing units unlike their corporate counterparts were governed by the registrar state cooperatives; in order to unshackle the cooperatives the Companies (Amendment) Act 2002, were amended to incorporate producer companies based on the principle of cooperation into its coverage.

Most indicators of dairy development have maintained an increasing trend around the third period. The increasing trend in some of the indicators of dairy development such as milk throughout and milk productivity have become robust during the period. This period may be referred to as a phase of qualitative growth.

It is clear from the above discussion that dairy development in the country has graduated into another phase in the 70s; for example, milk production has started growing exponentially, milk availability has also increased significantly, sources of milk production have also undergone expected changes in favour of crossbred cattle. Despite the robust trends in the dairy development of the country, milk productivity is yet less than one-fourth that in many developed countries, the proportion of milk throughput in production has been as low as 13 percent in the year 2000.

The total milk production in India more than doubled from 38.8 million tonnes in 1983-84 to 81 million tonnes in 2000-2001. The annual growth rate of total milk production from 1950/51 to 2000/2001 is shown in Table 5.3A. Table 5AII.1 in Annexure II indicates State/Region wise milk production from 1973-74 to 2001-2002. Annual average and annual

Table 5.3A: Growth in Milk Production: All India: 1950/51 – 2000/02

Period	Percent per year
1950/51 to 1960/61	1.64
1960/61 to 1973/74	1.15
1973/74 to 1980/81	4.51
1980/81 to 1990/91	5.50
1990/91 to 2000/02	5.00

Source: Ministry of Agriculture: Directorate of Economics & Statistics; Agricultural Statistics At A Glance 2002.

compound rate of growth of milk production in important Indian states during the period (1977-78) is also appended (Table A5.3B). The method of measuring and inferring trend growth is also placed at Annexure-IV. A time series data for buffalo and cow milk separately are not readily available from national sources. However, as per the Report of Sub-Group XIII Dairying constituted by the Planning Commission for formulation of 10th Five Year Plan, milk production in India is growing at 4.16 per cent Compound Annual Rate of Growth (CARG) (1996-97/1999-2000) annually as against the rates of growth of population (1991-01) and per capita real net national income (1996-97/1999-2000, at 1993-94 prices) of 1.93 (exponential) and 4.33 per cent respectively. That there have been no large-scale imports would suggest that milk production is matching the demand. However, the growth rate in milk production during the nineties has come down as compared to the growth rates in eighties.

Per capita availability of milk/milk products is presently about 221 gm per day (2000-01). But it appears that growth of milk production is slowing down even before the per capita availability of milk can match the minimum daily nutrition that should be obtained from milk consumption as per the recommendations of the nutritionists in this regard. It is interesting to note that though there has been a higher rate of increase in cow milk production, buffalo milk still accounted for almost 52 per cent of the total milk output. In 1992/93, the latest year for which data is available, the milk yield per day per animal in milk for India was 3.46 kg. per buffalo compared to 2.1 kg. for cow. There is, however wide variation in milk production per animal among different states due to difference in species, feeding pattern, health and hygiene of animals. About 85 per cent of Indian cows give less than 1 kg milk per day and cows giving more than 2 kg. of milk per day are only about 5 per cent. An average Indian cow milk yield ranges from 200 to 500 kg. per lactation of 300 days compared to 4154 kg. in the USA, 3950 kg. in the UK and 3902 kg. in Denmark. A major proportion of indigenous stock is also plagued with longer ages of first calving i.e. 36 to 50 months and inter-calving period of 14 to 22 months. The situation with buffaloes is a little brighter as 10 per cent of the buffalo population yields a little less than 1 kg. milk per day and about 25 per cent yield more than 2 kg. milk per day. On an average an Indian buffalo gives about 650 kg. per lactation. In a nutshell, poor yields are direct reflections of poor breed, feed and management.

India is one of the fastest growing milk economy in the world today. Already the single biggest milk producer — canning more than the annual output of Australia, New Zealand, Brazil, Pakistan and the Russian Federation added up, India's production is expected to rise by a whooping three million tonnes in 2003, to reach 85 million tonnes. With total world supplies pegged at 600 mn tonnes, India will thus contribute almost 15%. Adding an extra dash of cream to profits, India's ghee and skimmed milk exports are set to rise on the back of a bullish world market. To put India's growth trajectory in perspective, this is a year when milk production is expected to remain virtually static in other large producers like the European Union, Russian Federation, Ukraine and Poland. It will be marginally higher in the United States, Pakistan, Brazil and New Zealand; and lower in Argentina and Australia, which are suffering from the aftermath of droughts.

Overall, while the global milk production is rising only by 1%, India's output will be up by as much as 3.5%. As this surpasses the 2% annual increase in population, there will be a net increase in the per capita availability. According to the FAO, India's increased milk output in 2003 is expected to be largely due to better feeding of cattle and genetic improvements rather than herd expansion. From sturdy like Sahiwal germplasm for poorer farmers to exotic Holsteins capable of producing milk in the range of 12,000-14,000 litres, with a fat content of more than 4.8% and SNF (solids non fat) of 8.8%, better cattle breeds will hold the key to growth. With tightening exportable surplus in the global market, prices of all milk products are sharply on the rise. Milk powder prices have increased most strongly, by about 60% in the first quarter of 2003. Butter and casein prices rose by 30% and cheese prices registered a 20% growth. This provides a good opportunity for India to boost its ghee and skimmed milk powder exports. But India's total foreign exchange earnings from dairy products will remain far below its potential due to continued problems with quality and processing. Consequently, despite a total production which is lower than India's, the biggest gainers from an increase in world prices this year will be the EU, the USA and countries of eastern Europe.

Interestingly, with rising world prices, export subsidies paid by some high-cost producing countries have also fallen. For example, average United States monthly export subsidies for skimmed milk powder declined from a high of $864 per tonne in March 2002 to $142 per tonne in March 2003. In a related policy development, in November 2002, the US adjusted the levels of government support purchase prices, reducing the prices of skimmed milk powder by 11% and increasing that of butter by 26%. These adjustments were felt to be necessary to bring support prices more in line with prevailing domestic prices, as the previously relatively high price for skimmed milk powder had resulted in a substantial build up of government stocks and necessitated increased use of export subsidies. In the EU, export subsidies for milk powder dropped from Euro 850 per tonne in mid-2002 to Euro 440 per tonne by the end of January 2003. Skimmed milk powder subsidies were subsequently raised to Euro 510 per tonne in February 2003, to reflect an increase in the value of the Euro against the US dollar.

Rough estimates indicate that milk use pattern in India include liquid milk (45%), ghee (28%), dahi (7.0%), khoa (6.5%), butter (6.5%), milk powder (2.6%), channa, cheese and paneer (2.0%), cream (0.5%), ice-cream (0.2%), and others (1.7%). It is estimated that 20-25% of the milk is retained by the rural people. Surplus milk is converted into the products like ghee, khoa, channa, paneer etc. Milk products fetch higher price than liquid milk and the traditional dairy products and sweetmeats are in great demand than the western products like butter, ice-cream, cheese, yoghurt etc. NDRI, Karnal developed scraped surface concentrators for khoa-making. Efforts are on to mechanise traditional dairy products processing.

Crossbreeding Technology for Increased Milk Production

Increasing milk production has been one of the major goals of livestock development policy in India. Crossbreeding of cattle and upgrading of buffaloes have been the main thrust for improved breeding, the rationale being that new breeds are more productive and unit cost of milk production is lower than the local nondescript breeds. Systematic crossbreeding research in cattle started during mid-1960s. The focus of crossbreeding research has been mainly on cattle because of their role of milk production and also use as draught animals in the agriculture sector. Crossbreeding projects like Indo-German project in Himachal Pradesh, Indo-Swiss project in Kerala and Punjab, Indo-Danish project in Karnataka, Indo-Australian project in Haryana and Assam and Indo-Newzealand project in Tamil Nadu were initiated under bilateral collaborations. The Indian Council for Agricultural Research launched an All India Coordinated Research Project on crossbreeding of cattle with research units located in different agroclimatic regions of the country. Some important crossbreeds in the country include Haryana X Friesian, Haryana X Jersey, Haryana X Brown Swiss, Rathi X Jersey, Gir X Jersey, Gir X Criesian and Sahiwal X Jersey.

Adoption of crossbreeding technology has, however, been slow. As per Livestock Census, 1992, only about 7.5 per cent of the cattle population consisted of crossbreeds. Between 1982 and 1992, population of crossbreed cattle increased at the rate of 5.6 per cent a year. Female population increased at a faster rate than males. On the other hand, indigenous stock seemed to be approaching stabilization. Annual growth rate of indigenous cattle stock was 0.52 per cent, although the female population witnessed a slightly higher growth. Low milk yield and decreasing demand for animal draught services were the main factors for slow growth in indigenous stock.

Regional Pattern of Adoption of Crossbreeding Technology

It is evident from the above that despite decades of research and extension efforts, diffusion of crossbreeding technology has been very slow. However, the extent of diffusion of this technology varied considerably across the states. The proportion of crossbred cattle in milch cattle ranged from minuscule 0.27 per cent in Rajasthan to 48 per cent tin Kerala. Punjab ranked second in transforming the local cattle into crossbred ones (37 percent), followed by Haryana (13 percent), Tamil Nadu (10 percent) and U.P. (9 percent). On the other hand, in Rajasthan, Madhya Pradesh and Gujarat, the percentage of crossbred cattle was less than one till 1982.

In the subsequent decade (1982-92), at the all India level due to rapid growth of adult crossbred females (compound annual growth rate 6.30 per cent) and marginal decline of breedable indigenous cows (annual growth rate –0.02 percent), the share of the former in total milch cattle population nearly doubled to 9.8 percent in 1992. In the majority of the states also, the population of breedable cattle increased significantly. It is interesting to observe that in all the states except Uttar Pradesh and Bihar, the share of crossbreds has increased not only in milch cattle population but also in total milch bovines, due to their faster growth as compared to buffaloes.

The spread of crossbreeding during the 1980s has been particularly notable in Gujarat and Jammu and Kashmir, where the number of crossbred females increased more than 5 times between 1982 and 1992. The other states which have registered high rates of growth in breedable crossbreds are Maharashtra, Madhya Pradesh, Rajasthan, Orissa and Himachal Pradesh. However, despite high growth rates, in Rajasthan and Madhya Pradesh, adoption of crossbreeding technology continues to be very low. Only about one percent of female cattle population is crossbred in these states.

The share of states in the increment of crossbred cows between 1982 and 1992 provides magnitude of concentration of change across states. The states of Maharashtra, Punjab and Tamil Nadu together account for nearly half (47.68 per cent) of the total increase in crossbred milch cattle in India. The share of Maharashtra alone is as high as 23.82 per cent. In contrast, the share of majority of the states is below 5 percent.

Interestingly in northeastern region of Gujarat, from where the concept of 'Anand Pattern Dairying' has originated, there are more indigenous female cows than crossbred cows; but the phrase 'Anand Pattern' is associated with recommendations of crossbred cows in policy documents. The Operation Flood programme though resulted in the increasing acceptance of crossbred cows, still indigenous cows and buffaloes are dominant in the milch stock in Kaira District, of which Anand is a tehsil.

Gains from Crossbreeding: Impact on Milk Production

Bovine milk production in India was 20.58 million tonnes in 1972, it increased more than 2.5 fold in 1992 to 55.38 million tonnes, registering a growth rate of 5.07 percent per annum. The rate of increase in cow milk production (6.36 percent) was higher than that of buffalo milk production (4.25 percent). In 12 of the 17 states, growth in cow milk production was higher than buffalo milk production. In three states, Andhra Pradesh,

Madhya Pradesh and Orissa, milk production of both the bovine species increased at roughly similar rates.

The National Dairy Development Board and Milkfed have joined hands with Cooperative Resources International, USA to streamline animal breeding services in Punjab. The National Dairy Development Board (NDDB) and Cooperative Resources International (CRI), USA, have signed a consulting agreement calling CRI to evaluate the existing systems to providing animal breeding and advisory services by the dairy cooperatives in India to dairy farmers and give recommendations to modernise the system with a view to achieving higher and faster progress in increasing productivity of cattle and buffaloes in the country.

CRI is currently examining the systems of semen production, sire evaluation, distribution of semen and liquid nitrogen, artificial insemination services, data collection and information generation, advisory services, etc. in order to suggest measures to improve efficiency and quality in providing these services to farmers. They will also study the existing institutional arrangement and recommended changes that need to be made to make it more responsive to farmers' needs. Two experts from CRI, Mr. Herb Rycroft, vice-President and Dr Robert Bower, consultant among with experts from the NDDB were on a study visit to Punjab between January 31 and February 3,2003 The team had meetings with the Chief Minister of Punjab, Parliament Secretary (Cooperation), Financial Commissioner (Cooperation), Secretary (Animal Husbandry and Dairy Development) and Managing Director of Milkfed when the purpose and objective of this study was discussed.

Dairy Perspective

Despite rapid strides in all other sectors of the economy, agriculture and animal husbandry in India still continue to employ the greatest number of people. With recent advances in technology, these sectors now offer a range of truly varied and remunerative career options. There are several career avenues within the agricultural industry, ranging from farm management to careers in related areas like horticulture, dairy farming, poultry farming, and many others.

The People for Ethical Treatment to Animals (PETA) has come forward with reasons and research reports to apprise people the undesirable consequences of consumption of milk products. In particular, it emphasises that milk is a product loaded with cholesterol and fat, low in iron and there is no protective effect of its calcium on bones. Dr John Mc Dougal, Advisor to Bill Clinton calls cow's milk "liquid meat". Dr Benjamin Spack, leading authority in child care, opines that milk can cause anemia, allergies in human infants. Milk with too much Vitamin D can be toxic. Individuals who do not have enzymes that digest milk lactose develop gastrointestinal symptoms. Milk containing residues of antibiotics, hormones, dyes and germs is a health hazard for consumers. We cannot controvert the above opinion and findings by the Physicians Committee for Responsible

Medicine without specific reasons. A fact-finding committee of eminent experts and physicians of India needs to review the latest data on the milk consumption. If in the opinion of the committee the reports are of any benefit to the public, these must be circulated widely among the public to know the other side of the coin.

The dairy sector is concerned with producing milk and milk products and raising and breeding of cattle. The dairy industry produces a range of milk products—milk, butter, cheese, ghee, condensed milk, powdered milk, yoghurt, etc. While providing raw material for many other industries. India, which enjoys a locational advantage, in the international market, is the largest producer of milk and the second largest producer of milk products in the world. Incidentally, India also happens to be the lowest cost producer of milk per litre in the world at 27 cents (*vs.* 63 cents in the USA and $2.8 in Japan). If the present trend continues, like the mineral water industry, the milk processing industry is poised for exponential growth. With production expected to triple in the next 10 years, India will easily emerge as the world's leading producer of milk products. This in turn will result in a consequent spurt in the number of jobs in the sector.

Those who train to be dairy technologist have to be not only technologically trained but also adept at managing a farm, as this constitutes the major part of the job. In fact, they are trained and work more as dairy managers. A typical dairy manager's work would include selection and purchase of animals, housing and feeding of animals, looking after dairy hygiene, supervising the milking process and monitoring the processing and sale of dairy products. Incidentally, India also has the largest cattle population (with some 20 recognised breeds) in the world. However, despite being the world's largest milk producing country, our yield per animal is very low. Although Punjab surpasses the national average, increasing the yield is a major challenge.

Regional Indicators

The report of National Commission on Agriculture (1976) identified breeding, feeding, management, animal health, dairy education, dairy research, incentives and credit as the factors which affect the pace of dairy development of any region. In order to study the regional imbalances in livestock development, seven indicators, viz., distribution of bovines in various States, adult females not calved once, adult bovines neither used for breeding nor for work, pressure on draught animals, availability of grazing area, veterinary facilities, and level of milk production and per capita milk availability are important. These factors were responsible for temporal and spatial imbalance in livestock status of India.

Similarly, some scholars have identified five indicators while discussing 'Drift in the Dairy Development'. These were dairy productivity, buffalo-cattle ratio, level of agricultural development, cooperative bondage and farm level resource capacity. The findings based on dairy development indices divides the Indian Union into most developed group (Gujarat,

Haryana and Punjab), moderately developed group (Rajasthan, Karnataka, Maharashtra and Uttar Pradesh), less developed group (M.P., Andhra Pradesh, Tamil Nadu, Bihar and Kerala) and least developed group (Jammu & Kashmir, Orissa and Assam). Powar (1983) in his study entitled 'Differential Dairy Development in Selected States of India' took the help of nine, which were more or less similar to those mentioned above.[1]

An analysis has been made here on differential scenario of dairying in India, keeping in view the indicators/parameters as suggested by Patel (1993) and Pandey (1995). These indicators are more comprehensive than those used by earlier authors. Further, for ease in discussion, entire country is subdivided in the four regions as under: [2]

(a) Northern Region : Chandigarh, Delhi, Haryana, H.P., J & K, Punjab, Rajasthan, U.P.

(b) Western and
Central Region : M.P., Maharashtra, Gujarat, Goa, Dadra,
& Nagar Haveli.

(c) Southern Region : A.P., Karnataka, Kerala, Pondicherry,
Tamil Nadu.

(d) Eastern Region : Bihar, West Bengal, Orissa, Assam,
Arunachal Pradesh, Nagaland, Sikkim, Tripura, Manipur.
Meghalaya,

Powar also found poorest dairy development index in the State of Orissa (2,856.7) as compared to Punjab. Bovine density, cattle-buffaloes ratio, crossbred population, number of cooperative societies and producer members per society and milk procured per society per day, A.I. routes per 1,000 breedable bovine population, cattle feed production and productivity of milch animals were found as an important decisive indicators responsible for imbalance in diary development in different regions.

The discussion also revealed that Eastern region though having enough bovine resources is still lagging behind the other regions and thus indicating a lot of scope for improvement in this region. The high stocking rate in this region should be recognised as the strength and opportunity, rather than a threat.

Milk productivity is also found to be most crucial indicator of dairy development. This goes without saying that there is a need to motivate farmers to reduce dry-milch cattle ratio, to rear few good animals rather than larger unproductive and less productive animals and also, to cull the unproductive stock to increase average milk production per milch cattle unit.

---

[1]Powar. R.K. (1983); A study on differential dairy development in selected states of India. Ph.D. Theses, NDR/Deemed university), Karnal, Haryana.

[2]For details refer to Shantanu Kumar, Agricultural Situation in India, September, 2000.

Similarly, C-B ratio was also identified as an important determinant of dairy development. Northern region was found to have highest number of buffaloes per thousand of cattle and thus, putting this region at better place in dairy development. From, this it could be implied that high quality buffaloes need to be supplied to the underdeveloped region, but particularly to those States where there are good irrigation facilities and in the States having poor irrigation facilities, it is not suggested to increase crossbred population.

Procurement, Processing and Marketing

The average milk procurement during April – December 2002 was 24 million kg. per day, about 3 per cent higher than the same period last year. During 2002-03 (April – December), an average of about 13.70 million of milk per day was marketed as against 13.51 million litre per day during the responding period last year (Table 5.3B).

Table 5.3B: Physical Progress

Particulars	1999-2000	2000-01	2001-02	2002-03*
Societies Organized ('000)	83.7	98.0#	100.56#	101.24 # $
Farmer Members (Million)	10.52	10.83	11.05	11.23 $
Avg. Rural milk Procurement (million kg pd)	15.74	16.55	17.60	17.24 @
Liquid milk marketing (million litre per day)	12.90	13.40	13.42	13.70 @

-   Cumulative
\#   Includes conventional societies and taluka unions formed earlier.
*   Provisional
$ Refers to December 2002
@   Refers to April – December 2002.
   Source: Annual Report 2002-03, Deptt. of AH&D, Min. of Agriculture, Govt. of India, New Delhi.

Delhi Milk Scheme (DMS) is processing and supplying toned milk containing 3.0% fat and 8.5% SNF, double toned milk containing 1.5% fat and 9% SNF and full cream milk containing 6% fat and 9% SNF to a network of 1506 outlets spread all over the city. These outlets (milk booths) are manned by students engaged as senior depot agents /depot agents and ex-service men/retired government/semi government servants as concessionaries. DMS is selling double toned milk, toned milk and full cream milk, at of Rs. 11 per litre, Rs. 14 per litre and Rs. 17 per litre respectively with effect 01.03. 2000 DMS is also supplying milk to 148 institutions such as Hospitals, Government Canteens, Schools and Hostels. In order to promote the sale of milk, DMS has converted its 158 depots All Day Milk Stalls. Capacity utilization for milk processing is as given in Table 5.4.

Table 5.4: Capacity Utilization of Milk Processing

(Lakh litre per day)

Year	Processing/ Packing capacity for distri- bution	Quantity of milk processed	Quantity of milk sold	Percentage capacity of utilization
1997-98	5.00	3.45	3.36	69.0%
1998-99	5.00	3.71	3.61	74.2%
1999-00	5.00	3.97	3.82	79.4%
2000-01	5.00	2.42	2.15	48.4%
2001-02	5.00	2.38	2.06	47.6%
2002-03 up to Oct.'02	5.00	2.21	1.97	44.2%

Source: Annual Report 2002-03, Deptt. of Animal Husbandry and Dairying, Ministry of Agriculture, Govt. of India, New Delhi.

Besides, the DMS is also manufacturing and selling ghee and butter out of surplus fat available. The production and sale of ghee and butter are shown in Table 5.5.

Table 5.5: Production and Sale of Ghee

(In metric tonnes)

Year	Ghee production	Sale	Butter production	Sale
1997-98	815.00	899.00	70.00	66.00
1998-99	805.61	742.84	75.22	72.50
1999-00	918.21	857.43	41.20	52.10
2000-01	648.36	760.83*	69.43	70.84
2001-02	718.02	666.94	83.70	86.96
2002-03 (up to Oct.'02)	336.06	413.11*	36.36	45.70*

Note: * Sale includes sale of previous year's stock also.

Source: Annual Report 2002-03, Deptt of Animal Husbandry & Dairying Ministry of Agriculture, Government of India,. New Delhi.

Further, DMS is also manufacturing and marketing Yoghurt cups & *kullars*) and Flavoured Milk (in pouches) for the citizens of Delhi Quantity of Flavoured Milk and Yoghurt manufactured and sold since 1998-99 are indicated in the Table 5.6. The production and sale of Paneer in 200 gm pack has also been introduced with effect from 1.11.2001.

Table 5.6: Production and sale of Flavoured Milk and Yoghurt by DMS

(in thousands numbers)

Year	Flavoured milk (in 200 ml. pouches)		Yoghurt (in 100 gm cups & kullars)	
	Production	Sale	Production	Sale
1998-99	—	—	700	683
1999-00	83 **	81**	725	713
2000-01	512	500	962	1130*
2001-02	892	879	1321	1300
2002-03 (up to Oct.'02) 618		613	858	851

Note: * Sale includes sale of previous year's stock also.

       ** The production and sale of flavoured milk (in 200 ml pouches) was introduced with effect from 4.8.1999.

Source: Annual export 2002-03, Deptt of Animal Husbandry & Dairying, Govt. of India

Physical Targets and Achievements

DMS's targets and achievements regarding procurement of milk production/ Sale of milk and milk products for 2001-02 and 2002-03 are indicated below:

Table 5.7: Target and Achievements of Procurement and Sale of Milk by DMS

Year	2001-2002		2002-03	
	Target	Achievement	Target	Achievement up to Oct. 02
1. Procurement of Milk (lakh kg)	766.50	706.02	766.50	387.73
2. Production/Sale of				
a) Milk (lakh litres)	766.50	753.53	766.50	422.52
b) Ghee (in MT)	800.00*	718.02	800.00*	336.06
c) Table Butter (in MT)		83.70		36.36

Note: *The values are combined for ghee and table butter

Source: Annual Report 2002-03, Department of Animal Husbandry & Dairying, Govt. of India

Annual production of butter totals about 1.2 million tonnes, most of which is produced by small businesses and households.[1] Annual production of milk powder and infant food is estimated at 160, 000 tons, malted milk food at 45,000 tons, cheese at 3,000 tons and condensed milk at 8,500 tons has increased impressively in per cent terms. In the coming decade the products that are likely to enter the market in a big way will be the fermented products like dahi (yoghurt) and acidophilus health drink, health foods

---

[1]Indian Agricultural Situation: 1994: AGR No. IN 4084: and Department of Animal Husbandry: Basic Animal Husbandry Statistics: 1997, p. 101.

like milk with fruits, calcium rich and low fat dairy products. Lastly there is also immense potential for the Indian milk sweets like the traditional rasogollas, pedhas, halwas, and payasam in ready to consume form. The combined market of these products exceeds Rs. 100 billion and organized dairy sector perhaps today accounts for less than 10 percent of market share. The Government is attaching great importance to the processing industry. During 1991-2001 investment in the livestock processing industry increased to Rs. 385.3 billion (Table 5.8).

Table 5.8: Investment in the Processed Food Sector (Since liberalisation in July, 1991)

(Rs. in crores)

SL. No.	Sector	Industrial Entrepreneur Memoranda		Industrial Approvals (l00% Export Oriented Units Industrial Licenses (till Nov. 2001)		Total		Foreign Investment out of total Investment
		No.	Invest.	No.	Invest.	No.	Invest.	
1.	Grain Milling & Grain Based products	368	5801	104	1078	472	6879	1207
2.	Fruits & Vegetable Products	1723	3314	421	5177	2144	8491	1089
3.	Meat & Poultry Products	89	384	59	1394	148	1778	267
4.	Fish Processing & Aquaculture	113	460	192	2228	305	2688	548
5.	Fermentation Industry	672	9301	211	2073	883	11374	1094
6.	Consumer Industry Including Soft Drinks / Waters / Confectionery etc.	853	7438	78	5814	931	13252	4423
7.	Milk & Milk Products	1104	13751	26	1082	1130	14833	1004
8.	Other including food additives, flavours etc.	-	-	71	934	71	934	535
9.	Edible Oil/oil seeds	1675	13416	-	-	1675	13416	-
	Total	6597	53865	1162	19780	7759	73645	10167

Source: Government of India, Ministry of Food Processing Industry: Annual Report 2002-03.

As regards regional distribution of milk production in India, the Central region consisting of UP and MP accounts for around 26% of the total output. This is followed by Western region (22%), Southern region (21%), Northern region (18%), and Eastern region (11%). The dairy business in India is currently estimated at Rs. 80,000 crore. India dairying has several in-built competitive advantages which, if exploited, would lead to the manifold growth of the industry. A large bovine population, strong procurement infrastructure, skilled manpower, cheap labour and a large number of processing and allied facilities are some of the advantages which India enjoys. With the present growth rate of around 4 per cent per annum, India is expected to produce around 182 million tonnes of milk by 2030, more than one-third of the projected global production of 620 to 650 million tonnes.

Considering that the dairy market in the developed countries had reached a saturation point and emerging milk markets were expected to be Asian and African countries, India had yet another advantage, India's geographical location is an advantage when compared with other dairying countries like the Scandinavian nations, the US, Australia and New Zealand, with increasing awareness of the importance and better values of buffalo milk, it will gain prominence at the global level. India has a vast milk procurement and distribution system with 90,000 village cooperative societies, 170 district unions and 23 state federations. With nine dairy science colleges, 31 veterinary colleges and 80 agricultural research institutes, India has large number of professionals working in the industry. One of the greatest challenges before Indian dairying is improving the quality of milk which may be attributed to lack of hygiene and sanitation at the production level.

Dairying as an Instrument of Change

Introduction to dairy development programme will lead to better utilization of land, water and human resources. Dairying is reckoned with as an instrument of social and economic change. The lack of appreciation by farmers who are traditionally crop-oriented to pursue animal agriculture on a large scale, the lack of capital and, in most cases, lack of incentives, have been included among the major setbacks in developing an economic oriented dairy enterprise. The dairy industry may be considered in relation to its component segments, viz., production, organisation, processing and marketing. Thus, the programme has to depend upon the maximum use of available resources, utilization of manpower, provision of incentives, existing organisation and administrative machinery and social and religious dogmas of the people in these areas. Further, the dairy development aims not only to improve economic output, but also to improve the nutrition of the people both rural and urban by making available a ready source of balanced nutrients.

Because of recent technological advancements in the field of Agriculture and Animal Husbandry a perceptible change has occurred in the farming community which as a whole gradually drifted from traditional low productive livestock to modern high productive potential livestock farming system. Today the candid opinion is that the adoption of mixed farming is the salvation for the problems of the rural folk who are generally poor, underemployed and unemployed. There is an imperative need for development of integrated livestock production involving improvement of genetic makeup, adequate nutrition, health programme, institutional credit facilities and an efficient marketing system.

The animal and plant components should be complementary instead of competitive. The development of Animal Agriculture would be a great asset to crop production and would add to the prosperity of the small farmer. In one sense the small land holdings in the developing countries may be an asset rather than a liability in as much as they would act as a buffer against large areas of land suitable for cereal production being taken away for animal production.

The human element as a factor in animal or dairy development is important as purely economic one although the latter is always credited with miraculous potentialities. The production of dairy cattle in small land holdings in the rural areas in conjunction with primary cereal production creates employment and contributes substantially to domestic income. This could be a worthwhile occupation of women and possibly young people in these areas and any increase in their buying power so achieved is bound to produce far-reaching effects in the long run that could be accomplished otherwise.

Dairy farming has been considered as a subsidiary occupation for the village farming community with a view to improving the potentialities in gainful employment and to ensure regular supplementary income to the small and marginal farmers and landless labourers in rural areas. Raj Krishna, eminent economist, has impressed that dairying is one of the most effective instrument for generating income and employment in the rural sector. He added that dairying can help fight poverty in this country. He observed that dairying required one million rupees to create an employment potential of 290 person years as against 120-200 person years for crop production. Of the targeted employment generation in the country, the dairy sector can safely assume responsibility for a substantial production. Expressing dissatisfaction with the present rate of growth in this sector, he pleaded for a greater share for rural landless and the small farmers who own 53 percent of the milch cattle population in the country and contribute about an equal share of the total milk production.

Based on data collected from 113 households of various resource situations in rural Karnal, by Patel and Kunbhane, the human labour utilisation in dairy enterprise, by man, woman, and child it is reported that landless households take about 40 percent of total time spent on dairy enterprise was contributed by female family labour. Dairy activity has a large potential for gainful employment of underemployed and unemployed female labour especially belonging to weaker sections in rural areas. Dairy enterprise, if practised on scientific and commercial lines could offer gainful employment to rural folk especially women. A large number of women hailing from landless labour households and small and marginal families would be able to supplement their income and employment potential through dairy enterprise besides providing better nutrition to their family members. Secondly, a constant and regular flow of income from milk production throughout the year is welcomed by the households. Under the new strategy of rural development milk production will not only contribute to national health and wealth but also provide substantial employment opportunities in the rural areas to solve the problems of rural poverty and rural employment.

Punjab has become the first state in the country by deciding to enact the Punjab Herds Legislation act, that would ensure the registration of animals in the state to improve the quality of animals and milk products subsequently. The Act, waiting for President's approval, was aimed to revolutionise the whole milk processing sector by modernising milk production. The state government is determined to give a big boost to the production of milk and milk products as per international standards. The Act would take a holistic view, to restructure the dairy sector. Since, the dairy sector was contributing about 20 percent to the state GDP, but due to lower quality of milk and higher production costs of the cooperative milk plants, the share of state in exports was limited. The share of India, in the total US $12000 million world trade was just one per cent, despite the fact India was the largest milk producer in the world.

One of the important factors responsible for placing so much emphasis on dairying as a measure to improve the conditions of the rural poor, or to use this as one of the safeguards against accentuation of interclass disparities in rural areas, is the impression that dairying fits with the farm level infrastructure of the small farmer. This impression is strengthened further by the Kaira District Cooperative Milk Producers Union, Anand, and more importantly by the presence of dairy animals even on the smallest holdings in different parts of the country. Thus, there exists a nucleus of dairying even on small farms. Further, this enterprise, compared to some other activities, has a distinct initial advantage in terms of the store of traditional skill in maintaining dairy production, which is available with the small farmers. The nucleus of dairy farming and the traditional skill accompanying it, may be profitably used in promoting the enterprise on a more scientific and commercial basis. These are the basic premises underlying and the whole approach to dairy development through small farmers. However, it would be misleading to infer too much from the mere presence of a few milch cattle on the small farms. Unless relevant details about operations of dairy farming and their economic significance are properly understood a worthwhile planning for promoting dairy farming on small farms may become absolutely difficult. Thus the financial institutions engaged in developing dairying as a rural enterprise will have to arrange or supply the necessary inputs, besides credit to deploy the funds in the most suitable and remunerative manner.

The concept of modernisation in dairy cattle production has to be discussed in relation to land use, energy input and in terms of human or social factors. The importance of any rural change should be assessed by its capacity to increase the buying power of the producer. The highly specialised large-scale dairying, as practised in Western countries, is not applicable to developing countries because of the high capital investment, technical speciality and enormous energy input. Dairy production by the small farmer as an adjunct to primary crop agriculture is more likely to increase milk production in the country as a whole and enhance milk consumption eventually than the modern large scale dairying. The establishment of large government and institutional farms should, therefore, be supplemented with an active programme to stimulate the small farmer to accept dairying as part of the rural activities. Unless efforts are concentrated to appeal to the 'human element' involved in the process of this change, handling of dairy production in large modernized units can only be a partial answer to the problem. Initiatives to introduce this concept of animal agriculture should include on the farm demonstration of green fodder production and preservation. Experience in the past has shown that there is no miracle solution to the complex problem but manipulation of the human factor at the small farm level may be closer to reality than modernization at the suburban level.

Government Intervention in Dairy Sector

To ensure adequate supply of milk to consumers at affordable prices and ensure reasonable prices for dairy producers, the Government of India implemented two major programmes. The first was the setting up of City Milk Schemes in the 1950s and the second was the launching of the Operation Flood Programme in 1970.

City Milk Schemes

City milk schemes were introduced in the 1950s to ensure a cheap and stable supply of milk to urban populations. The first programme was established in Delhi in 1955 with a large dairy plant supported by a network of rural milk and chilling centers. This programme was subsequently replicated in about 100 towns and cities throughout the country. By the 1960s, however, the sourcing of milk from the urban peripheries became more difficult because of increasing competition from the *dudhias* (milk traders) who collected milk from farmers and delivered it directly to customers. In many cases, the city milk schemes started handling milk supplied by the dudhias. The inflexibility and inefficiencies associated with the government operation of milk schemes prevented the milk schemes from adjusting to changing market prices and conditions. Consequently, as market prices increased producers started supplying milk directly to consumers or to vendors instead of selling it to the milk schemes. To cope with the short milk supply, the schemes began importing and reconstituting milk powder. At the same time, milk-rationing programmes, intended to control the heavy demand for cheap, subsidized milk, gave rise to milk cards (vouchers) and milk queues.

Dairy Cooperatives

The Animal Husbandry and Dairying Department of the Government of India has been making concentrated efforts for promoting dairy activities in non-Operation Flood areas with emphasis on building up cooperative infrastructure, revitalization of sick dairy cooperative federations and creation of infrastructure in the states for testing the quality of milk and milk products. In 1999-2000, the country had about 80,000 organized primary village dairy cooperatives with an aggregate membership of 1.1 crore producers. These primaries are federated into 183 district cooperative milk unions and state cooperative dairy federations. During the year the dairy cooperative network collected about 16 million litres milk per day and paid an aggregate amount of about Rs. 6000 crore to the milk producers.

Post-Operation Flood-III (which coincided with the first four years of the Ninth Plan, 1996-97/1999-00), milk procurement by cooperatives registered a Compound Annual Growth Rate (CAGR) of 8.3 per cent (Table 5.5). The number of organized village cooperatives during the Ninth Plan registered a growth of 3.81 per cent per annum. By 1999-2000, over 20,000 village cooperatives were covered under single/cluster Artificial Insemination (AI) centers. During the year, nearly 4.8 million AIs were performed and more than 1.3 million MT of cattle-feed was sold. All these efforts were effective in enabling producers to sustain both milk production and income from milk during the Ninth Plan.

Table 5.9: Key Physical Performance of the Dairy Cooperatives

Particulars	96-97	99-00	CARG per cent
Procurement (LKGPD)	124.01	157.41	8.27
Milk Sale (LLPD)	106.75	128.95	6.5
DCS Organized	74862	83747	3.81
Total Farmer Members ('000)	9721	10516	2.65
Cattle Feed Sale: BCF + BPF (lakh MT)	9.66	10.32	2.23
AI done (lakh)	40.46	47.87	5.77

Source: NDDB, Anand.

During the Ninth Plan, milk marketing by dairy cooperatives grew at a CARG of 6.5 per cent. Currently, cooperatives market about 13 million litres per day (MLPD) in over 750 cities and towns. Even as they continued to assign the highest priority to fulfilling the demand for liquid milk, the cooperatives produced about 131000 MT milk powders of different types, 76000 MT butter, and 61000 MT ghee during 1999-2000. To meet the growing demand for value added milk products, they also manufactured a variety of cheeses, curd, gulab-jamun, ice-cream, peda, etc.

The market share of city milk schemes has been gradually declining (Mumbai and Kolkata) or posting slower growth (Delhi and Chennai), with the advent of the regional and National Milk Grids operated under Operation Flood (OF). In large cities the milk schemes coexist with the Mother Dairies established under OF[2].

Joint Ventures and Cooperatives

It all began in December 2002 when Mother Dairy Foods Limited (MDFL), a Companies Act-registered subsidiary of NDDB, signed a joint venture (JV) agreement with the Kerala Cooperative Milk Marketing Federation (Milma) to market milk products in the coastal state. It was a break from the straight and narrow path followed so long by the NDDB, and a miffed Kurien, who had no role to play in the process, soon afterwards went public with his warning that JVs would make the cooperative federations redundant.

Cooperatives run more on sentiments than hardcore business principles have no role in the dynamic economy India aspires to become. The cooperatives have to come out from the clutches of the state government. The challenge in the marketplace from the MNCs is so strong that if we don't wake up now, it will be too late. If we look at the equity of any state cooperative federation today in any state outside Gujarat, it varies from 55 to 98 percent state government equity. Is that what a cooperative is supposed to be? We are merely trying to free cooperatives from government control.

"NDDB was set up as a government body to rescue dairying from the government", in 1965, when Dr. Kurien said this, Amul was the only true cooperative. In every other state, dairying was under the control of the government.

If we want cooperatives to stand on their feet, it is absolutely essential they become economically independent. Economic independence will only come about if cooperatives can independently market their products. We believe that in the future, when the JVs are strong and able to perform, they will appoint efficient marketing teams. There is, however, a provision that once the JVs become strong, the federations can disengage themselves with all infrastructure, entire staff and brand. They can simply pull out. If, 10 years hence, the cooperative becomes a producer's company under the Companies Act, then MDFL will simply pull out of the joint arrangement. The marketing company has not been produced for the sake of profit alone, it has to provide expertise in marketing

For the Gujaral-cooperative milk marketing federation (GCMMF) — the success of which led to the establishment of the NDDB, with a one-point brief of replicating Amul's success elsewhere in the country — though,

---

[2] The Mother Dairy is a marketing mechanism developed under Operation Flood involving the installation of milk vending machines in major cities.

the parting of ways couldn't have come at a worse time. Undisputed market leaders for close to half a century, Amul today fights for shelf-space alongside products of MNCs like Britannia, Nestle and Hindustan Lever Limited (HLL), not to mention various regional cooperatives.

Notwithstanding the criticism, MDFL is already in talks with federations in other states, including Andhra Pradesh (Vijaya), Punjab (Verka), Rajasthan (Saras), Karnataka (Nandini) and Uttar Pradesh (Parag) for the formation of similar marketing ventures. Independent marketing of their products is the only answer for cooperatives seeking to stand on their own feet, instead of government crutches.

Milk market is expected to grow to Rs. 100,000 crore in the next five years — and in areas as varied as butter, ice-creams and dahi, the GCMMF is already feeling the heat. Till a few years ago, Amul had 55-60 percent share of the 9,000-tonnes annual cheese sales. Britannia, which entered the market in July 1997, now accounts for more than 20 percent of the market, thanks to its aggressive marketing techniques. A threatened Amul has countered by launching new variants such as Emmentha, Gouda and Mozzarella, and plans to introduce cheese sauces and dips. Even its traditional stronghold of milk is under MNC threat, with Britannia's Milkman and Nestle's UHT Milk and Slim Milk venturing into the market. Amul, in response, has entered the Nagpur and Pune markets — earlier, its polypacks were available only in Gujarat and Mumbai — and its long-life tetrapack milk is said to be doing very well in milk–deficit areas like Kolkata, the Northeastern states, Andamans, etc.

Health concerns may have led to a sluggish 6-7 percent growth in the butter market, but that hasn't deterred Britannia from taking on the Amul bull by its horns. Amul still commands nearly 75-80 percent of the national market as the only all-India brand, while local products like Parag (Uttar Pradesh), Verka (Punjab), Vijaya (Andhra), Vita (Haryana), etc. account for between 3-6 percent. Though a senior Amul official refuses to recognise Britannia as competitor, the GCMMF is trying to protect its turf by launching new varieties like salt- and colour-free cooking butter.

If the Amul presence in these three product categories — as also the slow growth milk powder sector, where its Amulya brand has competition from Britannia's Milkman and Nestle's Everyday—is well entrenched, areas like ice-creams and chocolates present pictures less in its favour. The chocolate market, for instance, is heavily tilted in favour of Cadbury. More than 60 percent of the 20,000-tonnes, Rs. 3.5 billion chocolate market belongs to the MNC, while another 32.8 percent is bagged by Nestle, leaving just five percent for Amul.

Then there's ice-creams. According to an independent market research agency, A C Neilson, HLL's Kwality-Walls has 38.6 share of the market in five metros (Delhi, Mumbai, Kolkata, Hyderabad and Bangalore) that account for more than 60 percent of the Indian ice-cream market, compared to Amul's 16.5 percent. Under an agreement between the GCMMF and the NDDB, Amul initially stayed away from the Delhi market, though used

Mother Dairy's manufacturing facilities to cater to the northern market. Then suddenly, one day, Kurien decided to enter the Delhi market. A simple incident, but it probably tells the story that few care to analyse. Not high ideals, not management philosophy, not even farmers' interests vs market forces. This could just be a turf war with terribly high stakes.

Milk and Milk Product Market

Cooperatives, the world over, have started restructuring themselves. The McKinsey Quarterly of 2002, volume 3, has a detailed analysis on how cooperatives in other parts of the world are performing. The message is that the road ahead will be rocky, and cooperatives should strengthen their vehicles to be able to take this journey, rather than be obsessed with the road behind. The article called "A value culture for Agriculture" says "cooperatives (in the United States) handle $ 121 billion annually…With a few notable exceptions, they destroy value — nearly $ 2 billion in 1999 and 2000 — and the destruction continues through both the high and low phases of the agricultural cycle. Cooperatives must create value to survive. Successful cooperatives focus on a clear need or a discrete customer group, use scale to deliver their products and services efficiently to their target markets, and hold themselves to high performance targets. Performance management and reformed operations promote a virtuous cycle of value creation. Combined with new-generation approaches to equity trading and a new, competitive mind-set, these measures can ensure that cooperatives adapt to and thrive in the changed agribusiness industry."

One of the examples of reform the article talks about is the "Fonterra Co-operative Group, created in 2001 through the merger of New Zealand's largest dairy coops and the Dairy Board (also ultimately owned by farmers), shows the power of consolidation. In the 1980s, New Zealand had more than 50 coops, but by 2000 consolidation had cut their number to 4, bringing improvements in productivity and farmers' earnings. Dairy farmers recognised that further mergers could provide the scale of investment required to complete in global markets. With aggressive move such as a joint venture (announced in March 2002) with Nestle, Fonterra is expected to have annual sales of some $ 1.4 billion. It is poised to become a leader in the global dairy industry." The Fonterra model is not necessarily the model for Indian cooperatives to adopt, but it is a pointer to radical steps that cooperatives are taking in order to survive and create value for their members. NDDB has crafted its own model, taking the realities of the Indian situation into account. This is obviously not the most perfect solution, but all in business know the imprudence of waiting for the most perfect solution to emerge, in the fullness of time — while competition steadily gains ground, and achieves the critical mass it needs to destroy others business! NDDB has to try hard to invest and implement the new cooperative model for the new competitive world.

It would not be out of place to mention here the example of New Zealand where dairy industry is based on a cooperative structure, with some 14,000 farmers owning the processing plants. The Dairy Board, which is the sole exporter has a network of 80 countries through which the Board markets one million tons of milk products each year. Interestingly, New Zealand has only two percent share in world milk production, but is still the largest exporter of dairy products. Their manufacturing technology is advanced and they are already marketing more than 800 different dairy products. The New Zealand Dairy Board sees tremendous potential in India in the future for finished specialised milk products, milk proteins, substitutes for vegetable proteins, gelatine, egg-whites, and the high-calcium nutritional 'Analine' at an appropriate time.

Gujarat Picture

The branded fresh milk market is on the boil. While the entry of MNCs like Britannia and Nestle is heating up the estimated Rs. 10,000 crore fresh milk market, cooperatives venturing out across the state borders are posing tough competition to the existing players. The eight-nine lakh litres per day Ahmedabad market is already in the midst of a milk-war, with existing players slashing prices and offering freebies to the consumers to counter entry of new players.

While the MP cooperatives 'Sanchi' and Mumbai-based Mahanand Dairy's 'Mahanand' brands have firmed up an entry, Rajasthan Cooperative Dairy Federation's (RCDF's) 'Saras' brand hit the city in May 2002 and ice-cream manufacturer Dairy Den's brand entered in August. Now, Ahmedabad has over a dozen brands. Market leader Amul has presently reduced prices of its toned milk 'Taaza' by Re. 1 per litre from Rs 14, while Dairy Den cut prices of three variants by Re. 1 to Rs 13 per litre.

Liquid milk is the biggest product category in food and has the largest share of the consumer's monthly food bill. Recently, cooperatives across the country have adopted a common brand design to differentiate their products from the private players. Though dominated by cooperatives, fresh milk is a lucrative business. It's a major cash generator. Being a perishable necessity commodity, it has no inventory cost and is unaffected by seasonal variations. Even though margins are low, the volumes are high and one can easily generate a good turnover.

With almost 35-40 percent of the milk market being catered to by loose milk, it offers a huge potential for new players. With growing consumers awareness, the milk market is seeing a shift from loose to pouched milk. Amul, which already has a presence in Mumbai, has made a foray into some cities of Rajasthan and Maharashtra and is eyeing Delhi. Britannia's Milkman, which has a presence in Delhi and Kolkata, is planning to enter Mumbai and other cities. Nestle, which has a presence in UHT long-shelf life milk, is also eyeing Delhi its Everyday brand. Nestle is learnt to be already present in and around Moga in Punjab, where it has a milk processing facility.

OPERATION FLOOD—A SUCCESS STORY

In the 1960s, India's major priority was to safeguard food supply for its rapidly expanding population. Annual milk output had stagnated at around 20 million tonnes. In the government's five-year plans, the development programmes initially focused on the urban conurbations. The buffaloes and cows required for milk production were brought in from the rural regions and housed in large production units on the edges of the cities, with the result that milk production in the rural regions continued to decline.

Twenty years earlier, a lively but still largely obscure cooperative movement, known as "Amul", had sprung up in Gujarat state around the city of Anand. In 1946, farmers there protested against their exploitation by middlemen, who bought low-price milk from the poor and generally landless milk producers in order to supply the city of Bombay 400 kilometers away. On the initiative of a respected local citizen of Anand — Sardar Vallbhbhai Patel, who later became deputy prime minister of India — 200 smallholder farmers set up a cooperative and began to market their milk themselves. The movement, which began with 250 litres of milk in 1946, has led to the establishment of a modern network of cooperatives with its own dairies and marketing structures.

In the mid 1960s, the central government in Delhi also became aware of the success of the Amul cooperatives in Gujarat. Following a visit by the Prime Minister to Anand in 1965, the National Dairy Development Board (NDDB) was set up with the task of launching the AMUL model nationwide. This marked the inception of "Operation flood". With support from the World Bank and especially the European Union, it evolved into what is probably the largest and most successful development programme, with India ultimately becoming the largest milk-producing country worldwide.

Over the years, OF has developed an infrastructure that harnessed the productive energies of about seventy million milk producers of India spread over 267 districts in 25 States and Union Territories (UTs) through a cooperative network covering above 70,000 village societies. Beneficiaries now, add over Rs. 50,000 million farmers every year, through the milk sale to village cooperatives. The spectacular achievement in the field of dairying during the last decade have disclosed that Indian dairy farming no longer is merely a traditional farming. Despite the best efforts and excellent outcome thereupon, the accomplishment of the task is skewed and unevenly distributed and the dairy development is showing inequity and imbalance from one region to another. For instance the per capita milk availability is as paltry as 20 g/day in the parts of the Eastern region as against a high of 400 g/day in Northern region while the bovine density in those regions is quite the reverse (Dairy India, 1997).

Operation Flood I (1970-81)

Operation Flood (OF) was the result of an organised attempt directed towards the development of the dairy industry in India. The programme laid emphasis on setting up of "Anand Pattern" rural milk producers' cooperative organisations to procure, process and market milk and to provide some of the essential technical input services for increasing milk production. In setting up dairy cooperatives, the OF sought to capitalize on the beneficial features of cooperatives. The cooperative would (i) provide farmer members an assured market for their output which is critical for a perishable commodity like milk, (ii) a farmer controlled support mechanism for delivering essential support services and (iii) enable farmers to directly share the benefits from the returns generated by the cooperative. The National Dairy Development Board (NDDB) was established to oversee the planning and implementation of the programme.

OF-I was launched in 1970 following an agreement with the World Food Programme (WFP), which undertook to provide as aid 126,000 tonnes of skim milk powder (SMP) and 42,000 tonnes of butter oil (BO) for financing the programme. The programme involved organising dairy cooperatives at the village level, providing the physical and institutional infrastructure for milk procurement, processing, marketing and production enhancement services at the union level and establishment of city dairies. The main thrust was to set up dairy cooperatives in the milksheds, so as to link them to the four metro cities of Mumbai, Kolkata, Delhi and Chennai, in which a commanding share of the milk markets were to be captured. The overall objective of Operation Flood I was to lay the foundation of a modern dairy industry in India which would adequately meet the country's need for milk and milk products.

Funds for Operation Flood I were generated by the sale of SMP and BO. A total of Rs. 116.54 crore was invested in the implementation of the programme. The achievements of Operation Flood I are indicated in Table 5.10. By its end, about 13,300 dairy cooperative societies (DCS) in 39 milksheds were organised, enrolling 18 lakh farmer members. It achieved a peak milk procurement of 34 lakh litres per day (llpd) and marketing of 28 Lakh lpd.

Operation Flood II (1981-85)

The background of the institutional framework of OF-II essentially comprised the successful replication of the Anand Pattern – a three-tier cooperative structure of societies, unions and federations. OF-II was designed to build on the foundation already laid by OF-I and the IDA-assisted dairy development projects in Karnataka, Rajasthan and Madhya Pradesh. The programme was approved by the Government of India, for implementation during the Sixth Plan period, with an outlay of Rs. 273 crores. About US$ 150 million was provided by the World Bank and the balance in the form of commodity assistance from the European Economic Community (EEC).

OF-II helped to market milk in about 148 cities and towns, with a total population of 15 million, through a national milk grid, linking these towns and cities to 136 rural milksheds. The project expanded the number of village cooperatives societies to 34,500, covering 36 lakh farmer members.

The peak milk procurement increased to a level of 79 lakh litres per day and milk marketing to 50 lakh litres per day. The achievements of Operation Flood II are provided in Table 5.10.

Table 5.10: Operation Flood at a Glance

Parameters	1971	Phase I	Phase II	Phase III			Target
		1981	1985	1990	1994	1995	1996
Number of milksheds	5	39	136	170	170	170	170
Number of DCS ('000)	1.6	13.3	34.5	60.8	67.32	69.60	70.0
Number of farmer members (lakh)	2.8	17.5	36.3	70.0	86.9	90.0	**
Average milk procurement (lkgpd)	5.2	25.6	57.8	98.1	111.45	102	115
Peak milk procurement (lkgpd)	6.5	34.0	79.0	120.0	130.0	116	140
Processing Capacity:							
Rural dairies (llpd)	6.8	35.9	87.8	140.3	167.5	167.5	193.7
Metro dairies (llpd)	10.0	29.0	35.0	37.9	38.8	52.30	72.40
Milk Marketing:							
Metro dairies (llpd)	NA	21.8	29.5	30.6	32.34	35.0	38.0
Other cities & towns (llpd)	0.9	6.1	20.6	41.9	53.90	59.0	62.0
Total marketing	NA	27.9	50.1	72.5	86.24	94	100.0
Milk drying capacity (t/d)	NA	261.0	507.5	663.0	831.5	842	974
Milk powder production ('000 tonnes/year)*	22.4	76.5	102.0	165.0	185.0	195.0	**
Technical Inputs:							
Number of AI Centres ('000)	NA	4.9	7.5	10.9	15.12	16.28	16.50
Number of AI done (lakh)	NA	8.2	13.3	30.1		37.9	39.5
Cattle feed capacity ('000 tonnes/day)	NA	1.7	3.3	4.3	4.7	4.9	5.0
Investments (Rs crore)	NA	116.54	277.17	411.59	690.60	896.21	1303.10

* Including production by cooperative and other dairies.
** Target already achieved.
Source: Basic Animal Husbandry Statistics, 1997

Operation Flood III (1985-96)

The third phase aimed at consolidation of the gains of earlier phases. The main focus of the programme was on achieving financial viability of the milk unions/state federations and adopting the salient institutional characteristics of the "Anand Pattern" cooperatives. The OF III programme was funded by a World Bank credit loan of US $ 365 million, Rs. 222.6 crore of food-aid (75,000 tonnes of milk powder and 25,000 tonnes of butter/butter oil) by the EEC and Rs. 207.7 crore by NDB's own resources. The programme covered some 170 milksheds of the country by organising 70,000 primary dairy cooperatives societies. The World Bank has granted provisional extension of OF-II credit up to April 30, 1996. Its major emphasis was to consolidate the achievements gained during the earlier phases by improving the productivity and efficiency of the cooperative dairy sector and its institutional base for its long-term sustainability. Investments in OF-III were focussed on strengthening the institutional management aspects of dairy cooperatives at its various levels to establish financially strong farmer owned and managed organisations.

Table 5.11 Resources and Fund Outlay of Operation Flood III (1987-96)

Rs. crores

Resources	
NDDB's own resources	207.7
External Assistance	
World Bank	872.8
EEC	222.6
Total	1,303.1
Component-wise fund outlay	
Processing facilities	634.6
Technical input for milk production	89.4
Milk marketing systems	359.7
Support to village cooperatives	101.2
Planning, information system, market promotion, training & research	52.5
National milk grid and stabilisation	34.8
Disease control and progeny testing etc.	30.9
Total	1,303.1

The OF-III also had provision for productivity-enhancement inputs and institutional strengthening in the form of training, research, market promotion, monitoring and evaluation. Particular emphasis was placed on institutional and policy reforms. Efforts were made to expand infrastructure in all major markets, linking them to milksheds through the National Milk Grid (NMG) to ensure year-round stable milk supply. Marketing thus becomes the driving force to improve procurement and strengthen the financial viability of the unions. The role of NMG is crucial in ensuring the availability of milk to consumers and a remunerative price to milk producers by levelling out regional and seasonal imbalances in supply and demand. Marketing of indigenous milk products forms an important part of the overall marketing strategy.

Operation Flood was a movement of some 9.88 million rural families, who were the primary members of milk cooperatives, and who by their income from milk were progressively able to improve their standard of living. As in March 1998, about 77,531 dairy cooperatives societies (DCS) had been organised in 170 milksheds which procured 12.9 million kg of milk per day and marketed over million litres per day of liquid milk in over 600 cities and towns. Milk processing capacity of 168 litres pd and milk powder production capacity of 842 tonnes/day had been established. To operate the NMG and balance regional and seasonal fluctuations in milk procurement and marketing, some 1,108 road/rail milk tankers have been provided for long distance transportation of liquid milk. Adequate storage facilities have also been set up (33,750 tonnes for milk powder and 4,280 tonnes for butter) to facilitate the operation of the NMG. With the increase in the production of milk and milk products, the country has been achieving a greater degree of self-reliance than before. To stabilize the domestic prices of milk and milk products, and exploit any export potential for Indian dairy products, the Government has recognised the NDDB as the canalising agency for export.

For improving the productivity of dairy cattle and thereby milk production, the OF programme provided animal health and breeding facilities. Nearly 40,313 DCS have been covered with the animal health programme, while 16,280 DCS are provided with artificial insemination facilities. The bypass protein feed, developed by NDDB, has now been increasingly adopted by farmers. This increases the protein conversion efficiency of the cattle feed by 33 per cent and dry matter conversion by 30 per cent and minimises the dry matter requirement for milk production by 24 per cent. The treatment of straw with urea, a cheap and simple technique to raise the nutritional level of the straw, is being promoted. Feeding of urea-treated straws reduces the concentrate requirement by 33 per cent, minimises wastage of straw and improves animal health. These technologies have implications on lowering the cost of milk production and, thereby, maximising returns to farmers. Balanced cattle feed compounding capacity of 4,905 tonnes/day has been set up and currently some 34,576 DCS are marketing cattle feed to their farmer members. The bypass protein technology has been introduced in 17 cattle feed plants, the feed being marketed through 5,943 DCS. In addition, eight urban molasses block plants with a total capacity of 72 tonnes/day have been established.

Processing Facilities

It is estimated that by 2000, some 290 llpd equivalent of rural milk processing facility with about 1075 tonnes/day of milk powder manufacturing capacity was created. To facilitate the procurement of milk from the hinterland milksheds, an additional chilling capacity of 28 llpd has been set up either by expansion or creation of new chilling plants. Milk conservation facilities have an important role in balancing seasonal fluctuations in production. The experience of both a good and a bad year has brought out the need to provide buffer stock of conserved milk solids. Processing and conservation facilities must not only precede procurement buildup, but must be at a higher level than any anticipated peak procurement. This alone can ensure the member's confidence in the cooperatives since milk offered by them must be collected.

Marketing Infrastructure

Marketing facilities for milk and milk products has been expanded to 100 llpd by the end of third phase. An incremental 44 llpd capacity has been set up by expanding the existing rural and metro dairies. As the fluid milk markets expands through the cooperative sector, it has become necessary to progressively provide the consumers greater choice and convenience in terms of packaging. With this objective, the cooperatives will be marketing milk in a variety of packages and qualities. The mode of liquid milk distribution will be mainly through sachets and bulk vending system. Financial viability and sustainability of the cooperative structure would depend upon more efficient marketing and distribution of milk and milk products by developing a suitable product mix.

Village Cooperatives

The milk production is largely the domain of the economically weaker sections of the rural population, and they stand to benefit more from Operation Flood. More and more farmers are becoming member of the milk producers cooperative societies, and there is an upward trend in the overall milk procurement (Table 5.12). This phenomenon indicates that dairy farmers are being offered remunerative prices. The producer price of milk has increased by 10 per cent per annum during the period from 1991-

Table 5.12: Trends in Overall Milk Production

Particulars	1991-92	1992-93	1993-94	2000-01 (target)
Milk production (million tonnes)	55.7	57.8	60.6	81.4
Average milk procurement (lkgpd)	93.66	105.67	111.45	157.2
Farmer-members (lakh)	79.45	83.71	86.90	108.07
Producer price (Rs/litre)	5.13	5.96	6.17	N.A
Wholesale price index (for all commodities) at 1981-82 prices	207.5	228.7	247.8	363.1*

lkgpd: lakh kilogram per day.
*Till December, 2000 relates to 1999-2000.
Source: Govt. of India, Ministry of Agriculture, Deptt. of Animal Husbandry & Dairying: Annual Report 2000-2001.

92 to 1993-94, as compared to only 9.7 per cent in the increase in wholesale price index. Of has been successful in spreading the dairy cooperative concept and providing an important demonstration effect on the potential for dairy development in India.

Technical Inputs

Efforts have been made through a Technology Mission on Dairy Development to optimise the use of available inputs and infrastructure facilities established through the OF programme and the State Governments. Animal health care and cattle feed are the inputs most readily accepted and adopted by rural milk producers. OF has been successful in spreading the dairy cooperative concept and providing an important demonstration effect on the potential for dairy development in India. In its 25 years, Operation Flood has replicated the cooperative model in more than 200 districts. As on 31 March 1998, 9.9 million member farmers (estimated to be more than one third of the total dairy farmers) were supplying 12.9 million tonnes of milk to 77,531 milk cooperative societies, who in turn delivered the milk to 170 milk unions for processing and marketing.[1] In addition, the programme provide training, extension, animal health, and artificial insemination services to its members and the NDDB, through its research institutes, conducts livestock research.

The OF-III programme has set up an additional cattle feed production capacity. Considering the current rate of increase in cattle feed utilisation, seven new plants have been set up and five existing ones expanded. The use of urea molasses block (UMB) as feed supplement increases the digestibility of fodder and reduces quantity of concentrate feeding. All the new DCS organised have been covered with the first-aid programme and efforts were made to improve the training and supervision of the village-level first-aid workers.

Artificial Insemination

Similarly, the AI network of the State/Central government was linked to the cooperatives. Through Operation Flood, the AI facilities were expanded to an additional 16,280 DCS. Semen production stations strengthened and the liquid nitrogen production and distribution system expanded. In the area where AI services cannot be reached, arrangements were made to provide quality bulls for breeding purposes.

Breeding

The existing bull mother farms for producing exotic and crossbred bulls were strengthened to produce adequate number of breeding bulls. The programme also undertakes a sire evaluation programme for crossbred and

---

[1]National Dairy Development Board: 1999.

buffalo bulls at 10 semen production centres. A bull-calf rearing programme has been undertaken to speed up the availability of superior breeding bulls for AI and natural service.

Fodder Development

The programme also envisaged implementing silvipasture schemes for improvement of fodder availability. Silvipastures were developed on about 18,652 hectares of land. The silvipasture programme was implemented both on community waste lands (Gram vans) and on the marginal lands of individual farmers (Kisan vans). About 1,670 hectares of community land and 16,982 hectares of farmers' individual land were developed through this programme.

FMD Control

A provision has been made in the programme for Foot-and-Mouth Disease (FMD) control in selected milksheds to minimise economic losses to milk producers. The programme supports vaccination campaign against FMD and supply of FMD vaccine by creation of cold chain facilities for vaccine storage and handling and for extension service for increased farmers awareness. The Government programme covers a very limited area and vaccines are provided free of cost. Through Operation Flood the cost of vaccines is being progressively recovered from the farmers availing this facility. The facilities created in the FMD Control Laboratory at the Indian Immunologicals, Hyderabad have been strengthened. The programme also continues to support the FMD control project in the Southern States.

Applied Research and Development

The applied research and development activities in animal productivity, product development and dairy process engineering were focussed towards ensuring better returns to the farmers. In order to progressively minimise the input costs and, thereby, the cost of milk production, the programme will carry out applied research for better management of dairy animals, reared by cooperative dairy farmers in rural areas.

Financing Operation Flood III

Financial support for Operation Flood was generated largely through the sale of recombined milk (processed from skim milk powder and butter oil) provided by the Food and Agriculture Organization of the United Nations and the European Union, five World Bank project loans, and government expenditure. During 1971-92 the food aid received by the NDDB included 411,170 tonnes of skim milk powder, 15,380 tonnes of whole milk powder, 110,940 tonnes of butter oil, and 34,000 tonnes of butter (Table 5.13). Valued at world market prices, these contributions total at least US$ 1.15 billion in 1990 dollar terms (Table 5.14). The programme also received World Bank loans for dairy projects, which in real terms (1990 dollars)

Table 5.13: Total Volume and Estimated Value of Food Aid to NDDB, 1971-1992

Year	Skim milk powder			Whole milk powder			Butter oil			Butter		
	Vol. 000 mt	Price/mt	Value $000	Vol '000 mt	Price/mt	Value $'000	Vol 000 mt	Price/mt '000 mt	Value $000	Vol '000 mt	Price/mt	Value $000
1971	6.28	595	3734	0		0	2.29	Na		0		
1972	9.98	610	6090	0		0	2.45	Na		0		
1973	11.98	692	8290	0		0	3.71	Na		0		
1974	9.05	965	8730	0		0	4.28	Na		0		
1975	10.56	1243	13125	0		0	3.21	Na		0		
1976	26.86	1102	29597	0		0	7.17	Na		0		
1977	17.63	1464	25814	0		0	1.78	Na		0		
1978	7.82	708	5534	0		0	4.68	Na		0		
1979	22.40	386	8654	0		0	6.04	Na		0		
1980	31.15	975	30367	0		0	12.29	1875	23046	1	1525	1955
1981	18.81	1035	19470	0		0	9.37	2400	22495	1	2125	1806
1982	77.44	938	72600	0		0	14.04	2353	33017	4	2146	8514
1983	37.57	745	27992	0		0	9.33	1975	18429	3	1771	6123
1984	7.70	663	5098	0		0	0.60	1580	946	1	1360	816
1985	48.97	666	32626	0		0	15.86	1283	20339	6	1013	6501
1986		738	0	9.52	930.00	8849.88	2.81	1200	3376	3	1000	3492
1987		840	0	5.86	962.50	5639.29	0.34	1200	413	1	1000	800
1988	22.00	1588	34925	0		0	3.03	1481	4491	6	1250	7574
1989	17.99	1750	31483	0		0	1.66	2013	3331	7	1775	12982
1990	14.99	1425	21362	0		0	0.00	1625	0	0	1375	0
1991	0.00	1425	0	0		0	1.00	1669	1669	0	1413	0
1992	11.99	1681	20165	0		0	0.00	1644	0	0	1363	0
Total	411.17		315924	15.38		14489.17	110.94		131551.46	34		50564

Source: Volume of food aid are from NDDB, Commodity prices are from FAO (1971-79) and GATT, "The World Market for Dairy Products, International Dairy Arrangement" various issues. GDP deflators (1990-100) are from the IMF, International Financial Statistics Yearbook, various issues.

amounted to US$ 1.13 billion. Since the loans covered only 70 percent of programme costs, the NDDB received an additional grant from the government of about US$ 480 million (1990 dollars). During 1974-90, government diary expenditures (under the 5th through 7th Five Year Plans) amounted to equivalent of US$ 1.5 billion (1990 dollars). NDDB projects had also privileged access to preferentially loan terms and interest rates and other grants from the Government of India. Not counting the interest on state subsidies, Operation Flood had received at least US 3 billion, in real terms subsidies (US$ 1.5 billion in food aid), US$ 480 million in grants and US$ 1.5 billion in government spending).[1]

Table 5.14: Food Aid Received by the NDDB (millions of 1990 dollars)

Year	Skim milk powder	Whole milk powder	Butter oil	Butter	Total
1971	18.27	0.00	NA	0.00	18.27
1972	26.75	0.00	NA	0.00	26.75
1973	31.05	0.00	NA	0.00	31.05
1974	27.72	0.00	NA	0.00	27.72
1975	42.58	0.00	NA	0.00	42.58
1976	90.36	0.00	NA	0.00	90.36
1977	75.43	0.00	NA	0.00	75.43
1978	15.89	0.00	NA	0.00	15.89
1979	21.56	0.00	NA	0.00	21.56
1980	67.67	0.00	51.36	4.36	123.39
1981	39.36	0.00	45.47	3.65	88.49
1982	136.65	0.00	62.15	16.03	214.82
1983	48.55	0.00	31.96	10.62	91.13
1984	8.23	0.00	1.53	1.32	11.08
1985	49.00	0.00	30.55	9.76	89.32
1986	0.00	12.48	4.76	4.92	22.17
1987	0.00	7.33	0.54	1.04	8.90
1988	42.00	0.00	5.40	9.11	56.51
1989	34.85	0.00	3.69	14.37	52.90
1990	21.36	0.00	0.00	0.00	21.36
1991	0.00	0.00	1.47	0.00	1.47
1992	16.09	0.00	0.00	0.00	16.09
Total	813.37	19.81	238.88	75.18	1147.23

NA = Not available.
Source: World Bank India Livestock Sector Review: Enhancing Growth and Development.

---

[1]World Bank: India Livestock Sector Review: Enhancing Growth and Development: Report NO. 14522-IN, May 23, 1996.

Impact of Operation Flood and Role of Dairy Development in Alleviation of Poverty and Hunger in Rural India

The inauguration of Operation Flood corresponded to a turnaround in per capita incomes, which had been falling to a period of sustained, if modest, growth. Rising per capita incomes, together with rising population and a high-income elasticity of demand for milk, resulted in a rapid growth in the demand for milk (technically, a rapid shift in the demand function for milk). In the absence of supply side adjustment this would have led to a rapid escalation in the price of milk or the need for extensive imports. In fact, the shift in the supply function from policy changes introduced with Operation Flood resulted in an even larger shift in the supply (function) and declining real prices.

The overall expansion of the dairy industry from the early 1970s has been comparable to the more widely recognized Green Revolution crops of wheat and rice. Two key policy changes which accompanied the decision to provide direct financial assistance to the cooperatives to develop the dairy industry were the ending of direct efforts by the public sector to promote dairy production and the decision to sell dairy food aid at commercial prices within India. Both of these changes reduced the price risks for farmers, small-scale milk traders and private processors. Crossbreeding of local cows with specialized dairy breeds provided the technology for rapid increases in the milk production, and Operation Flood provided the example of large scale modern milk processing fed by a well-organized milk shed procuring milk from a large number of producers in very small amounts (1 and 2 liters). The actual volume of milk handled by Operation Flood remains a small fraction of the increased supply. It is thus not possible to attribute increased production simply to the dairy processing, marketing infrastructure, and technical support provided by Operation Flood directly (important though these contributions have been). Rather, one has to look to the changed dairy policy environment that accompanied the decision supporting Operation Flood. The policy was promising because of its probable production impact, but even more because of its capacity to reach the poor. Present position regarding Dairy Development is shown in Table 5.15 & 5.16.

A byproduct impact of Operation Flood and the accompanying dairy expansion has been the establishment of an indigenous dairy equipment manufacturing industry (only 7 per cent of dairy equipment is now imported) and an impressive body of indigenous expertise that includes animal nutrition, animal health, artificial insemination (AI), management information systems (MIS), dairy engineering, food technology, and the like. For AI, milk-testing, and village society sectoral services, Operation Flood trained villagers to a high degree of competence and thus controlled costs. It capitalized on rural India's ample supply of very low cost labour. This indigenous infrastructure explains in large part why milk processing and marketing costs of Operation Flood have not exploded in the face of having to procure and account for minute quantities of milk.

Table 5.15: Achievement of Some of the Key Components of Dairy Development in Different States Under Cooperative Sector As On 31-3-1998

S.l	Name of the state	DCS organised (no.)	Farmer members ('000)	Rural Milk procurement ('000 kg./Day)	Milk marketing ('000 LD)	Processing capacity Liquid Milk ('000L/Day)	Powder (MT/D)
1.	A & Nicobar	–	–	–	–	5	–
2.	Andhra Pradesh	5108	710	748	623	2397	126.0
3.	Assam	123	2	3	6	60	–
4.	Bihar	2737	143	211	242	586	12.5
5.	Delhi	–	–	–	1199	1150	–
6.	Goa	155	17	25	71	75	–
7.	Gujarat	12132	2039	3989	1576	6960	453.0
8.	Haryana	2630	166	199	62	530	25.0
9.	Himachal Pradesh	254	15	16	22	30	–
10.	J & K	–	–	–	–	10	–
11.	Karnataka	7871	1499	1474	1299	2030	37.0
12.	Kerala	1509	419	317	366	410	10.0
13.	Madhya Pradesh	4601	237	196	227	1030	30.0
14.	Maharashtra	6387	1174	2210	2168	3970	60.0
15.	Nagaland	35	1	1	1	–	–
16.	Orissa	1268	92	77	92	125	–
17.	Pondicherry	85	24	31	39	50	–
18.	Punjab	6175	362	739	373	1460	100.5
19.	Rajasthan	5413	390	661	361	1050	60.0
20.	Sikkim	162	5	7	7	15	–
21.	Tamil Nadu	7775	1888	1156	1381	2421	70.0
22.	Tripura	84	4	1	5	10	–
23.	Uttar Pradesh	11568	597	673	356	1140	60.0
24.	West Bengal	1459	91	160	650	1570	10.0
	Total	77531	9875	12894	11126	27084	1054.0

Source: Dairy Division DAH&D

Table 5.16: Number of Dairy Plants, Statewise, Registered Under MMPO as on June 1, 1996

(Capacity '000 litre per day)

Sl	States	Cooperative		Private		Others		Total	
		No.	Capacity	No.	Capacity	No.	Capacity	No.	Capacity
1.	Andhra Pradesh	13	2905	12	1068	1	200	26	4173
2.	Bihar	6	485	0	0	0	0	6	485
3.	Delhi	0	0	0	0	9	1600	9	1600
4.	Goa	1	30	0	0	0	0	1	30
5.	Gujarat	17	6280	2	300	7	670	26	7250
6.	Haryana	5	400	34	4050	2	130	41	4580
7.	Himachal Pradesh	3	44	2	345	0	0	5	389
8.	Karnataka	12	1733	4	395	1	400	17	2528
9.	Kerala	10	570	0	0	2	35	12	605
10.	Madhya Pradesh	8	1230	3	650	2	20	13	1900
11.	Maharashtra	29	2819	43	3956	38	3395	110	10170
12.	Orissa	8	212	0	0	0	0	8	212
13.	Pondicherry	1	50	0	0	0	0	1	50
14.	Punjab	12	1530	21	3090	0	0	33	4620
15.	Rajasthan	12	1190	8	800	0	0	20	1990
16.	Sikkim	1	15	0	0	0	0	1	15
17.	Tamil Nadu	22	2242	3	130	1	0	26	2372
18.	Tripura	1	10	0	0	0	0	1	10
19.	Uttar Pradesh	31	2246	115	9558	0	0	146	11804
20.	West Bengal	2	216	3	90	2	820	7	1126
	Total	194	24207	250	24432	65	7270	509	55909

Source: Dairy Division, DAH&D

For those landless people who own or have been able to purchase a milch animal (a cow or buffalo), it has been a boon. Of course, those who are both cowless and landless have only been slightly affected by some of the social programmes supported by the village Dairy Cooperative Societies (DCSs) out of their profit and by the increased prosperity of the village economies. Operation Flood, in collaboration with NGOs, has established 6,000 women's dairy cooperative societies (WDCSs) and generated higher incomes for some women. Indirectly, it has increased the number of children attending school because of the high-income elasticity of demand for education in Indian villages. This project has produced diverse results on the ground and a few clear signals.

1. A well conceived investment project in support of an already adopted and appropriate policy change can help achieve results out of all proportion to the investment involved. This occurs in part because it solves the "ownership" problem, in part because it avoids having to

create an institution at the same time that the new institution is being expected to implement the project.

2. By raising incomes, an apparently simple single commodity project can have multiple beneficial effects, including nutrition, education (especially of girls), and job creation.

3. By focusing a project on a predominant activity of the poor, "self selection" is likely to result in a major portion of the beneficiaries being poor. This provides an alternative to "targeted" projects for reaching the poor.

The lessons from the Operation Flood in India stand out and point to an approach different from the traditional and conventional one of exclusive species and discipline oriented approach in livestock programmes. The production of some five lakh villages flows as a flood of 100 million liters for urban consumers every day. The flood has empowered producers at the grassroot with 70 million farmers maintaining an almost 100-million strong milch herd (57 million cows and 39 million buffaloes). Per capita availability of milk, which was 132 gm a day in 1950, has reached around 233 gm a day now.

In 1994-95, milk became India's number-one farm commodity in terms of value of output. Out of every 100 liters of milk produced, 44 was retained by the rural folk, 56 liters was the marketable surplus for the urban areas. Out of these 56 liters, only 10 liters was handled by the organized sector (cooperative, public and private) and the remaining 46 liters by the traditional sector. Which means there is still scope for progress not just in terms of quality and productivity but also distribution patterns.

It is estimated that 70 to 75 percent of the households possessing milk cattle belong to the vulnerable category of small and marginal farmers and landless agricultural labour. A bulk of the total rural dairy households own one or two milch animals. A survey by the National Council of Applied Economic Research in 1991 found that 43 percent of the number of households of milk producer cooperative societies in "Operation Flood" areas has only one milch animal and almost 75 percent of the members belonged to the category of landless labourers and marginal and small farmers. These households contributed over 60 percent of the milk output in the "Operation Flood" areas.

A village enumeration survey conducted by the National Dairy Development Board in 1984 covering nearly six million households in 20,386 dairy cooperative villages spread over 108 milksheds in the country, also confirmed the importance of the landless, small and marginal farmers in the ownership of the milch animals. Some 72 percent of the families owning milch animals belonged to landless and marginal and small farmers. The vulnerable group of families accounted for about 61 percent of the total buffaloes and cows in the survey area. Nearly 60 percent of the total rural households owned generally two or three milch animals. Only the large farmers having 4 hectares or more of land holding kept more than four milch animals.

Operation flood was not an all-purpose poverty removal programme. It could not be, because it focused clearly on a single activity, dairying, while the ranks of the rural poor include many different categories of the disenfranchised: the old, the infirm, the tribals, the landless, the small farmers, the artisans and so forth. Similarly, Operation Flood is not all-purpose development programme, aimed at removing economic and social inequalities existing in rural India for centuries at one stroke. However, the Operation Flood programme has achieved immense success as revealed in the expansion of the dairy industry in India. In addition to the assured market for milk produced by small farmers under the Operation Flood, several other factors have contributed to its success. These include increased demand resulting from increasing incomes and population, improved technology including increased availability of straw from the Green Revolution and the adoption of crossed bred cattle.

Much of the milk collected under the Operation Flood programme initiated in 1974 would otherwise have been processed in the village. Of course, some milk comes from one or more additional cows being kept by farmers (or more accurately, their wives) or as a result of better husbandry. However, a proportion of the extra production came from women who were enabled to stay home to look after a newly purchased cow or buffalo and thus avoid the necessity to go out for work. Each such change opened up a job for someone else needing work. According to the World Bank's Impact Evaluation Report if even 5 percent of producers made this switch (unfortunately data to properly quantify this point is not available), this would represent the creation of 175, 000 jobs under the First and Second National Dairy Projects. According to the NDDB's estimates about 6.3 million were direct beneficiaries of Operation Flood. If however, beneficiaries were taken to include the families of these poorer the number would be about 32 million. Some of the benefits of the Operation Flood were undoubtedly enjoyed by larger farmers still in most cases (poor by any absolute standard), but there is strong evidence that the majority of beneficiaries were small and marginal farmers and was from "other backward castes".

Since 1974, there has been a tremendous impact of policy changes associated with Operation Flood on milk production in the country. More than 50 million tonnes more milk were produced in 1998 than would have been produced if the pre-1971 growth rate had continued. It has also a nutritional impact. Under the new policy, per capita milk consumption has risen from 107 grams/day in 1970 to 193 grams/day in 1994. The programme has also had clear benefits for the poor and women. For those landless people who own or have been able to purchase a milk animal (a cow or buffalo), it has been a boon. Operation Flood, in collaboration with NGOs, has established 6,000 women's dairy cooperative societies (WDCSs) and ensured higher income for some women. Indirectly, it has expanded the number of children attending school because of the high-income elasticity of demand for education in Indian villages.

Operation Flood, which helped develop the dairy sector in India, as mentioned above, was not designed an all-purpose poverty removal programme. However, by focusing on a predominant activity of the poor, the programme encouraged "self-selection. This seems to have resulted in a major portion of its beneficiaries being poor. The beneficial effects of higher incomes received from sale of milk by the landless, small and marginal farmers helped in relieving the worst aspect of poverty. The income flow from Operation Flood to villages is now massive. The annual payment by the cooperative system to farmers now averages about Rs. 3, 450 crores per annum. Allowing for both cash costs of milk production (especially cattle feed) and switching, perhaps a quarter of this (say Rs. 870 crores per annum) is net increased income. The village studies have identified faster growth of incomes in Operation Flood villages and higher levels of milk production. Operation Flood only handles about 6.3 percent of production, the extra cash flow to villages from the higher dairy growth rate approximates about Rs. 55,200 crores per year.[1] Investment in diary stock and recurrent cash costs are involved in the generation of this gross revenue at the village level. However, clearly cash flows of this magnitude can be expected to generate real poverty alleviation and linked benefits. Studies have shown that a many as 70 percent of milk suppliers belonged to the marginal and small farmers, together with some landless, so a large part of these benefits are reaching the very poor.

Based on these data and the NSSO's survey estimated on the number of in-milk cattle in rural India, an attempt is made here to indicate in broad terms the gross financial benefit derived by the vulnerable group of families in rural India from the dairy development programme in 1997/98. Total gross income from sale of milk for the 70 million vulnerable group of households consisting of landless labour, marginal and small farmers in rural India out of 130 million rural households, is estimated at Rs. 98, 000 crores in 1997/98.[2] Net profit per milch animal per year comes to Rs. 5,700 and per milch animal per month at Rs. 475. These are rather conservative estimates. This is clear from the Economics of New Dairy Unit consisting of 3 cow and 2 buffaloes, worked out by the VET HelpLine India, Pune. Their estimates indicate net profit per animal per year of Rs. 7,602.40 and net Profit per animal per month of Rs. 633.50 (see Annexure I).

---

[1]World Bank: Impact Evaluation Report on India-Karnataka and Rajasthan Dairy Development Project and the Madhya Pradesh, First and Second National Dairy Projects: Report No. 16848, 30 June 1997. P.11

[2]This rough estimates is based on the following assumptions: in 1997/98, total milch animals were 96 million, consisting of 57 million cows and 39 million buffaloes, of total milch animals about 90 percent were in rural areas. Total rural households were 130 million, of these 60 percent owned milch animals. Vulnerable group constituted about 75 percent of the total rural households and each vulnerable household owned on an average two milch animals each. The sale of milk of these groups is assumed to be 90 percent of each household milk output (3 percent is taken to be fed to calves and 7 percent for family consumption).

Livestock rearing seems to have played an important positive role in the alleviation of poverty and hunger in rural India. A study conducted on the subject revealed that the percent of population Below Poverty Lines as well as of undernourished reduces with those households who own cow, buffalo and cow & buffalo. This is true for submarginal, marginal and small farmers. For instance according to the NSSO 50th Round data (1993-94) in the case of submarginal farmers, those with no milching cattle, the proportion of persons Below the Poverty line was 42 percent, compared to 37 percent for those who have a cow, 30 percent both for those who possessed a buffalo and those who owned cow & buffalo (Table 5.17). In the case of small farmers, the respective figures were 24, 23 and 14 percent. Similarly the percent of undernourished population declined among all the three classes of farmers.

Table 5.17: Impact of Dairy Stock on Alleviation of Poverty and Hunger by Farm Size Group: Rural India

Farm Size	Livestock	Percent of Population		Food deficit of under-nourished (kcal./person/day)	Diet composition (Share of cereals in total dietary intake
		Below poverty line	Under -nourished		
Sub Marginal	None	42	40	325	78
	Cow	37	28	285	76
	Buffalo	30	22	276	71
	Cow & Buffalo	30	21	286	70
Marginal	None	33	32	307	77
	Cow	28	23	272	76
	Buffalo	21	17	232	69
	Cow & Buffalo	20	15	275	69
Small	None	24	25	302	75
	Cow	23	21	279	74
	Buffalo	14	12	236	66
	Cow & Buffalo	14	13	227	67

Source: National Sample Survey 50th Round: 1993-94: P. Kumar: F.A.O. Regional Office for Asia and the Pacific: Bangkok

DOMESTIC PROTECTION OF THE NASCENT DAIRY COOPERATIVE SECTOR

The Government of India undertook three measures to promote the development of the nascent dairy cooperative sector. Protected as an "infant industry", diary product imports were canalized through the NDDB until

1994 to shield the sector from competition from cheaper imports. Only imports in the form of food aid were allowed to enter the country and proceeds from the sale of food aid were appropriated exclusively by NDDB to finance its cooperative development efforts. In addition, domestic competition from the noncooperative private sector was limited by the Industrial Development and Regulation Act 1951, which restricted entry into the diary industry through licensing. In the context of liberalization, the licensing requirement was abandoned in 1991, only to be reintroduced in 1992 under the Milk and Milk Products Order (MMPO), in response to political pressure.

However, by the 1990s many cooperatives were performing poorly. A 1994 review conducted by the World Bank of 117 cooperatives receiving assistance under the World Bank National Dairy Project II found that 52 percent incurred losses (Table 5.18). Rajasthan recorded the worst performance, where all 17 cooperatives incurred losses. Cooperative losses amounted to Rs. 553 million in 1993 and Rs. 583 million in 1994 (Table 5.19). A major factor, which exacerbated the poor performance during 1993 and 1994, was the milk production surplus and the resulting crash in prices.

Table 5.18: Performance of Milk Cooperatives

State	Total no. of cooperatives	No. of cooperatives incurring losses	Percent incurring losses
Andhra Pradesh	11	9	81.8
Gujarat	20	2	10.0
Karnataka	14	7	50.0
Punjab	13	6	46.2
Rajasthan	17	17	100.0
Tamil Nādu	11	4	36.4
Uttar Pradesh	31	16	52.1
Total	117	61	52.1

Source: World Bank data

Table 5.19: Financial Performance of Sample Cooperative Unions: 1993 and 1994

Region	No. of unions		Losses (million rupees)	
	with losses	Total	1993	1994
Northern	16	61	- 151	- 302
Southern	19	37	- 336	- 232
Western	24	35	- 53	- 45
Eastern	3	14	- 13	- 4
Total	62	147	-553	-583

Source: World Bank Data

Inventory and interest costs and sales below production costs contributed to substantial losses in Punjab, Haryana, Uttar Pradesh, Rajasthan, Andhra Pradesh. Dairies with good liquid markets were less affected, and some capitalized on the low prices of skim milk powder to produce milk (Orissa, Mother Dairies, Kolkata and Delhi).

Government Policies Contributed to Weak Performance of Cooperatives

In order to protect both producer and consumer welfare, many states exercised considerable control over cooperative operations, including controls over input and output pricing and the appointment of state officials to cooperative management operations. These interventions, and thus the diversion from the original farmer-controlled concept, contributed to the poor performance of many cooperative unions. Social pricing policies implemented in some states resulted in negligible or zero processing margins. For example, government pricing of milk supplied to the cooperative federation in Tamil Nadu prevented profitable operations and the move to reduce the producer price in Karnataka in order to maintain profitable operations was blocked by the state government. In Maharashtra, the selling price was fixed if the union delivered supplies to the government dairy. In Andhra Pradesh and Karnataka, selling prices of the cooperative federations required government consultation.

Moreover, the poor management of the Cooperatives also contributed to poor performance. Besides state interventions, weak management and poor market orientation resulted in the poor economic performance of some cooperatives. Lack of flexibility in adopting to changing market conditions, poor quality control, overstaffing, underutilization of capacity due to the limited milk market, processing inefficiencies and weak marketing and commercial orientation further contributed to the poor financial performance of these cooperatives and resulted in their continued dependence on state financial transfers/subsidies. In some federations and unions, the frequent turnover of state appointed officials in Cooperative Boards and top management contributed to poor incentive structures and weak management commitment.

Nevertheless, Cooperatives have considerable potential to improve their performance. Continued protection of cooperatives will only sustain the inefficient operations of the poorly performing cooperatives, which in the long run will hurt both farmers and consumers. Introducing incentives that improve cooperative management and performance would help ensure the sustainability of cooperative operations and the continuous stream of benefits for farmers. Elimination of state interventions and closer adherence to the Anand Model, with greater farmer control of operations (rather than government control), and upgrading of skills in production, marketing, and financial management would help cooperatives meet the new marketing challenges. Improved cooperative performance would lead to increased profits for the cooperatives and permit greater returns to the member's investments. It will ensure sustainable operations and generate earnings for further productivity improving. This would enable cooperatives to compete on an equal basis with private entrepreneurs. It would also strengthen the cooperative's capacity to continue providing production-related and associated social services demanded by members.

In fact, the NDDB had tried to improve the management of cooperatives under the Cooperative Development Programme. By 1999, more than 100 unions had participated in the programme, which included problem-solving workshops, field-level training and orientation, and leadership training programmes. The NDDB had also created a marketing group to help unions develop in-house expertise and carried out market surveys to assess consumer preference and demand as it formulated a marketing strategy. The Board also provided financial and technical assistance to dairies for consumer education campaigns and was increasing efforts to market higher-value-added products. In view of the large number of poorly performing cooperatives, upgrading their management continues to be a major task requiring significant resources.

Delicensing of Dairy Processing Sector

In the late 1980s OF and the NDDB had come under increasing scrutiny as the private sector had lobbied for free entry into the dairy processing industry and reduced protection for the diary cooperatives. In July 1991 the GOI exempted the dairy processing industry from the 1951 Industries Development and Regulation Act. The Act had blocked the entry of private entrepreneurs and multinationals. Delicensing attracted considerable private investment into the dairy sector. By May 1994, 694 applications for investment had been received and 141 approvals were issued. As new private enterprises began operating some of the new entrants were accused of poaching into cooperative territory. Moreover, concerns about excessive capacity and charges of private trade misconduct (mainly the sale of adulterated or contaminated milk) prompted calls for the reintroduction of market controls. Consequently, in June 1992 the GOI promulgated the Milk and Milk Products Order. The enactment of the MMPO in June 1992 compromised the GOI's policy on liberalization. The MMPO reintroduced controls on the entry and operation of participants in the dairy industry. Several key features of the MMPO have important economic implications, as mentioned below:

1. All plants handling more than 10, 000 litres or producing milk products containing more than 500 kg., of milk solids a day are required to obtain a license from the MMPO controller. Those processing between 10, 000 litres and 75,000 liters/day or greater than 500 kg. but less than 3,750 kg of milk solids a day require state permission, while enterprises processing more than 75,000 litres/day or greater than 3,750 kg a day of milk solids require central government approval, with the license renewed every three year. In May 1993, the GOI amended the MMPO. The registration requirement was abolished for all units handling less than 75,000 liter a day or

3,750 kg a day of milk solids. The amendment also increased the license renewal term from three to five years.

2. New processors must develop their own milkshed or milk collection area and cannot encroach on cooperative milk sheds. If shortage of milk occurs in one area and milk needs to be procured from other areas, it can only be sourced through cooperative unions or the cooperative federation at prices set by the union or federation.

3. The processing of milk into higher-value products is banned during the lean summer months.

4. Licensed processors must submit information on stock, procurement, production and marketing to the government and allow it to enter and inspect private premises, with the power to seize stocks if necessary.

5. A Milk and Milk Products Advisory Board was set up to assist, aid and advise the central government on any matter concerning the production, manufacture, sale, purchase, and distribution of milk and milk products. Members of the board include representatives from the Ministry of Agriculture, Ministry of Industry, Ministry of Food Processing Industries, Ministry of Health and Family Welfare, National Dairy Development Board and National Cooperative Dairy Federation. The Board's powers range from managing supplies across regions and establishing standards to approving license applications for new dairy processing plants. As the Advisory Board was widely perceived as having an over-representation of farmer cooperative, in the May 1993 amendment, greater representation was allowed of the state government and consumer bodies in the implementation of the MMPO.

MMPO maintains barriers to increased competition and market efficiency. Though the increase in capacity threshold and other modifications have changed somewhat the perceptions of MMPO, several critical components of the order militate against operational efficiency and provide higher prices to milk producers.

First, the delineation of milksheds, or areas from which milk is collected, creates local monopolies (for cooperatives or for any new private enterprises). This reduces the incentives for increasing operational efficiency. For farmers, the local monopoly prevents access to higher prices that come with greater competition. Competition would increase producer prices and encourage processing firms to increase their operational efficiency. The producer prices would improve the incentives for farmers to undertake investments to increase productivity and product quality, such as genetic upgrading and improved feeding. The resulting increase in milk supply and quality in the long run will enable processing firms to diversify their product lines and process more higher-value-added products to meet increasing consumer demand. The implementation of MMPO has led to several problems. In U.P. for instance, despite the fact that cooperative processing capacity in some areas was far below the milk supply capacity of its milkshed, other private processors were not allowed to buy the excess milk.

Second, the condition that new entrants set up and develop their own milksheds imposes a higher investment cost on new firms, thus limiting the number of potential entrants to those with access to large amounts of capital. This provides an unfair advantage to cooperatives, who in the past have received considerable resources from the public sector in developing their own milksheds. Third, imposing barriers to private entry is not an efficient way of addressing problems regarding the sale of contaminated or adulterated products by private producers. Rather, more stringent enforcement of hygiene and sanitation standards will better address product quality problem directly. These require strengthening the regulatory and enforcement agencies for hygiene and sanitation. Finally, the provision of allowing government to dictate stock levels and to seize stocks during emergencies reduces the capacity of entrepreneurs for inter-seasonal arbitrage and enhances market uncertainty. Given that trade liberalization has increased domestic access to world markets and supplies this restriction does not seem legitimate.

The achievements and contributions of cooperatives to the development of dairy sector in India are laudable and remarkable indeed. However, after 25 years of their operation, the dairy cooperatives should no longer be treated as an **infant industry.** As in any sector that has reached maturity, promoting market competition it needed to ensure the development of a sustainable and efficient industry. Thus ensuring a level playing field for all participants and the elimination of any barrier to entry for any firm are necessary. It is essential to create the level playing field for all market participants in the dairy industry. For this the Government of India must take a package of measures. These include (I) Lifting of MMPO: (2) Eliminating all State Intervention in Cooperative operations and transfer full control of Cooperatives to farmer members. (3) Establish mechanism to monitor milk market to ensure fair competition and (4) Strengthen Public monitoring and enforcement of Hygiene Standards.

The issue of repeal of MMPO should be thoroughly discussed with all the parties concerned before taking the final decision. However, the arguments put forward by some politicians that the interest of the farmers and consumer will suffer and that the MMPO ensure partial safeguard on quality front, do not hold ground. The decision should be based on economic rationale rather than be influenced by the pressure of the vested cooperative lobby. The dairy industry needs to be liberalized and the Government should repeal the MMPO. The status of registrations under the MMPO as at Dec' 2000 is given in Table 5.20.

NESTLE MODEL

Another milk procurement model is that of Nestle, a Multinational Company, which is operating in Punjab and Haryana. Although there are no Cooperatives like the Anand system, Nestle model is more transparent, has motivated milk collectors, provides better extension service and the farmer is looked after much better. The future dairy development may find

*Table 5.20: **Status of MMPO Registrations***

Registering	Cooperatives		Private		Others+		Total	
Authority	No	Capacity*	No	Capacity	No	Capacity	No	Capacity
Central	138	257.9	100	196.19	34	63.90	272	517.69
State	74	26.04	290	104.95	30	9.10	394	140.09
Total	212	283.94	390	301.14	64	72.70	666	657.78

*Capacity in LLPD. + Include government dairies and the Mother Dairy Delhi
Source: DOAH&D, GoI

this model better replicated. The company has been allotted two milkshed areas for their two different factories at two different locations- one in Punjab for the Moga Unit and other for Samalkha Unit (Panipat) in Haryana under Milk and Milk Products Order, 1992 (MMPO) for the purpose of milk development and procurement. Moga Milkshed is having about 850,000 LPD (Lit. Per day) in flush season from 85,000 farmers and Samalkha 60,000 LPD (in flush) from about 6000 farmers. Samalkha Operation is small and new (4, 6 years old).

In each potential and viable village (of the allotted area) one farmer from every village is selected for the purpose of milk collection, called Agent who after a brief training is allotted the village 'milk agency'. All the materials for milk collection are given by the Nestle except the milk collection room. Agent is given a commission of about 2.5% of the value of milk collected. Milk is collected twice daily morning and evening at the centre in the farm coolers or aluminum cans. About 400 farm coolers at about 900 Agencies have been installed in Moga whereas there are 25 in Samalkha milkshed. Milk is lifted in double-jacketed tanker from bulk farm coolers and in LCVs (Light Commercial Vehicles) from about 150 agencies. It is then chilled at a centralized chilling centre in rented ice factory as a stopgap arrangement and then transported to the factory (after chilling at/below 4°C in double jacketed tankers. Proper record is generated for each activity to keep control for measurements purpose.

The System is upgraded on a continuous basis to improve working transparency, control and reduce the cost/expenses incurred on milk collection. Emphasis is given to provide best comparable milk prices with speedy payments. Other feature is farmer services. The Company provides most of the inputs required by the dairy farmer at the farmer's doorstep. Some inputs are provided at actual cost while others are subsidized or even free. All inputs like Veterinary Medicine, cattle feed, fodder seed, FMD Vaccine that are charged, directly procured from reputed companies thus eliminating the middle person's margin. While services for AI, Bull calves etc., are given on subsidy, farmer tows to animal fairs/ agricultural institute etc. are free of cost. Apart from this, focus is on the dissemination of farm tech know-how.

In conclusion, the government policy along with the efforts of the government, particularly the departments concerned with dairying, animal husbandry and veterinary services have played an important role in raising the productivity of Indian milch herd. The contribution of the cooperative sector has also been of great importance both in creating a market and in supporting farmers with technical inputs, e.g. feed, breeding and veterinary services. These technical inputs, made available under programmes like Operation Flood provided an impetus for the higher growth of dairy sector.

Foreign Students

"One end is moo, the other milk", Ogden Nash wrote rather dismissively about the cow. However, India's achievement on the dairying and other farm fronts is now attracting research students from the reputed international agriculture and rural development course at the American university of Cornell. A 40-member strong team comprising of 30 students and 10 faculty members from Cornell is crisscrossing the country which is the world's largest producer of milk and other agricultural products. While Cornell's course in international agriculture and rural development started over three decades ago, this is the first time students from the programme have come to India as part of their field work.

Hitherto, the two-week study course which is part of the curriculum was largely restricted Latin countries. Proximity and cost had influenced this decision, admits Prof Robert Blake, professor at the department of animal science and director of graduate studies. The course has an international mix of students coming from countries like Malaysia, Korea, the US and Europe. The visit to India would help the students gain a close view and appreciation about issues relating to Indian agriculture. Based on the interaction with a cross-section of farmers, agricultural scientists and others, there is a possibility for Cornell's students to explore collaborative research projects with agencies in India. India can provide inputs to the students to explore and this trip should throw up something interesting.

The success of both the cooperative sector (notably in milk and dairy products) and contract farming (through the experience of multinationals like Pepsico) indicates the potential in this field using two diametrically-different approaches.

DAIRY INDUSTRY AND WTO AGREEMENT

Of the total world trade of $10,000 million in milk and milk products, the share of India is a meagre $10 million only. This is despite the fact that cost of production of milk in India is the lowest in the world (about $ 21/- per 100 litres) followed by New Zealand. Incidentally, India and New Zealand are the only two countries without any subsidy component while most other countries subsidises the production of dairy products in one form of the other. Hence, there is an urgent need for the government to look into its policy of zero duty on the import of dairy products. The conventional indices of dairy industry suggest that our domestic dairy industry cannot survive in a regime of duty- free imports. Factors such as international prices of dairy products, producer and export subsidies offered by many advanced nations, exchange rates and cost of milk are the important parameters that have an influence on the competitiveness of the industry, and India has no control over them.

India had committed zero per cent base and bound rates of duty on imports of skimmed and full cream milk powders and 40 per cent on butterfat, cheese and whey under the WTO agreement. In contrast, the bound rate of duty for fresh milk and creak buttermilk and yoghurt was fixed at 100 to 150 percent. No other country except Singapore has agreed to zero duty. Bangladesh has tariffs on dairy products bound at 200 per cent, Pakistan at 100 per cent, Sri Lanka at 50 per cent, New Zealand at 12.8 per cent, Brazil at 31.5 per cent and Poland at 102 per cent with a weighted average base rate for 43 countries of 144 percent.

In addition to skim milk powder and whole milk powder, which are already under the OGL, India has shifted cheese, butter milk, whey, whole milk, curdled milk and acidified milk and cream to the OGL list. This means that subsidised exports from the advanced dairy nations of North America and Europe that depress the world market have already begun to depress our domestic prices, adversely affecting producers and the processing industry. Hence, it is imperative that we renegotiate India's base and bound rates of duty for all dairy products (SMP, FCMP, butter, butter oil and cheese in particular) on the one hand and work vigorously with those committed to free trade to reduce export subsidy by developed countries. Failure to do so would lead to slowing in the rate of growth in milk production, starting a vicious cycle where increased gaps between growing demand and supply will force India to import. As an emerging dairy nation we should press for the following in the renegotiations of the next round of WTO.

Import Duties There is a need to renegotiate our bound rates of duty of zero per cent on skimmed and whole milk powder to about 50-60 percent, keeping in view the global trends.

Special Safeguards (SSG) As most of the developed nations have SSG provisions for dairy products which they can impose either when prices fall below the trigger level or imports surge above a level, India should negotiate for SSG clause.

Export Subsidies During the reference period (1986-90) in the developed countries export subsidies on dairy products were much higher than during the 1990s; therefore, a 36 per cent reduction in subsidies does not result in significant reduction in subsidies. Therefore, there is a need for further reduction in the export subsidies to ensure a level playing field in international trade of dairy products.

SPS Measures Sanitary and phytosanitary measures have been used by countries as non-tariff barriers. Different countries use different scientific criteria and standards to decide about the quality and safety of the imported products. There is a need for common standards, which are not unnecessarily raised to unscientific level so as to become internationally mandated non-tariff barriers.

Multifunctional Role   Dairy for Indians is not just producing another litre of milk. A vibrant dairy industry ensures an alternate source of income to the farm families. It leads rural socioeconomic development.

India has a zero tariff for SMP and FCMP and comparatively low tariff for other dairy products. Cheap, subsidised imports of dairy products from developed countries are a matter of great concern. There is an urgent need for India to impose import tariffs for milk powders and other dairy products.

India's milk production is increasing annually by 5 per cent. With the availability of milk at very economical prices, many large MNCs have entered into the dairy segment in India. The only thing which needs to be looked into is the basic quality of produce. Efforts are being made by the domestic dairy industry to improve the basic quality as it is going to play a major role in the competitive market. Majority of the Indian dairies are preparing to obtain quality certification like ISO and Hazard Analysis Critical Control Point (Haccp). At least nine dairy units have already succeeded in obtaining the necessary quality certification. With this beginning being made on maintaining quality, perhaps India will be able to launch its products in other continents in a big way during the coming decades.

If we are to enter the world market India has to move from the 'White Revolution' to the Quality White Revolution. What success we have achieved has been because conditions were created where dairying became potentially remunerative for large numbers of our rural people. We did things that the mandarins of the international financial institutions and their acolytes in Delhi now feel are immoral or worse. We denied the market its role. It seems, from the record, that the dairy industries of the industrial nations are fairly well insulated from market forces. But what is good for the goose appears not good enough for the gander. We did insulate our market by channelling all dairy commodity imports through the Indian Dairy Corporation and then the National Dairy Development Board. This system has to be protected lest the goose that lays the golden egg be killed. Indian dairying has succeeded because it has deliberately evolved in a way that it is complementary and not in competition with agriculture.

Dairying employs those who are underemployed in agriculture. Our animals feed off the waste and byproducts of agriculture. Our milk-producing animals often produce the draught animals that till our fields. As a consequence, our dairying is energy-efficient, labour intensive and ecologically sound to sum up.

The world's finest milk and milk products can be achieved without tinkering with the basic structure. Research has to be focussed on every stage from the udder to the consumer to build in quality. Processes have to be developed to produce the products that Indian consumers want and that can be sold abroad. There is a need to develop knowledge of the markets, not just the international market but the Indian one. The Indian industry has to be encouraged to produce equipment and machinery of world quality and at competitive prices.

Quality assurance of milk and milk products would be the main thrust in sustaining the Indian dairy industry in the next millennium, as the international trade would be strongly regulated by WTO regime, which was framing stricter sanitary standards for regulating the quality. Going by recent developments at the WTO's meet to define Codex standards for International trade in milk and milk products, exports from India could be rather difficult. For one thing the minutes of the meeting stipulated that products like cheese should be derived from cows and not buffaloes (where India has a majority population). For the other, the Codex standards also spelt out that the cows should be milked by machines under covered conditions. All of which seems to guarantee the dominance in international trade of the advanced dairying nations.

Annexure I

Economics of establishing New Dairy unit consisting of 3 Cows and 2 Buffaloes.

ASSUMPTIONS

1. Cows:
- Production level: 3000 lits. Per lactation
- Cost: Rs.15, 000/ each
- Period between successive calving : 14 months
- Pure milk sold @ Rs.10 per lit

2. Buffaloes:
- Production Level: 2400 lit.
- Cost: Rs.20, 000/ each
- Period between successive calving: 16 months
- Pure milk sold at Rs.14 per lit

3. Feed Cost: Dry fodder @ Rs.1.50 per Kg, Green fodder @ 0.70 per Kg, Concentrate @ Rs.8.00 per Kg

4. Feeding: Dry fodder @ 5 Kg / day; Green Fodder @ 20 Kg /day; Concentrate @2 Kg /day (Maintenance ration, needs to be adjusted with production, general thumb rule for Cow: Milk production / 3 Buffalo: Milk production / 2.5); Mineral Mix @ 30 gms per day (Rs.50 per Kg.)

5. Insurance: Crossbred cow @ Rs.800 per animal per year; Buffaloes @ Rs.600 per animal per year.

6. Depreciation: @ 20% year for animals; 10% per year for equipment; 20% per year for building

7. Veterinary Care: @ Rs.200 per animal per year.

8. Labor (Mostly family): @ Rs.5000/ year for 5 animals

9. Interest: @ 15%

10. Cost of Construction: @ Rs.70 per sq. ft; Cow shed and Store cost Rs.5000 per animal.

(A) Capital Investment

	Cross bred cows 3 numbers	Buffaloes 2 numbers
Cost of Animals	Rs. 45,000	Rs. 40,000
Buildings	Rs. 15,000	Rs. 10,000
Equipment	Rs. 3,000	Rs. 2,000
Total	Rs. 63,000	Rs. 52,000
Capital Investment Grand Total: Rs. 1,15,000/		

Fixed Expenses

	Cross bred cows 3 numbers	Buffaloes 2 numbers
Interest on Capital @15%	Rs. 9,450/	Rs. 7,800/
Depreciation of Livestock @20% per year	Rs. 9,000/	Rs. 8,000/
Depreciation on Building @10% per year	Rs. 1,500/	Rs. 1,000/
Depreciation on equipment @ 10% per year	Rs. 300/	Rs. 200/
Insurance	Rs. 2,400	Rs. 1,200/
Total	Rs. 22,650/	Rs. 17,300/
Total Fixed Grand Total: Rs.39, 950/		

Recurring Expenses

	Cross bred Cows 3 numbers	Buffaloes 2 numbers
Green fodder @20kg /day Cost 0.70 / kg	Rs. 15,330/	Rs. 10,220/
Dry fodder @ 5kg/day Cost1.50/kg	Rs. 8,212.50	Rs. 5,475/
Cost of Concentrate (Maintenance feeding) Cost Rs.8 per Kg	Rs. 17,520/	Rs. 11,680/
Labor	Rs. 3,000/	Rs. 2,000/
Veterinary care @Rs.200 per animal /year	Rs. 600/	Rs.400/
Misc. Expenses Rs.500/animal	Rs. 1,500/	Rs. 1,000/
Total Recurring	Rs. 46,162.50/	Rs. 30,775/
Total Recurring Grand Total = Rs.76,937.50/		
Total Expenses (B + C): Rs.1,16,887.50		

Income from Sale of Milk

	Cross-bred cows	*Buffaloes*
Total Milk Produced	9000 Lits.	4800 Lits.
Fed to calves	300 Lits.	265 Lits
Total Milk Sold	8700 Lits	4535 Lits
Milk Sold as Pure Milk	@ 60% (5220 Lits)	@30% (1360 Lits.)
	Rs.52,200	Rs.19,040
Milk Sold as Mixed Milk @ Rs.12 / lit	@40% (3480 Lits)	@ 70% (3175 Lits)
	Total: 6655 Lit.	Amount : Rs.79,860/
Total Income From Milk	Rs. (52,200 + 19,040 + 79,860) = Rs. 1,51,100/	

1. Sale of Calves

	Cross-bred cows	*Buffaloes*
Calves available for sale	2 Female + 1 male	1 Male + 1 Female
Amount	Rs.900/ (@Rs.300/ calve)	Rs.600/ (@Rs.200 for male Rs.400 for female)
Total income from sale of calves	Rs.1,300/ (Rupees Thirteen hundred only)	

2. Sale of Manure @ Rs.500/ animal / year

Cross Bred Cows	*Buffaloes*
Rs.1,500	Rs.1,000
Total income from sale of manure : Rs.2,500/ (Rupees two thousand five hundred only)	
Total Income	Rs.(1,51,100 +1,300 + 2,500) = Rs.1, 54, 900

Profit : Net Income: Total income – Total Expenses (Fixed + Recurring) = Rs. 38,012.50 Rupees thirty eight thousand and twelve and fifty Paise.

Profit per animal: /year Rs.7, 602.40

Profit per animal /month: Rs. 633.50

Annexure II

(in '000 tonnes)

Table 5AII.1: Milk Production Region/State-Wise

Region State/UT	1973-74	1979-80	1980-81	1981-82	1982-83	1983-84	1984-85	1985-86	1986-87	1987-88	1988-89	1989-90	1990-91
NORTH													
Haryana	1344	1950	2187	2275	2262	2427	2441	2556	2624	2558	2785	3151	3200
Himachal Pradesh	64	304	315	339	358	376	404	431	459	478	500	529	573
Jammu & Kashmir	180	235	250	260	270	285	342	379	406	400	450	487	557
Punjab	2122	3059	3221	3494	3599	3758	3876	4093	4355	4365	4626	4972	5142
Chandigarh	15	N.E.	18.6	19.2	19	20	21	23	25	30	28	31	33
Delhi	136	N.E.	157	163	168	175	179	221	255	219	223	224	244
Sub Total	3861	5518	6148.6	6550.2	6676	7041	7263	7703	8124	8050	8612	9394	9749
SOUTH													
Andhra Pradesh	1850	1802	2010	2127	2303	2375	2668	2783	2783	2807	2814	3030	3010
Karnataka	909	1375	1425	1590	1655	1758	1839	2013	2070	2189	2248	2291	2389
Kerala	414	854	908	982	1078	1150	1220	1282	1334	1426	1513	1600	1690
Tamil Nadu	1036	1860	1738	1886	1788	2562	2846	3118	3295	3109	3238	3410	3375
Lakshadweep	—	N.E.	0.24	0.35	0.46	0.7	0.7	1	1	1	1	1	1
Pondicherry	13	N.E.	8.3	14.55	14.5	14.5	14.5	18	23	26	26	27	27
Sub-Total	4222	5891	6089.54	6599.9	6838.96	7860.2	8588.2	9215	9506	9558	9840	10359	10492

Table 5AII.1: Milk Production Region/State-Wise (Contd.)

(in '000 tonnes)

Region State/UT	1973-74	1979-80	1980-81	1981-82	1982-83	1983-84	1984-85	1985-86	1986-87	1987-88	1988-89	1989-90	1990-91
CENTRAL													
Madhya* Pradesh	1679	2210	2282	2390	2510	2640	2784	2891	3530	4272	4382	4529	4700
Uttar Pradesh	4904	5665	5728	6461	6666	7004	7723	8015	8417	8595	8824	9145	9692
Sub Total	6583	7875	8010	8851	9176	9644	10507	10906	11947	12867	13206	13674	14392
WEST													
Maharashtra	1013	1506	1756	1909	2009	2228	2358	2466	2459	2657	2800	3266	3735
Gujarat	1716	2115	2153	2228	2529	3093	3239	3270	3246	2997	3041	3351	3532
Rajasthan	2394	3085	3250	3300	3400	3544	3884	4146	1168	3911	4036	4217	4339
Dadra & N. Haveli	1	N.E.	1.00	1	1	2	2	2	2	2	3	3	3
Goa, Daman & Diu	—	N.E.	18.5	19	20	25	27	27	25	25	27	25	25
Sub Total	5154	6706	7177.5	7457	7959	8891.8	9509.85	9911	9900	9592	9907	10862	11634
EAST													
Bihar [x]	1744	1860	1942	2035	2133	2235	2330	2702	2814	2648	2826	3000	3123
Orissa	200	238	310	316	322	344	386	394	401	423	434	455	470
West Bengal	955	1231	1282	1782	2013	2107	2210	2400	2597	2664	2704	2805	2912
Andaman & Nicobar	2	N.E.	9.47	11.23	10.35	12	13	17	17	18	18	18	19
Sub-Total	2901	3329	3543.47	4144.23	4478.35	4698	4939	5513	5829	5753	5982	6278	6524

Table 5AII.1: Milk Production Region/State-Wise (Contd.)

(in '000 tonnes)

Region State/UT	1973-74	1979-80	1980-81	1981-82	1982-83	1983-84	1984-85	1985-86	1986-87	1987-88	1988-89	1989-90	1990-91
NORTH EAST													
Assam	318	460	464	469	482	498	512	526	539	610	603	617	653
Arunachal Pradesh	20	30	31	32	33	34	35	36	37	37	38	40	41
Manipur	51	58	60	62	63	64	66	69	73	77	80	82	82
Meghalaya	42	54	56	58	60	40	44	46	47	41	47	47	48
Nagaland	2	3.25	3.05	3.04	4	4	4	4	5	30	33	32	43
Sikkim	—	14.2	17	18	19	19.6	20.2	22	22	22	25	27	28
Tripura	13	15.5	16.5	17.5	18	19	22	23	25	26	27	27	29
Mizoram	1	N.E.	2.7	2.85	2.95	4.28	5.5	7	7	8	8	9	8
Sub Total	447	634.95	650.25	662.39	681.95	682.88	708.7	733	755	851	861	881	932
All-India	23168	29984	31619.36	34264.72	35810.3	38817.88	41515.8	43981	46061	46671	48408	51448	53723

Table 5AII.1: Milk Production Region/State-Wise (Contd.)

Region State/UT	1991-92	1992-93	1993-94	1994-95	1995-96	1996-97	1997-98	1998-99	1999-00P	2000-01P	2001-02A
NORTH											
Haryana	3565	3715	3850	4062	4055	4204	4373	4527	4679	4849	4976
Himachal Pradesh	597	610	654	663	676	698	714	724	741	760	810
Jammu & Kashmir	581	937	780	641	869	902	1167	1232	1286	1037	1088
Punjab	5395	5583	5970	6215	6424	6755	7165	7394	7700	7984	8375
Chandigarh	34	37	38	39	43	42	43	43	42	44	46
Delhi	230	235	251	257	261	264	267	290	290	292	321
Sub Total	10402	11117	11543	11857	12328	12955	13729	14210	14738	14966	15616
SOUTH											
Andhra Pradesh	3650	3103	3766	4221	4261	4471	4473	4842	5122	5521	5145
Karnataka	2461	2590	2736	3003	3190	3460	3970	4231	4473	4598	5357
Kerala	1780	1889	2001	2118	2192	2258	2343	2420	2673	2771	2907
Tamil Nadu	3357	3468	3524	3695	3791	3976	4061	4273	4574	4899	4629
Lakshadweep	1	1	1	1	1	1	1	2	1	1	1
Pondicherry	27	27	32	33	33	38	36	36	36	37	38
Sub-Total	11276	11078	12060	13071	13468	14204	14884	15804	16879	17827	18077
CENTRAL											
Madhya Pradesh*	4806	4879	4975	5047	5125	5224	5377	5442	5600	5806	6091
Uttar Pradesh**	10200	10649	10991	11321	11877	12387	12934	13618	14153	14840	16506
Sub Total	15006	15528	15966	16368	17002	17611	18311	19060	19753	20646	22597

Table 5AII.1: Milk Production Region/State-Wise (Contd.)

Region State/UT	1991-92	1992-93	1993-94	1994-95	1995-96	1996-97	1997-98	1998-99	1999-00P	2000-01P	2001-02A
WEST											
Maharashtra	3955	4102	4250	4812	4991	5127	5193	5609	5706	5850	6024
Gujarat	3386	3795	3935	4459	4608	4831	4913	5059	5255	5317	5573
Rajasthan	4474	4586	4958	5103	5449	5874	6487	6923	7260	7455	6330
Dadra & N. Haveli	8	10	7	1	1	1	1	1	1	1	1
Goa, Daman & Diu	25	31	34	44	40	41	42	49	53	54	58
Sub Total	11843	12524	13184	14419	15089	15874	16636	17641	18275	18677	17986
EAST											
Bihar x	3240	3195	3227	3250	3321	3410	3420	3440	3740	3878	4068
Orissa	505	542	565	584	648	687	672	733	847	875	865
West Bengal	3019	3023	3095	3250	3340	3376	3415	3441	3465	3470	4079
Andaman & Nicobar	23	24	25	25	21	21	22	22	23	24	25
Sub-Total	6787	6784	6912	7109	7330	7494	7529	7636	8075	8247	9037
NORTH EAST											
Assam	704	658	676	698	699	714	719	725	733	738	894
Arunachal Pradesh	41	21	21	22	42	44	43	45	45	45	55
Manipur	95	83	84	64	57	61	62	65	67	69	73
Meghalaya	50	52	53	54	57	58	59	61	62	64	71

Table 5AII.1: Milk Production Region/State-Wise (Contd.)

Region State/UT	1991-92	1992-93	1993-94	1994-95	1995-96	1996-97	1997-98	1998-99	1999-00P	2000-01P	2001-02A
Nagaland	44	44	45	43	44	46	46	48	50	50	54
Sikkim	29	30	30	32	33	34	35	35	35	36	46
Tripura	32	34	35	38	39	44	57	76	49	51	53
Mizoram	10	9	9	9	9	9	17	20	18	14	11
Sub Total	1005	931	952	960	980	1010	1038	1075	1059	1067	1257
All-India	56319	57962	60607	63804	66197	69148	72147	75426	78779	81430	84570§

* Including Chattisgarh,
* Including Uttaranchal,
† X including Jharkhand,
P-Provisional, A-Anticipated
Source: Basic Animal Husbandry Statistics, 1999 and 2002,
Ministry of Agriculture, Department of Animal Husbandry and Dairying.

Annexure III

Table 5AIII.1: *Annual Average and Annual Compound Rate of Growth of Milk Production in Important Indian States during the period (1977-8 to 1997-8)*

States/Union	Annual average growth rates	Annual compound growth rates	Coefficient of determination linear exponent	Inferences for trends in ACGR based on CoD
Andhra Pradesh	4.6	4.1	0.88	Increasing
Assam	3.1	3.0	0.89	Increasing
Bihar	3.7	3.6	0.96	Decreasing
Gujarat	4.5	4.2	0.91	Inconclusive
Haryana	5.1	5.0	0.97	Increasing
Himachal Pradesh	5.5	5.2	0.99	Inconclusive
Jammu and Kashmir	10.0	8.3	0.86	Increasing
Karnataka	7.9	6.2	0.59	Increasing
Kerala	6.5	6.3	0.98	Increasing
Madhya Pradesh	6.2	6.1	0.93	Inconclusive
Maharashtra	8.4	7.3	0.96	Increasing
Orrisa	6.1	5.8	0.99	Decreasing
Punjab	5.1	4.9	0.98	Increasing
Rajasthan	3.2	3.9	0.97	Inconclusive
Tamilnadu	4.7	5.2	0.90	Decreasing
Uttar Pradesh	4.9	5.2	0.99	Decreasing
West Bengal	5.9	6.3	0.95	Decreasing

Annexure IV

Views on Milk Consumption

Milk's great value stems from it being a source of calcium, which provides structure to our bodies; 99 percent of the calcium in our bodies is stored in bones and teeth. The rest is found in blood and other tissues. We get calcium from two sources: the food we eat (see box) and from our own stores of calcium in the bones. In other words, if you were to follow a diet that had absolutely no calcium from your bones. Unless you are able to pay back that calcium, your bones, at some point, will become weak. But, according the Harvard School of Public Health, bone loss is an inevitable part of aging. Even if you were to gulp gallons of milk and other calcium-rich food, you would still lose bone. Various factors – genetic makeup, sedentary lifestyles and lower hormonal levels contribute to bone loss.

There are ways of minimising the risk: getting enough vitamin D (in India we get plenty from the sun), and vitamin K (found in green, leafy vegetables), weight-bearing exercises (walking is best) and cutting down on caffeine, smoking and alcohol. But we can also start by building strong bones early in life. How? By consuming enough calcium. American health authorities recommend 1,000 mg of calcium a day for pregnant and lactating woman as well as for people between 19 and 50 years of age and 1,200 mg a day for those over 50. But where should the calcium come from? Here's where the pro and anti-milk lobbies get each other's throat. The pro-milk lobby-primarily dairy organisations and some researchers – can't stop talking about the virtue of milk. But a long-term study of Harvard health professionals found that people who drank more than two glasses of milk a week were just as likely to suffer fractures as those who had less than a glass.

Personality traits for someone wishing to enter this profession as a dairy technologist would include a scientific bent of mind and willingness to experiment and innovate. To that add loads of patience, especially in research-related work areas, willingness to roll-up one's sleeves and work with one's hands, ability to handle workers tactfully, good and effective communication skills as his ideas and directions will have to be effectively put across to those who will be actually executing the task. Relevant knowledge of agriculture, economics, animal husbandry, chemistry, mechanics and bacteriology is essentially required. Though dairies are increasingly being located in large cities, a majority of them are located either in the outskirts of large cities or in the countryside, so this is a job for those who don't mind staying in rural environs. As in any other scientific job, good observation and an eye for detail is also essential.

For those employed in the management or sales and marketing divisions of this sector, some knowledge of the field, even its technical aspect is necessary. A dairy manager generally combines administrative work with practice in his day-to-day work. His job includes recruiting the staff, supervising the overall work in the dairy, taking decisions about buying of feed, machinery, livestock and also overseeing the marketing of the produce. In large dairies, specialist managers are in charge of different sections of the dairy.

The Case For and Against Milk

Why milk is good for you

- Milk is a rich source of calcium which goes a long way in preventing osteoporosis.
- Milk is additionally a source of protein. In a largely vegetarian society, milk should be the important part of any diet.
- Milk contains the vitamins B12 and riboflavin and also vitamin D.
- Those with a cholesterol problem or those with a high coronary heart disease risk should have skimmed milk and low fat dairy products which have the same calcium and protein benefit as full fat milk.
- Milk could possibly help prevent certain types of cancer—breast and colorectal, for instance.
- Breast milk contains antibodies that help develop immunity to various diseases.
- In India, milk is an important farm commodity that supports one million households.

Why it can be avoided

- Calcium from dairy sources could increase the risk of fractures since animal protein leaches calcium away from the bone.
- Milk and other dairy products contribute significant amounts of cholesterol and saturated fat to diets, increasing the risk of coronary heart disease.
- Milk consumption could increase the risk of some types of cancer— ovarian and prostate.
- A majority of Asians are lactose intolerant and do not have the enzymes that digest milk sugar lactose leading to gastrointestinal distress, diarrhea and flatulence.
- Milk could aggravate asthma.
- Milk proteins, sugar and fat could pose health risks for children by leading to the development of obesity and diabetes. Babies fed with cow's milk are likely to be colicky; breast-feeding mothers who themselves drink cow's milk could also have colicky babies.

Where to train

Various universities and institutes in the country offer course in dairy technology. BSc/BTech (Dairy Tech). The eligibility for admission to most of these courses is merit in the BSc. degree (with mathematics in plus two). Some institutes conduct entrance tests. The duration of the courses ranges from two to four and a half years, although most courses are of four-year duration.

Postgraduate courses in dairy sciences/technology can be pursued by graduates in dairying or related fields of agriculture, veterinary sciences, pure sciences, engineering, food technology, etc. However, an entrance exam has to be cleared for seeking admission to a PG course. These courses are offered at:

- Gujarat Agriculture University, Gujarat.
- Rajasthan Agricultural University, Bikaner.
- University of Agricultural Sciences, Bangalore.
- West Bengal University of Animal and Fishery Sciences, Kolkata.

Specialisation is offered at the Master's level — dairy technology, dairy chemistry, dairy microbiology, dairy engineering, dairy extension education, food technology, genetics and breeding, dairy quality control, animal biotechnology, livestock production and management, dairy production and many others.

One can even pursue academic (teaching and research) by doing a PhD, for which he will again have to take an all-India level entrance exam (JEST).

Besides, diploma courses are also offered at some universities. The National Dairy Research Institute, Southern Regional Station, Bangalore, offers a two-year diploma in dairy technology.

Job Prospects

Job opportunities exist in both government and nongovernment sectors. The National Dairy Development Board (NDDB), a multi-locational organisation involved in planning, implementing, financing and supporting farmer-owned professionally agribusiness enterprise is the core PSU in this field, although with almost every state aping Amul's 'cooperative' success, employment opportunities have increased manifold for both technologists as well as managers, both in production as well as marketing.

With the entry of multinational giants like Nestle, Cadburys, Britannia, Kelloggs, Heritage Foods, KFC, HLL, etc. into the Indian market, employment opportunities as well as salaries have received a further boost. Traditional Indian market leaders like Mother Dairy, Indana Milkfood, Amul, Dalmia, Dabur, Cadburys, Vadilal, Parag, Vijaya and Milkfed (Verka) are also modernising and diversifying their operations and exploring nontraditional channels to boost demand.

For young people looking at a career away from the hurly-burly of urban life, this could be one of the most attractive choices available.

6

Poultry Development

Unlike most other countries, the definition of poultry, in India, is pretty narrow. It does not take into account turkey, quail, fowl, ducks and geese which are part and parcel of the poultry industry in other countries. For Indians, the poultry industry is restricted to broilers and eggs and for good measure, our *desi* variety too. That's about it. However, even in this segment alone, the Indian industry has a long way to go. This was accentuated by the fact that till a couple of decades ago, there was no poultry industry worth the name. It was the age old problem – a lack of solidarity. The industry was fragmented. It still is.

Poultry is known to exist in India for over 5,000 years. Most contemporary breeds in Western countries were developed from Red and Silver Jungle fowls which originated in India. Before the advent of the Planning era, commercial poultry production was practically nonexistent. Poultry farming was then fairly extensive but limited to backyard poultry keeping with low productive *desi* fowls maintained under peasant husbandry practices. The benefits derived were, therefore, only a small fraction of what could be obtained from scientific poultry farming. Superior exotic poultry breeds with high egg productivity were introduced in the country from time to time for improving the indigenous stock but in the absence of a systematic large-scale development programme such efforts proved abortive.

The poultry industry is one of the fastest growing sector in the country. The overall growth rate of the poultry industry is 15-20% per annum. At present the total turnover of Indian poultry industry is Rs. 12000 crore and the industry has set of target for achieving a total turnover of Rs. 30,000 crore by the year 2005. Poultry industry provides employment to 2 million people. The reported turnover in 2001 was Rs. 10,000 crore.

Early Development

In fairness, the credit for pioneering action for poultry development should be given to a few Christian missionary organizations and some British

---

*Then named as Imperial Veterinary Research Institute.

people who brought some superior exotic breeds into India like Leghorns, Minorcas, Anconas, Sussex, Rocks, Rhode Island Red and Australops in the beginning of the 20th century. The objective was to establish their own poultry farms and to make cocks available to the neighbouring farmers for crossing and improving the indigenous stock. The farmers appreciated the help of the missionaries in Etah (Uttar Pradesh), Katpadi (Tamil Nadu) and Martendum (Kerala). These activities created amongst them some awareness of the advantage of raising better quality fowls.

The first major step towards scientific poultry management in the country was the establishment of the Poultry Research Division at the Indian Veterinary Research Institute (IVRI)[*] in March 1939. The Poultry farm of the Division maintained 4,000 layers and had facilities for hatching, brooding and rearing of birds. The farm was stocked with exotic breeds like White Leghorn, Rhode Island Red, Australops, Black Minorca, New Hampshire and Light Sussex. The flocks were simply multiplied or crossed to improve egg production.

The breeding programme in the early stages was limited to multiplication of pure stock and some crossbreeding for improved egg production. The IVRI also supplied hatching eggs and cocks to the neighbouring villagers for obtaining better-quality chicken and made available cockerels of improved breeds to poultry farmers for mating the indigenous stock owned by them. These steps taken by the IVRI generated considerable amount of interest. Possibly the most important single contribution of the IVRI for poultry development in India was the evolution in 1942, of an effective vaccine against Ranikhet disease by its Pathology and Bacteriology Division. This disease was the greatest obstacle to successful poultry farming in the country. The control over this disease built confidence in farmers

---

A Few Facts

- According to Indian history, the first fowl was domesticated as early as in 3200 B.C. Egyptian and Chinese records show that fowls were laying eggs in 1400 BC.
- Research Indicates that chicken feather can be used to make products ranging from paper to diapers and high-quality animal feed.
- Unfertilised eggs, like milk, are of animal origin but not non-vegetarian. Most of the eggs (about 90 percent) available are unfertilized eggs.
- Milk is good for chickens. Recent studies show that milk products have a positive effect on the performance and health of chicks.
- A hen requires 24 to 26 hours to produce an egg. Thirty minutes later she starts all over again.
- Egg yolks are one of the few food items that naturally contain Vitamin D.
- White shelled eggs are produced by hens with white feathers and white ear lobes. Brown shelled eggs are produced by hens with red feathers and red ear lobes.

and a number of poultry units were then established by the Government. Because of these developments a number of model poultry farms were established in the forties by different State Governments for demonstration, training and multiplication of improved poultry stock. Most of the states appointed Poultry Development Officers to promote poultry production. During the Second World War, the demand of the army for egg and table birds increased manifold. To meet this demand the military authorities set up 10 poultry farms with improved exotic stock, each of 10,000 birds capacity. From time to time some poultry stock and eggs for hatching were distributed by the military poultry farms to the neighbouring farmers for raising poultry stock of improved variety. These steps helped to popularize the rearing of better quality poultry stock amongst a small section of rural people.

The foundation on which poultry farming grew in India was truly laid in the fifties with the introduction of the Five-Year Plans. Since then number of poultry birds has increased manyfold. Under the First Plan, an All-India Poultry Development Programme aiming at establishment of Poultry Extension-cum-Demonstration Centres was launched. A beginning was made with 33 centres having facilities of poultry houses and staff under the State Animal Husbandry Departments. Some State Government poultry farms were also strengthened to take up large-scale multiplication and acclimatization of exotic stock and subsequent propagation. The scope of the programme was enlarged during the Second Plan (1959) by establishing 5 Regional Poultry Farms, 1 each at Bangalore, Bhubaneswar, Mumbai, Delhi and Shimla (Kamlahi) by the Ministry of Agriculture. The farms at Mumbai, Bhubaneswar and Bangalore were redesignated as Central Poultry Breeding Farms. The nucleus stocks for these projects were imported from the USA. Substantial aid was received from the US Technical Cooperation Mission (TCM) in 1956 which supplied 30,000 day-old chicks of White Leghorn and Rhode Island Red breeds, and the requisite equipments. The TCM chicks were distributed among the Central and State Government poultry farms, which in turn provided chicks and technical guidance on poultry management to the farmers. This helped to augment substantially the breeding programmes that were already in progress. As a result, the number of Poultry Extension-cum Demonstration Centres were increased ten fold.

POULTRY TODAY

Livestock and poultry contributes 28% of agriculture GDP & 8% of national GDP. Annual egg and broiler production in India has been estimated as 37 billions and 800 millions (2001-02) respectively. There is an estimated annual placement of 135 million layer and 1,200 million broiler in the country. Poultry sector contributes more than Rs. 11,000 crore and provides direct employment to 1.6 million people. The growth rate in poultry industry in the last 15 years has been estimated to 8 to 10% (egg sector) and

(NABARD). In world map, India stands 4th in Egg Production & 18th in Broiler Production (FAO estimates).*

In spite of this achievement, the annual per capita consumption of 32 eggs and 1.0 kg meat is very low than 180 eggs and 10.8 kg meat recommended by national committee on human nutrition (ICMR). In other words, the industry has a potential to grow at about 5 times in egg sector and 10 times in meat sector. There is little doubt that eggs and poultry meat are one of the finest source of bio-available protein for human consumption in India.

Having faced the recent bird flu crisis successfully, India is poised to emerge as a major player in poultry. The flu may have affected the poultry sector in other countries, but it has rather benefited the Indian sector, which has shown its strength in the global market after the initial setback. With an annual turnover of over Rs. 800 crore, the Pune based group (Venkateshwara Hatcheries) has interests in the total product chain, including eggs, broilers, breeding, medicines, vaccines, equipment for hatchery and poultry, egg processing, poultry feed, technical consultancy, health and nutrition products, chicken-based food products, human resources and training.

During the past two decades, the Indian poultry sector has turned up as the most advanced one with the lowest production costs in the world. If the developed countries withdraw subsidies to their poultry farmers; we can emerge as the top player in next few years. Unlike the dairy and fisheries industries, Indian poultry is much more advanced and systematic in its approach.

Presently India is exporting poultry products like the table eggs, egg-powder, SPF eggs, hatching eggs, breeding stock and vaccines to the tune of Rs. 400 crore annually. The world chicken markets are estimated to be $18 billion. In future, India would play an important role in chicken exports. The annual turnover of the sector was over Rs. 29,000 crore. It has the potential to solve the problems of malnutrition and unemployment in the country to a great extent.

Breeds of Poultry

The Red Jungle fowl (gallus gallus) has been recognised as the ancestor for a number of present day poultry breeds of the world. The famous jungle fowl lived in the jungles of India and in the forests of neighbouring countries like Burma, Ceylon, Malaysia, Java and other South Asian countries.

The poultry population in India consists of indigenous (desi) and exotic (improved) birds. Mostly indigenous birds are active and are able to subsist on meagre food available in the backyards of Indian villages. They are strong enough to withstand the diversified agroclimatic conditions in India. The hens of indigenous birds are poor layers of small sized eggs but they are ideal sitters and good foster mothers.

---

*Poultry Planner, January 2004.

Commercial Poultry

The chicken production systems of India are divided into 2 production systems.

    (i) Industrialized or the sophisticated production system.

    (ii) Primitive/rural/traditional/backyards system sixties proved to be the turning point in the history of poultry production in the country.

The concept of backyard poultry keeping, yielded place to poultry farming as a commercial enterprise. Grandparent stocks of reputed companies were imported. The growth of the industry was initially slow but got impetus after Green Revolution due to availability agricultural byproducts. First commercial chick was hatched in November 1962 at the Delhi-based Rani Shaver Poultry Breeding Farms Pvt. Ltd. Commercial production of balanced compounded feed as well as of modern veterinary medicines and vaccines – so very essential for successful poultry production- were also started at the same time. Also came in its wake, the indigenous production of equipments for hatching and incubation, feed mixing and commercial housing.

Initiation of an Intensive Egg and Poultry Production-cum-Marketing Programme, popularly known as the Intensive Poultry Development Project (IPDP), in the sixties with an area development and package approach, was the most important factor for bringing about the favourable development. Introduction of deep litter system of management and further importation of high quality stock and mass preventive vaccination against common avian diseases, income-tax exemption for the poultry sector in agriculture, progressive industrialization with resultant higher purchasing power of people, were among other major contributing factors.

Scientific poultry breeding programmes were launched during this period by the Indian Council of Agricultural Research and in the Central Poultry Farms as the first step towards attaining self sufficiency in the production and supply of high quality chicks. At the Central Poultry Breeding Farms, poultry layer strains like HH-260, BH-78 and Kalinga Brown were evolved and released to the commercial farms. The training programme for the farmers was extended. Financial assistance for supply of poultry house materials and rearing equipment at concessional rates, and subsidy for purchase of incubators was extended. Sizable international assistance was also available during this period for promotion of poultry farming.

During the Fourth Plan period, poultry production continued to progress satisfactorily. To give additional support to the training programme a High Level In-service Training Institute was established at Hessaraghatta near Bangalore with the assistance of the FAO. The selective breeding programme initiated earlier at the Central Poultry Breeding Farms was modified and a Coordinated Poultry Breeding Project (CPBP) was launched in which 3 Central and number of selected State poultry breeding farms participated. The IPDP was further enlarged. Poultry disease control measures and disease diagnostic services were strengthened and mobile veterinary clinics were established. During this period the Central

Government launched a special project (SFDA/MFAL) to help the small and marginal farmers and agricultural labourers. Poultry development formed an important component of this project.

Though broilers were introduced in India in early seventies, the growth was spectacular surpassing the egg-type stocks. The growth rate of broilers is estimated at 20% annually as compared to 10% of layers. The number of commercial birds has thus increased fast and the contribution of poultry in the GNP has increased nearly 12-fold during the last 15 years (Table 6.1). During the Seventh Plan, egg and broiler production registered a compound growth rate of 7.3% and 18% respectively. Poultry production achieved a faster rate of growth during the Eighth Plan and egg production increased at the rate of 8.2%. Even with this growth, per caput availability of eggs was at the rate of 32 only, as against recommended and desirable level of 180 eggs per person per year.

Today almost all strains of poultry stock of international repute are available in India. Strains of both egg- and meat-type birds have been developed in the country, and dependence on import of grand parentstock from outside has almost been eliminated. Availability of quality chicks would be required to be encouraged by providing incentive and easy flow

Table 6.1: Value of Poultry Products at Current Prices Between 1980-81 and 1999-2000

(Rs. million)

Year	Eggs	Poultry meat	Total poultry
1980-81	3,510	4,440	7,950
1981-82	4,060	5,590	9,650
1982-83	4,490	6,070	10,560
1983-84	5,480	8,080	13,560
1984-85	6,390	9,970	16,360
1985-86	7,370	10,870	18,240
1986-87	8,290	13,050	21,340
1987-88	9,030	15,350	24,380
1988-89	10,260	18,200	28,460
1989-90	12,020	22,760	34,780
1990-91	13,430	24,060	37,490
1991-92	17,360	31,650	49,010
1992-93	18,400	34,020	52,420
1993-94	22,820	44,860	67,680
1994-95	26,030	51,090	77,120
1995-96	28,340	58,460	86,800
1996-97	31,680	62,170	93,850
1997-98	34,190	69,160	1,03,240
1998-99	35,160	68,080	1,20,380
1999-00	38,530	81,850	1,20,380
2000-01	40,670	85,820	1,26,490
2001-02	44,380	86,980	1,31,360

Source: CSO National Accounts Statistics: 2003

of institutional finance and appropriate training and guidance. Poultry feed accounts for over 70% of the total cost of production. The quality of feed has a major bearing on the efficiency and health of the bird. A national policy on poultry feed is required to be evolved to supply different feed ingredients at reasonable price.

Most of poultry-rearing activities in the country are in the unorganized sector. Poultry development needs to be organized and developed on cooperative basis on Anand Pattern cooperatives. A viable and efficient cooperative structure needs to be established at the village, district, state and national levels, which apart from ensuring remunerative prices to the producers, would help in providing all the requisite inputs to the producers including credit, training, processing and marketing facilities. Processing, marketing and storage infrastructure facilities would have to be strengthened in selected districts along with input supply like chicks, balanced feed and health care. Disease surveillance, production of quality vaccines for poultry and duck, and statutory provision for strict quality control of all the vaccines produced in the private and public sectors need to be instituted as part of the national policy of disease control of birds and animals.

Poultry Associations along with the National Egg Coordination Committee (NECC) take care of pricing, etc. The expanded scope of NECC includes the following.

1. The fixing of remunerative egg prices across the country.
2. Price support operations in cooperation with the National Agricultural Cooperative Marketing Federation of India (NAFED).
3. Market intervention through Agro-Corpex India Ltd., a marketing company with only poultry farmers as shareholders promoted by the NECC.
4. Rural market development by promoting distribution channels.
5. Including eggs in the Noon-Meal Programme for school children.
6. Mass communication programmes to promote egg consumption.

Potentialities

With a poultry population of over 100 million layers (to be precise, one that lays eggs) and 150 million broilers (a young chicken suitable for cooking), India is among the top ten producers in the world. The industry is growing at a rate of 15% per annum. India is the fifth largest producer of eggs in the world, with an estimated production of around 32 billion eggs in 2000. Ironically, however, per capita consumption of eggs in India is just around 32 per person per year as compared to 120 in developed countries. In 1970, the figure in India was 10 eggs per person per year.

Poultry meat, today, accounts for 27% of all meat consumed in the world. But considering the rate at which consumption is growing, the equations can change within the next 20 years or so and will account for 45% of meat consumption globally. Why? Is it cheaper, more readily available, more nutritious or less prone to the mad cow type scares? India is not isolated from these developments and the poultry industry appears ready to rake in the benefits. Industry sources point out that they have set themselves a target of 180 eggs per person per year by 2015 and they intend to raise the per capita consumption of chicken to six chickens/nine kg of meat per annum per person. The pertinent point screaming for attention is the fact that India has the potential to develop poultry into an industry which can rake in money. More important, this industry has the potential to provide cheap food and a source for livelihood for millions. It has been estimated that an increase in per capita consumption of one egg can create 25,000 additional jobs. Similarly, an increase in consumption of 50 gm poultry meat, per capita, can generate 20,000 additional jobs. All these facts point towards one thing – to highlight the kind of potential the Indian poultry industry has.

EGG AND BROILER

India is known to be the home of modern hen, which owes its ancestry to the Indian Red Jungle fowl (Gallus murghi). Found in the jungles of South and South-East Asia, it is regarded as the ancestor of the present-day chicken breeds of the world. The earliest records of domesticated jungle fowl are found in the Harappa and Mohanjadaro civilization, going back to 2500 BC. The Indian Red jungle fowl is mostly confined to the northern and southeastern parts of the country, and the grey variety to western and southern parts. An endangered species, it has been successfully bred in captivity at the National Zoological Park, New Delhi.

The sport of cockfighting contributed largely to the domestication of the fowl in South and South East Asia, and its subsequent distribution elsewhere. Desi breeds found in India include Aseel, Chittagong and Ghagus. Aseel (meaning real or true), a well-known breed of India, is famous for its endurance power and fighting qualities. Pure Aseel is an aggressive bird. It has an upright and majestic gait. Pure specimen of this breed is now rare and is available only with a few fanciers in part of Andhra Pradesh, Karnataka and Uttar Pradesh. Several varieties, mostly crosses between Aseel and local fowls, are known in other parts. Chittagong Malay, originally a native of the Malay peninsula and largely bred in Chittagong (Bangladesh), is found in some parts of eastern India. Ghagus, a big and hardy breed, is fast becoming scarce in India. Good specimens are found with the nomads in parts of Andhra Pradesh and Karnataka. Busra, a minor breed of this class, can be found in small numbers in parts of Gujarat and Maharashtra, particularly around Mumbai.

Egg

Egg poultry all over the world was more or less a family affair – a sort of a backyard enterprise, managed under the traditional system. It was in 1939, following the VII World Poultry Congress at Cleveland, Ohio, that the fancy poultry industry was separated from the commercial side of the business in the USA. Although they continued to have many dual-purpose flocks, by 1960 the USA was well on its way into the second poultry revolution – towards a totally commercial egg industry. In 1950, there were 4.2 million laying flocks in the USA from which eggs were sold. This dropped to 3.4 million in 1954. That was the start of a major transition in the production of commercial eggs in the USA.

While talk was going on in the USA during the mid-fifties about the future egg factories with heating and air-conditioning and all of the birds in cages with mechanical feeders and automatic waterers, and eggs being gathered and processed automatically and manure removed automatically to a fertilizer processing station, the developing world remained more or less unaffected in this regard. The production of eggs in India was 1.8 billion during 1950-51. It rose to just 2.88 billion by 1960-61. The first commercial egg was produced in a private farm near Delhi in 1962. Since then there is no looking back. The production of eggs was 5.34 billion in 1971 and 10.06 billion in 1980. During the last two decades, the production of eggs had an annual growth of 8% and touched 31.77 billion mark in 2000. Per caput availability went up from 7 eggs in 1961 to 32 in 2000 (Table 6.2). India is the fourth largest egg producer in the world. The industry provides employment to over two million people and contributes Rs. 120 billion to GDP. The poultry sector has a high employment potential.

Table 6.2: Annual Production and Per Caput Availability of Eggs, Boilers and Poultry Meat, 1961-2002

Year	Production			Per caput availability per annum	
	Egg (million)	Broiler (million)	Poultry meat ('000 tonnes)	Eggs (No.)	Poultry meat (gm)
1960-61	2,881	0	81	7	188
1970-71	5,340	4	121	10	220
1980-81	10,060	30	179	15	266
1985-86	16,128	75	274	21	365
1990-91	21,101	190	412	25	498
1991-92	21,983	215	440	26	521
1992-93	22,929	210	382	26	433
1993-94	24,167	235	454	27	505
1994-95	25,975	275	507	29	554
1995-96	27,198	330	479	30	513
1996-97	27,496	400	479	29	510
1997-98	28,689	450	527	30	552
1998-99	29,476	500	540	30	557
1999-00*	30,629	550	559	32	566
2000-01*	31,770	600	575	32	575
2001-02**	34,034	700	NA	34	NA

* Provisional ** Anticipated achievement

Source: Government of India, Ministry of Agriculture, Department of Animal Husbandry and Annual Reports of Ministry of Food Processing Industries: Basic Animal Husbandry Statistics, various issues.

Herbal and Branded Eggs

Tagma Agrotech launched herbal and low cholesterol eggs under the brand Organegg Priced at Rs 22 for a pack containing six eggs, the odourless Organegg is enriched with natural vitamins, proteins and minerals. It not only possesses many health promoting, immunostimulating therapeutic and functional properties but is also low in cholesterol with 80-120 mg per egg as compared to 200-240 mg in conventional egg, and that makes it heart-friendly. The innovation has been brought about by feeding hens exclusively on a vegetarian diet fortified with herbs galore, a few of them being cholesterol-lowering. Organegg is not a medical egg but a food supplement to maintain the body's defence system. The product has no side effects as only herbs which are consumed by human beings are used. The Rs. 4 crore firm eyes five per cent of the overall egg market by year-end and expects to triple its turnover by 2005.

Chandigarh-based Toubro Industries are poised to offer branded eggs and one can be sure it is farm fresh, with date of hatching and shelf life specified clearly. Once Toubro Industries' biggest ever investment of Rs. 600 crore on eggs is complete, east and northeast promises to turn 'eggetarian'. The project is aimed also to correct the falling farm income in rural West Bengal. The Tourbo group will set up a training institute to provide training to farmers in poultry farming. The company which has a financial services arm, is also open to act as an angel investor to enable farmers set up their own units at a later stage and have a 100% buy-back arrangement with it. Clearly the state government has a taste for eggs. Land had already been allotted to the company on war footing and six units of Tourbo will come up in Durgapur, Siliguri, Contai, Kalyani and Raichak. The company will pump in Rs. 145.5 crore in the first phase to set up integrated table egg production facilities at these six places. Another Rs. 460 crore will be put in subsequently by way of assistance to 7500 contracted small farms across the state, over a period of five years.

State Level Scenario

The growth of the Industry has, however, been quite uneven among different states. Andhra Pradesh and Tamil Nadu, the two southern states accounting for only 13% of the population, are responsible for producing 31% eggs in the country. Next come Maharashtra and Punjab with a share of 10% each in total production, but have fastest growth rate (Table 6.3). With regard to per caput availability also, Punjab tops the list (128 eggs/year), followed by Andhra Pradesh (77 eggs/year) (Table 6.4).

The problem can also be looked at on a regional basis. The region-wise production of eggs and broilers differed a lot. The southern region had the maximum production of eggs, followed by the eastern, central, northern and western regions. The respective contribution of these regions on per caput basis comes to 45.1, 20.6, 20.2 and 14.1 per cent during 1994. Southern region also produces maximum number of broilers (105 million)

Table 6.3: *Regional and State-wise Share in Production of Eggs (%)*

States	1983-84	1984-85	1985-86	1986-87	1987-88	1988-89	1989-90	1990-91	1991-92	1992-93	1993-94	1994-95	1995-96	1996-97	1997-98	1998-99	1999-2000	2000-01	2001-02
North																			
Haryana	1.64	2.18	2.12	1.98	1.48	1.58	1.65	1.52	2.33	2.25	2.20	2.44	2.32	2.34	2.23	2.32	2.48	3.41	3.42
Himachal Pradesh	0.23	0.24	0.24	0.24	0.24	0.25	0.24	0.25	0.27	0.30	0.30	0.26	0.27	0.26	0.26	0.26	0.26	0.26	0.26
Jammu & Kashmir	1.79	1.51	1.41	1.40	1.13	1.37	1.32	1.35	1.35	1.25	1.40	1.22	1.40	1.44	1.44	1.76	1.82	2.07	1.43
Punjab	6.03	5.79	6.11	7.20	7.48	7.69	8.01	8.67	8.75	9.44	9.64	9.38	9.23	9.94	10.19	8.92	9.08	9.33	9.83
Chandigarh	0.23	0.21	0.19	0.18	0.21	0.20	0.19	0.17	0.17	0.17	0.21	0.13	0.13	0.11	0.07	0.06	0.07	0.05	0.10
Delhi	0.53	0.43	0.39	0.37	0.38	0.38	0.26	0.25	0.27	0.27	0.27	0.25	0.25	0.25	0.24	0.16	0.18	0.16	0.24
Sub-total	**0.45**	**10.36**	**10.45**	**11.38**	**10.92**	**11.37**	**11.68**	**12.22**	**13.14**	**13.68**	**14.02**	**13.68**	**13.60**	**14.34**	**14.43**	**13.48**	**13.89**	**15.28**	**15.28**
South																			
Andhra Pradesh	18.53	21.55	19.44	18.17	18.07	18.14	18.36	18.24	17.03	17.28	18.35	20.92	22.16	20.58	20.13	20.10	20.71	21.40	18.56
Karnataka	7.25	6.92	6.65	6.52	6.64	6.51	6.33	6.12	6.15	5.93	5.86	5.66	5.73	5.93	6.34	6.57	6.50	6.27	6.83
Kerala	9.85	9.21	8.43	8.07	8.11	7.77	7.43	7.34	7.37	7.74	7.63	7.37	7.30	7.36	7.48	6.93	6.71	6.40	7.24
Tamil Nadu	7.79	7.47	12.82	11.99	12.37	12.11	12.18	12.15	12.45	12.41	12.08	11.74	11.21	11.06	10.68	12.17	12.55	12.37	10.87
Pondicherry	0.04	0.06	0.07	0.05	0.06	0.05	0.05	0.05	0.06	0.05	0.04	0.04	0.03	0.03	0.03	0.03	0.03	0.03	0.03
Lakshadweep	0.01	0.01	0.01	0.01	0.01	0.01	0.01	0.01	0.01	0.02	0.02	0.02	0.02	0.02	0.02	0.02	0.02	0.02	0.02
Sub-total	**43.47**	**45.22**	**47.42**	**44.81**	**45.26**	**44.59**	**44.36**	**43.91**	**43.07**	**43.43**	**43.98**	**45.75**	**46.45**	**44.98**	**44.68**	**45.82**	**46.52**	**46.49**	**43.55**
Central																			
Madhya Pradesh	4.72	4.91	4.59	4.51	3.41	4.55	4.98	4.83	4.79	4.66	4.54	4.41	4.39	4.55	4.72	4.75	4.61	4.55	4.54
Uttar Pradesh	2.67	2.62	2.33	2.23	2.24	2.18	2.45	2.47	2.47	2.47	2.49	2.41	2.47	2.54	2.53	3.38	2.62	2.30	2.93

Table 6.3: Regional and State-wire Share in Production of Eggs (%) (Contd.)

States	1983-84	1984-85	1985-86	1986-87	1987-88	1988-89	1989-90	1990-91	1991-92	1992-93	1993-94	1994-95	1995-96	1996-97	1997-98	1998-99	1999-2000	2000-01	2001-02
Sub-total	7.39	7.53	6.92	6.74	5.65	6.73	7.43	7.3	7.26	7.13	7.03	6.82	6.86	7.09	7.25	8.13	7.23	6.85	7.47
West																			
Gujarat	1.85	1.83	1.56	1.46	1.42	1.70	1.91	1.96	1.57	2.06	2.09	1.80	1.78	1.82	1.78	1.58	1.56	1.09	2.03
Maharashtra	10.55	10.02	9.36	9.18	9.65	9.52	9.69	9.99	9.87	9.99	9.67	9.63	9.57	9.77	9.68	9.96	9.92	9.75	9.54
Rajasthan	1.18	1.12	1.22	1.21	1.20	1.20	1.14	1.33	1.46	1.52	1.64	1.61	1.60	1.75	1.75	1.81	1.82	1.80	1.74
Dadra & N Haveli	0.02	0.02	0.02	0.02	0.02	0.02	0.02	0.02	0.02	0.03	0.03	0.03	0.01	0.02	0.01	0.02	0.01	0.01	0.02
Goa, Daman & Diu	0.57	0.53	0.48	0.45	0.49	0.49	0.46	0.44	0.42	0.44	0.42	0.40	0.39	0.39	0.39	0.38	0.38	0.41	0.37
Sub-total	14.17	13.52	12.64	12.32	12.78	12.93	13.22	13.74	13.34	14.04	13.85	13.47	13.35	13.75	13.61	13.75	13.69	13.06	13.70
East																			
Bihar	7.28	7.02	6.82	6.79	7.38	6.78	6.57	6.36	6.35	6.02	5.75	5.38	5.15	5.13	4.97	4.85	4.69	4.55	4.60
Orissa	2.45	1.96	2.01	1.57	1.93	2.14	2.07	2.00	2.21	2.30	2.35	2.21	2.15	2.18	2.89	2.59	2.12	2.30	3.45
All India	100.00	100.00	100.00	100.00	100.00	100.00	100.00	100.00	100.00	100.00	100.00	100.00	100.00	100.00	100.00	100.00	100.00	100.00	100.00

Source: Report of the Technical Committee of Direction for Improvement of Animal Husbandry

Table 6.4: Per Caput Production of Eggs—State-Wise

(Nos)

State	1979-80	1980-81	1981-82	1982-83	1983-84	1984-85	1985-86	1986-87	1987-88	1988-89	1989-90	1990-91	1991-92	1992-93	1993-94	1994-95	1995-96	1996-97	1997-98
North																			
Haryana	13	14	14	15	15	22	23	23	17	19	21	20	31	30	31	36	35	35	34
Himachal Pradesh	5	5	6	6	6	7	8	9	9	10	10	10	11	13	13	13	13	13	13
Jammu & Kashmir	38	34	33	37	36	33	35	36	29	37	37	39	39	36	43	43	45	45	46
Punjab	29	31	35	37	44	46	54	67	70	75	83	91	94	104	110	114	116	124	128
South																			
Andhra Pradesh	33	33	38	39	42	54	54	53	55	55	59	59	56	58	64	77	84	77	77
Karnataka	21	21	22	23	24	25	26	27	28	29	29	29	30	29	30	31	32	33	37
Kerala	39	38	40	45	47	49	49	50	51	51	52	53	55	59	61	63	64	64	67
Tamil Nadu	18	17	19	18	20	21	40	39	41	42	45	46	48	49	61	53	52	52	51
Central																			
Madhya Pradesh	8	10	10	10	11	12	13	13	10	14	16	16	16	15	16	16	17	17	18
Uttar Pradesh	3	3	3	3	3	3	3	3	3	3	4	4	4	4	4	4	5	5	5
West																			
Maharashtra	3	3	3	3	4	4	4	4	4	4	5	5	4	28	28	30	30	31	31
Gujarat	31	34	36	37	38	39	41	42	44	46	49	52	52	11	12	11	11	11	11
Rajasthan	4	4	4	4	4	5	5	5	5	5	5	6	7	7.6	9	9	9	10	10

Table 6.4: Per Caput Production of Eggs—State-Wise (Contd.)

(Nos)

State	1979-80	1980-81	1981-82	1982-83	1983-84	1984-85	1985-86	1986-87	1987-88	1988-89	1989-90	1990-91	1991-92	1992-93	1993-94	1994-95	1995-96	1996-97	1997-98
East																			
Bihar	10	11	11	12	13	13	14	15	16	16	16	16	16	15	15	15	15	15	14
Orissa	11	14	13	12	11	10	11	11	12	13	14	13	15	16	17	17	17	17	23
West	15	15	15	16	24	26	28	36	35	35	34	33	34	33	33	35	35	35	35
Bengal																			
Northeast																			
Assam	14	14	16	16	15	15	16	16	19	19	20	22	24	18	19	19	19	19	19
Manipur	22	19	21	24	25	25	26	28	34	36	36	51	44	35	35	54	29	29	29
Meghalaya	24	24	25	29	36	38	38	39	39	29	38	38	38	38	39	39	39	39	39
Nagaland	0	0	19	19	20	20	21	21	29	33	29	35	36	30	33	31	32	32	31
All-India	14	15	16	16	18	19	21	23	23	24	25	25	26	26	27	28	30	30	30

Source: Report of the Technical Committee of Direction for Improvement of Animal Husbandry and Dairying Statistics NE. Not estimated
Relates to the financial year (1979-80) and so on

followed by northern (72 million) western (59 million) eastern and central (39 million) regions. Within the regions also, there are specific pockets where concentration of poultry is relatively higher (Table 6.5).

Another very interesting feature of the poultry industry is that 75% of eggs and 80% of broilers are produced in urban areas, accounting for just 26% of the population leading to a lopsided consumption pattern of eggs – 80 eggs per year for the urban areas (as much as 170 for Mega cities) and only 10 eggs/year for rural areas with an average of only 28 eggs per caput for the country as a whole (Table 6.6).

As for broiler, India is blessed with all the major inputs for the development farming: breeding programmes for quality chicks, raw materials for feed, technology, dynamic farmers, technical and training facilities, vaccines and veterinary products, etc. just a handful of countries enjoy these assets in the world. Nevertheless other Asian countries have developed and progressed far ahead of India. With these advantages, even the present impressive growth is expected to be outpaced in the coming years.

Regional Analysis

An analysis of the region-wise placement of broiler chicks in different parts of the country is presented in Table 6.7. These regions have been selected not on the basis of the geographic contiguity of different parts of the country, but on the demand and consumption pattern as well as income

Table 6.5: Region-wise Distribution of Human Populations, Eggs, Broilers and Per Caput Availability of Eggs, 1994

Region	Human population in million (% of total)	Eggs Production in million (% of total)	Per caput availability (% of All-India average)	Broiler production in million (% of total)
Northern	256.7 (28.6)	5,307 (20.2%)	21 (-27.6%)	72 (26.2%)
Western	128.6 (14.3%)	3,694 (14.1%)	29 (At par)	59 (21.4%)
Southern	208.5 (23.2%)	11,865 (45.1%)	57 (+ 96.5%)	105 (38.2%)
Eastern and central	301.0 (33.6%)	5,426 (20.6%)	18 (-37.9%)	39 (14.2%)
Total	894.9 (100%)	26,292 (100%)	29 (net. ave.)	275 (100%)

Note: Northern region: Chandigarh, Delhi, Haryana, Himachal Pradesh, Jammu & Kashmir, Punjab, Rajasthan, Uttar Pradesh.

Western region: Dadra and Nagar Haveli, Daman and Diu, Goa, Gujarat, Maharashtra.

Southern region: Andhra Pradesh, Karnataka, Kerala, Lakshadweep, Pondicherry, Tamil Nadu.

Eastern and central region: Andaman and Nicobar, Arunachal Pradesh, Assam, Bihar, Madhya Pradesh, Manipur, Meghalaya, Mizoram, Nagaland, Orissa, Sikkim, Tripura, West Bengal.

Table 6.6: Estimated Production of Eggs, Broilers and Poultry Meat in Urban and Rural Areas in India, 1993

	Population (million)	Egg production total (million)	Per caput (Nos.)	Poultry meat production		
				Broiler (million)	Total ('000 tonnes)	Per caput (g/year)
Urban						
Mega cities	70.6 (08%)	11,900 (40%)	170	14 (60%)	272 (60%)	3.852
Other cities	162.4 (18%)	6,700 (27%)	40	47 (20%)	91 (20%)	0.560
Total	233.0 (26%)	18,600 (75%)	80	188 (80%)	363 (80%)	0.558
Rural						
Deve-loped	215 (24%)	4,100 (17%)	20	40 (17%)	77 (17%)	0.358
Deve-loping	430 (50%)	2,100 (08%)	5	7 (03%)	14 (03%)	0.33
Total	645 (74%)	6,200 (25%)	10	47 (20%)	91 (20%)	0.141
Grand Total	878 (100%)	24,800 (100%)	28	235 (100%)	454 (100%)	0.517

Note: Figures in parentheses represent per cent of total

Source: Indian Poultry Industry Yearbook, 1994

level. Not surprisingly, Region I in the north has the highest per caput production and availability of broilers, over two times the national average. This is so because of the higher income levels and a larger proportion of people who prefer non-vegetarian food. Even the current demand can be stepped up, but the prevailing weather is hostile to the rearing of broiler parents with high summer and low winter temperatures. Also, the expansion of poultry in Punjab was checked on account of the nebulous law-and-order situation in eighties.

Now that the conditions are quite normal, there is a scope for the Region to achieve higher growth. Another popular trend here is the emergence of integrated broiler projects. This is more so in northern India where large broiler producers have set up in-house facilities for the production of day-old chicks and feed. At times, they may have only a breeding farm and depend on custom-hatching, or have a hatchery and depend on hatching eggs from breeders. The integrator has the option of setting up an independent marketing network or enter into an arrangement with a national chain.

Andhra Pradesh (Region II) is the only state having annual surplus of an estimated 18 million broilers. This state mainly feeds the Mumbai area of Maharashtra. Given proper financial and marketing support, this region can produce a much larger number of commercial broilers on account of low production cost. It may well become the 'chicken bowl of India',

Table 6.7: Region-wise Production of Broiler Chicks and Per Caput Availability of Poultry Meat

Region	Population (million)		Annual broiler production (million)		Per caput availability (g)	
	1988	1994	1988	1994	1988	1994
I. Delhi, Haryana, Himachal Pradesh, Jammu and Kashmir, Punjab	54	62.2	36	59	680	948
II. Andhra Pradesh	62	67.3	29	49	470	728
III. Maharashtra	73	78.6	28	48	380	598
IV. Goa, Karnataka, Kerala, Tamil Nadu, Pondicherry	130	140.8	38	58	290	398
V. Assam, Sikkim and Eastern States, West Bengal	94	105	23	32	245	295
VI. Bihar, Gujarat, Madhya Pradesh, Orissa, Rajasthan, Uttar Pradesh	379	429.1	14	29	37	65
Total	792	883	168	275	212	311

Source: Bansil, P.C & Bhat, P.N.: Poultry Development in India: Perspectives and Approaches: Special Number of India Journal of Animal Production.

complementing its role as the country's 'egg basket'. It is estimated that 35 – 37 million eggs are produced daily in the state and roughly only one-third of them are consumed within the state and the rest exported to other states, especially West Bengal, Orissa, Assam and Tamil Nadu, Of late, these states have also made rapid strides in the sector and offtake and prices have suffered as a result. With not many quality processing units, there seems to be little scope for export of egg products to the Gulf and other countries. Many experts blame the crises in the sector on haphazard expansion, so characteristic of the state in other sectors such as aquaculture and advocate cuts in production to revive the market.

Western India (Region III) is in the forefront of broiler development. Some of the biggest broiler farms in the country are located in the Mumbai-Pune area in Maharashtra. The state leads the country in terms of modernization and sophistication. They have the capacity to produce over 10,000-20,000 broilers per week. This pocket also has the distinction of having India's first chicken-based fast food projects, viz. 'Venky's', 'Tasty Bite', 'All Season' and 'Al-Kabeer'. A number of multi-product food-processing companies also operate in the Mumbai-Pune area. The chicken-based delicacies form a significant part of their product range. These developments have given rise to a new type of arrangement for broiler farming- contract growing where the poultry processor enters into contractual arrangement with broiler growers to the mutual advantage- the grower assured of his market, and the processor of birds.

The performance of the three southern states, forming Region IV, comes as a welcome surprise, particularly when taking into account the predominant percentage of vegetarian population and the limited urban markets of Chennai and Bangalore. It means that the broiler consumption is evenly spread throughout the region. Major production centers are Bangalore – Mysore-Mangalore and Namakkal-Salem-Coimbatore belts. A number of industrial townships dot the region. Bangalore has the unique distinction of being the fastest growing metropolis in the country.

Tamil Nadu is second only to Andhra pradesh in egg production. But the poultry farmers here are finding it hard to retain this position in view of rising input costs and the State Government's apparent lack of interest in helping them maintain the competitive edge. As of now, the Namakkal poultry farmer leads the south, with a virtual monopoly over Kerala and Tamil Nadu and a 25% share of the Karnataka market. But this may not be possible, if the problems posed by State policy are compounded by rising input costs. Chicken feed can no longer be referred to dismissively as 'chicken feed' as it is getting to be prohibitively expensive. Maize, an essential ingredient, is getting out of reach of the farmers. The Namakkal farmer needs a helping hand particularly because he has only recently recovered from a yearlong devastating epidemic of Ranikhet and Infectious Bursal Disease (IBD), which claimed 1.5 million chickens during 1994. Vaccination had to be given about 5 times and this costs money.

Namakkal, a calm village a couple of decades ago, has now turned into a 'Poultry Town' of Tamil Nadu with a turnover of more than Rs. 50 million a day because of the poultry and its allied activities. Namakkal zone is the fifth biggest poultry center in the world, second biggest in egg production in the country, next to Andhra Pradesh. This zone comprises Ahnamakkal, Rasipuram, Namagiri-pettai in Salem district, Erode and Palladam in Periyar district. It has more than 6,500 poultry farms with a bird population of 21.5 million. Of these, 30% are chicks and growers, and the rest are layers. The total egg production in the zone is around 9.5 million per day. The poultry industry there grew with hardly any assistance from the Government. Major reason for the development of this industry is the acute water scarcity, due to which, the farmers had to switch over from agriculture, which was unremunerative. The development of egg trade in Namakkal zone was the 'barter' system prevailing here. A trader would give a farmer chicks, feed, medicine, besides credit (whenever required) and would take back eggs from them.

In the southern region, broilers expanded rapidly from 4 million in 1980 to 64 million in 1988, representing a 16-fold gain. It accounts for almost 40% of the total broiler production in the country. Further, Andhra Pradesh has emerged as the leading producer of broilers in the country. Three major pockets in the region are: Hyderabad, Bangalore and Coimbatore-Erode. A bird's life in broiler farming is only 2 months compared to 17 months for layers. Being shorter, it seems to be a more attractive proposition. In some states such as Kerala, there is tremendous development in broiler farming and a negative development where layers are concerned. Perhaps, we would project that any state having an unpredictable labour situation such as Kerala and West Bengal would not have much development on the layer front.

Region V in the east is a highly deficit area in the country. Its percentage of non-vegetarian population is higher than even Region I, and so the potential for growth is enormous. But it suffers from constraints of high cost of production, inadequate long distance public transportation and strong trade union activities. Further, fish competes with the chicken in the region and scores over it, when parity in retail prices exists. The vast hinterland of Assam and other eastern states cannot be serviced because of poor air transport links. Kolkata is the Mecca of all markets in the eastern region, but tends to develop transport bottleneck in the absence of adequate linkages with hinterland it serves.

The eastern region has had a slow growth in the past, but is expected to make sizable gains in the coming years. It faces continuing broiler shortage. According to one assessment, the broiler production in West Bengal alone could double itself, if only the stock was available. In view of the broiler shortage, cockerel-raising is popular. An estimated 0.1 million cockerels are raised every fortnight in West Bengal. The small village poultry units form the core of poultry production in this region. The organized, intensive commercial poultry is confined to industrial belts like those around Kolkata and some pockets of Midnapore, Hooghly, Jalpaiguri and Malda districts.

Poultry industry in Orissa is still at a nascent stage in 1998-99, Orissa had produced 7,628 lakh eggs and 4 million broilers. A recent allegation that some of the large poultry breeding farms in Orissa were polluting the environment is not correct. This was being propagated by local vested interests with political backing. Otherwise, there would be no poultry farms in the environmentally-conscious developed countries. In Orissa per caput egg and meat consumption of 20 gm and 250 gm, respectively, as against the national and advanced countries averages of 32 eggs and 280 gm and 120 eggs and 15 kg meat respectively. The National Institute of Nutrition has recommended that a balanced diet should contain 60 gm of egg and meat per head per day, and this works out to 180 eggs and 11 kg of meat per annum. To achieve this goal, poultry industry in India, which produced 32 billion eggs and 400 million broilers per annum (98% of it in the private sector), has to grow 10-fold in the near future.

Region VI is the most disappointing. With almost half of the country's population, it accounts for less than 10% of the total broiler production. With easy availability of feed ingredients and low labour costs, this region has an enormous scope to meet the deficit of broilers in other areas –mainly Region I in the north and Region V in the east. Moreover, by 1995, the number of towns with population above 1 million in this region increased to be 14 – Bihar, 4; Gujarat, Madhya Pradesh and Uttar Pradesh 3 each;

and Rajasthan, 1. In the coming decade, this region promises to see a spectacular growth. Considering the scope, opportunities and constraints in various regions, the production targets that can be aimed by 2005 are presented in Table 6.8. Despite the regional variations in production, per caput poultry meat availability has been steadily rising in the past 4 decades. The increase was substantial during the decade of eighties – a period of broiler boom.

Table 6.8: Estimated Laying Stock and Egg Production (1961-2005)

Million

Year	Layers			Eggs		
	Desi	*Improved*	*Total*	*Desi*	*Improved*	*Total*
1961	63	1	64	2,861	20	2,881
1971	50	12	62	2,280	3,060	5,340
1980	64	37	101	2,875	9,625	12,500
1985	72	50	122	3,325	12,903	16,128
1990	78	76	154	3,495	19,805	23,300
1991	79	77	156	3,549	20,111	23,660
1992	76	74	150	3,411	19,329	22,740
1993	66	84	150	2,974	21,826	24,800
1994	70	89	159	3,154	23,136	26,290
1995	75	350	550	5,455	21,820	27,275
1996	73	400	650	5,800	22,362	28,162
1997	72	450	725	6,000	24,000	30,000
1998	70	500	800	6,200	24,800	31,000
1999	72	550	870	6,500	25,500	32,000
2000	70	600	950	6,640	25,860	32,500
2001	75	700	1,100	6,655	26,345	33,000
2002	72	800	1,200	6,250	28,750	35,000
2003	70	850	1,275	6,200	28,800	36,000
2004	70	890	1,370	6,250	30,250	36,500
2005	75	930	1,430	6,500	30,750	37,000

Source: (i) Till 1994 - Indian Poultry Year Book 1994.
(ii) 1995 to 2002 – Ministry of Food Processing Industry, Govt. of India, Annual Report 2002-03
(iii) 2003 to 2005 – Projection made by Authors

PRIVATE SECTOR AND VOLUNTARY AGENCIES

Prior to sixties, practically all the poultry services in the country were provided by the public sector, primarily through the Animal Husbandry Departments of various state governments. Other than production (which was also in the nature of backyard poultry), private sector had practically no hand in research, breeding and disease control. There were hardly any feed-manufacturing units, or even testing laboratories in the country.

It was just about two decades ago, that someone actually made a foray into the sector in a planned manner—the late Dr. B.V Rao, who conceived Venkateshwara Hatcheries Ltd (VHL). He was followed by a few others like Agritech Hatcheries Ltd (AGL), set up by the Damanias, and Srinivasa Hatcheries. But the fact is that none of these corporates have really managed to make any tangible mark on the industry, with the possible exception of VHL which currently has a turnover in the region of over Rs. 3500 million. The group has quite a few companies in the industry, which are involved in every aspect of the industry - right from breeding the pureline varieties to specific pathogen free eggs (SPF eggs), automatic feed machines and branded poultry products.

Private sector has by now done a wonderful job in increasing the production and raising the level of poultry to that of an independent full-fledged industry. Commercial GP and parent stocks were introduced in the Indian market during the sixties when 2 large hatcheries in collaboration with foreign parties in the USA and Canada were set up, one near Pune and the other near Delhi, with the objective of propagating hybrid stock developed in those foreign countries through a great deal of research and experimentation. Most of the companies received grandparents of broilers as a part of the package. Again during the Third Plan 2 more collaboration hatcheries were set up in the private sector one in Haryana (Karnal) and the other in Delhi, for propagation of stocks received from the USA and Czechoslovakia.

The Pioneer

The late Padmashree Dr. B.V. Rao, along with Jagapati Rao, planned and set up the Venkateshwara Hatcheries (VH) in 1971. In 1980, they took up breeding research. The VH has set a trend. Its breeds dominate the market both in layers and broilers. The VH became an instant success, and in its first year of operation, the turnover touched Rs. 10 million. By 1996, when Dr. B.V Rao died, the turnover was Rs. 3.5 billion, which increased to Rs. 10 billion by 2002. Dr. B.V. Rao's daughter, Anuradha Desai, took over as the chairman and managing director of the VH. She is striving hard to bring international recognition to the Indian poultry industry. She organized the World Poultry Congress in 1996 at New Delhi. Dr. B.V Rao and Jagapati Rao had conceived a national body for the industry. Thus emerged the National Egg Coordination Committee (NECC) in 1982. Later, as a trading wing of NECC, Agro complex India Ltd., was started for doing egg business. Today, the NECC, with a membership of more than 25,000 farmers, is the single largest association of poultry farmers in the world. In 1993, the VH Group, with a view to uniting broiler farmers, promoted BROMARK, the all India broiler Farmer's Cooperative Marketing Society Ltd., It seeks to increase broiler production, organize the farmers on a cooperative basis, provide technical assistance and help them market their produce at remunerative prices.

People in India were not aware about the qualities of broiler meat and it was difficult for the companies to push the commercial broiler chicks in the market. Slowly when it became popular, broiler industry started growing at a rapid pace so much so that by 1990 the population of broilers rose to the level of 200 million which is now (2002) estimated at 330 million.

FARMING SECTOR

In India, we have the intensive farming sector with a high degree of technological competence, as well as the small traditional farmers, coexisting without any unhealthy competition with each other. On the one hand, we have, during the last two decades, established international standard pureline breeding farms, vaccine production units, high-tech incubators, ultramodern processing units and state-of the-art technology in the production of specific pathogen-free eggs, most of the developments having come about through private enterprises.

On the other hand, we have small farms with capacity as low as 100-200 birds or even a few birds almost in the backyard of the entrepreneur, managed and looked after by himself or his family. Since time immemorial, these backyard farms have been a means of supplementary income to small and marginal farmers, whose land holdings alone could not sustain them. This again is a sector which is primarily controlled by the private sector without much of technical assistance from the public sector. Under the peculiar Indian conditions, it is this traditional sector which will call for immediate attention.

In nutshell, the industry in India has a population of 170 million layers and 330 million broilers spread over 100,000 farms employing nearly 700,000 people. Another feature of the Indian poultry is that 90% of poultry farms are owned and operated by agriculturists themselves who, more often than not, use the poultry manure on their own lands.

Experience from Abroad

We have the example of other countries with different experiences. The USA, for example, with a layer population of 250 million, which is estimated to be owned by just 25 or fewer firms. With the type of automation in the USA, one can imagine how many people this industry can employ. Similarly, Malaysia's 18 million laying birds are reared in some 2,500 poultry farms, which translates approximately to about 7,000 birds per farm, the largest flock size being 200,000. Malaysia has not only achieved a per caput consumption of 240 eggs per annum but has also started exporting sizeable volume of eggs. There is, however, the experience of China, the largest egg-producing country in the world. Here 80% of the birds belong to local breeds and only 20% to improved breeds. The yield per layer of the local breeds was merely 120 eggs per year. Yet, China could not only become the world's largest egg producer but could also achieve a per caput consumption of 6.5 kg or approximately 130 eggs, which is really commendable when compared to most other developing countries.

Poultry in Bangladesh includes chicken, duck, and a small number of pigeon, geese, guinea fowl and quail. About 89% of the rural household keep poultry and the average number per household is 6.8. The number of poultry in the country is estimated to be about 129.94 million (chicken 116.47 million and ducks 13.47 million), which grew at an annual rate of 6.49% over 1990-1994. The share of poultry in the animal protein component of human diet is estimated to be 30% in 1995. In the last few years, small commercial poultry farming is expanding in the country in the peri-urban areas as layer and broiler farming and cockerel raising. In the rural areas, small scale farming of poultry, duck and mini hatchery are developing by the support of institutional credit, NGO and public sector technical support. The number of poultry farms is 1,11,608 out of which 89,702 farms raise a maximum 50 birds per farm. The number of duck farms is 20,223. Almost all farms are small enterprises except a few large farms.

Importance of Traditional and Free Range Poultry Farming

The earliest system of egg production in India was an extensive sector comprising a large number of small units estimated at 100,000 scattered in rural areas having flock strength of 25 to 250 birds in their backyard. Before 1960, practically the whole of poultry production was in the form of backyard farming where standard feeding or housing practices were not followed. The birds moved freely, scavenging for their food and also received the table scraps from the household. They were quite often provided with minimum shelter. Sometimes they sought shelter on trees or walls, laid a few eggs. Eggs were smaller than of commercial birds. The expenditure involved was nil. This sector fulfilled and still fulfills the socioeconomic needs through improved nutrition, and by providing some supplementary income from the sale of eggs and birds.

The traditional system of poultry keeping although still prevalent in tribal and rural areas of the country is losing its importance day by day under the impact of modernization and industrialization. Indigenous desi fowl which is poor in growth and productivity, still continues to be the mainstay of backyard poultry keeping. About 100,000 farms of varying flock sizes ranging from 5 to 250 birds are located in rural areas which follow backyard or semi-backyard system of poultry keeping. (Table 6.8).

India has nearly 70% of its population living in the villages. However, more than 75% of eggs and about 100% of broilers produced commercially are consumed in the cities and towns. The demand of the rural areas is therefore, to be met by backyard poultry. Backyard poultry keeping has been practiced by the rural people since time immemorial. The need to adopt commercial exotic crossbreds was emphasized as development. The rural people with scarce resources take to practising commercial poultry in the backyard. These improved birds obviously do not perform to their full potential in these conditions. High motility rate; malnutrition and adverse environmental conditions in many areas are antagonistic to the successful raising of heavy weight or high producing types of poultry.

In traditional farming system it is more important to minimise the risks than to increase outputs. Generally rural people identify themselves with the local breeds; free-range eggs fetch a premium price and help to ensure better Nutritional Status of the people in the villages. The introduction of the exotic breeds has lead to an increase in the per capita availability of eggs and meat 5.7 and 4.78 times respectively from 1961 to 2000 AD. Although there has been a substantial increase, its availability to the rural people is limited and at a very high cost. At present, most of our poultry production units are located near urban areas, catering to urban needs and when a fraction of this production reaches the villages, it costs the rural consumer at least 50% more what it costs the urban consumer. The higher price to the rural consumer leads to the lower consumption and low volume of trade itself acts as an inhibiting factor to higher production in villages.

An essential requirement to meet village needs is to find a methodology by which eggs can be made readily available to them at affordable prices. This will call for a new approach. Village poultry production offers one hope. By setting up a local unit to serve a cluster of villages, the birds will be scavenging in the backyard supplemented by kitchen waste and feed containing locally available ingredients. At night, the birds can be provided shelter through small low-height houses constructed with cheap wood or bricks utilizing some corner of the house. It is obvious that villages with small population cannot really sustain industrial approach to poultry production. The clue perhaps lies in developing egg production in villages not as an occupation but as a supplement methods which even if they do not lead to high levels of production per bird, do enable eggs to be produced at least possible cost. One must remember that the cheapest egg is the backyard egg which is produced by a foraging hen, scavenging in the backyard and feeding on nothing specific. The output of these birds can be sold readily within the village or in its neighbourhood. Such flocks certainly cannot be left at the mercy of nature altogether, as the traditional backyard flocks were.

The task is to induct a small dose of appropriate husbandry technology which will permit effective management of small flocks of say, 20-25 birds. For example, improved birds may be distributed to villages within the periphery of a breeding farm. Also free-range poultry products command a higher price than factory-farmed ones. Organic farming has a bright future both for home as well as external markets. The important thing is to strike a right balance between making poultry production profitable for the backyard producer and affordable to the rural consumer. Such a step would also help to increase the purchasing power of village farmers. It is true that backyard poultry raising may not result in as many eggs as the intensive system does about 270 eggs per layer per year. The village poultry units may be expected to yield, at best, 60-70 eggs per bird per year. In a way, this is a blessing in disguise because demand in rural areas is quite low, and so avoids the glut that it would otherwise cause.

There is a need to develop a low-cost shelter, a minimal health cover programme and may be some low-cost feed supplement based on local ingredients so that the birds can both be protected and induced to lay substantially more eggs than if they were left totally to forage in backyard conditions. Such methodology if developed by our scientists can extend poultry production to villages where most of India lives and where these eggs are perhaps even more needed.

The facilities in the backyard poultry will not permit the rearing of broilers as the chicks are costly and due to rapid growth rate, require ideal feed and management. If chicks of medium-type dual-purpose breeds like Rhode Island Red (RIR) or crosses of White Leghorn X RIR are supplied as straight run, the males so reared can be used for meat. Already some people buy male chicks from layer hatcheries and sell them in the rural areas. In spite of slow growth and poor liveability, these birds provide some meat to the village folk.

India produces annually around 90 million male day-old chicks as a byproduct of the egg industry. These are sold through a complex distribution channel, mainly to rural households. These cockerels, which serve villages and small towns, are grown on least-cost backyard basis and, therefore, despite their poor growth rate and possibly poorer survival rates, most of what they fetch represents net income for the grower.

The challenge once again, as in case of eggs, is to devise a total production system, including appropriate type of bird as well as a health and nutritional supplementation programme so that village households can increasingly take up raising meat birds as a supplementary activity.

The latent demand for such a product exists as is evident by high prices paid in villages and small towns for chicken of whatever description a price which is generally much higher than that in metro cities.

The prime tasks before poultry scientists and industry personnel are:

(i) Including non-conventional ingredients in feed to overcome the constraints of feed availability;

(ii) evolving more cost-efficient feed formulations, bearing in mind the Indian crop profile and availability scenario, to minimize the increase in production costs; and

(iii) devising appropriate methodology and poultry stocks for semi-range/backyard type poultry production as supplemental household activity in village to enable mass production of eggs and meat for the interior and rural markets.

Improvement of Village Backyard Chicken

In our country the government has attempted to improve the village chickens by using commercial hybrid chickens either by introducing commercial birds directly or introducing males of improved stock for crossing. Since, these villages chickens are not fed properly, they act as scavengers, feeding on food waste as well as various insects and worms. Their egg production mostly is less than 100 eggs/bird and eggs are entirely for family consumption under backyard chicken keeping system, farmers do not spend even a rupee on feed and medicine including vaccines.

Due to the above reasons, the rural farmers do not accept exotic breeds or its crosses in their traditional system to backyard poultry production. They prefer the native breeds because these breeds have acquired considerable adaptability to local climatic environments, stress of feeding and management and considerable resistance to tropical diseases. They are good foragers, efficient mothers, require less cost and less care to grow and thus have characteristics essential for raising poultry under village conditions. Hence, there is urgent need to improve the production potential of some of the native breeds of chicken, which will be accepted by the rural mass for backyard poultry production.

Strategies for Backyard Poultry

There are some institutions or private breeding farms like Central Avian Research Institute, Izatnagar; and some State Governments where the work on improvement of native breeds is in operations. It is general practice in traditional backyard poultry production that once the pair of chickens are purchased, the replacement is taken from the mating of the offspring from generation to generation. In scientific term full sib mating is practiced which is most effective method of in breeding. As a result there is marked decrease in egg production, fertility, hatchability and increase in mortality. Further the hatching of chicks from the hen throughout the year is one of the major causes of low production in desi fowl. To avoid the above mentioned two most important reasons of low production of backyard poultry, replacement of birds from out-source is very essential. Hence one of the problems demanding urgent and careful consideration is the establishment of breeder stock of native poultry populations capable of producing large number of hatching eggs. To fulfill this goal, establishment of a research center in each State for improvement of native breeds of that particular state would be crucial, as the particular breed has acquired adaptability for the particular environment. Such institution would evaluate, conserve and improve the productivity of native breed and provide improved native patent stock to the villagers.

To improve the diet of scavenging birds, farmers need to be able to identify the main nutrient supplied by each scavenged material. Many of these materials are byproducts of human food processing, but they may need further processing like drying or fermentation. There is need to acquire the ability to recognize other material that are not normally used for human food and to prepare them into a suitable form for poultry. The chicken shelter shed should be constructed with locally available materials, which are available even in rural areas, like jungle wood in place of steel for pillars, trusses and ridges etc., and tiles for roof, ordinary chicken-mesh wire along sides lengthwise taking care to prevent entry of predators into the shed. These types of sheds will be cheaper for rural farmers.

The need for research on small-scale poultry farming is not generally recognized but small-scale poultry farming is promising in developing countries as the demand of poultry products in developing world is growing very rapidly and it requires less investment. To meet the increasing demand of eggs and meat, research efforts need to be directed towards the small-scale poultry farming in developing countries as the problems in these countries are different than in the developed countries. The transfer of technical know how in different stages of skills and adoption of techniques are the major constraints in village backyard poultry production. The research efforts are also needed to be undertake the problems of backyard poultry.

Role of Poultry in Rural Development

In India poultry production which has remained as backyard venture till 1960 has emerged into an encouraging enterprise for rural folk especially for small farmers, landless labourers and educated unemployed and also for big entrepreneurs maintaining the birds on large scale in thousands. Poultry rearing is no more considered as low prestigious occupation fit for only weaker sections of the society. It has become a full-time job for many and the size of flock maintained ranges from 100 to 50,000. After achieving self-sufficiency in cereal production the attention has been diverted to plan and develop potential arena for better and protective foods such as eggs, poultry meat, milk and milk products. Poultry industry with about 1500 million population producing 35 million eggs annually has been deemed to be commercially viable enterprise contributing more than Rs. 400 crore to the Gross National Product (GNP). India actually requires nearly three times more eggs against the present (2002) availability of about 35 billion eggs a year. Thus, it is warranted that the egg production should be increased by 3 times to reach the level of recommended requirements of half an egg per day individual for half of the country's population comprising of non-vegetarian group.

Poultry production has an appreciable advantage of being relatively easy to raise and at the same time the enterprise can be adopted under the diversified agroclimatic conditions of our country. The initial requirements of land and capital required to initiate this enterprise on a moderate scale are within the limits of the rural sector of our country. The agricultural farmers who are generally not engaged throughout, Poultry industry with about 1500 million population producing 35 million eggs annually has been deemed to be commercially viable enterprise contributing more than Rs. 400 crore to the Gross National Product (GNP). India actually requires nearly three times more eggs against the present (2002) availability of about 35 billion eggs a year. Thus, it is warranted that the egg production should be increased by 3 billion eggs a year. Thus, it is warranted that the egg production should be increased by 3 times to reach the level of recommended requirements of half an egg per day individual for half of the country's population comprising of non-vegetarian group will be occupied all the year round and the income derived from egg and meat production will be continuous process throughout the year. The manure obtained from the poultry having more essential nutrients of Nitrogen, Phosphate and Potash (NPK) than the other organic manures, can supplement the synthetic fertilizers which have become costlier due to hike in the price of petroleum products. The poultry farming finds a source for utilising the surplus and coarse grains which form the bulk of the poultry mash. Poultry development by utilising these coarse cereals helps in stabilising the prices of the coarse grains in the long run, which otherwise do not fetch decent price to the agricultural producers. Poultry farming creates a demand for agro-industrial by products and wastes which are utilised and incorporated in the poultry feed. Poultry industry helps in promoting ancillary industries and as on today there are nearly 200 standard feed manufacturers all over the country producing 5 lakh tonnes annually. One of the salient features of the rapid progress of the poultry industry has been the remarkable growth in the production of egg and meat which cannot be compared by any sector of agriculture.

Considering the large number of unemployed, more than ten millions and an equal number, if not more, may be unemployed in rural areas who may not come in the Live Employment Register, it is essential to find out suitable occupation for the poor rural sector. With greater attention towards rural sector than urban sector the Government now stress more towards generating employment in the rural area which is the nerve centre of Indian Economic Progress and Prosperity, where most of the people comprise mostly small and marginal farmers with small holdings and landless labourers depending on manual labour for their livelihood. Therefore it becomes imperative to improve the lots of small farmers, marginal farmers, landless labourers, artisans, tribals, backward and depressed classes who form large segment of rural population. The small fragmented holdings possessed by the small and marginal farmers do not bringforth enough remuneration to meet their family requirements. Lack of funds at appropriate times for implementing improved methods of agriculture, besides the limitation in the productive capacity of the land render the pattern of generating employment in rural area to remain static. Bearing this in mind the National Commission of Agriculture has suggested poultry programmes on massive scale which can generate employment and improve the income of the rural poor through production of eggs and meat on small holdings.

Poultry farming fits in squarely with the primary objectives envisaged in the integrated rural development programmes. The main objective of various plans of eliminating unemployment and significant underemployment can be attained to a large extent by means of poultry farming which, by virtue of its employment potential may become the most popular medium of self-employment among the rural masses.

NDDB may Assist in Poultry Farming

The National Dairy Development Board (NDDB) had agreed to examine whether it could use its vast infrastructure to help small farmers and landless rural workers to do backyard poultry farming. The NDDB's now-legendary establishment of a national grid of milk cooperatives ensures its presence almost everywhere. It also boasts of year of expertise Duck farming in helping small farmers to organise production and marketing.

DUCK FARMING

There is need to exploit water resources for production of fish and ducks to meet the requirements of animal protein. Ducks are proliferating layers and the people living in costal belts relish their meat. Ducks can be raised in both intensive and extensive husbandry practices along with fishponds for better production. Duckery and fishery are two separate systems (avian and aquatic) but can maintain symbolic relationship when integrated together. The raising of ducks with fish in the same pond is more rational as compared to any other system of integrated farming. The pond provides both living and foraging area for duck and fish. The duck manure for primary and secondary production (plankton and plants) and serves as high protein source for better growth of fish.

Extensive inland watershed areas serve an excellent habitat for the ducks. These watershed areas besides the ponds and lakes provide natural food viz. algae, fishes, earthworms, insects, fungi, snails, waterweeds etc. for the ducks and reduce the feed cost. Hence to augment duck production in the rural areas there is still need to popularize duck farming so that economic viability of duck farming is made known to the people. Following facts should be made out before duck farming:

(a) Ducks have a natural tendency to forage; hence they are widely reared in rice growing areas, as the expenditure on rearing is negligible. On the other hand these birds help to enrich the soil by their droppings with nitrogen and minerals.

(b) The rearing cost of ducks as compared to chicken is further reduced as they lay 40-50 eggs more than the chicken. They are proliferating layers and can lay for 2 years or more.

(c) Unlike chicken the duck has virtually no cannibalism problems.

(d) Ducks are quite hardy and are resistance to many diseases. However, they are susceptible to diseases like duck-cholera, duck-plague and duck-viral hepatitis. Thus the expenditure incurred on medication is also lower in duck farming.

(e) The ducks usually lay the eggs before 9:00 am, which saves the labour cost in collection of eggs.

(f) Ducks are less sensitive to extreme weather as thick layer underneath their feathers protect them against cold and heat.

(g) In some parts of the country like West Bengal, Assam and Tripura duck eggs fetch good revenue.

Extensive duck farming is common in India and that is considered as the main duck-breeding tract. The number of duck population depends on the availability of water sources like rivers, ponds, canals, basins and low-lying lands. The water resources fed these birds with balanced feed. Duck accounts about 7% of the total poultry population of India. Ducks are not only prolific layers (280-300 eggs/year) but also produce bigger-sized egg when compared with hen. Duck meat and eggs are equally tasty and nutritious.

The major states for duck population include West Bengal, Assam, Kerala, Tamil Nadu, Andhra Pradesh and Orissa, followed by Bihar, Jammu and Kashmir, Tripura, Uttar Pradesh and Karnataka. The natural resources like water bodies are plenty in this region. Majority ducks are indigenous variety with low productivity. Various states have identified some local variety and named them. In Assam the local ducks are known as Patti, Deo Hanh, Raj Hanh, Nageswari, etc. Likewise in Kerala they are known as Chara and Chemabelli. However, systematic reporting is still missing. Some of the local breeds/varieties have good production potential with better disease resistance as well.

Since the requirement of ducks is minimum there is a vast scope for the introduction of high-yielding exotic duck and their crosses to achieve visible changes in enhancement of production of duck eggs and meat. Among the high-yielding varieties of ducks, Khaki Campbell, Indian runner, Cherry valley, Muscovy and Pekins are common.

Where there is big natural water basin and swampy areas. The water resource feeds these birds with high valued aquatic weeds, snails, insects, fingerlings, tadpoles and frogs for their optimum growth and production thus the expenditure for feed is practically less. An attendant allows ducks for foraging the whole day in open field and are shifted from one area to other. In the evening they are allowed to stay under a netted enclosure, which protect them from predators. This also helps for easy collection of eggs as the ducks generally lay in the early morning.

Integrated Farming System

Integrated farming system is an age-old practice in India. Now scientific research considered it as most profitable and efficient enterprise. Attention is paid to utilize the natural resources like water bodies for composite farming. Integration of duck into fish culture is gaining its popularity in India.

The main features of the Integrated Farming System are as follows:

(a) best utilization of the waste of ducks as an input of protein source for the fish;

(b) economic utilization of the space in which the 2 subsystems occupy part for all space required for individual system;

(c) there is increased productivity, more income generation, gainful employment and cheap availability of animal protein with minimum expenditure; and

(d) above all these 2 systems usually help each other in maintaining ecological balance and best utilization of the natural resources in and around the pond area.

Advantages

The advantage of integrated ducks and fish farming are as follows:

(1) The droppings of ducks are rich in nonprotein nitrogenous substances (urea) which serve as readymade feed for the fishes thus minimize the expenditure of artificial feeding which is about 70% of the total input.

(2) Duck /consumes weeds, grass and green algae.

(3) Ducks consume the grasshoppers, beetles and snails in and around the ponds as protein rich natural feed source.

(4) During summer the ducks help in reducing the heating of surface water due to regular swimming.

(5) The enhancement of the fish ponds is preferably used and as duck sheds thus no additional land is required for duck-houses.

(6) Fish and duck together ensure higher profit due to higher production of fish yield, duck eggs, and duck-meat within an unit time and limited water area through minimum investment.

The profit margin in duck and fish culture depends on the density of the duck population and also on the availability of natural feed resources to reduce the feed cost and inputs for ducks. Higher density of ducks helps in optimum utilization of natural resources. For more profit the duck farmers should adopt extensive, semi-intensive and intensive methods for Duck rearing along Farming. Fishes raised on Integrated duck farming are fed in the semi-intensive mode whereas the reverse is not true.

Now some of the progressive farmers started integrating farming. They prefer to keep ducks in their fish ponds for better profit from fish and additional income from the ducks. This is gaining popularity day by day. These progressive fish farmers prefer to keep flocks of high-yielding ducks in semi-intensive mode. Small amount of duck feed is provided depending on natural feed resources. The number of ducks may vary from 300 to 1000/ha of water area. This is best suited for Indian conditions.

The intensive duck farming in fishponds is more profitable as ducks are confined in higher numbers per unit of pond area. The dropping of ducks serves in fertilizing the pond water for more vegetation. This vegetations serves as natural food for the fish. Besides some amount of duck feed is also dropped into the pond as feed for these fish. This will be more profitable, if the stocking density is increased up to 3000/ha. The approach of integration of duck farming is practical, profitable and acceptable to the farmers in the developing world for maximum utilization of land and water resources.

FUTURE PROGRAMME

Besides the Ministry of Agriculture, the ICAR and State Governments, there are a number of other organizations like the Ministry of Rural Development, NCDC, Department of Women and Child Development and Small-Scale Industries, which are also engaged in Poultry Development in the country. None of them has, however, succeeded to either develop a rural market or establish a proper system for such supplies. Therefore, the demand is being curbed in the absence of a regular supply channel. The number of desi birds in rural areas are not enumerated separately; hence, it is difficult to know the relevant details. In fact nothing is known about the present demand and supply situation of eggs in the rural areas, although it is conjectured that there is a huge untapped potential.

It is recommended that a comprehensive survey to find out the real ground situation should be conducted as early as possible in rural India to enable us to evolve an appropriate policy frame in this respect. We would suggest that the present Central Poultry Breeding Farms can be utilized. Study of the 4 Poultry Breeding Farms shows that 3 of them (excluding Chandigarh) are engaged in breeding egg poultry. Although each of them has the capacity to produce over 50,000 (parent stock) birds, they are producing hardly 20,000 birds each, which are being supplied to State Farms to produce commercial birds. Although these birds are being sold at half of the market price, there is no demand for them. All this indicated that the scientific poultry breeding programme taken up by these farms during 1971-72 has not kept pace with genetic improvement in production by birds in the private sector.

A question which arises is should the farmer continue to raise whatever is available or should try to introduce a bird which is just replica in physical characteristic of indigenous hen but has potentiality to produce 100% more eggs under scavenger system of management? An answer is provided by Krishna-J breed, a replica of desi fowl (Table 6.9). Krishna-J is a synthetic bird developed by introducing sex-linked gene (dwarfing) on Z-chromosome and autosomal light bar gene. One of the major factors was to produce pullet weighing 0.9 kg at 20 weeks and 1.4 kg at 72 weeks of age. Krishna-J has white barring on black background or solid black, with low frequency of 'ld' sex linked gene imparting blackish colour to beak and shank.

Substitution of dw gene in the first generation delayed sexual maturity from 11.6 to 12.8 days. Backcrossing to broiler and layer genome resulted reduction in sexual maturity from 218 days to 163.8 days. Egg production increased 100% in Krishna-J layers compared with the base population. Under scavenger system of raising it produced 110-120 eggs, i.e. twice that of the indigenous breeds, and laid heavier eggs. Krishna-J pullets utilize protein less and energy more efficiently for growth and egg production. Chick ration must contain 24% protein and for the egg production the diet must contain 18% crude protein, and 2,600 kcal metabolizable energy. Hen consumes 72 g feed in summer and 86 g in the optimum season. Crude

Table 6.9: Perfomance of Krishna-J Coloured Layer Hen

	Base population	*VI generation*
Body weight (g)		
20 weeks	594	926
40 weeks	N.A	1258
72 weeks	800	1330
Egg Production (no.)		
280 days	41	82.4
448 days		216.0
Scavengers system (Annual)		110-120
Sexual maturity (days)	218	163.8
Egg weight at 40 weeks (g)	40.1	50.6
Egg colour	Tinted Brown	Tinted Brown
Feed consumption (g)	72-86	

fibre tolerance is about 1.5 times more in Krishna-J and can also withstand starvation better than normals. Superior viability and increased fitness in summer was due to higher level of sodium concentration in the blood of Krishna-J than normal (1.77.0 meq/litre *vs* 130.75 meq/litre) which helps better water retention by dwarfs than normal sibs under stress.

In spirochaetosis infection the regeneration mechanism of red blood cells was quicker in Krishna-J and was the cause of less mortality. Similarly, dwarf chick suffers from coccidiosis, weight loss but the percentage of natural recovery was high. Backyard poultry is integrated in socioeconomic and cultural habits of rural and hilly tribes. In such cases improved birds such as Kadaknath and Krishna-J should be introduced.

The present proposal would mean multiplication of indigenous poultry breeds which are supposedly relatively disease-resistant and have tremendous ability to survive on inadequate nutrition and still produce 60-70 eggs in production cycle. The problems of brooding would be handled through modern hatchery management and day-old chicks would be provided to the farmers at subsidized rates so that they do not have to brood their own chicks. The hatchery would also vaccinate the day old chicks after vaccination against RD. This would ensure a large spread of desi poultry as backyard enterprises.

An organizational framework for implementing this programme would involve Ministry of Rural Development, the Department of Women and Child Development, Small-Scale Industries. NCDC and Programme Implementation Department in the PMO. The Programme could be run through NGOs to avoid bureaucratic hassles in dealing with the individual farmer, cooperatives and community groups. This programme would also be integrated with other social development programmes currently run under the Jawahar Gram Samridhi Yojana (JGSY) and Swarnajayanti Gram Swarozgar Yojana (SGSY), etc.

The research programmes of ICAR (CARI, Izatnagar and PDP, Hyderabad) have not shown any better performance than CPBFs in comparison to private poultry breeders. A time has come, that the money invested by the ICAR in its poultry breeding programmes should be invested only on indigenous poultry breeds and their improvement. They should be directed to produce pureline, GP stock and parent stock in their research facilities. The 4 central poultry breeding farms of the Department of Animal Husbandry and Dairying (DAHD) should serve as multiplication and supply centers for the 4 regions and the facilities should be effectively utilized.

As soon as the result of the survey suggested above are available, e.g. the number of indigenous birds and their type, egg and meat producing capacity of various breeds, growth potential for broiler, likely potential of village markets, and demand elasticity for birds, meat and eggs, a comprehensive work plan can be chalked out both for development as well as for market strategy for day-old chicks, birds, meat and eggs. A stage will then reach when just like commercial poultry, private sector will take over the production and distribution of poultry products for the rural areas.

The whole scheme can be taken up as a joint venture with all the concerned organizations. For example, ICAR farms should supply the parent stock, NCDC should form cooperatives, IRDP beneficiaries should join the training programmes, APEDA should try to create an export market and Small-Scale Industry may join to provide infrastructure facilities. Training and supply of day-old chicks would in that case be the function of the DAHD. A Committee under the chairmanship of Secretary, Animal Husbandry and Dairying with membership of all the concerned departments would be basically the implementation agency for this purpose. It would be worthwhile to set up this committee immediately before the recommended programme is initiated.

While we recognize that commercial poultry breeding is likely to improve the status of this industry and become globally competitive based on exotic germplasm, indigenous poultry is also likely to be a force to reckon with for the coming decades, particularly when dealing with small and marginal farmers, landless labourers, handicapped gender, and poorer section of the society. This proposal is basically targeted to them for their nutrition, employment and wealth generation so that they are able to enjoy the fruits of equity and justice under our system.

The poultry industry must undergo radical changes to compete with international competitors. The WTO is not a threat to the industry but a challenge which should be met successfully. New challenges on poultry sector include market access, SPS measures and food safety. There is the need to modernize abattoirs and processing plants. Eggs and chicken meat are among the cheapest source of protein and could be of immense help in fighting protein malnutrition in India. The per capita consumption of eggs in the country is only 32 and poultry meat 1 kg against a recommended consumption of 180 eggs and 10.8 kg poultry meat person per annum.

It would be appropriate for India to have a food authority to include and cover all food standards and food-related issues. The proposed food authority would end multiplicity of agencies doing similar work in different directions haphazardly. This would ensure food safety and hygiene in the country.

Opportunity exists in poultry, dairy, pet food and aquaculture, where issues of biosecurity, probiotics, toxin binders and nutritionals are some of the areas of focus for vetcare in India. With the world becoming a global village, human health and animal welfare are the important market trends. Today's consumer demands a high quality of eggs. With the layer industry growing particularly in Asia, more layer breeding companies are required, calling for genetic solutions to breed hens according to requirements.

At present majority of the people in India are vegetarian and do not eat even egg because of the orthodox thinking that like meat, egg has also life. They are not fully educated about the present system under which egg produced is lifeless—it is of animal origin like milk. In addition they contain constituents that help in the treatment of a wide range of human health problems. Annexures I and II provide detailed information in these two aspects.

Targets

The physical target and achievements for some of the important items during the last two years are indicated below:

Item/Unit		2001-02		2002-03
		Target	Achieve	Target
Parent chicks to be supplied (in thousand)	Egg type	60	43	45
	Meat type	40	46	25
Production of ducklings (in thousands)		100	81.7	100
Feed sample to be analysed	(in nos.)	300	2998	2000
No. of persons to be trained		100	60	500
No. of random sample	Layer	4	4	1
Tests to be conducted	Broiler	3	3	1

Centrally Sponsored Scheme "Assistance to State Poultry/Duck Farms

The centrally sponsored scheme – Assistance to State poultry farms including other species like ducks, turkey, quails, guinea fowl etc., are now being implemented in all the States and UTs. The pattern of assistance is 100% in the case of North Eastern States including Sikkim whereas it is 80:20 in respect of other States between Center and State respectively, at the rate of maximum Rs. 6.00 lakhs for each farm. While calculating the State share, the cost of land and other inputs provided will also be included as their share. In the existing premises of State farms poultry, guinea fowl, quail, turkey can also be taken up as a new activity. The scheme will also apply to the farms of the State Governments who may run in collaboration with cooperatives/private sector/NGOs, etc. One time assistance is provided to suitably strengthen them in terms of hatching, brooding and rearing of the birds with provision for feed mill and their quality monitoring and in-house disease diagnostic facilities. These farms will strictly maintain the parent stock of low input technology birds duly identified by this department in consultation with ICAR and State Government. Necessary in built provision has been made in the proposal for revolving fund for purchase of replacement breeding stock, feed ingredients, transportation, medicines and vaccines etc., The amount so spent has to be recouped from the sale proceeds of eggs, chicks and culled birds etc., and may be in turn used for the farm year after year making it a financially self sufficient unit.

Middleman's Exploitation

Poultry sector has become an easiest prey and of the middlemen and they are very much active by dint of their illusion and influence upon the poor producers. Needless to mention that broiler farmers particularly have become their easy targets in most of the parts of our country, except some areas where full form integration is going on with their retail outlets, or in some places where the farmers have united to form a strong society/association/cooperative by themselves with the mission Self help is the best help. The most glaring example of such cooperative is in Madhya Pradesh which is running successfully in the broiler market. In south India the growth in the broiler market has been encouraged by creating a line of bromark shops. This is a new initiative where the farmers have been able to do away the middlemen by putting the farmer and the retailer in direct touch.

How they act: It is obviously a tactical activity of the middlemen traders to create artificial less demand in the market, and farm gate price falls even below the production cost of a kg of broiler meat. Farmers on the other hand cannot retain the broiler in his farm as broilers are perishable goods and when it has attained the marketable age, it should be marketed as early as possible, otherwise the farmer has to sustain a heavy loss for not marketing it. While the retail market price which is paid by an end customer remains unchanged. Hence the lion share of the profit margin goes into the hands of the middleman trader, depriving the farmer. The farmer on his part, being unable of lower down the production cost finds no other way than to stop his business. In this way the pressure ultimately goes to the hatchery that produces broiler chicks which are purchased by the farmer. Due to this crisis the hatchery men are also bound to reduce the price of Day-old chicks even much below the production cost, in order to dispose of the large number of chicks already produced. To save the industry from the crisis of stagnant chicken market, the hatchery has to roll out a production cut plan by culling broiler breeders at 65 weeks instead of culling birds at 70th weeks. The chicken producers representative body, the Broiler Coordination Committee (BCC) has to take this contingencies initiated to counter "the continued weakening prices of chicken in the live bird market". Same is the case with egg markets and the egg producing farmers are also in a losing concern. Due to fall in market egg prices, they are bound to sell eggs to the dealer at or even below the production cost.

Broiler Cooperatives

Poultry farmers of the northern region are all set to form cooperative societies to achieve the twin objective of making fresh chicken available at an affordable price as well as reducing malpractices in the trade. Though Bromark—All-India Broiler Farmers Marketing Cooperative—has already evoked good response from both poultry farmers and consumers in Andhra Pradesh, Maharashtra and few other states, it will soon be spreading its operations in Chandigarh, Punjab and Haryana markets.

If one looks at the price at which a poultry farmer sells a bird and the rate at which a consumer buys it, one will find the difference unacceptably high. For example, the prevalent rate that farmers get is Rs 32 to Rs 35 a kg, while in the retail market it is sold for Rs 75 to Rs 80 per kg Chandigarh is a big market. The average consumption is about 15,000 birds a day. If we make chicken available at an affordable price, say Rs 60 to Rs 65 a kg, it will push up sale and help both consumers and producers.

The idea is that both farmers and consumers should benefit and prevent trade malpractices. Once this cooperative movement is in place, the market scenario will improve. This cooperative should have its own outlets so that consumers are assured of quality as well as affordable price. One of the challenges facing the poultry industry is establishing credibility. Because of the big variation in the price of chicken, at times consumers get the impression that they are being supplied diseased or dead birds.

The endeavor of the new cooperative federation would be to build credibility and promise consumers that they would get healthy birds. All outlets will have a standard design and each outlet will have to maintain hygiene and cleanliness standards. Regarding low prices, the increase in consumption will offset the decreased margin of profit of traders and retailers. The idea is not to replace the existing trade channels in any manner, but to ensure quality products at affordable price.

The new concept is modelled on the National Egg Coordination Committee (NECC), which ensures that the egg prices are remunerative to the producer and fair to the consumer. With its various activities and promotional campaigns, it has been successful in keeping the gap between the farmgate price and the consumer price at not more than 30 percent. In the present-day chicken industry, the difference is 100 to 110 percent. Once farmers join the cooperative, things are expected to change markedly.

What is the Drawback on our Part!

1. The producers on their part are unable to lower down the cost of production both in egg as well as chicken meal sector due to hike in input cost. Feed cost alone comprises about 65-70% of total

production cost. The feed ingredients price hike day by day makes the feed costlier and so the cost of output goes upward.

2. The volume based production of eggs and meat has led to this situation and created opportunity for the middle-traders to exploit the market.

3. We have failed to keep a balance between demand and supply, which is virtually controlled by the retailers.

4. The industry has failed to create a market in this country with vast population by increasing food awareness specially protein rich food like egg and chicken meat.

5. Although egg is cheaper than even a cup of tea, still the egg consumption has not increased as per our assumption since majority of the population believe egg is a non-veg item. They consume milk and libitum considering these veg. food. This is one of the main reasons for the crisis in the industry.

What Measures Should We Take?

1. Creating market for the end products like eggs and meat and retail marketing should be done by the producers.

2. Formation of strong association of cooperative marketing society as in some states to promote retail marketing products. In some cases, it has been seen that retail outlets have been opened by the Association/Society where the producers come in touch with the end consumers directly.

3. Integration in the poultry production has come a great way in solving this problem. In this case the farmers are under the contract farming system and they are paid for their products by the integrator irrespective of profit or loss to the company. Farmer has not to worry about the marketing of his broiler, no middleman will be involved to market the product. Above all the farmers become free of all worries and engage fully on the hygienic production of broilers and eggs.

In our country the integration is coming up at snail's pace. Still the farmers under contract are relieved of marketing problems. In other developed countries there are marketing companies or food companies to market processed chicken. There are just five companies in India who have organized processing facilities. There are small players with semi organized facilities marketing here and there.

Finally, the effort should be made to improve the broiler quality and should reach the customer level at affordable price. The hatchery people and farmers together come with a product which would be taken up by the consumer, who is puzzled by extreme disparities in price-, sometimes selling at Rs. 80 per kilo and sometimes selling @ Rs. 50 per kilo of dressed chicken. Consumer is taken by confusion and is clue less why so much of fluctuations. Hatcheries produce chicks, farmers rear them and public consume-but who is the decider of the fluctuation rate ! Is it not the terrorist middle man?

BIOTECHNOLOGY AND POULTRY VACCINES

Poultry industry all over the world has made significant progress in production efficiency due to innovative management practices and the regular use of vaccines' to reduce disease related losses. But, the diseases (bacterial and viral) still remains one of the most important hurdle in development of poultry sector not only in India but throughout the world. Annual losses due to various diseases in poultry industry in India are to the tune of Rs. 300 crores. In the International scenario, for instance, the losses due to latest outbreaks of Newcastle disease (NDV) in California (US) have been estimated to the tune of US $ 300 million, while the outbreaks of Avian influenza (AI) in Virginia (US) cost losses of about US $ 130 million. Yet, it is quite reasonable to acknowledge that the incidence of many poultry diseases has been lowered through the use of currently available vaccines consisting of either attenuated (live) or inactivated (killed) vaccines. Today the annual market for poultry vaccines in India is to the tune of about Rs. 140 crores and looking at the growth rate @8% in the industry, it is expected to rise to the tune of Rs. 240 crores by the yr. 2010. However, most of the present day vaccines are produced using age old technologies and therefore have their own pros and cons. Some of the most important drawbacks associated with these vaccines include –

1. Highly expensive production processes.
2. Conventional live vaccines : require maintenance of cold chain up to the point of vaccination, has a possibility of contamination with adventitious agents or other cells, chances of reversion to virulent state, need for refrigeration temperature for storage and limited shelf life. Apart from these, there is a potential hazard to personnel working with large amounts of live microorganisms like *Salmonella sp.*
3. Killed vaccines also has its own drawbacks like need to ensure complete inactivation, presence of cellular debris, repeated injections and the period of immunity offered by most of these vaccines at the field level are still questionable.
4. Most important factor contributing to the reducing of efficacy of conventional vaccinated and infected birds or animals.
5. Methods used for quality control of vaccines are time consuming and laborious. For instance, detection of mycoplasma spp. as a contaminant in vaccine product requires weeks to months for isolation and identification.
6. The standards fixed by the international bodies such as OIE, FAO, WHO also limit the use of the number of vaccines. Since poultry and poultry products finally enters human food chain, the residual effects of chemicals used in vaccine production, excretion of virus in vaccine production, excretion of virus in case of live vaccines, effect of vaccine strains or ingredients on meat and egg quality are some of the burning issues of the hour linked with conventional vaccines.

During the last two decades, a new subject called biotechnology has emerged as a possible remedy to such problems. Biotechnology is an amalgamation of subjects like microbiology, biochemistry and molecular biology. The use of advanced molecular biology techniques, identification of immunogenic component of organisms, better understanding of avian immune system and pathogenesis of diseases has mandated that introduction of a number of new approaches to develop and deliver vaccines. Therefore, poultry industry is in favour of developing new generation vaccines that will party if not completely replace the conventional vaccines.

To attest to that statement, the first genetically engineered fowl pox virus vectored vaccine against New Castle Disease (NDV) virus infection in chicken has been licensed for use in the US. A recombinant avian influenza (AI)- fowl pox (FP) vaccine has been approved for use in Mexico following an outbreak of a highly pathogenic avian influenza (HPAI) virus in 1995. Recently, a live gene deletion mutant Salmonella enteritidis vaccine has also been approved for use in poultry. Various biotechnological approaches have been used for development of poultry vaccines. For better understanding, these modern biotechnologically designed vaccines can be classified into two major categories.
    a.   Killed / inactivated vaccines
    b.   Live vaccines

a. Killed / inactivated vaccines
    i.   Conventional sub unit vaccines
    ii.   Recombinant DNA (DNA)
    iii.   Synthetic peptide vaccines
    iv.   Anti-idiotype vaccines:

b. Live vaccines
    i.   Gene deletion/mutant vaccines :
    ii.   Live vectored vaccines:

BIRD FLU HITS ASIA'S FEED TRADE

Asian nations following the outbreak in early 2004 of the bird flue disease are bracing for a sharp drop in commercial feed demand following a lack of orders from the poultry sector, forcing feed makers to restrict production. As governments in Thailand, Indonesia, Vietnam, Japan, South Korea, Cambodia, Pakistan, Taiwan and Laos battle to contain the spread of the virus, the feed trade is fearing the worst. "We are hearing a new country reporting bird flu everyday. Surely, the impact on the feed business is going to be bigger than what we initially thought," said one grains trade official. Regional grain traders said feed makers in countries such as Thailand, one of Asia's leading poultry exporters, and Indonesia, were asking suppliers to hold back shipments. In Vietnam, feed ingredient buyers were shying away from placing fresh orders. The spread of the virus, which has killed six people in Vietnam and two in Thailand, came as Asia's feed trade is also struggling with high ingredient prices in the absence of Chinese offers and surging freight rates.

In Thailand, the poultry sector accounts for about 55% of the commercial feed consumption, while it's 35% in Vietnam and 80% in Indonesia. Poultry feed formulation needs about 20% soymeal and at least 50% corn. Southeast Asia's feed demand has been growing steadily in the past three years, with some nations expecting before the outbreak double-digit demand growth in 2004 following a year of healthy growth in 2003. "Nobody is asking about soymeal right now. Importers are struggling to find out to what extent feed demand might be hit. Everybody is a bit confused and nobody is willing to guess," one regional trader said. "And getting corn at competitive rates is anyway difficult as China is not offering. With so much uncertainty surrounding demand prospects, people have reason to be hesitant in bringing in corn at high prices from the United States".

Feed makers could buy Chinese corn at about $125 a tonne, on a C & F basis, early last year. US corn is currently offered about $165. Some trade officials are fearing that the soy crushing industry in countries such as Thailand might have to face losses. "Some crushers expanded operations only last year, anticipating good growth in demand. Now, they have to slow down their operations," said John Lindblom, regional director for Southeast Asia of the American Soybean Association. Trade officials said it could take up to five months for Southeast Asia's poultry industry to return to its normal health. "They will have to go through the massive culling exercise to depopulate and disinfect the farms. There are no vaccines or antibiotics. The process will be long," Lindblom said.

Indian Scene

The Rs. 24,000 crore odd domestic poultry industry has reason to worry. Although no single case of bird flue has so far been reported from anywhere in the country, the government, went into full alert to prevent an outbreak of high pathogenic avian influenza. After having officially issued a ban on import of poultry feed from any country and sounding a red alert in Pakistan-bordering districts of Punjab, Rajasthan and Gujarat as well as north eastern states abutting Myanmar, the agriculture ministry asked the MEA to issue a priority travel advisory to passengers bound for the affected countries.

In addition, the environment ministry has been asked to both monitor and report urgently to a special panel set up in the animal husbandry department any unusual deaths observed among migratory birds.

Conclusions

The intensive poultry industries rely heavily upon the use of vaccines for disease control. The use of biotechnology to create recombinant DNA vaccines, viral vector based vaccines and gene deletion vaccines offer new avenues for the development of modern vaccines for effective disease control in poultry. ND, AI, ISD and MD antigens expressed recombinant fowl pox virus have been shown to be effective vaccines for poultry. Although, only few products have seen market place, we may see many more in near future since biotech vaccines are novel, safer, more efficacious and less expensive to produce in order for them to gain a niche in the market place. It may not be an exaggeration if we say that biotechnology promises revolution in poultry industry.

US INDUSTRY STATISTICS

During the period from 1992 to 2002 the average size of America's laying flock expanded from 234 million birds to an estimated 278 m. In the early nineties only 18% of flocks yielded a hen-housed average to 60 weeks to age, of 230 eggs or more, today, that percentage has risen to around 35%, while the best flocks average almost 250 eggs between 21 and 60 weeks of age. This and a mass of other statistical information can be abstracted from United Egg Producers 2003 Production Planning Calendar.

In the year 2003, production is expected to amount to around 205 million cases of which 122 m (59.5%) will be sold retail, almost 31% will go for breaking, while 9% will be traded to the institutional markets with less than 1% going for exports. The most striking figures show that the quantity of eggs broken out has jumped from 41.3 million cases (24.5% of the total) since 1992 to the estimate for this year of 63 million.

Since 1992 the human population in the US has grown from 255 million to an estimated 288 million for 2003. Relating these figures to egg production indicates that the quantity of eggs produced/person has climbed from around 238 back in 1992 to around 257 in recent years. The volume consumed in shell has fluctuated from 177/person to a 'low' of 170 in 1995. At that time the industry was wrestling with the cholesterol issue but uptake has since increased, as a result of excellent promotional work by the Egg Nutrition Center and the American Egg Board. Per capita production of eggs in product forms has shown a steady climb form around 58 in 1992 to over 78 last year. The estimate for the year 2003 was a further rise to almost 79 eggs. Total average egg consumption per person has improved dramatically in the past few years to around 254. This compares with 235/person just six years ago.

EGGS ARE VEGETARIAN

Egg and milk are more common food of animal origin. The nutritionists have ranked the egg and milk proteins as number one and two, respectively; among hundreds of animal and vegetable foods consumed by human beings; based on their biological value, digestibility, net protein value, protein efficiency ratio and chemical score. Moreover, they are easy to cook and digest, compared to cereals, pulses (legumes), vegetables, nut, meat and cheese.

Egg *vs.* Milk

The lacto-vegetarians accept milk and milk products in their menu as a vegetarian food; but not the egg; why? They consider milk as a secretion of the udder, having no life; which is true. On the other hand, they think that the egg is having embryo, which will come out as chick. This is true in olden days, when the hens and cocks are roaming freely in the open yard, producing fertile eggs. However, in modern layer farms, no cocks are reared; hence the hens will produce lifeless eggs only.

Even well educated people think that the egg is produced only when the hen is mated with a cock or by artificial insemination; but this is not true. The fact is that the egg production is a normal physiological reproductive cycle in hens; from the time they attain sexual maturity, similar to menstrual cycle in women. In women, during every menses cycle, one unfertilized ovum will come out, once in about four weeks period. Similarly in hens, without any contact with cocks or artificial insemination, an unfertilized egg (ovum) will come out once daily. Chicks will not come out of these table eggs, even if they are incubated in an incubator or under broody hen; because these eggs are not fertilized and lifeless. Only in the presence of cocks or by artificial insemination, the egg will become fertilized and chicks will come out of such eggs, when incubated. For table purpose, no farm will produce fertile eggs, because it is very expensive to produce fertile eggs.

Vegetarianism

In countries like India, Nepal and Bhutan, the per capita egg consumptions are very low, compared to rest of the world; because nearly 25% are lacto-vegetarians, about 20% are ovo-lacto-vegetarians and the remaining 55% are semi-/anti- vegetarians (old name "non-vegetarians" is not proper, because they are not against vegetarian foods).

Even these so called-vegetarians do not consume meat for many days in an year due to poverty, religious, socioeconomic and other reasons. Hence, their egg and meat consumption will be less than one egg and 40 g of meat per week, compared to 3-5 eggs and 0.5-3 kg meat per week in developed and developing countries. Hence, they are basically lacto-vegetarians and their health related problems cannot be attributed to egg and meat consumption. This vegetarianism (veganism) is mainly due to improper understanding about the nutrition, religion and sin. All religions have benevolence; but none have banned consumption of lifeless eggs.

Food of Plants *vs.* Animal Origin

A person can survive entirely on foods of plant origin during his/her entire life period; but it is not possible to depend on foods of animal origin alone; because even for cooking animal foods, we need spices and condiments of plant origin. Moreover, human needs carbohydrates (starch and sugar); which form 50-70% of their food, to supply energy and 25-30 grams fibre/day, for easy bowel movement; which are absent or scanty in animal foods. Hence even in the diets of rich semi-vegetarians, nearly 80% will be foods of plant origin only. However, foods of animal origin are preferred due to the following reasons.

1. Foods of animal origin are more tastier than foods of plant origin .
2. Animal foods are more easily and completely digestible than plant foods.
3. Plant foods have more anti nutrients, naturally occurring toxicants and mycotoxins than
   animal foods.
4. Animal foods have higher levels of high quality protein, with balanced amino acid profile, than plant proteins.
5. Animal foods are rich in B-complex group of vitamins. Vitamin E, D and certain essential minerals. Vitamin B_{12} is presently mainly in animal foods; hence it is also called as "animal protein factor" previously. Folic acid, which is rich in all animal products prevents anemia. Recently the scientists have identified the folic acid deficiency, as a risk factor for cardiovascular disease (CVD.).

Is Egg Consumption a Sin?

Unlike plants, animal including humans have to depend on plants and animals for their food. Both plants and animals are having life and human beings cannot survive, without taking these foods having life. Hence consuming these foods is not a sin; but killing or harming plants and animals for pleasure, fun and other selfish reasons, may be a sin. The anatomy (presence of canine teeth) and physiology of humans suggest that they are born omnivorous. Hence they are consuming foods of both plant and animal origin, since time immemorial.

Nuts, cereals and pulses, which are nothing but seeds of plants having life, will be killed when consumed. Milk is a secretion of udder and natural food for the calf, hence, by consuming milk and its products, we are partly starving the calves and committing a sin. On the other hand, by eating the table eggs, which are secretion of ovary and oviduct having no embryo or life, we are not killing or starving any life. If such table eggs are not consumed, they are going to be wasted. Even the father of India, Mahatma Gandhi has stated that a sterile table egg will never develop into a chick. Therefore one who can take milk should have no objection in taking the sterile table eggs also.

Hence a strict vegan, and a 'sin' fearing person, in order to avoid killing/ starving of other lives, can eat only fallen leaves, fruit pulp without seeds, table eggs and naturally dead plants, trees and animals but shall not eat grains, nuts seeds and milk, because they can germinate and develop into live plants and milk will feed the calves fully. However, this is not at all practicable. Moreover, such lifeless foods are available in small quantities, not sufficient to feed the entire human population. Hence we have to depend on the foods of plant and animal origin for our survival. Therefore, consuming of sterile, infertile table eggs, a natural, safe secretion of ovary and oviduct, is not at all a sin; whereas not consuming it, leads to wastage of valuable food.

Eggs Cholesterol and Health

Many persons have restricted the consumption of eggs, due to its higher cholesterol levels. However, the latest research carried out throughout the world, has proved beyond doubt that there is no significant correlation between dietary and serum cholesterol levels. Moreover, by denying eggs due to cholesterol scare; we are forgoing many valuable nutrients, antioxidants, anti-carcinogenic principles, immuno modulators and antiinflammatory, antimicrobial agents present in the eggs. Based on these findings, the egg consumption in many countries, which has fallen since II-world war, has picked up again from 1990 onwards.

Cholesterol is Essential

All vegetarian foods are free from cholesterol; but even vegans (pure vegetarians, not taking even milk) are also having elevated serum cholesterol levels, like others and they are not exempted from CVD. This has clearly indicated that there is 100% cholesterol biosynthesis in vegan. Cholesterol is essential for the body; but not dietary essential; because our body can synthesize as much as 3,000 mg of cholesterol per day; whereas the daily requirement is about 1200 mg only. Nearly 0.14% of our body weight is cholesterol; which is the basic material for various hormones, vitamin D_3, cell membrane and nervous tissue.

In a healthy individual, the cholesterol biosynthesis is controlled by a feed back mechanism, based on the dietary cholesterol and actual cholesterol requirement. However, in hypercholesterolemic individuals, the body mechanism to control cholesterol biosynthesis or excretion of cholesterol has failed (just like insulin failure), leading to hypercholesterolemia.

Major Risk Factors

Many nutritionists, researchers and the National Cholesterol Education Programme (NCEP) have identified several risk factors (Table below) for elevated serum cholesterol levels and consequent cardiovascular diseases (CVD). Recently, chronic constipation has been identified as one of the risk factors for elevated serum cholesterol levels, because the only route through which the cholesterol is excreted from the body is through stools, via bile. In case of constipation, there will be more reabsorption of cholesterol. Hence it is not wise to ignore these major causes for hypercholesterolemia and simply avoiding cholesterol rich foods, having other benefits.

Moreover, epidemiological evidences had also provided that there is no association between dietary and serum cholesterol levels. Eskimos, who are consuming the highest cholesterol and animal fat daily are having the lowest incidence of CVD. Similarly in France, Spain, Mexico and Japan, where the annual average per capita consumption of eggs are more than 300, with daily cholesterol intake of more than 400 mg from different sources, are not showing any elevated serum cholesterol levels. On the other hand, the African blacks and the lactovegetarian Indians, consuming less than 100 mg of cholesterol per day, are having higher LDL (bad) and lower HDL (good) serum cholesterol levels; leading to higher incidence of CVD. Hence it can be safely concluded that there is no significant association between dietary and serum cholesterol levels.

How Many Eggs Per Day are Good for Health?

No country or health authorities have restricted or banned the consumption of eggs. Only the American Heart Association, in consultation with the NCEP and American Dietetics Association, to be on more safer side, has advised the high risk group to restrict the weekly consumption of egg yolks up to four; but there is no such restriction on consumption of egg whites.

In fact, persons having more than 60 mg/dl HDL-C (good cholesterol) can consume more number of eggs, for a longer period, without any risk. In the New England Journal of Medicine, Kern (1991) has reported normal serum cholesterol levels in few persons consuming up to 25 eggs a day. The World Health Organisation (WHO) and several other health authorities have recommended a minimum of half an egg per person per day, in a balanced food, for healthy living. Based on all these evidences, a healthy person can consume at least an egg a day and those doing more physical work as well as those having higher HDL-C, can consume two eggs a day; without any risk or sin; for prolonged good health.

Table 6AI.1: Factors Responsible for Elevated Serum Cholesterol Levels and CVD Along with their Approximate Share (%)Total Causes

I Non-dietary causes	*= 75%*	*II Dietary causes*	*= 25%*
1. Heredity	= 14	1. Over eating and excess calorie intake	= 6
2. Obesity (over weight)	= 11	2. More consumption of sugar and refined carbohydrates rich foods like, sweets, soft drinks, bakery product etc.,	= 3
3. Hormones and enzymes imbalance	= 8	3. More saturated fat consumption especially myristic acid	= 3
4. Emotional stress, socio-economic insecurity and unsatisfied life	= 8	4. More consumption of trans-fatty acids (claidic acid) rich fried food (chips etc.)	= 3
5. Hypertension	= 7	5. Imbalanced food lack of fibre and nutritional deficiency	= 2.5
6. Diabetes mellitus	= 6	6. Chronic alcoholism	= 2
7. Lack of exercise (sedentary habits)	= 5	7. Irregular food habits	= 1.5
8. Smoking	= 5	8. High dietary cholesterol (>300 mg/day)	= 1.5
9. Environmental pollution	= 3	9. Folic acid deficiency	= 1
10. Low birth weight	= 1.5	10. Other dietary causes	= 1.6
11. Chronic constipation	= 1.5		
12. Age, sex, chronic diseases and other causes	= 4		
Total	**= 75%**	**Total**	**= 25%**

Usually a single cause may not be responsible for elevated serum cholesterol levels; but a combination of many dietary and non-dietary causes are responsible for it.

Annexure II

CURE DISEASES FROM EGG

There's more to eggs than just a good nutrition. They also contain constituents that help in the treatment of a wide range of human health problems from wounds and rashes to cancer and cardiovascular disease.

Besides excellent nutritive value, the egg possesses several health-promising, immunostimulating, therapeutic and functional properties, which make it a versatile product.

- Egg albumen is used as an antidote to counteract some toxins and irritants consumed accidentally. It protects the mucous membrane of the stomach and intestine and prevents ulcer formation.
- Due to its water holding and binding properties, it counteracts the enteritis caused by several toxic substances and microbes. Egg white is a good natural remedy for gastritis, enteritis, diarrhoea, dysentery and dehydration.
- Studies have revealed that egg contains three substances lumiflavin, lumichrome and sulphoraphane – that are capable of restraining the multiplication of cancer inducing viruses and also prevent normal cells turning into cancerous cells. These compounds are also natural antioxidants.
- The lysozyme (GI – globulin), G2 and G3 globulins, ovoma-croglobulin, antibody 1gY and other natural antimicrobials and immunostimulants in the egg prolong the life of AIDS patients, due to high nutritional value, as well as their immunostimulating and antimicrobial properties.
- The carotenoid pigments present in the egg yolk are natural antioxidants that eliminate free radicals as well as anti-carcinogenic agents, natural pigments and precursors of vitamin A. They also reduce the serum LDL (bad) cholesterol levels and thereby prevent cardiovascular disease (CVD).
- Intralipid, a parenteral fat emulsion prepared from egg yolk, is used as a carrier of fat soluble drugs.
- The yolk phospholipid, lecithin-conjugated with vitamin-B 12, when given to rats, premature babies and persons suffering from Alzheimer's disease, resulted in better nervous tissue development and mental abililty.
- The yolk protein, phosvitin, is a potent natural antioxidant that is safer than synthetic compounds. Ethanol-extracted yolk lipid showed anti-oxidative effect on dicosa-hexaenoic acid (DHA), an omega-3 fatty acid that quickly becomes rancid. It also prevents premature ageing.
- Lecithin of egg yolk is more stable and has higher entrapment efficiency than soy lecithin.
- The toxicity of diamidine and other drugs used against protozoal diseases was significantly reduced when encapsulated in egg yolk lecithin.

- The yolk lipoprotein YLPp 17.5 promotes the growth of several types of mammalian cells, including human hepatic cells in biotechnology and genetic engineering experiments.
- This lipoprotein and other high biological value proteins in the egg act as excellent growth promoters in children and animals.
- The egg yolk and chalaza are rich sources of sialic acid, mainly Neu-5-Ac, patented and sold as SLEX in some countries. It has powerful antimicrobial, antiinflammatory and antiviral properties. Hence it is used in the treatment of *H. pyroli* and other microbial infections causing ulcers, colon cancer, gastritis and enteritis.
- Chicken egg is abundant in antibodies like IgY, which is cheaper and better than mammalian immunoglobulin IgG. Over a six-week period, a hen produces about 298 mg of specific antibodies, compared with only 17 mg from a rabbit. This IgY can be used to treat human rotavirus, E. coli, Streptococcus. Pseudomonas, Staphylococcus and Salmonella infections.
- For burns and cuts, insect bites and rashes, the application of egg white (especially chalaza) followed by pasting of shell membrane over the affected skin, reduces inflammation and infection and promotes healing.
- The Indian systems of medicine (Ayurveda & Sidda) recognised the antiinflammatory, healing, binding, antomicrobial and immunogenic properties of the egg thousands of year back. The eggs are used for burns and fractures, after mixing with other herbs, for quick healing. A paste made from eggs, herbs, sesame oil and green mung bean paste is applied over fractures before the plaster of Paris bandage for quick healing of fractures.
- Unlike milk, meat, fruits, vegetables, and other high-moisture foods, eggs can be stored at room temperature for 2-4 weeks because the lysozyme, ovomacroglobulin and other components of the egg. These have antimicrobial properties that prevent microbial spoilage.
- Eggs provide a cheap but good medium for immunoglobuliln and vaccine production. In 2002, scientists at India's Vittal Mallya Science Research Foundation produced an anti-snake venom from chicken eggs. Compared to an anti-snake venom product from horse serum, it was 100 times cheaper because a hen can produce about 300 eggs per annum; which contains anti-snake venom present in 6 litres of horse serum.
- The taurine present in the eggs, milk and meat prevents the antherosclerotic plaque formation in the arteries and thereby prevents CVD.
- Conjugated linoleic acid present in the egg yolk reduces the risk of certain heart and cancer problems.
- Yolk lipid is one of the richest source of the monounsaturated fatty acid (MUFA), oleic acid, having about 42% of total yolk lipids.

- Nutritionists have concluded that MUFA is better than PUFA (polyunsaturated fatty acids) for human health.
- A high level of homocysteine in the blood vessels, leading to the deposition of plaques and CVD. Betaine a methyl donor present in sugar beet, egg, red wine and other food products reduces the plasma homocysteine concentration and prevents antherosclerosis, CVD and stroke.
- So-called "designer eggs" are rich in omega-3 fatty acids (linolenic, eicosapentaenoic and docosahexaenoic acids) as well as carotenoid pigments, vitamin E, organic selenium and chromium. The omega-3 fatty acids reduce hypertension, LDL and VLDL cholesterol and triglycerides levels, prevent thrombosis, platelet aggregation, angina, atherosclerosis and stroke.

7

Role of Sheep and Goat in Rural Economy

Down through the centuries, rearing of sheep and goat has remained a subsidiary occupation of a vast segment of the rural population in India. Incidentally, these small ruminates need very little investment and provide more meat and milk per unit weight per year than cows and buffaloes. Traditionally, rural women have been contributing significantly to goat and sheep rearing. Nomadic or migratory groups in North West India have evolved their own management practices for maintaining herds of sheep and goats. In recent years, a number of corporate houses in India have taken to goat and sheep rearing and the state of Maharashtra takes a lead in this area.

Despite a huge goat and sheep population (123 million goats and 51 million sheep) in the country and their contribution to the national economy—there is till now no organized central body to improve the prospects of goats and sheep rearing in the country. Livestock experts are of a view that a body patterned after the National Dairy Development Board (NDDB) whose singular efforts over the years have helped turn India into a numero uno milk producer in the world, could go a long way towards boosting the productivity of the sheep and goat population in India.

In the wake of the rapid deforestation and progressively shrinking grassland, the continued grazing by ever growing herds of sheep and goat is being viewed as an ecologically unsustainable proposition. Of course, while the sheep grazes on grassland, goat could easily survive on available hardy shrubs under diverse harsh environment in low fertility areas. However, because of their small body size and docile nature, both goat and sheep pose least management problems in so far as their rearing requires low initial investment, rural poor and marginal farmers earn supplementary income from the tending of ruminates. No wonder, sheep and goat constitute an inseparable part of the agricultural ecosystem in India.

Sheep like goat is a small ruminant with a high adaptability to extreme climate. Sheep by nature is a gregarious uniparous unlike goat which produces more than one young at the time of kidding. Sheep plays an important role in the animal production and rural economy in arid and semiarid regions and largely in marginal and submarginal holdings. Of the total 1043 million sheep in the world in 1975 more than one-third of the world sheep population in the topics consist of indigenous breeds with poor yields. The animals are kept almost exclusively for domestic purposes, by the nomads of Africa, Saudi Arabia and the Near East, and provide meat and milk. Sheep production accounts for 75 per cent of meat eaten in Afghanistan, Iraq, Iran, Jordan, Pakistan and Saudi Arabia. Though India accounts for 17 per cent of total goat production in the world, its share in sheep population is only 4 per cent of the world total (Table 7.1). Population of sheep in India continued to be unaltered and remained between 39 and 40 million for the past three decades. The production potential of sheep in India is estimated to be around Rs. 140 crores of rupees per annum. This is based on yearly production of about 34.5 million kg of wool, 101 million kg of mutton, 14.6 million pieces of skin and 20 million tonnes of manure.

Role of sheep rearing in improving the rural economy is well established. In the event of failure of seasonal rains, the rearing of sheep gives a helping hand to the farmers at a time of crisis arising from crop failure. Therefore, sheep is affectionately labelled as 'mortgage lifter' by the rural poor.

Sheep rearing can be recommended as an occupation to the rural people especially to the weaker sections of the group in hilly, drought prone and desert areas. In the north and northeastern hilly regions comprising Jammu and Kashmir, Himachal Pradesh, Uttar Pradesh, Assam, Meghalaya, Nagaland, orchards and cereals are raised in combination with sheep rearing. Sheep farming through small and marginal farmers and landless agricultural labourers will provide employment opportunities for most of the unemployed and underemployed in the rural areas. Sheep raising can be recommended as a subsidiary occupation. When mixed farming is practised, sheep forms an effective complimentary component in improving the economy of the farm. Sheep can thrive well in all agroclimatic conditions excepting in rainfall areas. Sheep can subsist on low set and sparse vegetation, whereas, other species of farm livestock may be struggling to thrive. This is possible because of their inherent capacity to browse very close to the roots of herbage. Sheep manure excels cattle manure and penning of sheep in harvested fields enhances the fertility of the soil by richness of nutrients in the faecal materials voided. Penning of sheep in the field bring in additional income to the flock owners. Since sheep rearing does not warrant any large investment in buildings and equipments, it opens good scope for exploitation by the small, marginal farmers and landless agricultural labourers. In the drought prone and desert areas shepherds are compelled to lead a nomadic life for welfare of their sheep. The system of migration in search of grazing area not only tells upon the illiteracy among these weaker sections of people but also on their children who have no chances of education because of the constant shift of their family. The children are compelled to become as caretaker of sheep flocks while grazing. As such sheep husbandry remains primitive among these illiterate sheep

Table 7.1: Trends in Livestock Population and Meat Production 1975 - 1999

Livestock Species	Population in millions				Slaughter rate in %				Caracass weight in kgs.				Meat production in 000 tons.				Share in total Production in %			
	1975	1985	1995	1999	1975	1985	1995	1999	1975	1985	1995	1999	1975	1985	1995	1999	1975	1985	1995	1999
1. Cattle	180.1	182.4 (1.3)	194.6 (6.7)	214.9 (10.4)	4.9	6.1	6.4	6.4	82	80	103	103	724	890 (22.9)	1365 (53.4)	1421 (4.1)	35.3	34.0	31.8	31.3
2. Buffaloes	60.5	64.5 (6.6)	79.5 (23.3)	92.1 (15.8)	9.3	11.0	11.0	11	139	138	138	138	780	980 (25.6)	1351 (37.9)	1380 (2.1)	38.1	37.5	31.5	31
3. Sheep	40.1	41.3 (3.0)	45 (9.0)	57.6 (28.0)	31.9	35.8	31.3	30	9	9	10	10	117	141 (20.5)	194 (37.6)	228 (17.5)	5.7	5.4	4.5	5
4. Goat	69.7	81.5 (16.9)	119.4 (45.5)	122.5 (2.6)	42.5	42.9	39.7	38	9	9	10	10	269	358 (33.1)	450 (25.6)	466 (3.5)	13.2	13.7	10.4	10.3
5. Pigs	7.0	8.8 (25.7)	11.9 (35.2)	16 (34.4)	25.7	30.0	75.3	83.7	31	32	35	35	56	85 (51.8)	420 (394.1)	469 (11.6)	2.8	3.2	10	10.3
6. Poultry	141.0	161.0 (14.2)	498 (209.3)	587.7 (18.1)	-	-	-	-	-	-	-	-	101	161 (59.4)	507 (214.9)	551 (8.7)	4.9	6.2	11.8	12.1
7. Total	498.4	539.5 (8.2)	948.4 (75.8)	1106 (16.6)									2047	2615 (27.7)	4287 (63.9)	4545 (6.0)	100.0	100.0	100.0	100
8. Total meat production other than poultry meat													1946	2454	3708	3994				

Figures in brackets are percentage increase over the previous decade.
Source: FAO Production Yearbook: Various issues.

owners. Migration and grazing practices have profound effect on the present neglected state of sheep husbandry in the country. Studies on economics of sheep rearing show that the sheep population is subjected to considerable fluctuations on account of drought, diseases, wild animals, fluctuations prices of mutton and wool and uneconomic holdings and soil erosion over which the Indian sheep farmer has little control.

Compared with an average annual production of 3.5 to 5.5 kg of quality wool per sheep in Australia, New Zealand and USA, the yield is 1.4 kg in India and largely in Asian countries. Poor management, feeding and health care mean that only about 20 per cent of the possible meat yield per ewe is obtained. The maximum concentration of the wool yielding sheep remains in the arid regions of northern Indian plains and Joria region, comprising the area of Rajputana, Kutch, Saurashtra and North Gujarat. The Deccan plateau extending from Vindya mountains possesses the largest number of flocks in India and this is especially on the eastern sides of Hyderabad, Andhra and Tamil Nadu States. The majority of sheep in this area are hairy and produce little wool. Kashmir and adjacent districts of Himachal Pradesh, Garhwal hills and Nilgiri hills of Tamil Nadu are specially suited to raising superior wool types of sheep. The Lohi breed of the Punjab is well-known for its large size and milk and meat producing traits. The hairy types of southern Deccan is mainly for meat production.

Sheep has carved a niche in the agricultural economy of the country by effective utilization of the uncultivable wastelands and unwanted shrubs and weeds from the fields. Due to the great adaptability of sheep to widely varying biological and socioeconomic environmental conditions, there are varying methods of sheep farming. They include nomadic or partial nomadic or permanent rearing systems which in their turn, can have a subsistence or a commercial character to their production aims.

In an attempt to obtain the best possible combination of the existing–the mostly extensive–natural and economic influence factors, utilization alternatives have developed for particular locations, to which special production results can be attributed. While the production, purely of wool and fur, can be developed into a profitable system in the tropics and subtropics because of low fodder requirements and relative intensity to climate, meat and milk productions very quickly come up against the natural limitations of poor feed supplies and the low performance potential of native breeds. Only a favourable market position justifies the increased cost of pasture management, providing food, breeding and marketing. Adoption of modern techniques of breeding, improvement in the feed and fodder resources, better management practices and provision of health cover, will promote the sheep development and in turn improve the rural economy. In order to meet the nutritional requirements of sheep population, it is essential to develop arid and semirigid waste land into pastures and supplement with leaves of fodder trees by programmed planting of suitable fodder trees preferably leguminous variety like Sesbania, Ipil Ipil or *Leucaena leucocephala*. Grass can be stepped up or initiated through development of land, fencing, manuring, reseeding, soil conservation and water management. By controlled grazing, the forage yield can be maximised by hundred per cent in about 3-5 years of time. The development of village grazing lands could be managed by the village panchayats or sheep breeders cooperative societies which should be assisted to develop and manage village pastures.

However, in the backdrop of the rapidly shrinking grassland and the ongoing ecological disruption over a large part of the country, rearing of sheep which is mainly dependent on the grassland has become less profitable as compared to goat rearing. In fact, subsidiary farming makes sheep dependent on crop production activities. As such, farmers feeding sheep on crop residues are on the look out for a breed of sheep whose yield and quality of wool is high. In this context, Bharat Marino, an excellent wool sheep bred indigenously by the Central Sheep and Wool Research Institute in Rajasthan, has become the most favoured sheep variety. The sheep breed inherits the excellent qualities of imported and native sheep varieties.

BREEDS OF SHEEP

The sheep in India are believed to have been influenced by tahr, from the Himalayan and Nilgiri regions, and urials (*Ovis ammon–Orientalis gamlin*) which predominate in Punjab and adjoining areas of the west. Sheep found in three geophysiographic division of the country, viz., temperate Himalayan region, dry western region and southern region are types of sheep which differ greatly.

Sheep may be grouped as per the factors one wishes to emphasize. They may be classified in accordance with the area from which they originate, such as Bikaneri, Kutchi, and Mandya. Sheep farmers may stress about wool classification, western or native sheep, wool or mutton sheep, white face or black face, polled or horned. Sheep found in temperate Himalayan region, there is considerable admixture of different types of sheep. Sheep in the region predominantly produce coloured fleece, admixture of fine and coarse wool. Examination of fleece from these sheep has revealed that the wool is comparable to that obtained in Britain. Sheep breeds in north Indian plains of dry western region yield very coarse, long staple fleece, besides producing quality meat. The wool from this region is mostly suited for carpet manufacture. Southern region extends from the Vindhya mountains to the Nilgiris, have a large sheep population with a greater density than in the north Indian plains. Sheep in the region produce meat and about half coarse, low quality, pigmented, carpet wool and some yield hair but no wool at all.

Temperate Himalayan Region

Gurez This breed of sheep is found in Gurez Tehsil situated in the high elevated zone of Kashmir State. This breed is famous for long stapled and lustrous wool which is mostly white and less hairy. The average wool production per sheep is about 1.5 kilograms. Poonch, Karnah and Kashmir valley breeds of sheep are distinct breeds in Kashmir State. The first two breeds yield heavier and softer fleece. The colour of this fleece is generally white. Kashmir valley sheep are small, with predominantly coloured fleece, yielding admixture of fine and coarse wool.

Bhakarwal This breed of sheep originated in the lower hills of Himalayas and later migrated to Kashmir, Kangra and Kulu valleys, the flocks in the higher altitude possessing fine under coat. The average wool yield per sheep is 1.5 kilogram. The wool is long and mixed with coarser staple.

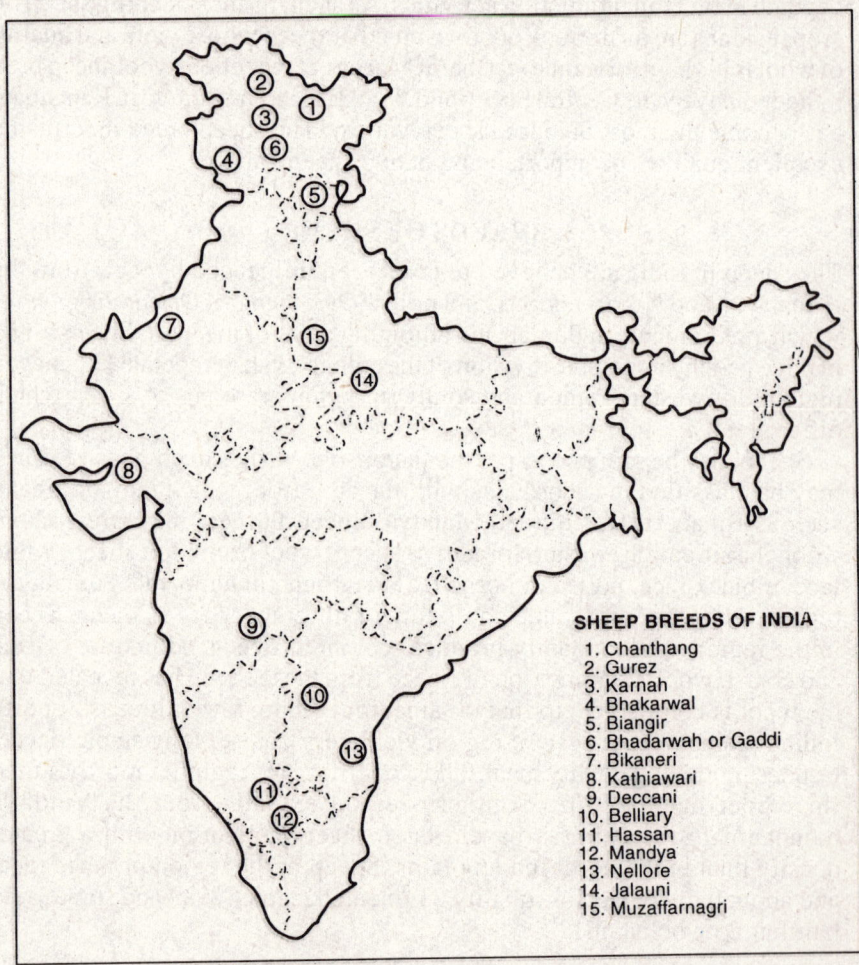

SHEEP BREEDS OF INDIA
1. Chanthang
2. Gurez
3. Karnah
4. Bhakarwal
5. Biangir
6. Bhadarwah or Gaddi
7. Bikaneri
8. Kathiawari
9. Deccani
10. Belliary
11. Hassan
12. Mandya
13. Nellore
14. Jalauni
15. Muzaffarnagri

Fig. 7.1: Map showing sheep breeds of India.

1. Chanthang; 2. Gurez; 3. Karnah; 4. Bhakarwal; 5. Biangir; 6. Bhadarwah or Gaddi; 7. Bikaneri; 8. Kathiawari; 9. Deccani; 10. Belliary; 11. Hassan; 12. Mandya; 13. Nellore; 14. Jalauni; 15. Muzaffarnagri.

GOAT DEVELOPMENT AND RURAL ECONOMY

Goat is capable of integrating itself into dissimilar socioeconomic situations prevailing in our country. Despite indiscriminate slaughter of goats, the total goat production of India accounting for 17 per cent of world population had gradually multiplied from 47 million in 1951 to 70 million in 1979. Sheep population in India had only marginal increase of one million between 1951 and 1979, the population is remaining at a static level of 40 million. Perceptible increase in the population of goat is because of its prolificacy in producing more than young one at the time of kidding and of short generation interval. Being a prolific breeder, the unique ability of the goat, kidding twice in 14 months and of producing seven female kids in eight years cannot be achieved either by a cow or buffalo in their life period.

The importance of goat in the rural economy is evidenced by its unparalleled economic traits; ability to get acclimatized under diversified agroclimatic conditions; unfastidious type in choosing of available forage; high fertility and short generation interval; practically no religious restrictions for goat and its products among the diversified religious people in rural area. Economically goat is ideally suited for poorer rural folk especially for marginal and landless labourers by its low cost maintenance, short-term return on capital with low risk capital investment. No involvement of extraneous labour, as such the entire rural family members especially woman folk and children are brought into the gamut of activity; thereby the health status is bound to improve with availability of cheap and good quality protein through goat milk and mutton. Goats thrive and add to the rural economy even in areas where it is difficult to raise cows or buffaloes. The multifarious methods of utility of goat render the animal to be labelled as a 'Poor Man's Cow'. Perhaps it is the only farm livestock which fits well for effective utilization in the diverse socioeconomic situations of the rural India.

Goat is a unique small ruminant reared by landless, small and marginal farmers in the country. Goat is the only livestock species that lives on ecology where grazing material is virtually not available and survives under diverse harsh environments in low fertility, degraded areas and uncultivated wastelands. Goat rearing requires low initial investment as compared to cattle and buffalo. It is the only meat animal, which in spite of several developmental setbacks and prejudices, has been able to maintain its positive growth rate with human population. Goat rearing has been proved to be most remunerative enterprise amongst various livestock activities. For small households, surviving on subsistence farming small ruminates like goats act as a buffer. They constitute an important disposable asset to tide over times of stress and yet the small farmers retain a part of the asset for continuing the enterprise. Hence the goat is called 'the bank of hooves'.

Indian goats contribute nearly 10 per cent of total meat production. 2.7 per cent of total milk production (0.7 million tonnes), 35 million skin pieces,

300 tonnes of hair and 50 million tonnes of dung annually thereby contributing about Rs. 400 crores towards national income. Considering the economic importance of goats in the national economy, the Union Government has set up the National Goat Research Institute near Mathura in Uttar Pradesh.

Stall-fed goats can ideally fit into the intensive integrated farming system (IIFS). The small animals are the most efficient converters of farm and crop residues into excellent organic manure. Several farmers have successfully run stall-fed goat farms, and they have found that such an integrated farming venture was more productive and profitable as well. Goats relish the stalks and residues of most of the nutritious cereals, and they do well particularly when mixed with green fodder such as grasses and subabul. Special goat feeds can be formulated using farm-grown millets and oilcakes. As the cost of the feed and also the labour gets distributed over other farming operations, the actual cost of raising the goats becomes minimal. The rich goat manure is a deal for fertilizing fishponds and all other crops. It is also a good base material for vermin-composting.

Goat farming needs less capital when compared with dairying, and the animals can be raised in small farms. The floor space requirement per adult animal is about one square metre. Stall-fed goat farming is an ideal occupation for the small, marginal and landless agricultural labourers. A properly fed and managed milch goat will yield at least as much milk (on an average two litres per day) as low yielding desi cows. The she–goat will deliver 2-4 kids at each parturition after a short gestation period of 150 days. A few exotic goats such as Saamen, Toggenburg, Angora, Anglo-Nubian, British Alpine, French Alpine have been found to be well adapted to Indian conditions, and they are crossed with superior Indian breeds to get good progeny. The popular Indian breeds are Jamnapari, Surti, Tellicherry, Beetal, Malabari, Barbari and Gujarati. The milch-type animals are ideal for integrated farming system.

A small shed with good cross ventilation is enough to keep a small herd. A deep-litter system with paddy husk and groundnut shell as bedding material is ideal material   for raising goats. The biological activity in the litter keeps the housing warm in winter and cool in summer. The bedding material will last for about six months, and after that it will have to be changed. The bedding has to be turned periodically to remove the foul odour in the pen. The bedding material collects all the dung and urine and it is found to be an enriched organic manure. An adult goat will add about a tonne of rich manure to the farm every year.

Though the goats are robust animals and are resistant to many diseases, they need to be vaccinated against foot and mouth disease, rinderpest and tetanus regularly. The animals need to be dewormed at least twice a year to keep in good stead. Goat farming with stall-feeding can be managed in small yards just like poultry, and it will prove to be an economical and rewarding enterprise for the small, marginal and landless farmers.

Production Potential

Goat, as stated earlier, popularly known as "Poor Man's Cow", is as hardy as it is versatile. Its most striking features is its admirable adaptability to diverse climatic situations. However, both the sheep and the goat are being blamed for ecological ills like soil erosion and deforestation. But, then, the field studies carried out in various parts of India have recognized the ground reality that goat or the sheep need not be the cause of ecological degradation. On the other hand, they are quite useful in eliminating some of the obnoxious weeds which are otherwise difficult to get rid of. Moreover, their ability to thrive on scanty vegetation in wasteland, could be exploited to reclaim barren stretches of land. As such, the bad reputation of these ruminates originates from the poor management by man rather than lay in the inherent nature of the animal. Significantly, the goat milk accounts for nearly 3% of the total milk production in India. The skin of the goat is an excellent raw material for leather production. Nutritional experts drive home the point that goat's milk contains smaller fat globules which is naturally homogenized and easily digested by the infants. In- depth studies of the economic viability of animal farming with various species of milk yielding animals vis-à-vis goat proves that the best benefit—cost ratio is provided by the goat.

Goat's contribution in terms of meat production is better than its share in milk production. In India goats contribute 458, 000 MT of meat, which constitutes approximately 10 per cent of total meat production. But there is an alarming deterioration in its contribution to the total meat production from 41 per cent in 1981 to 20 per cent in 1990 and further down to 10 per cent in 1998. This is not due to the less production of goat meat in recent years rather than the phenomenal increase in production of poultry (chicken) meat in the last decade. Above all the low productivity of Indian goats in absence of organized farming unlike poultry sector may be cited as the main reason.

Some Indian breeds have very high rate of multiple births, like Black Bengal, Barbari and Beetal. Dressing percentage (meat output of the animal) ranges from 38.80 for Gaddi to 58.40 per cent in Kutchi breed. Indian goats produce about 10 kg meat on an average per animal in comparison to 25 kg in UK and Oman and 18 kg in Germany. For higher productivity in Indian goats, improvement in body weight at slaughter is essential. The higher body weight at early age, however, depends on multiple factors like breeds, nutrition management, environment, health and their interactions. While growth rate is a genetic expression of the trait of the breed concerned, the level of nutritional management system, physical environment and health coverage are concomitant determining factors for a slaughter weight at any stage. Though in India larger breeds like Jakhrana, Jamunapari and Beetal produce more than 10 kg of meat per animal at slaughter age, the average production is lower due to more numbers of medium and small breeds spread across the country. Hence, the introduction of larger breeds in different regions of the country other than their home tract and rearing those with available scientific knowledge will improve upon the production potential. The spiraling prices of goat meat have encouraged indiscriminate slaughter; especially of males at early age with lower body weight. This needs to be avoided.

While cow and buffalo are playing a dominant role in India's milk production, goat milk has remained a minor statistics. Farm households having mixed herds of livestock, during the production season, market the cow/buffalo milk and retain the goat milk for domestic consumption. Since the household consumption of goat milk does not enter the commercial channels, its economic importance often goes unnoticed. Major dairies do not accept goat milk and it is mostly mixed with cow or buffalo milk during lean season. The contribution of goat towards milk production, therefore, largely remains unrecognized. However, the importance of goat milk providing nutrition for poor families cannot be ignored.

Breeds

India has about 20 well-known breeds of goat like Jamnapari, Surti, Beetal, Marwari, Sidhi, Barbardi, Deccan, Malabari, Bengal, etc. Some of these are milk breeds while others are meat types. Himalayan breeds like the Pashmina goat are important for their coat. Angora goats are famous for their 'Mohair' (Fig. 7.2). However, livestock experts have expressed concern over the indiscriminate breeding and the maintenance of impure breeds by nomadic tribes. The large sized Jamanpuri goat has a reputation for high milk yield. Dual purpose breeds like Barbardi, Sidhi and Marwari are also widely distributed in various parts of India. Goats with distinct characteristics of productivity in India are found in different agroclimatic regions of the country. This reflects the farmer's perceptions and testifies the useful role of goat plays in different farming systems. However, the economic impact of goat remains largely unassessed. The attitude of policy-makers towards the goat has always been for its elimination or reducing its numbers. The attitude has discouraged the formulation of a meaningful policy or programme for useful management of goat population.

Goats are energetic, inquisitive and versatile in the art of food gathering. They have a greater tendency than cattle and sheep to change their diet, with changing season. Goats spend over half of their total grazing time eating leaves and shoots of trees and bushes and also have special preference for inflorescences of grasses. The small size, large surface area relative to body weight, and limited subcutaneous fat cover, adapt them poorly to cold climates, but make them relatively more adapted to areas of high temperatures. The humid topics present problems of diseases and parasites. Most important, the goat appears to have a superior adaptation to the arid tropics, because of its ability to conserve water, travel well, graze selectively and to take willingly a wide variety of vegetation. Indigenous goats also trend to be resistant to many of the diseases which plague other livestock species.

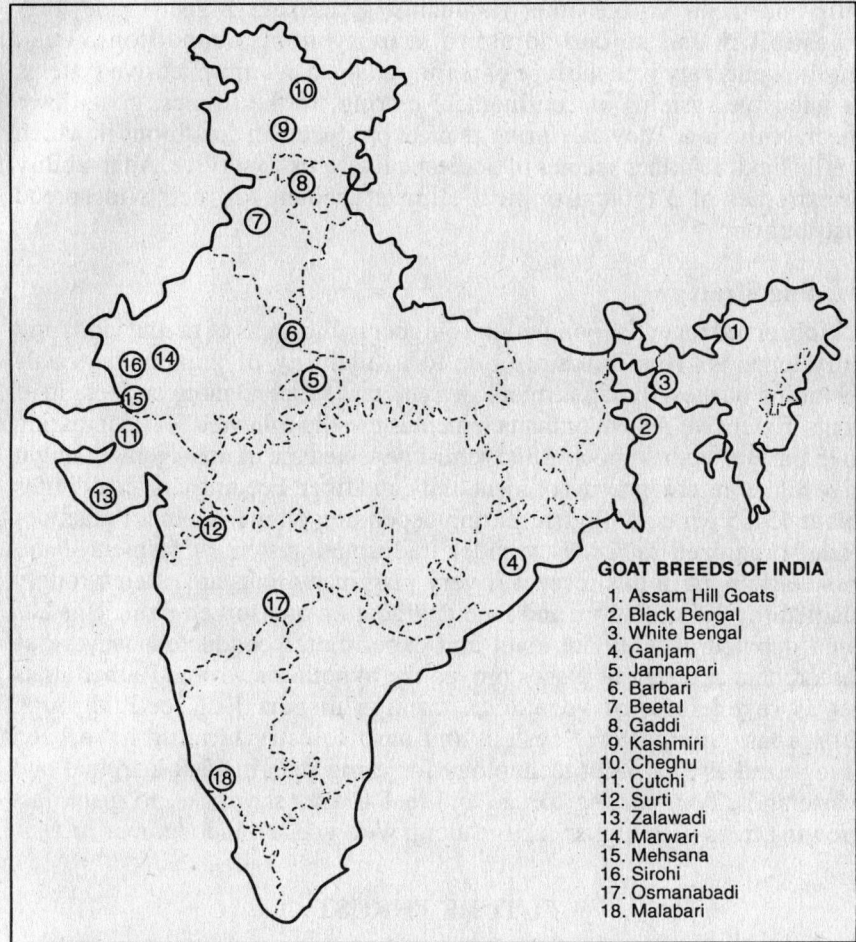

GOAT BREEDS OF INDIA
1. Assam Hill Goats
2. Black Bengal
3. White Bengal
4. Ganjam
5. Jamnapari
6. Barbari
7. Beetal
8. Gaddi
9. Kashmiri
10. Cheghu
11. Cutchi
12. Surti
13. Zalawadi
14. Marwari
15. Mehsana
16. Sirohi
17. Osmanabadi
18. Malabari

Fig. 7.2: Map showing goat breeds of India.

Semi arid areas with sparse vegetation, bushes and shrubs cannot support cattle but, suit the browsing taste of goats even more than sheep. Mountainous areas with steep slopes (above 30° and higher than 2,000 m above sea level) cannot be used safely by cattle, but may be used by goats. Depending upon the availability to climatic conditions, the breeds differ in body conformation, varying from those long rather large animals with long legs, fine skin and narrow bodies suited to desert life, to the smaller, shortlegged stocky type fitted for the easier life in humid climates or restricted surroundings.

Special feeding habits are exhibited by goats. This is made possible by their mobile upper lips and very prehensile tongues, goats are able to graze on very short grass and to browse on foliage which is not the common feed of other livestock. Goats can be profitably utilised to browse plants into milk and meat. Unlike other ruminants, goats have higher crude fiber digestibility and so can adjust to scarcity fodder conditions. Feed requirements vary with the type of rearing adapted to semi-intensive systems or intensive systems of confinement rearing. In the tropics, goats have special function. They can thrive as meat producers in conditions in which it is difficult for other species of domestic livestock to survive. Adaptability to extremes of a typical tropical climate account for their widespread distribution.

Feeding Strategy

It is observed that goat population is higher in the areas of ravine lands and hilly terrains. This is mainly due to availability of grazing materials including bushes. Indian farmers are reluctant to spend more on feeding of goats. Extensive system of management is usually followed for goat rearing in India. But studies showed that semi-intensive type of management might give higher return in terms of meat, milk and fiber. Feeding cost constitutes about 45-65 per cent of goat rearing depending on management practices under organized sector. But under traditional system at farmers' level monetary input in this respect is very marginal. Goats are often wrongly blamed for deforestation, and land degradation and soil erosion. This has been debated at National level and experiments conducted by various researchers at different places proved the hypothesis wrong. Rather goats act as regenerator of vegetation through dispersal of seeds through droppings. Silvipastoral system and agro forestry farming have been recognized as low input technology for using marginal/submarginal and wastelands. For meeting forage and leaf fodder shortages, to grow fast growing trees with higher foliage along with grasses and legumes.

FUTURE THRUST

The present trend shows that the demand of goat meat and meat products in the Indian market is increasing and expected to increase further due to several reasons. Though in India goat, sheep and pig are the principal meat animals, goat meat has a universal appeal over other meats due to its juiciness and aroma. The goat meat production has increased from 227,000 MT in 1981 to 466,000 MT in 1999 (Table 7.2). But this is due to population rise of goats and not due to the increase in productivity. The prevailing production system, mostly dependent on common property resources, is not healthy for their future sustainability. Nor it is conducive for conservation of nation's natural resources base. In the backdrop of above problems, the organised goat farming may be encouraged. Specialised farming system for goat production with semi-intensive management on commercial lines or cooperative movement can make goat industry a success. Unlike poultry, the commercial goat farming needs to be encouraged to maximize the profit from this untapped vast resources. Training on commercial goat farming is the need of the hour for our farmers.

Table 7.2: Meat Production in India and the World: 1981 to 1999: (In Thousand Tonnes)

Year	INDIA							WORLD						
	Beef & veal	Buffalo meat	Mutton & lamb	Goat meat	Pig meat	Poultry meat	Total	Beef & veal	Buffalo meat	Mutton & lamb	Goat meat	Pig meat	Poultry meat	Total
1981	78	127	125	227	75	120	802							
1982	80	130	132	298	80	130	850							
1983	80	132	134	302	80	137	865	46,096	1,760	6,076	1,920	55,661	28,916	144,049
1984	149	148	135	346	82	150	1,010							
1985	150	152	141	358	85	161	1,040							
1986	160	163	147	370	86	180	1,106	50,885	2,002	6,220	2,110	61,474	33,331	159,407
1987	239	207	162	380	80	193	1,261	50,972	2,014	6,350	2,294	63,526	35,904	164,546
1988	232	290	148	378	357	225	2,891	51,397	2,119	6,640	2,383	67,088	37,697	170,862
1989	845	936	160	385	359	289	2,974	51,717	2,210	6,834	2,540	68,173	38,660	173,677
1990	1,270	1,048	173	410	360	334	3,595	51,732	2,216	7,040	2,700	70,064	40,376	177,937
1991	1,185	1,176	168	455	364	362	3,710	52,146	2,375	7,138	2,816	71,155	42,368	181,835
1992	1,216	1,182	167	456	397	382	3,800	51,141	2,435	7,042	2,885	72,924	41,611	174,757
1993	1,276	1,182	169	466	403	454	3,950	51,706	2,457	6,863	2,948	75,370	41,937	186,240
1994	1,292	1,204	171	470	408	507	4,052	52,778	2,534	7,204	3,114	78,589		
1995	1,365	1,351	194	450	420	479	4,259	53,352	2,593	7,099	3,304	83,539		
1996	1,370	1,382	199	454	435	479	4,319	52,986	2,812	7,226	3,394	78,548	55,841	204,882
1997	1,378	1,403	222	458	533	527	4,521	55,169	2,986	7,400	3,647	82,731	59,017	214,934
1998	1,401	1,380	226	462	469	540	4,478	55,316	3,001	7,519	3,795	88,000	61,243	222,917
1999	1,421	1,410	228	466	469	551	4,545	55,867	3,083	7,474	3,821	88,430	63,249	225,945

Source: FAO Production Year Book: Various issues.

Krishi Vigyan Kendra (KVK) personnel and professionals directly related to the animal husbandry practices may extend their help to the farmers in this regard. Though the movement has already been started in that direction, the thrust at policy makers level will do a lot of good to the goat industry in foreseeable future.

The Union Agricultural Ministry has launched a new centrally sponsored scheme for the conservation of threatened breeds of small ruminants, pigs and pack animals. A provision of Rs. 15 crore has been made available for the scheme in the 10th Plan. Union Agriculture Minister Rajnath Singh addressing a meeting of the consultative committee of his ministry said the central assistance will be provided as 100 per cent grant to state government and NGOs. Small ruminants, pack animals, equine and pigs are being maintained by six million small and marginal farmers and agricultural labourers in the country. The preservation of these threatened breed of livestock and improvement in their productivity can play an important role in proving rural employment and meeting the international obligation of conservation of such breeds for future generations.

Efficient Sheep and Goat Production

For efficient sheep and goat production, there is need to follow the enumerated points:

- Rear only those animals of a breed that are best suited for the prevailing environmental conditions. Market demand and supply of the produce may also be considered and exploited through rural cooperatives.
- To establish sheep/goat farm one should purchase the animals from organisations and other societies after satisfying with the purity of the breed, past records of the animals in respect of pedigree, production performance, disease occurrence profile etc. The emphasis while purchasing the animals should be given either to newly kidded does of first and second parity or the heifers of breedable age. Animals should be purchased preferably during August-October or February-March.
- Farmers should organize their flocks in such a way that at least 15 to 20% breedable females could be added every year as a replacement of old and low producer animals. The flock size should not be more than 150 or so, as that becomes unmanageable in availability of inputs and proper care. Flock should consist of animals of all age groups and there should be 2-3 improved breeding rams in flock of 100 size.
- It is essential of protect all the animals from inclement weather conditions. Pay more attention to grower and older stock in extreme cold as they are more susceptible to cold and there is a chance to get infection of pneumonia etc. During summer, flock should be grazed early in the morning and late in evening (allowed to take rest

during the day), graze the flock near the canals and pounds so that they may get water easily and got cooling effect to reducing the heat stress.

- During crucial physiological stages (growth, pregnancy and lactation, etc.) animals should be grazed on fresh pastures and if feed is not available farmers should make arrangements for supplement feeding by some concentrate mixtures or with some lopping of locally available tree leaves. Feeding schedule is as per Table 7.3.

Table 7.3: Feeding Schedule at Different Physiological Stages to Attain Higher Growth and Production Level

Category	Period	Quantity (g/head/day) ad lib
Pre-weaned	0-3 months	
Up to yearling	3-12 months	200
Breedable female	20 day (before breeding)	250
Pregnant female	Last 30 days (Pregnancy)	300
Lactating	First 60 days	300
Breeding males	Breeding days	350

- Lambing/kidding in peak summer and winter may not be obtained to avoid higher lamb/kid mortality. Breeding should be managed as sufficient grazing material is available during advance pregnancy/lactation. Maintenance of such ewes on inferior pasture and poor feeding may result into abortion, parturition complexity, poor health and low birth weight etc. No female that is stunted or underweight should be allowed to breed.
- The lambing shed including floor and structure should be ready in microbial disinfections, which can be done either by spreading lime after scraping or changing the old soil and white washing of the walls. Refilling should be done with the soil having no linkage with livestock. Sufficient bedding material like *bhusa*, dry grasses or leaves should be provided in the pan during lambing/kidding.
- Pregnant animals, expected to lambing within days, should not be sent for grazing at a longer distance, to avoid any risk. They should be kept in individual lambing pans before a day of lambing and 2–3 days after lambing for their proper care and to avoid the chances of mismothering.
- During breeding and lambing period the surrounding genital parts should be cleaned by cutting the hair of those parts or ensuring successful mating without any infection and physical interruption. It will also reduce the infection in the lambing pans.
- As soon as lamb or kid is born the whole baby along with face should be cleaned with a clean cloth to ensure proper respiration and blood circulation in lambs. The newborn kid should be fed colostrum within

half-an-hour to provide them immunity against the various diseases. If some lambs are orphaned and no ewes are available for fostering, it will be necessary to feed them on milk. Goat can also be used as foster mother.

- The navel cord of the newly born kids should be cut at about 3-4 cm with sterilize blade/scissor and should be dipped in tincture iodine for disinfections. Liquid paraffin @ 4-5 ml/lamb may also be given to the new born for soothing effect.
- Newborn kids should be protected from adverse climatic conditions to avoid the risk of mortality. Special care should be given to the kids born with low birth weight and with multiple birth.
- After 2-3 days of birth lambs should be kept separately and allowed suckling at 6 hr intervals up to 15 days from the birth. The lamb should be allowed to suckle milk ad lib up to 3 months of age, and provide ad lib. concentrate mixture along with tender green forage for ensuring higher growth rates. Shift over process at the weaning should be adopted slowly so that kids may get accustomed with creep ration and other managerial changes.
- Teaser male should be allowed in the adult female flocks for heat detection. Never use breeding males in heat detection of females. Avoid inbreeding in the flocks for that never mate the closely related animals. Bucks should not be mixed with the adult milch goats to avoid goaty smell of the milk and to avoid stray mating. Supplementary feeding of breeding males (300-400 g concentration) is must during breeding season to ensure proper libido, semen quality and health of the animal.
- The animals of different age groups, viz. newborn kids, weaner, hogget, adult females and males should be kept in different flocks for their proper care and easy management. At least 9-10 hr grazing is essential under semi-intensive system of management for ensuring good health and production level.
- The prophylaxis is better than cure motto should be adopted without any hitch. Timely and effective prophylactic measures should be followed to ensuring disease free flock.
- At least 2 dipping annually in 0.2 to 0.4%. Cythion must be attempted for ectoparasites. For endoparasites 1-2 deworming with proper deworming agent (Panacure or Nilane @ 10 mg/kg body weight) must be done particularly in June/July and December/February. Sulmet drenching should be done to prevent occurrence of coccodiosis in the flock. During monsoon the animals should be passed through copper sulphate solution for foot bath. This will prevent foot rot.
- Shearing of sheep should be performed on a clean place free from dung, straw, water and soil. Shearing should not be performed in extreme hot or cold weather. The coarse hair and dirty wool should be removed from the fleece to maintain good quality wool. Washed sheep should be shorn.

- For the profitable sheep and goat farming proper breeding, feeding, kidding and production records should be maintained and advanced planning done.

There is need to check sheep and goat at each and every level of age and production. Culling of surplus, old, low producer, weak and abnormal animals must be done strictly at regular interval to avoid the extra expenses of rearing of these animals, which also reduces the average performances of the flock.

8

Meat Production and other Livestock Products

Basic physical dimensions of meat eating are quite fascinating than are its quite environmental social, and health impacts. Meat consumption has no bounds of size or species: wild and domesticated animals that are killed and eaten belong to every mammalian family and also include thousands of avian, reptilian, and amphibious species, animals ranging from birds that fit into the palm of a hand to bulls weighing nearly one metric ton. Porcupines and giant rats (*Cricetomys*) are cherished foods in Cameroon: domesticated guinea pigs become temporary pets around the kitchens of Peruvian houses before they are roasted; Cypriots use illegal mist nets to trap and kill more than 15 million migrating songbirds a year, discarding the unwanted ones and grilling and pickling the prized ones; and Congolese pick off meat from the seared scalps of nearly extinct mountain gorillas. And, of course, all modern societies have made mass-produced meat, particularly ground beef, one of the most readily available foodstuffs thanks to the now ubiquitous fast-food eateries and to increasingly generous servings in restaurants.

Meat eating is a part of evolutionary heritage world over. Recent field studies have shown that chimpanzees, our closest extant primate ancestors, are eager omnivores that supplement their plant-based diet by eating meat. Chimpanzee males hunt small monkeys and share the meat to reinforce social bonds within a group as well as to attract females. Similarly, meat acquisition is still considered a sign of success, and meat sharing still creates personal bonds in most cultures. And our carnivorousness continues to evoke strong emotions, being not only a nearly universal symbol of affluence, well-being, satiety, and contentment but for a minority also an object of scorn and moralistic disapproval.

There is little that is neutral about meat: it has been revered by *bons vivants* of all eras and it is seen as a high-prestige food of choice by America's obese weekend barbecuers peasants whose recent migration of the cities of Asia, Africa and Latin America has brought them closer (physically though not necessarily in terms of income) to the planet's meat-based fast-food outlets. But for millennia meat eating has also been abhorred and renounced by ascetics around the world, be they Dominican *fratres* or Brahmin *sadhus*. For centuries meat was seen as the essential food to energize marching armies and today it is the cornerstone of voguish high-protein diets. This despite the fact we do not have to eat any meat, indeed any animal foodstuffs, in order to lead healthy and active lives and to look forward to generous life spans.

Another meat related development of major evolutionary importance was the domestication of many animals species that began about 11,000 years ago with sheep and goats and then progressed to cattle , pigs, horses, and camels. These carefully husbanded deferred harvests of high-quality foodstuffs constituted a valuable resource that acted as a buffer against failures of field crops, but their management required a great deal of strategy, planning, cooperation, and sudden problem-solving, qualities that are uniquely human.

Extremes of daily intakes of animal protein among the remaining foraging populations that were studied by modern methods after 1950 confirm the wide range of per capita meat, and hence protein, intakes. Healthy and active adults require daily about 60 g of good-quality protein, but more than 300 g of protein were available to Alaskan Inuit feeding on whales, seals, fish, and caribou, while the foragers in arid African environments, subsisting mainly on nuts and tubers, had at their disposal often less than 20 g of protein per day.

As it is used in standard nutritional and agricultural writings, the term meat is actually a misnomer. Meat's correct definition is muscles of animals, and muscles are nothing but wet protein tissues. This simple definition would, of course, embrace muscles of all vertebrates (mammals, birds, amphibians, reptiles, and fishes) and invertebrates, whether domesticated or wild. But meat of invertebrates (most of the nutritionally important ones are aquatic species ranging from mussels of scallops) and fishes is usually classes separately. Italians (followed by the French) sweep these meats into the poetically names *frutti di mare* (fruits de mer). Including the meat of amphibians and reptiles makes a difference only in quantifying the food consumption of some rural populations in tropical countries where a significant share of the relatively low intake of animal foodstuffs comes from such sources. For people in affluent countries meat means usually only the commercially produced flesh of domesticated (and to a much lesser extent wild) mammals and birds. Its production, supply, and consumption are measured in three basic ways, but, unhelpfully, many statistics leave their particular choice unidentified.

INDIAN SCENE

The meat industry in India has great economic potential, but so far it has received very little attention. The quantity of meat produced is far below the requirements, and suitable meat breeds of animals have not been developed. The hygienic condition in most of the slaughter houses are appalling, and in animal byproducts substantial value is being wasted. At present 62 per cent of the meat is from beef and buffalo, 15.3 percent for sheep and goats, 12.2 per cent from poultry and 10.4 per cent from pigs.

According to the Indian Council of Medical Research, a balanced diet for a meat-eating adult should include 34 gm of meat and fish per day. The present per capita consumption of meat in India is around 1.5 kg, poultry meat 620 grams and eggs about 34 annually. This gives an actual consumption is as low as 14 grams per day. Urgent steps have, therefore, to be taken to enhance considerably production of wholesome meat for human consumption. There is considerable scope for building up an export market for buffalo meat, especially to the countries in the Middle East. At present very little buffalo meat is being exported. There are 37 lakh breedable buffaloes in Punjab, producing about 9 lakh male calves every year. At least 33 per cent of these die prematurely for want of care. These should be saved to the extent possible, and along with others, fattened quickly by giving them cheap feed with supplements of molasses and urea. Meat from such animals will find a good foreign market. Unproductive buffaloes should also be slaughtered and their meat exported.

PRODUCTION OF MEAT

The use of national and the international data to estimate population of meat animals and meat production in India is fraught with uncertainty. In fact no official time series data concerning meat production are available for India. The values given by such compilation as that of the Central Statistical Organization, Department of Animal Husbandry & Dairying and the Food and Agriculture Organization are only as good as the field systems used to collect the data. The number of animals slaughtered may be estimated accurately where government controlled slaughterhouses account for majority of slaughtered stock or where an efficient meat-inspection service exists. However, the number of animal slaughtered for clandestine sale is difficult to estimate. Estimates of carcass weight are also subject to considerable doubt.

In fact, it is partly for this reasons that the Ministry of Agriculture, Department of Animal Husbandry and Dairying publishes only the FAO series. The official data for meat production pertain to only a single year or so and relates to the registered slaughter cases. Thus it underestimates the rate of slaughtering and consequently the production of meat and beef in India. The Central Statistical Organization uses its own estimates of meat production to arrive at its estimates of value of output and the Gross Domestic Product from the livestock sector. However, the Department does not publish either the unit value used or the numbers of animals slaughtered. Department of Animal Husbandry and Dairying does not accept CSO's estimates of output and thus do not permit them to publish these estimates along with the value of output.

FAO compiles these series for India along with other countries. However, its system of collection of these data are not based on any scientific basis, in fact, some of the estimates are quite ad-hoc. This is quite clear if one examines the FAO series for India. In the earlier series, which were revised in 1992, the FAO assumed a very low culling ratio (below 0.5 for both cattle and buffalo) for the period 1971 to 1988. In the revised series the earlier estimates have been retained. The inconsistency in the FAO data is shown below (Table 8.1). In the revised series no explanation is given for almost three-and-half time increase in one year in the production of beef and veal, or for buffalo meat from 1988 to 1989. The increase seems to be mainly due to a substantial increase assumed in the slaughtered rate from 1989 onwards.

Table 8.1: FAO's Estimate of Beef and Buffalo Meat Production in India

(In thousand tons)

Year	Beef & veal	Buffalo meat
1971	179	N.A
1976	70	116
1981	78	127
1985	150	152
1988	232	290
1989	845	936
1995	1292	1204
1996	1370	1382
1997	1378	1403
1998	1378	1403
1999	1421	1410
2000	1442	1421
2001	1452	1428
2002	1463	1444
2003	1490	1471

Source: FAO Production Year Book: Various Issues

Growth Pattern of Meat Animals

Despite India having the largest number of world's livestock population, meat production potential has not been fully achieved because (a) India has the lowest extraction rate even among the developing countries, the per unit production of meat is the lowest in the world. The major production constraints are the poor genetic material, inadequate nutrition (feed and forage), inadequate health services and inadequate extension system. Of the total bovine population, only 12% are covered under improved breeding system through AI. There is a shortage of improved bulls for both AI and natural service. There is an acute shortage of feeds and fodders to the extent of 62 and 31 per cent respectively. (b) The carcass yield of various meat animals is low as they are not bred for meat purpose and (c) buffalo calf meets its early death because of neglect at the farm level. Further, cow slaughter is banned in India (except in West Bengal and Kerala) and export of beef is not allowed which is in the negative list of export policy. Improved extension services have to be adopted for salvaging male buffalo calves from early death both to conserve germplasm and increased meat production and availability of draught animals. There is then a need to have first a breeding policy under which at least buffalo specie is bred for meat and milk specially.

There are about 159 meat processors engaged in production of meat products. Although processed meat sector is in existence since the British era, very little progress as well as growth have been made. In British era, Ham, Bacon, Salami and Sausages were manufactured from pork and Indian society was reluctant to consume such products because of social and religious taboos. On the other hand, in the State of Goa which was a Portuguese colony these products were patronized on large scale. Even after independence also, there were hardly any change in attitude to such products because of food habits of the masses. But Indian people have an affinity for consumption of fresh product. In 1997-98 the total quantity of meat products manufactured was 2443 MT which was lower than that of the previous year when it was 2602 MT. However, in 1998-99, again it went up to 2763 MT.

The competitiveness of the meat industry in general and each of the species types within it depends critically on production of quality and quantity of meat at the acceptable prices. In India, cattle and buffalo are raised exclusively for milk and work, some of which become available for meat after their useful productive life as milch or draught animals is over. Sheep, goat and pigs are mainly raised for meat though considerable emphasis on sheep is also given for wool fibre production. Due to emphasis on milk and wool production, the genetic research in India has been largely confined to crossbreeding programme of cow and sheep. Crossbred of these species are being produced continuously mainly under extensive conditions from more variable genetic material, with the main thrust on breed substitution and selection pressure aimed at yield and quality of milk and wool. No emphasis has been laid on meat production traits, viz growth rate, feed efficiency, carcass yield, meat–bone ratio, meat quality and their importance in relation to postmortem factors on commercial scale. Faced with these problems and the need to develop a strategy for production of meat-type animals, some co-coordinated trials were initiated in mutton, pork and poultry production. As regards broiler production better information is available and it is gradually being applied for commercial practices. Similar state-of-the-art projects for improved production through other meat species have not yet advanced. However, some small studies have been conducted for meat production at various academic institutions related to Animal Sciences.

Poultry Meat Grading System on the Cards

Indian integrated poultry producers are expected to take a focused approach on setting standards for domestically sold chicken and establishing a grading system for poultry meat, the two crucial steps that may give synergy to their drive in promoting processed chicken retailing in the near future. As the major poultry processors in the country are initiating action towards setting production standards for chicken, the organised poultry sector will simultaneously seek to secure proper legislation to discourage the slaughter of live birds on streets on hygiene considerations. This is to emphasis both the strengthening retail market for processed chicken and its promotion as safe food product.

To give a direction to these considerations the major integrated poultry producers have formed a task force that could prepare the standards for poultry meat and the grading system according to the Poultry Federation of India (PFI), the task force, involving members of the poultry processors' associations will analyse world standards for poultry products and make suggestions to the Government on evolving a national standard. It will result in a system of certification of poultry standards as well as identify a suitable agency to implement certification of the standards.

The Sri Lankan poultry industry has managed to expand the island nation's per capita chicken consumption from less than 1 kg to 3.9 kg in a span of 10 years, which compares with India's current consumption of around 1 kg. The Sri Lankan chicken industry has also shifted to processed meat marketing from a mainly live bird market during this period.

The task force is also seeking to expand consumer awareness about processed meat and creating cold storage chain facilities to improve its marketing. It will also look into the financial aspects of the poultry sector through Government grants launching generic branding of chicken and poultry products. Right now, it is estimated that the processed chicken marketing in India handles less than 4% of the total produce and hence, good scope is foreseen for the expansion of processed chicken/branded chicken. Recently, an incentive was given to the agri-business/food processing industries via the Ministry of Food Processing Industries providing a grant to chicken processing units to the extent of 25% of the asset value of the unit with a Rs. 5-million cap.

Buffalo

Buffaloes have been bred for milk production and as work animals for many years in the Asian countries, particularly in India, Pakistan, Nepal and Bangladesh. However, buffaloes for meat production gained popularity in the recent years and buffaloes have been recognized as triple purpose animals (milk, meat and draught) in most of the buffalo producing countries. Developing buffaloes only for meat production is practised in some European countries and Australia. The prospects of buffaloes for meat production are excellent in view of their triple function, efficiency for converting roughages into valuable products and superior quality of buffalo milk and meat.

Buffalo meat (carabeef) is normally the end product of buffaloes which are slaughtered in an emergency or when they are too old for work or milk production. Here, we must remember, however, that buffaloes are able to convert low quality rations into remarkable muscle growth and can live over lengthy periods of environments unsuitable for other species of domestic animals. They are generally of a placid disposition and respond to good management.

Researchers in several countries have been inspired by the knowledge that the water buffalo is able to maintain good bodily condition even when fed on a ration consisting wholly of coarse fodder. A number of experiments have been conducted to determine their growth rates and fattening capabilities under varied conditions of management and nutrition, ranging from poor pasturage to intensive systems utilising fodders and concentrates. Daily weight gain, food conversion efficiency and carcass yields have been compared with those of corresponding classes of cattle. The results have been, in many cases, quite surprising, generally substantiating the claim that buffaloes may be used effectively in suitable environments as a source of meat and meat products. The variation in size and weight between types, breeds and individuals (from 250 kg to over 1,000 kg) indicate the possibilities for selection of breeding stock for meat production. A great deal of more information is required, however, for a better understanding of their genetic potential for growth capacity.

There exists some knowledge gap on the variation existing among buffaloes with respect to meat production characteristics. In the absence of information on meat quality characteristics of different breeds of buffaloes it is not possible for developing effective breeding programmes for buffaloes for superior meat production and quality characteristics. Efficient use of carcass traits as breeding objectives is restricted by the lack of simple accurate live animal measurement techniques. Slaughter age, improvement of quality by increasing growth rate and processing procedures are used as effective means of altering carcass composition to meet specific markets. The buffalo meat is considered better since it is lean, with fat content lower than the beef. It contains low cholesterol, therefore, it is much healthier than beef. There is no report about the incidence of "Mad Cow Disease" in buffaloes in any part of Asia. Buffalo meat, therefore, has its own place in international trade.

It was reported by de Franciscis (1986)[1] that after many genetic crossings among various buffalo races (Murrah, Surti, Jaffrabadi, Nili and Badawari), a new type of buffalo called "Buffalypso" was obtained with a particular aptitude to meat production. Development of a variety of products from buffalo meat is important to create demand for all types of buffalo meat and efficient utilization of the meat and edible byproducts. The products developed from buffalo meat include sausages, patties, nuggets, meat balls,

---

[1]de Franciscis G. 1986: Buffaloe for Meat Production. Proceedings of the 3rd World Congress on Genetics Applied to Livestock Production. Lincoln, Nebraska, July 16-22 p. 703-704

ham, bacon, meat jersey and fermented sausage. Production of minced or emulsion based products is important for better utilization of tough meat from spent buffaloes.

Meat from buffalo is produced either from young male calves or from old and culled animals. In the first practice, quality is high, whereas in the second, quality is not up to the mark. In spite of the fact that buffalo meat is not of required quality due to unusual late slaughter over the age of 10 years, the demand has increased and is gradually increasing because of rise in price of other meats such as mutton and chicken. Buffaloes are generally considered as efficient user of roughages but their growth performance is not optimum when fed only on cheap fodder and byproducts. Roughages supplemented with concentrate have revealed that, as energy level of the ration was increased, there was also a parallel increase in daily gain and improvement in the feed conversion.

A few units in India producing value added byproducts like Dicalcium Phosphate, Ossein, Gelatin, other byproducts such as bone, bone meal, bone grit have export value. There is vast potential for utilizing blood, liver and certain glands from animals for pharmaceutical purpose from modern abattoirs. Intestines could be processed to casings, organs like liver, heart, lungs, kidneys are most suitable for pet foods. Skin and hides when processed suitably will further increase value of leather and leather products of good quality. As a matter of fact, profits from a meat factory comes from byproducts when utilized.

Sheep

In India 51 million sheep are almost equally divided between the plains and semiarid regions of the south and the colder hills and plains of north. There are six important meat-type sheep breeds in India, viz. Mandya, Nellore, Mecheri, Nali, Magri and Lohi. Due to low genetic potential of most of these breeds, attempts have been made to develop new meat-type breeds by crossbreeding with exotic meat breeds, like South Down, Suffolk and Dorset. Among Indian breeds, Bannur strain of Mandya has been considered, to certain extent, for its carcass quality. It is considered as butcher's ideal sheep.[1]

Goat

In India there are about 20 well-defined goat breeds apart from nondescript local ones. The bulk of the goat population is found in rural areas and primarily raised on grazing. Fast growth in goats from birth onwards is one of the most important traits for viable economy and larger returns to farmers. Together, sheep and goat annually produce around 2,30,000 tons

---

[1] Bhat, P.N. and Sharma, N: Meat Animals Available to India Meat Industry: Indian Journal of Animal Production Vol.21, No.1-4, 1998,p.89

of mutton and 4,60,000 tons of chevon (goat meat), accounting for over 15 percent of total meat production in the country. The foreign exchange earnings from small ruminants meat exports were Rs. 891 million in 1999/2000, or 11 percent of the total meat exports in 1999/2000. The foreign exchange earnings from exports of sheep and goat meat increased by 11 percent per annum during the last decade. Besides, live animals are often exported especially to the Middle East at the time of Haj. The pashmina of the Indian goat breeds is considered to be one of the finest in the world, though its production is low.

Rabbit

Rabbit farming was started by an entrepreneur in the early sixties at Kulu in Himachal Pradesh in 1986, German angora rabbits were imported in a farm near Palampur. The technology of the rabbit farming was adopted by small and marginal farmers and landless labourers in rural areas. There was a good demand of rabbit wool from Himachal Pradesh, which was easily sold at the rate ranging from Rs. 900 to Rs. 1400 per kg depending upon the quality. On an average 600 to 700 gms of wool is procured from each rabbit in a year, besides sale of kits at the price of Rs. 250 to Rs. 300 each as a female rabbit usually gives birth to eight to 10 kits, subject to the mortality rate of 20 per cent, thrice a year after the gestation period of between 29 to 35 days and the process is known as "kidling". Being a burrowing animal, rabbit has short reflexes and grooms in a peaceful environment. The ideal temperature for rabbits is from 10°C to 26°C and can survive even at 0°C and the maximum 33°C. They are sensitive to humidity below 55 per cent but feel comfortable in the humidity level ranging from 60 to 70 per cent with exposure to light for at least eight hours in a day. The rabbits are usually kept in wire mesh cages of 3 ft. × 2 ft. size having 15 inches height under hygienic conditions to save them from the common "coccidosis" disease. Young rabbit's only food is mother's milk for 20-21 days after birth and thereafter they start chewing straws of grass.

Rabbit farming is becoming popular in northeastern hills region for increasing demand of meat, wool and pelt. But the major constraint faced by farmers in this area is non-availability of standard feed which costs about 70% of the total production cost of rabbit up to 12 weeks of age after weaning. Farmers always have to depend on transportation of concentrate feed from other states, which ultimately increases the cost of concentrate feeds and as a result feeding expenditure become too high to be afforded by small-and marginal-farmers. Generally pelleting involves about 10% more cost than non-pelleted concentrates as it requires grinding, steaming and passing through pelleting machine. But in cold process there is no involvement of any heat and pelleting machine and as a result cost of cold process pellet feed is cheaper when compared with produced through hot process machine in feed mill.

Preparation of Pellet Feed Through Cold Process

Pallet feed preparation through cold process requires ingredient which are having binding/gelling properties or which helps in binding process (Table 8.2). Main binding agents are molasses, bentonite and lime powder. To meet the mineral and vitamin requirement, mineral mixture, vitamin and salt are used. To meet protein and fiber requirement, some filler material like dried tree leaves, grass, maize cob, wheat-bran, rice bran and different oilcakes/meal can be incorporated. In coccidiosis prone area anticoccidial agent may be incorporated in pellet feed.

Table 8.2: Physical and Chemical Composition of Pellet Feed Prepared at ICAR Complex, Sikkim Centre

Physical composition		Chemical composition	
Ingredients	*Parts*	*Parameter*	*%*
Molasses	40	DM	93.44
Mustard cake	30	OM	77.28
Nevaro (Ficus hooked) leaves	15	CP	8.69
Mineral mixture	4	CF	7.17
Sodium bentonite	4	EE	2.60
Lime powder	5	Ash	22.72
Common salt	2	NFE	58.82
Solidification time		24 hr	

As a complete feed an adult rabbit can consume on an average 115-120 g/day cold process pellet feed on dry matter (DM) basis. DM and organic matter digestibility of this pellet feed is 79.44% and 83.18% respectively which are at par with concentrate mixture and higher when compared with hot process pellet feed. However, pellet feed for rabbit should be of 3-4 mm diameter and 10-15 mm length but this pellet feed of 1.5 cm diameter and 6.0 cm length does not affect the feed intake of rabbit. This complete feed can sustain growth rate of rabbit at par with concentrate mixture (maize 42 parts, mustard-cake 30 parts, wheat-bran 25 parts, mineral mix 2 parts and common salt 1 part) and hot process pellet feed for rabbit available in market and reduce the feed cost per kg weight gain when compared with those feeds.

The production of meat animals is not an organized business. The production system, feed, slaughter weight and slaughter practices vary to a great extent in India. These situations lead to unreliable and non-consistent raw materials. Usually carcasses are either overlean or overfat. No serious effort has been made to develop meat animals of various species. The data of growth rate, feed efficiency and carcass quality have been collected by way of experiments on breeding and nutrition and not through purposeful planned study on meat production and quality. However, these information can be used as guideline to develop organized experimental trials for meat production. Meat quality has received relatively little attention from breeders. Considering the vast economic dimension of livestock industry, there has recently been some awakening of interest in the quality. It is hoped that the availability of improved meat animals will still increase in the years to come; major meat production will however, depend on adequate availability of raw material.

Trends in Livestock Population and Meat Production

Data on livestock population, slaughter rate (number slaughtered as % of population), carcass weight and meat production in India for 1975, 1985, 1995/1999, 2000 and 2003 are shown in Table 8.3. The data have been revised based on the new series. In India more than six percent of cattle and eleven percent of buffalo are slaughtered each year. This is equivalent to about one-third of the potential cattle offtake and about two-thirds of the potential buffalo offtake. With increasing mechanization, the demand for draught animals in states such as Punjab, Haryana, and Uttar Pradesh is declining, resulting in surplus of male buffaloes, which often are slaughtered at birth. The slaughter of these young male calves is a waste of productive capital.

India accounts for a mere 2 percent of the world total meat production. However, its share in buffalo meat is as high as 46 percent, and only 2.5 percent for beef. India's share in world goat meat production is 12 percent, and for sheep meat it is 3 percent. For pork and poultry meat India's share is insignificant. FAO's time series data for meat production in India and the world from 1981 to 2003 are shown in Table 8.4.

The slaughter weight of buffalo of 138 kgs., corresponds to the world average, although it is below that of Thailand, Philippines and Nepal. In the case of cattle, 103 kgs., slaughter weight is almost half of the world average. This is due to the fact that only old and decrepit cattle and calves and young animals that have been at the threshold of starvation reach the slaughterhouses. The productivity in the case of goat and sheep carcass weight at 10 kgs., per animal is almost two-third of the world average and one-third of USA. Total meat output increased by an average of 3.5 percent per year during the last 24 years. The rate of increase accelerated during 1985 to 2003, largely due to outstanding increase in poultry meat output. Beef output increased by 2.9 percent a year during the same period, while buffalo meat, mutton and goat meat rose by 2.5 percent a year. The annual increase was highest during the decade 1985 to 2003 and appears to have been slowed down considerably during the last six years. In 1999, despite the fall in buffalo meat share in the total meat production, its contribution was the third highest (25 percent). Beef output also followed the same trend its share declined from 31.8 percent in 1995 to 25.3 percent. The share of poultry meat increased from around 5 percent in 1975 to 27 percent, while that of pork increased form about 3 percent to over 11 percent. Goat meat accounted for 10.3 percent and sheep meat 4 percent in 2003 (Table 8.3).

Table 8.3: Trends in Livestock Population and Meat Production 1975-2003

Livestock species	Population in millions						Slaughter rate in %						Carcass weight in kgs					
	1975	1985	1995	1999	2000	2003	1975	1985	1995	1999	2000	2003	1975	1985	1995	1999	2000	2003
1. Cattle	180.1	182.4	194.6	214.9	218.8	226.1	4.9	6.1	6.4	6.4	6.4	6.4	82	80	103	103	103	103
2. Buffaloes	60.5	64.5	79.5	92.1	93.6	96.9	9.3	11.0	11.0	11.0	11.0	11.0	139	138	138	138	138	138
3. Sheep	40.1	41.3	45.0	57.6	57.6	59.0	31.9	35.8	31.3	30.0	33.0	33.0	9	9	10	10	10	10
4. Goat	69.7	81.5	119.4	122.5	123.5	124.5	42.5	42.9	39.7	38.0	38.0	47.3	9	9	10	10	10	10
5. Pigs	7.0	8.8	11.9	16.0	17.0	18.5	25.7	30.0	75.3	83.7	90.0	90.0	31	32	35	35	35	35
6. Poultry	141.0	161.0	498.0	587.7			–	–	–	–	–	–	–	–	–	–	–	–
7. Total	498.4	539.5	948.4	1105.8			–						–					

Table 8.3: Trends in Livestock Population and Meat Production 1975-2003 (Contd.)

Livestock species	Meat production in 000 tons						Share in total production in %					
	1975	1985	1995	1999	2000	2003	1975	1985	1995	1999	2000	2003
1. Cattle	724	890	1365	1421	1463	1490	35.3	34.0	31.8	29.0	27.9	25.3
2. Buffaloes	780	980	1351	1410	1421	1472	38.1	37.5	31.5	28.8	27.1	25.0
3. Sheep	117	141	194	228	229	234	5.7	5.4	4.5	4.6	4.4	4.0
4. Goat	269	358	450	466	467	473	13.2	13.7	10.4	9.5	8.9	8.0
5. Pigs	56	85	420	560	578	630	2.8	3.2	10.0	11.4	11.0	10.7
6. Poultry	101	161	507	821	1081	1600	4.9	6.2	11.8	16.7	20.7	27.0
7. Total	2,047	2,615	4,287	4,906	5239	5899	100.0	100.0	100.0	100.0	100.0	100.0
Total meat production other than poultry meat Annual growth rate previous period (percent)	1,946	2,454	3,708	4,085	4,158	4,299						

Source: FAO Production Yearbook: Various issues.

Table 8.4: Meat production in India and the World: 1981 to 1999

(In thousand tonnes)

| | INDIA | | | | | | | WORLD | | | | | | |
Year	Beef & veal	Buffalo meat	Mutton & lamb	Goat meat	Pig meat	Poultry meat	Total	Beef & veal	Buffalo meat	Mutton & lamb	Goat meat	Pig meat	Poultry meat	Total
1981	78	127	125	227	75	120	802	46,096	1,760	6,076	1,920	55,661	28,916	144,049
1982	80	130	132	298	80	130	850							
1983	80	132	134	302	80	137	865							
1984	149	148	135	346	82	150	1,010							
1985	150	152	141	358	85	161	1,040							
1986	160	163	147	370	86	180	1,106	50,885	2,002	6,220	2,110	61,474	33,331	159,407
1987	239	207	162	380	80	193	1,261	50,972	2,014	6,350	2,294	63,526	35,904	164,546
1988	232	290	148	378	357	225	2,891	51,397	2,119	6,640	2,383	67,088	37,697	170,862
1989	845	936	160	385	359	289	2,974	51,717	2,210	6,834	2,540	68,173	38,660	173,677
1990	1,270	1,048	173	410	360	334	3,595	51,732	2,216	7,040	2,700	70,064	40,376	177,937
1991	1,185	1,176	168	455	364	362	3,710	52,146	2,375	7,138	2,816	71,155	42,368	181,835
1992	1,216	1,182	167	456	397	382	3,800	51,141	2,435	7,042	2,885	72,924	41,611	174,757
1993	1,276	1,182	169	466	403	454	3,950	51,706	2,457	6,863	2,948	75,370	41,937	186,240
1994	1,292	1,204	171	470	408	507	4,052	52,778	2,534	7,204	3,114	78,589		
1995	1,365	1,351	194	450	420	479	4,259	53,352	2,593	7,099	3,304	83,539		
1996	1,370	1,382	199	454	435	479	4,319	52,986	2,812	7,226	3,394	78,548	55,841	204,882
1997	1,378	1,403	222	458	533	527	4,521	55,169	2,986	7,400	3,647	82,731	59,017	214,934
1998	1,401	1,380	226	462	469	540	4,478	55,316	3,001	7,519	3,795	88,000	61,243	222,917
1999	1,421	1,398	228	466	560	821	4,894	56,334	2,966	7,371	3,614	88,430	65,145	225,945
2000	1,442	1,421	229	467	578	1,081	5,218	56,859	3,004	7,571	3,787		69,054	233,963
2001	1,452	1,428	230	469	595	1,251	5,425	56,138	3,069	7,587	3,896		71,556	237,845
2002	1,462	1,443	233	470	613	1,401	5,622	58,134	3,125	7,728	4,048		76,645	246,257
2003	1,490	1,471	234	473	630	1,560	5,859	58,741	3,180	7,734	4,091		75,921	249,851

Source: FAO Production Year Book: Various issues.

Production of red meat is increasing at a lower rate due to the following factors:

i. The turnover for broilers is much faster, i.e. within 6-8 weeks the broilers are ready for consumption whereas in the case of goats it takes much longer time before they are ready for consumption.

ii. The requirement of land to produce 1 kg of red meat is far higher than for the production of poultry meat.

iii. Even on health grounds, doctors advice people to consume white meat.

In India, buffalo population increased proportionately higher than cattle population and they contribute significantly to total milk output production (about 55 percent) though systematic improvement of buffaloes through breeding did not take place. However, the meat potential of the buffalo remains largely unexploited so far.

The concept of fattening young buffaloes is largely unknown. Mostly infirm or diseased animals are brought to abattoirs. The buffalo keeper gives away the animal against a nominal charge or even free and thus feels relieved of the burden of the act of killing, for which he has to overcome his religious sensibilities. He does not seek to ameliorate his economic condition by such means. However, the buffalo meat processing has developed into a full-fledged business and relevant products are marketed at various stages to meet domestic as well as the export demand (canned meat). The Brooke Bond meat industry in Aurangabad illustrates the role of an efficient system of meat production. Buffaloes are bought directly from the individual farmers, thus avoiding the animal markets and middlemen. The Company guarantees the buffalo keepers who are willing to sell their animals, quite at a reasonable price. It also makes its own arrangements for transporting the animals to the slaughter facilities, where they are processed into canned meat. The processing capacity finds use of all edible and non-edible products.

Except in a few export-oriented units, unsophisticated slaughtering practices contribute to poor meat quality and low recovery of various byproducts such as hide and skins, tallow, blood, viscera and organs. Most meats are sold without the benefit of sanitary inspection. Butcher shops often lack chilling equipment, further contributing to product deterioration and increased marketing losses. Poor enforcement of hygienic standards constrains India's export competitiveness. Capital investment in existing slaughterhouses would contribute significantly to the collection of byproducts. For example, blood and other offals could be used as animal feed supplement. Political and social pressures, however, continue to impede efforts to modernize the slaughtering sector.

Buffaloes and buffalo meat have a promising market in the neighbouring Asian countries. This provides a better basis for qualitative improvements. Buffalo meat exports exhibited tremendous growth. Export almost trebled between 1988 and 1994, rising from 51,205 tons to 95,000 tons and reaching a value of $ 96 million. Still, total buffalo meat exports only account for

12 percent of domestic output. Some private slaughterhouses and processing plants have established footholds in foreign markets for buffalo meat; major markets include Malaysia and Middle Eastern countries (Bahrain, Jordan, Kuwait, Oman, United Arab Emirates). The removal of the minimum export price for frozen and chilled buffalo meat (formerly set at $ 750 per ton) should help increase exports. There is considerable potential for buffalo meat export due to the meat price competitiveness.

Taking advantage of export incentives scheme, several modern export-oriented meat-processing plants have been established with technical assistance from foreign firms. Unlike most slaughterhouses in India, the export-oriented slaughterhouses are modern, hygienic and have proper storage and processing facilities to meet export quality standards.

It has been mentioned earlier that the prospects of buffaloes for meat production are excellent in view of their triple function, efficiency for converting roughages into valuable products and superior quality of buffalo milk and meat. An immense potential exists for an organized buffalo meat industry on scientific and modern lines. The following approaches are recommended for development of buffaloes for meat[1]:

(1) The recommendations made by the National Commission on Agriculture in 1976 on development of buffaloes in general and for meat production for domestic and export trade are appropriate even today and need to be implemented. These recommendations include: (i) a fresh review and a study in greater depth should be carried out for a more satisfactory breed classification of the Indian buffalo stock; (ii) the buffalo should be developed not only for enhancement of milk production but also for making it a source of production of quality meat; (iii) attempts should be made to develop distinctly separate milk and meat breeds or types of buffaloes; (iv) a number of seed stock farms with at least 150 breeding she-buffaloes should be established; (v) in buffalo farms and research institutes wide scale investigations and studies should be undertaken on early weaning of buffalo calves and their rearing on low cost calf starters; (vi) research studies on the effect of feeding and husbandry on fattening buffalo calves should be undertaken. Promotional activity for consumption of buffalo meat in the country and consumer educational programme should be undertaken on a countrywide scale; and (vii) a deliberate and energetic drive should be made to develop export trade in buffalo meat.

(2) Salvaging male buffalo calves from early death both to conserve germplasm, increased meat production and availability of draught animals. Improved extension services should be adopted for salvaging buffalo calves.

---

[1] Kondaah, N: Improvement of Buffaloes for Meat Production: Methods and Organization, Indian Journal of Animal Production: No. 1-4: January-December 1998. pp.57-58.

(3) Entrepreneurial programmes for salvaging buffalo calves from early death. Meat exporters need to provide the required assistance before the activity is adopted.

(4) Simple breeding programme for increasing availability of a large number of buffalo bulls for natural service.

(5) At least ten more integrated meat processing complexes should be established in the buffalo population rich states with backward integration of improved buffalo production programme with farmers adoption by providing input services and marketing of animals.

(6) Meat exporters should organize selection programme to identify superior buffaloes in the abattoir project area and provide necessary facilities for effective use of the superior animals in the overall improvement of buffaloes.

(7) The superiority of buffalo meat needs to be demonstrated through continuous experimentation for promotion of buffalo meat for domestic and export market.

(8) Fattening buffaloes through economical feeding to exploit compensatory growth phenomenon, and increased buffalo meat and hide production potential need to be actively adopted.

(9) Pragmatic approach in culling and utilization of spent buffaloes need to be adopted for better utilization of feed resources and sustainable buffalo production.

(10) Concerted efforts for defending and promoting meat exports by demonstrating the public interest involved are required in view of the demand raised for ban on meat exports.

(11) A review of the State Animal Preservation Acts for effective utilization of the buffalo resources in view of the changing agricultural practices and growing buffalo population.

(12) Quality assurance of buffalo meat for domestic and export market to promote buffalo meat.

Problems

One of the major hurdles in the production of wholesome meat is the primitive condition of slaughter houses. Most of these lack even elementary facilities for hygienic production and handling of meat. A scheme for modernisation of slaughter houses was taken up in Punjab State during Third Five-Year Plan with 100 per cent central assistance. However, due to then non-availability of technical knowhow, and also due to socio-political hindrances, the Punjab Government could not avail of the financial assistance.

Pig farming as a commercial venture is still to be established in the country. It is neglected because of a general prejudice against this occupation. Punjab has the smallest population of pigs as compared to other states. Feed conversion efficiency in the case of pigs is 1:4. An increase in the sale price of pork and pork products, and the price paid to primary producers need careful consideration to change pig rearing system.

PIG PRODUCTION IN RURAL DEVELOPMENT

Recently, greater attention has been drawn towards improving the economic conditions of rural small holdings which are renowned for extremely low level of production and barely sufficient to meet the requirements of the farmer and his family. In most of the cases financial resources are negligible and the farming community continues to live at a semi-subsistence or subsistence level. The farm family remains underemployed during off-seasons and is in a position to take up some subsidiary occupations to increase the income. Therefore, the rearing of livestock forms a suitable subsidiary occupation which should be encouraged along with crop production. Such integrated development of livestock in areas has demonstrated appreciable complimentary relationship, between cropping and livestock production, leading to improved social changes evidenced by better economy of the farmers. The adoption of latest technologies in crop and livestock production has enabled farmers in different parts of the country to appreciate the advantages of adoption of combined arable farming and livestock production for bettering their economic conditions.

Pig raising fits in very well with mixed farming. As any other livestock, pig raising can easily be complimentary to intensive crop enterprise. In India, pig production has an important role to serve as an effective instrument of social change in sizeable number of weaker sections of rural community. Pig excels other farm livestock by its efficient feed conversion and by its prolificacy in reproduction. Pigs are considered as 'mortgage lifters' by farmers in agriculturally developed countries. In future meat production from sheep, goat and cattle is not likely to meet fully the demand of increasing population because ruminants with a low prolificacy and prolonged generation interval will take a long duration of period to increase their numbers and productivity. It is obvious that sizeable portion of meat supply will have to be come from pigs and poultry.

Modern pig breeds can effectively help in improving the animal protein requirements of a large segment of rural population. The ever increasing food needs of man, particularly of animal origin have resulted in great expansion in livestock industry. The importance of inclusion of animal products in human diets to have balanced nutrition has been better understood than before. In these days of prohibitive cost of good quality mutton, availability of pork at a lesser price is really a boon to the common man who can alleviate to certain extent the animal protein deficiency in his diets by proper utilization of pork.

Out of 590 million pigs in the world, about 34 per cent are reared in tropical countries. In India, there are six million pigs. The pigs in India predominantly belong to dwarf type producing low quality pork. Pig rearing in our country continues to be primitive because they are raised by certain rural people who are educationally, economically and socially backward. They are too poor to provide nutrients to the pigs. They let loose the pig to seek its own food, which eventually becomes a scavenger. As a result of such continued poor management and neglect, indigenous pigs could not establish themselves as economically sound and visible component in Animal Agriculture.

Despite the fact that the cost of good quality pork is far cheaper than that of mutton, the religious restrictions and rearing of pigs under unhygienic surroundings still stand in the way of consumption of pork. Apart from traditional cultural practices prevailing in different parts of the country, insufficient capital for implementing innovations in pig husbandry, lack of appropriate technology, poor educational background of the pig farm operators and inadequate means of disseminating worthwhile changes in pig husbandry are the diversified problems that inhibit efficient pig production. The impetus in increasing pig production in India to a large extent depends on the acceptance of pork as a decent quality food capable of overcoming animal protein shortage in the diet of common man, and on the establishment of economic superiority of pigs in typical rural farms which practice mixed farming.

Production Potentials of Pig

The pigs are probably the most accommodative of farm animals. They can be managed in many different ways and brought on and sold off at different stages of growth.

Pigs can be reared economically with minimum expenditure on building and equipment. Since the generation interval of pig is short and pigs give birth to many offsprings at a time, the stock can be reduced or increased to the desired number. With a large stock, there is greater scope for proper selection for fattening and breeding purposes. The quantity of meat available per unit live weight of pig is larger than that with other meats per unit weight. Pig husbandry requires minimum labour and returns over investments are quick. Pigs utilize garbage, garden waste and discarded feeds very effectively. They are the most efficient convertors of feeds into edible meat. Considering the acute paucity of protein supply and the increasing demand for animal protein on the one hand, and the high production potentials of a well organized pig industry on the other, it is evident that the improvement of pig production in the poorer rural parts of our country has greater promise.

In the rural sector, pig husbandry is merely at subsistence level. Rural families maintain a few pigs feeding on domestic waste, swills and whatever the animals pick on free range including farm offals and night soil. Pig rearing has been continued in this manner traditionally for ages and it might be difficult to effect a change in the existing traditional system of rearing. There is no room for improvement in pig production in India, unless the entire traditional subsistence pig farming is changed into commercial pig production. Merely extensive hybridization of indigenous stock with fast growing exotic breeds without providing clean environment, health cover and sound management will lead to disastrous results in rural pig rearing under primitive methods. This is because, the exotic pigs in spite of possessing favourable genes for rapid growth rate, are unable to express their production potential under poor environmental condition. Further, the upgraded stock becomes highly susceptible to diseases when they start their scavenging career as any other indigenous stock.

Pig being a simple stomached animal requires grains which form bulk of its ration. Therefore, pig production on large scale is closely associated with the general development of agriculture in the concerned area. Pork can be popularised commercially only when there is favourable marketing, fetching remunerative price to the pork producer. Commercial pig production should be encouraged as an integrated part of peri-urban agriculture. Successful pig production envisages two main prerequisites (feed supply and good market). If commercial pig production fails in spite of availability of these inputs of feed and marketing it will certainly be a failure in more remote rural sector. The most suitable strategy is to choose bridgeheads near population centres or cities from where improved production techniques and better breeding stock can be gradually disseminated to rural pig farmers living in remote rural areas. Piggery farms in public sector should arrange to supply weaned piglets to the farmers who must be provided with basic inputs of feed and health cover through institutional credits. The pigs should be procured from the farmers after attaining the weight between 60 and 70 kg by the cooperative or government agencies and arrangements are made for profitable marketing in large population centres or cities, where there is greater demand for pork. The pig operators should be paid adequately for their management of pigs from weaning to the marketing age of pigs. The continuance of pig rearing in primitive stage is that, the rural pig operators are burdened with breeding, feeding and management of breeding stock-boar, sow and above all marketing of pigs. Unless the basic input, the feed, is supplied to the pig farmers, even the graded pigs will be stunted in growth by being driven to scavenge the available domestic waste. By arranging tie-up system between Government agencies and pig farmers who will be supplied with weaned piglets, feed and health cover, pig farmers will be made responsible for bringing the weaned piglets at a desirable body weight of 60-70 kg in 810 to 210 days of age which they will be accordingly paid. Thereby the pig operator is relieved of the multifarious aspects of piggery operation of breeding, management of breeding stock, procurement of feed and marketing and they will concentrate mainly·in bringing up the supply of weaned piglets to attain the desirable body weight for marketing.

Geese

Goose, the robust farm bird, is one of the fastest growing avian species commonly raised for meat. Goose rearing requires little attention and it ideally fits into intensive integrated farming systems (IIFS). Geese offer nutritious meat, large eggs and rich fat for cooking as well as soft down and feathers for bedding and clothing. Thee birds are particularly appropriate for providing farmers with supplementary income. Mature geese are independent, larger than other poultry species, and thus less vulnerable to predators. When kept in small flocks and allowed to roam in farmyard or field, they are adept scavengers, requiring less attention than any other domestic bird. Geese adapt easily to captivity and if small quantities of supplementary feed are provided in the evening they will even return home by themselves.

Geese are found all over the world, but their rearing is widely practiced as an economic enterprises in Asia and Central Europe. Most geese are well adapted to hot climates as long as shade is available and to high rainfall regions. They particularly flourish in aquatic regions and marshlands. They do exceedingly well in warm, shallow waterways. A Chinese goose, which is the most popular breed of goose in Southeast Asia, is ideally suited for ecologically friendly IIFS farmers. The Chinese geese are good layers, active foragers, and the most alert and "talkative" birds producing the leanest meat among the various breeds of goose.

Geese can play a crucial role in weed control and pest management in integrated farming systems. They relish grasses and shun most broad-leaved plants. They have shown particular preference to troublesome perennial grasses such as the nutgrass (*Cyperus rotundus*) and Bermuda grass (*Cynodon dactylon*). They feed voraciously on various crop residues and are effective in managing aquatic weeds as well. "Geese can be raised well by feeding with cooked rice and a host of other farm-grown commodities.

They are affectionate birds and are loyal to the masters. Geese with their sharp eyesight and wide field of vision, combined with their strident calls, make excellent guards against approaching intruders or predators. They will charge at strangers entering the farms ferociously and they cannot be calmed into silence by them. They are thus good unbridable watchdogs for the farms. They are known to be messy birds, and it is better to house them little away from the farmhouse. These birds do not require much of a veterinary care.

Geese lay about two clutches of ten eggs each in a year. The eggs on an average will weigh about 115 g each. The eggs can be hatched using a brooder hen or in incubators at a temperature of 37.8 degree Celsius, and they hatch in about 40 days. The young goslings can be reared in brooders generally used for rearing chicks. The young goslings should not be let in to ponds and pools for swimming. Only when they are over ten weeks of age, they should be let out to roam freely in the farm. Geese will be ready for mating in about two years, and they should be paired with ganders of same age. One gander is sufficient to fertilise five to seven geese.

QUAIL FARMING

Japanese quail (*Coturnix coturnix japonica*) farming, popularly called "Bater" in Hindi, is an untapped alternate farming to traditional chicken and has immense potentiality due to low capital investment and high profit. Although it is a dual purpose bird for both meat and egg but due to more popularity of meat than egg in country, quail farming is described here for meat only. It can provide a diversified, quality food having high protein but low in energy, fat and cholesterol to consumers whereas assured income to small as well as large farmers of both rural and urban areas. Although quail farming is gradually gaining popularity in many countries of Asia and Europe but its commercial potentiality is still not well-known around the globe.

Quail broiler farming yields quicker economic return compared to any other livestock including chicken broiler. Quail broilers are marketed at 5th week of age (185 g body weight), earlier than chicken broilers which are generally marketed between 6 and 8 weeks of age. The investment on land is less due to requirement of small floor spaces as 10 quails can be reared in the same space provided to one chicken. In a small house, 52 batches can be raised per year with low investment. The medical expenditure is also less as no routine vaccination; medication and deworming are practised here like chicken. Besides, quail farming is comparatively free from risk of epidemics.

The generation interval is shorter since 3-4 generations can be obtained per year compared to maximum 2 generations for chicken broiler. Incubation period is also shorter (16-18 days) when compared with chicken (21 days), and management is simpler and labour saving due to small size of the birds. The business competition is lesser when compared with chicken broiler as it is a new enterprise.

Nutritive Value

Quail meat is highly nutritious and gaining popularity as a table delicacy among consumers. The meat is tasty, juicy and tender due to cartilaginous structure with game flavour. Quail meat (6 weeks), like chicken broiler (8 weeks), also contains higher protein (20.1 *vs* 18.2%) but lesser energy (125 *vs* 129 cal/100 g meat), and fat (5.0 *vs* 6.2%) when compared with other red meats. The cholesterol content (51.8 *vs* 60 mg/100 g meat-quail *vs* chicken broiler) which is also lesser than most of the red meats is desirable to todays health conscious consumers. Meat is excellent source of vitamin B_6, niacin and good source of vitamins B_1 and B_2, pantothenic acid, minerals and essential fatty acid. Besides, various quail meat products developed by CARI for diversification include quail meat pickle, *tandoori* quail, etc. All these qualities along with its unique game flavour have made it ideal source for meat.

Feeding

Presently, the balanced feed is not easily available commercially like that of chicken, however, the large and experienced farmers can easily prepare quail feed themselves. The suggested practical level of protein (%) and metabolizable energy (Kcal/kg) for starter (0-2 weeks), grower (3-5 weeks), and breeder/layer (6 weeks and onwards) are 27% and 2,750, 24% and 2,750 and 22% and 2,650 respectively. For practical purpose, considering unavailability of quail ration, one can easily prepare quail ration from broiler concentrate available from reputed feed manufactures. The percentage of broiler concentrate, maize rich polish and wheat bran are to be included 56, 20, 12 and 12% for starter; 50, 24, 12 and 14% for grower and 45, 25, 10 and 15% along with 5% limestone for layers respectively. However, it is advisable to consult poultry nutritionists for preparation of feed. The ration for Japanese quail is shown in Table 8.5.

Table 8.5: Suggested Ration for Japanese Quail

Ingredients (kg/100 kg)	Starter and grower	Layer/breeder
Maize	42.0	45.0
Rice kernel	15.0	10.0
Rice bran		6.0
Groundnut-cake	15.0	12.0
Soyabean meal	15.0	10.0
Fish meal/meat meal	10.0	10.0
Dicalcium phosphate	1.5	1.5
Lime stone/oyster shell	1.0	5.0
Common salt	0.3	0.3
Vitamins + Mineral mixture	0.2	0.2
Total	100.0	100.0

Management

Quails can be reared either on deep litter or in cages or a combination of both, i.e. up to 3 weeks in cages and then in litter system. In litter system, only 10 cm of thick layer of litter is needed and the rest is same to that of chicken. In cage system, 5 to 6 tiered battery brooder made up of galvanized iron or wire netting or bamboo or any other materials locally at cheaper rate may be used. Each tier may be 160 cm × 80 cm × 25 cm with the capacity of rearing 100 quail chicks, i.e. a 5-tiered cage is sufficient for rearing 500 chicks. The all-in, all-out system should be followed, i.e. the quails of same age should grow and sold simultaneously. For commercial broilers, it's better to grow the chicks entirely in battery cages up to 5 weeks of age without shifting them in rearing cages during growing period (4-5 weeks). The unnecessary catching, handling and shifting will not only hamper growth but also increase injury and mortality. The requirements of space at floor (cm^2), feeder (cm) and waterer (cm) levels are 125, 2.5 and 1.5 in cages whereas 200, 3.00 and 2.0 in deep litter respectively up to 5 weeks of age for commercial purposes. The space for layer quails (6 weeks onwards) for floor (cm^2), feeder (cm) and waterer (cm) are 175, 3.0 and 2.0 in cage system while 250, 3.5 and 2.5 in deep litter respectively. The breeder quails are housed either in colony cages (180 cm × 60 cm × 25 cm) for mass mating or in individual cages (20 cm × 25 cm × 22 cm) for pair mating. In large farms, automation can be employed for time and labour saving as well as sanitation and convenience of management. Special attention is to be given regarding brooding temperature, lighting schedule, injury, overcrowding, power failure, nutritional and disease aspects during the first 2 weeks otherwise mortality and retarded growth may occur. The small chicks are very susceptible to environmental stress due to immature development of nervous and endocrine systems. After 2 weeks, they become hardier and get well adapted to the environment.

Health Cover

As per our experience, mortality may occur during the critical period of first 2-weeks due to chilling, overcrowding, heat stroke, cannibalism, power failure, etc. which can easily be controlled through proper management and sanitation. The common diseases encountered include pullorum disease, ulcerative enteritis (quail disease), omphalitis, quail bronchitis, aspergillosis, avian cholera, avian pox, etc.

Training and Extension

As people are mostly unaware about quail, it is essential to popularize quail farming through mass campaign using various media and involving private and public sectors, financing agencies, nongovernment agencies and local panchayats. Emphasis should be given on training, particularly on practical aspects, to develop experience and confidence among the trainees to start and run their farms smoothly. It is suggested to contact Central Avian Research Institute, Izatnagar, Bareilly, where training for quail production is organized once in a year.

The common disease preventive measures including sanitation are to be followed strictly to keep away from disease and increase income and employment.

WORLD SCENARIO

International meat market in 2001 witnessed rising prices for meats other than beef, particularly poultry, in the wake of animal disease outbreaks which closed some meat markets and, in the case of Bovine Spongy form Encephalopathy (BSE), has heightened human health concerns around the globe. In 2002, however, a return to past meat consumption patterns provided some support to international beef prices, as well as lower production in the US, the world's largest beef import market, and a resumption of high quality beef shipments from South America to Europe. Increasing exportable supplies for all meats, however, constrained any significant upward price movements. The general price outlook is also affected by the Russian Federation's import ban in early 2002 on chicken, which triggered a sharp drop in leg quarter prices. Lower chicken meat prices over the course of the year limited upward price movements for other meats.

Global per caput meat consumption in 2002 recovered by 1 per cent to 38.8 kg after declining in 2001 for the first time in nearly 30 years. In the developed countries, per caput consumption of meat rose marginally to

78.3 kg after declining in the past two years. The gain in consumption in developing countries, while not expected to reach the average growth rate of 4.1 percent achieved over the past decade, was nevertheless expected to strengthen by about 2 per cent, taking per caput consumption up to 28.2 kg caput.

Meat Supplies Rise As Impact of Animal Diseases Wanes

After the adverse impact of animal disease outbreaks in 2001, meat markets witnessed a sharp increase in meat supplies in 2002 due to a return to earlier consumption and trading patterns. As exporting countries put an end to the massive animal culls and FMD vaccination which characterized meat markets in 2001, global meat output in 2002 rose to 241 million tonnes (Table 8.6) up 2.4 percent from the previous year, which experienced the lowest output growth in two decades. All meats witnessed stronger output growth in 2002, with those other than beef supported by last years rising prices and stable feed costs.

Table 8.6: World Meat Production

(Million tonnes)

Meat types	2000	2001	2002	2003 estimate	2004 forecast
World Total	**232.5**	**235.2**	**245.9**	**249.1**	**253.1**
Poultry Meat	67.7	69.6	73.8	75.2	77.3
Pig Meat	89.6	90.9	94.3	95.8	97.3
Bovine meat	59.6	58.9	61.6	61.9	62.1
Sheep & goat meat	11.4	11.4	11.6	11.7	11.9
Other meat	4.3	4.3	4.5	4.5	4.6
Developing Countries	**128.0**	**131.5**	**138.2**	**141.5**	**145.0**
Poultry Meat	35.4	36.9	39.5	40.6	42.0
Pig Meat	52.3	53.6	56.3	57.5	58.6
Bovine meat	29.5	30.0	31.2	32.1	32.8
Sheep & goat meat	8.1	8.2	8.3	8.5	8.6
Other meat	2.7	2.7	2.9	2.9	2.9
Developed Countries	**104.6**	**103.8**	**107.6**	**107.5**	**108.1**
Poultry Meat	32.3	32.7	34.3	34.5	35.2
Pig Meat	37.3	37.4	38.0	38.3	38.7
Bovine meat	30.0	28.9	30.4	29.8	29.3
Sheep & goat meat	3.3	3.2	3.3	3.2	3.2
Other meat	1.6	1.6	1.6	1.7	1.7

Source FAO: Total computed from unrounded data

After slipping 1 percent in 2001, beef production recovered to a record 60 million tonnes in 2002, up 2 per cent. The developing countries were set to expand their share of global production further in 2002 following a 4 percent increase in their output. This was facilitated by lower output in the United States, the producer of one-fifth of global beef supplies, and continued strong growth in the largest developing country producers of Brazil and China. A resumption in normal slaughter patterns in the EC prompted a 4 percent jump in beef production there, while the decade-long output declines in transition economies continued to extend into 2002.

Sheep and goat production, despite declining supplies in developed countries, rose by 2.3 percent, driven mainly by strong growth in China, the major Asian producer, with additional gains in Pakistan and India. Some flock recovery occurred in Afghanistan, the Islamic Republic of Iran and Sudan; the latter prompted by increasing access to livestock markets in the Near East. Reduced supplies from Oceania were expected in response to flock rebuilding in New Zealand (Table 8.7).

Moderate feed prices and strong demand were expected to support respective output gains of 2.9 percent and 2.4 percent for the poultry and pork sectors, with the strongest gains realized by South America and Asia. Most of the poultry output gains were generated in developing countries, however, poultry's share of global output declined marginally in 2002 to 29.7 percent, as growths in other meats recovered.

Table 8.7: International Meat Prices

Year	FAO index of international meat prices (1990-92=100)	Indicative international meat prices (US $/tonne)			
		Chicken (1)	Pork (2)	Beef (3)	Lamb (4)
1994	102	921	2659	2384	2975
1995	99	922	2470	1947	2621
1996	96	978	2733	1741	3295
1997	96	843	2724	1880	3393
1998	83	760	2121	1754	2750
1999	84	602	2073	1894	2610
2000	85	592	2083	1957	2619
2001	84	645	2077	2138	2912
2002	82	579	1830	2127	3303
2003	87(5)	572(5)	1880(5)	2044(6)	3757(7)

Source: FAO: Food Outlook

Notes: (1) Chicken Parts, United States export unit value, (2) Frozen pork, United States Export Unit Value, (3) Manufacture cow beef, Australia, *cif* prices to the United States, (4) Lamb frozen whole carcass, new Zealand, wholesale prices London, (5) January-February 2002, (6) January-April 2002, (7) January-March 2002.

Meat Trade Prospects Favourable as Consumption Recovered and Prices Remained Sluggish

Expanding exportable supplies from countries restricted from exporting in 2001 due to animal disease concerns, specifically Uruguay, Argentina, some EC countries, and the Republic of Korea, were expected to push up meat shipments in 2002. Global meat trade was estimated at 18.7 million tonnes in 2002, 4 percent above the lackluster performance in 2001 (Table 8.8). Strong gains were expected for all meats, with the exception of ovine meat, which was constrained by reduced exportable supplies in Oceania.

Table 8.8: World Meat Exports

(thousand tonnes)

Meat Types	2000	2001	2002	2003 estimate	2004 forecast
World	17,327	17,663	18,773	18,930	19,578
Poultry meat	7,328	7,648	7,870	7,871	8,104
Pig meat	3,271	3,442	4,061	4,079	4,122
Bovine meat	5,715	5,520	5,876	5,991	6,338
Sheep & goat meat	768	809	721	700	723
Other meat	245	245	283	289	289

Source: FAO,

Note: Total computed from unrounded data.

(1) Includes meat (fresh, chilled, frozen prepared and canned) in carcass weight equivalent; excludes live animals, offals and EC intra-trade.

After declining by an estimated 3 percent in 2001, beef shipments reached a record 5.8 million tonnes in 2002, up 4.4 percent from the previous year's level. Many markets previously closed to meat products from those countries in South America and Europe afflicted with FMD were opened, implying a realignment in market shares in 2002. A 20 percent jump was reported for South American beef exports to regional markets in South America and selected countries in the EC, as Argentina and Uruguay were officially recognized as "FMD free with vaccination". This helped to move up the region's share of global beef markets to one-fifth of global totals. While EC exports witnessed strong export gains, the shipments of 600,000 tonnes remained significantly below their WTO export subsidy limits of 822,000 tonnes. In North America, herd rebuilding, high prices, and a strong US dollar led to US exports decline by an estimated 5 percent. As for imports, markets, such as Egypt, the Republic of Korea, the Russian Federation, Canada and the United States, registered strong import gains. By contrast, however, the impact of food safety concerns in Japan arising from outbreaks of BSE in late 2001 spilled over into 2002 with Japanese consumers, for the second consecutive year, reducing consumption of imported beef.

Considerable instability in the global poultry meat market had surfaced in the first quarter of 2002. Issues relating to poultry disease and escalating concerns regarding the use of unauthorized antibiotics in feed have led to numerous import bans and heightened border inspections and testing. These issues range from illegal antibiotics found in Thai and Chinese chicken, the ban on US chicken by the Russian Federation, and some other CIS countries, as well as bans related to the outbreaks of low-pathogenic avian influenza in the eastern United States and avian flu in China (Mainland) and Hong Kong (Special Administered Region). Despite this backdrop of uncertainties, global poultry trade increased by 4 percent to nearly 8 million tonnes in 2002. Many of these market disruptions were of short duration and import demand, disrupted over the first months of 2002, recovered quickly. Imports by the Russian Federation, after jumping 11 percent in 2001, went up by less than 11 percent. A nearly 30 percent fall in the price of US leg quarters as a result of the month-long Russian import ban helped induce strong buying by other markets, particularly in Asia and Central America. Meanwhile, BSE-related concerns in Japan supported increased poultry imports.

High demand for pigmeat in Asia, the recipient of nearly half of global imports, led to a nearly 5 per cent jump in pigmeat trade to 4.1 million tonne in 2002. The Japanese imposition, in August 2001, of a "safeguard" (higher tariffs in response to import surges) on pigmeat imports constrained imports in late 2001 and early 2002. However, BSE concerns and a shift in Japanese consumer preferences to meats other than beef, prompted a nearly 30 percent jump in pigmeat deliveries in late 2001, pushing up Japanese import prices by 25 percent. Imports by Japan, the largest pigmeat market, continued to be strong in 2002. Increased import demand was witnessed in Hong Kong, SAR, the Republic of Korea, Mexico and the Russian Federation. Strong competition from the Canadian pigmeat industry and the high value of the US currency reduced US export in 2002, while a moderation in prices in the EC and Brazil, in the context of higher output, facilitated product shipments. Meanwhile, a clean bill of health for the hog industry in the Republic of Korea resulted in a resumption of exports to Japan after a two-year FMD-related hiatus.

Meat Prospects in 2004

Continued short-term price recovery will likely prompt a slight rebound in production in 2004, with global meat output anticipated to increase 2 percent to 253.1 million tones. The low supply growth that characterized the poultry and pigment markets in 2003 is projected to abate as stronger economic prospects in both developed and developing countries strengthen demand for meat. However, the anticipated growth in pigmeat and poultry output will not be matched in the beef sector as herd rebuilding starts in the United States and Oceania. The tighter supplies typically associated with herd rebuilding are anticipated to limit their export potential growth in beef supply availabilities is expected to come from developing countries.

The influence of trade-restricting measures in Japan and the Russian Federation, two of the major meat importing countries, will persist in 2004 because it is anticipated that both countries will maintain restrictive tariffs and TRQs. However, overall meat trade is expected to grow 3 percent, supported by strong import demand from the United States as its meat supplies decline and a rising Asian demand for pigmeat and poultry, particularly in China. Continued tightened supplies of beef, combined with a recovery in trade, are likely to maintain upward pressure on beef prices in 2004. Some stabilization is expected for pigmeat and poultry meat in the context of higher production.

A Perspective

During the last four decades of the twentieth century, global meat production increased more than threefold. The increment between 1980 and 2000 was about 70 percent; the output rose by about 32 percent during the 1980s and by 30 percent during the 1990s, and the annual total surpassed 230 Mt a year by the year 2000. Continuation of this trend would see the global meat output at about 300 Mt by 2020, but a plausible argument can be made for a lower increase. There will be obviously be major differences between rich and poor countries. Meat is now the single largest source of animal protein in all affluent countries (Japan, with its extraordinary high fish intake, is the only exception) and this is not going to change in any radical way. Moreover, several circumstances will promote higher meat consumption: more single-person households, high rates of female employment, and reduced willingness to cook are the ongoing shifts that have brought a continuing rise in the consumption of fast, ready-to-serve or easy-to-prepare foods whose key ingredient is often fatty meat.

While fatty fast food is here to stay (albeit to get a bit leaner with time), there is little chance for any widespread adoption of vegetarianism in affluent societies. Interest in reduced intake of animal foods has grown, and various forms of quasi-vegetarianism (ranging from lactovegetarians who enjoy their yogurt and cheese to lacto-ovo-pisci-vegetarians who eat everything except the red meat) may be practised by 3–7 percent of Western populations. But the best available foodstuffs, numbered only about half a million (less than 0.2 percent) of the population in 1994.

Similarly reduction of high Western meat intakes due to higher costs of beef, pork, and chicken is not very likely in a world where commodity prices have experienced a long secular decline. But even suddenly rising prices would make little difference in societies where disposable incomes are now generally so high that demand for such desirable items as meat or gasoline is highly price-inelastic. Converting people to healthy nutrition through education is a Sisyphean task in a society where gluttony-promoting advertisements and Brobdingnagian restaurant servings are a norm, and where a ubiquitous lack of dietary discipline has led to a growing perception of obese people as victims. Still, there are clear signs that the West's high meat intakes are near or above, the saturation level: average supply grew only marginally during the 1990s in the United States and Britain, remained nearly the same in France and Finland, and actually declined in Germany and Canada. Future absolute growth of Western meat demand may then largely reflect a slow population increase.

In contrast, relatively low levels of average meat consumption throughout Asia and Africa, generally only moderate intakes in Latin America, continuing dietary transition driven by higher disposable incomes, and the globalisation of food distribution translate into potentially high growth of global demand. But this does not mean that today's modernizing countries are set to emulate the dietary pattern of the carnivorous West. The experience of the past two generations shows that although the per capita consumption of meat in most countries of Asia, the Middle East, and Africa has grown appreciably in relative terms, in absolute terms it has remained restrained even as incomes has risen substantially. Consequently, average annual per capita meat supply (in carcass weight) remains below 30 kg in Vietnam and the Philippines, below 25 kg in Turkey and Egypt, below 15 in Pakistan, below 10 in Indonesia and Nigeria and below 5 in India, Bangladesh and the poorest countries of Africa.

Despite the indisputable globalisation of tastes, national and regional food preferences still matter around the world and food taboos, remain strong among nearly 2 billion Muslims and Hindus. Their mass conversion to, respectively, pork and beef eating is not likely, and the common assumption of high income elasticity of demand for meat may not be realized. A few countries in East Asia have seen a stronger growth, with Taiwan's per capita meat supply now at more than 70 kg/year and South Korea's rate approaching 50 kg. But, as already noted, China's rate has stabilised during the 1990s, as did Japan's intake. Moreover, land constrains alone mean that neither China nor India will be able to replicate the Western levels of feed production, and economic constraints will prevent those countries from being such large importers of animal feed as Taiwan and Japan are. Still, increased demand for imported feed grains could eventually lead to appreciable price increases (and hence to less affordable imports by countries depending on foreign food grain) — or it could stimulate the development of considerable grain-production potential in Ukraine and Russia. In addition, high-quality feed can be used much more efficiently to produce complete protein in milk and eggs, as well as in herbivorous fish. Not surprisingly, Asian aquaculture, particularly in China, has seen a rapid expansion. As a result, the global growth of meat demand during the next generation may not be relatively as large as it has been since 1980. Whatever the actual future demand, it is clear what course should be followed in order to moderate various undesirable consequences of globally rising meat consumption. By far the most important strategy for making diets with a reasonable share of meat available to an additional 2–3 billion people during the coming two generations would be to combine maximized feeding efficiencies with moderated intakes in affluent countries, and with appropriate adjustments of specific meat shares.

Fortunately, there are many effective ways to increase the overall efficiency of meat production, including more efficient cropping and the use of supplementary amino acids in order to raise feed conversion efficiencies. Further ahead is a partial replacement of meat by novel plant proteins. It is calculated that a relatively modest addition of such proteins to ground and processed meat, whose recent global consumption has totaled roughly 40 Mt, or nearly 20 percent of global meat supply, could result in savings of about 70 Mt of concentrated grain feed, an equivalent of about 10 percent of recent annual global consumption of concentrated feeds . More distant still is a large-scale deployment of various bioengineering advances designed to increase the metabolic efficiency of domestic animals and to reduce the volume of their wastes.

Modernisation of high Western meat intakes has no known downsides as there are no scientifically demonstrable advantages to the prevailing intakes. For more than a generation the Mediterranean diet has been seen as the most appropriate alternative. At the same time, modern Mediterranean diets have been shifting rapidly toward the less desirable pattern of higher meat and fat consumption. As a result, Spain's meat consumption is now nearly 50 percent higher than the British mean, and Italians consume more meat than do the Germans. Moreover, as some researchers argue, the traditional Mediterranean diet works only as a whole, and adjustment of a single factor is an alternative diet (e.g., reducing the amount of meat) may be relatively ineffective. But there has been a clear correlation between Europe's aging populations and reformed diets: a further increase in the share of older, nutrition-conscious cohorts everywhere in Europe will undoubtedly help the shift towards more rational diets.

Advances in our understanding have made many matters clear. There is no scientifically defensible reason for strict vegetarianism. Ours is an omnivorous species, and meat eating is a part of our evolutionary heritage. Even the fundamental and undeniably correct food-chain argument in favor of plant foods has important practical exceptions. Feeding cattle corn and soybeans produced by intensive cropping is the most irrational meat-producing strategy, but feeding ruminants on appropriately managed pastures and on cellulosic crop- and food-processing wastes is a perfect meat-producing strategy. Conversely, there is no scientifically defensible reason for the extraordinary meaty diets now prevailing in most Western countries. These diets do not make people healthier and do not prolong their lives. Instead, to recapitulate, they have undesirable environmental impacts as they generate more soil erosion and lead to higher nutrient losses (above all, of reactive nitrogen) to the atmosphere and to ground and surface waters; to more preventively injected antibodies that will increase bacterial resistance; to higher emissions of greenhouse gases; and to concentrations of animals in giant feeding enterprises where excessive crowding leads to abnormal behavior and increases the opportunities for devastating. epizootics. These diets also contribute to an alarming incidence of obesity and to higher rates of several diseases of highly industrialized populations.

The challenge for low-income countries is not to increase specifically red meat and poultry production but rather to raise the consumption of animal foodstuffs in general so that various combination of meat, dairy products, eggs, and aquacultured fish assure a better quality of nutrition with fewer negative consequences than have been experienced in the West. Adjustments of relative animal food intakes produced by grain feeding are a highly effective way of reducing the environmental impact of carnivorousness. The most desirable meat shift (from beef to poultry) is made so much easier by the virtually global acceptance of chicken, the most efficient converter of feed to meat; and there are enormous opportunities for increasing the productivity of dairy animals, the most efficient converters of feed to protein, in nearly all low-income countries.

Given their high consumption levels, the affluent countries can do much more to reduce the negative impacts of carnivorousness simply by gradually lowering their average annual meat intakes and by reforming their animal husbandry. A rational society would aim to reduce its average annual meat intake to less than 50 kg/capita, to minimize grain feeding to cattle, to treat all domestic animals in more humane ways, and to resist further concentration of meat production with all of its attendant ills. Success in this combined endeavor would help to moderate the claims the world's animal husbandry makes on land and water, and it would reduce environmental impacts of modern carnivorousness while improving nutrition and health everywhere.

HIDES AND SKINS

From official sources little information is available with regard to the production of hides and skins. Even though India is the largest producer of hides and leather, we are not able to reap the full potential. This is because a good part of the hides are damaged due to poor flaying especially in the small and unregistered slaughterhouses. There is, therefore, a considerable scope for improvement of hides and tanning and using entrails and offal etc. that generally go waste. Though the quality leaves much to be desired, there is considerable demand for quality hides. The only source of information regarding hides and skins production in India and other countries is the FAO's Yearbook. Besides the Central Statistical Organization publishes the value of Indian hides and skins in their National Account Statistics, but does not give either the unit value or the physical output. Based on data available from these two sources, production of raw hides and skins and their value in the selected years are presented in Table 8.9.

Production of cattle and buffalo hides increased from an average of 736 000 tonnes during 1979-81 to 982 000 tonnes in 2002, representing an increase of about percent 33 percent. Sheep and goatskin increased by 74 percent to 195000 tonnes during this period. Goat skin contributed the bulk of this increase (about 76 percent). In term of value the increase for raw hides was only 23 percent, while the value of sheep and goat skins lose by 80 percent during this period. At present nearly 35-40 percent of leather goes waste. A Committee set up by the Government had recommended the utilization of hides from fallen animals, upgradation of lower grade hides and skins, and commercial cattle farming to increase the quality. According to the forecasts prepared by the Indian Council of Leather Exports, by the year 2003, nearly 30 percent of the total demand for leather in India were to be met through imports.

Leather Industry

India is one of the largest bovine leather producers in the world, accounting for 12 percent and 6 percent of global output of heavy and light bovine leather respectively. However, its share in the world trade for bovine leather is rather small, less than 2 percent for light leather and only 0.6 percent in heavy leather. During the period 1974-76 to 1992, the world trade in bovine heavy leather increased three folds, while India's exports

Table 8.9: All India: Production and Value of Raw Hides and Skins: Selected Years

Years	Hides	Sheep skin	Goat skin	Total	Value at 1993/98 prices (in million Rs.)		
					Hides	Skin	Total
	.... *000 tonnes*						
1979-81	736	37	75	848	5,027	2,560	7,587
1989-91	860	44	107	1,011	4,417	3,320	7,737
(Growth rate %)	(1.5)	(1.9)	(3.6)	(1.8)	(-1.3)	(2.6)	(0.2)
1991	841	38	108	987	4,460	3,470	7,930
1992	850	38	109	997	4,760	3,330	8,090
1993	915	39	119	1,073	5,060	5,030	10,090
1994	924	45	120	1,089	5,410	5,150	10,560
1995	933	49	122	1,103	5,240	5,010	10,250
1996	944	50	124	1,118	5,380	5,080	10,460
1997	953	51	126	1,130	5,670	5,160	10,830
1998	942	51	127	1,120	5,920	4,900	10,820
1999	954	52	128	1,134	5,940	5,060	11,000
2000	968	53	129	1,150	6,150	4,710	10,860
2001	975	55	131	1,161	6,030	4,580	10,610
2002	982	57	138	1,177	6,190	4,570	10,760

Source: 1. FAO: Production Yearbook various issues and World Statistical Compendium for raw hides and skins, leather and leather footwear: 1974-1992, Rome 1994.

2. Central Statistical Organization: National Accounts Statistics; 2003.

only doubled. More striking picture emerges for bovine light leather as the world trade in value terms jumped by more than eight times, while value of India's exports rose by only 94 percent during this period. India did not benefit fully from the fast expanding global market for bovine leather. Till 1980s, India was exporter of raw and unfinished leather. This has changed over the years. Share of value added products such as footwear, leather garments, and other goods has increased continuously. At present value added products account for 81 percent of the total leather exports, while the share of finished leather had declined from 22 percent in 1992/93 to 18 percent in 1996/97. The leather industry exhibited tremendous growth as a result of simplification of export procedures, the government's decision to encourage exports of value added leathers and the liberalization of imports of capital goods and component. Increasing costs of production (especially wages) and growing concern about the negative environmental impact of tanneries in developed countries helped improve the competitiveness of Indian leather products. India enjoys a competitive edge due to low wage rates.

The tanning industry faces serious problems, including sizable losses due to the defective curing, preservation, storage, and handling of skins and environmental pollution resulting from the improper disposal of waste products from the tanning process. To address the pollution problem, the government is restricting the establishment of new units and the expansion of existing tanneries.

Leather export is identified as one of the thrust areas. Leather and leather goods form 20 percent of the India's total exports and rank fourth among export products. Indian leather products are exported to 120 countries with major destinations being Germany, the USA, Italy, the UK and France. However, Indian leather goods have only a minuscule 4.5 percent share in the $ 41 billion (1995 estimate) global market. The industry is facing serious difficulty, as exports have declined during the last two years. Indian leather industry suffers from several weaknesses. The major ones include: (i) Lack of modernization; (ii) underdeveloped component industry; (iii) higher freight cost due to long distance to our major export markets; (iv) infrastructural bottlenecks; and (v) non-implementation of pollution control measures. There is an urgent need for a coherent policy to improve competitiveness and provide the right export thrust. This needs to be done urgently in view of the sharp depreciation of the southeast Asian currencies and emerging competition from the East European countries, especially, Poland, Romania, Czech and Slovak Republics and Macedonia, where new manufacturing facilities are being established. The latter countries can affect the European market for Indian leather products, as they are capable of providing goods at much lower costs.

9
Government Policies

Livestock sub-sector is clubbed with agriculture, which is mainly a state subject. However, the Government of India plays an important role in the growth and development of the livestock sector. The Central Government sets out the broad Policy Framework for development of livestock sector. Strategies for livestock development are generally incorporated into overall national Five-Year Plans, which become the responsibility of Ministry of Agriculture, with implementation responsibilities devolving to states, district and local offices.

The Department of Animal Husbandry and Dairying (AH&D) in the Central Ministry of Agriculture is responsible for matters relating to livestock production, preservation, protection and improvement of stocks and dairy development including Technology Mission on Dairy Development. The Department came into existence w.e.f. 1 February 1991, by converting two divisions of the Department of Agriculture and Cooperation namely Animal Husbandry and Dairy Development into a separate Department. A list of main Departments/Agencies taking care of livestock development at various levels is shown in Table 9.1. The Organizational structure of the major agencies of the central Government dealing with Livestock sector is shown in Annexure I.

> The Department of Animal Husbandry and Dairying came into existence in February 1991 and Fisheries was transferred to the Department in October 1997. Main focus of the activities is on (a) development of requisite infrastructure in States/UTs for improving animal productivity, (b) preservation and livestock health care, (c) strengthening of central livestock farms, and (d) expansion of aquaculture in fresh, brackish water and welfare of fisherfolk, etc. The Department has 44 field offices/subordinate offices spread over the country.

PRE-INDEPENDENCE PERIOD

Till the setting up Royal Commission on Agriculture (1927), there was no specific policy of the British Government on livestock development in India. Royal Commission on Agriculture (RCA) recognized the importance

Table 9.1: Major Departments/Agencies Taking Care of Livestock Development At Various Levels

Central department / agency	Area of development	Level of operation
Department of Animal Husbandry and Dairying (Ministry of Agriculture, Govt. of India)	General Livestock Development and Health care	State / Province: Department of Animal Husbandry, Director of Animal Husbandry
	Development of breeding infrastructure for cattle and buffalo	State / Province: Department of Animal Husbandry, State Implementing Agency.
	Dairy Development outside Operation Flood Areas	State / Province: Department of Animal Husbandry, Dairy Cooperative Federation / Director of Dairy Development
	Milk and Milk Products Order (MMPO)	State / Province: Department of Animal Husbandry, Dairy Cooperative Federation / Director of Dairy Development
	Other animal products	State / Province: Department of Animal Husbandry, Meat and Poultry Development Corporations, Wool Marketing Corporations, Municipal Corporations.
National Dairy Development Board	Dairy Development through Cooperatives	State / Province: Dairy Coop. Federation District : Cooperative Milk Union
Ministry of Rural Development, Govt. of India	Rural Development (including livestock oriented schemes)	State / Province: State Dept. for Rural Development District : District Rural Development Agency (DRDA)
National Bank for Agriculture and Rural Development (NABARD), National SC/ST Development Finance Corporation, National Minorities Development Corporation.	Institutional Finance/ Credit	Regional Offices of NABARD Commercial and Cooperative Banks, Special Development Corporations, Respective State Corporations.
General Insurance Corporation.	Insurance cover to Livestock	Four Subsidiaries operating at country level, with their respective state and district level branches.
Department of Agricultural Research and Education (DARE)/ Indian Council of Agricultural Research (ICAR)	Education and Research in Agriculture and allied sciences	Research Institutes and Regional Research Stations, Training Centres/ Extension Centres. State/ Province: State Agricultural Universities

of bullock power for agriculture and cow for supply of milk. However, the Commission was of the view that under the conditions commonly found in villages, it was unlikely that selling of dairy produce would be more remunerative to cultivator than raising crops. The RCA concluded that in the breeding of draught cattle qualities should be acquired only insofar as these were consistent with the maintenance of essential qualities which good draught cattle must possess. The Commission recommended that no crossbreeding programme should be taken up by the concerned departments of the Government and the departmental endeavours should centre around the improvement of milking qualities of indigenous breeds like Sahiwal and Sindhi or specially selected strains of breeds like Haryana.

Colonel Olver, Animal Husbandry Expert, Imperial Council of Agricultural Research (now designated as Indian Council of Agriculture Research) was also against introduction of European breeds of Cattle in India and suggested that sounder policy effecting systematic improvement in the indigenous stock should be adopted by means of selective breeding, better feeding and improved management. He also recommended giving greater attention to increase in milk production in cows under a system of mixed farming.

Mr. C. Norman Wright in his report on "The Development of Cattle and Dairy Industries in India (1937)" opined that only high yielding milch cows would be economical for city milk supply while in the rural areas, draught breeds were needed to produce good working bullocks. He also strongly opposed adoption of large scale cross breeding to improve the milk yield of local cattle under the prevailing conditions of animal husbandry and recommended that immediate steps should be taken in selecting and improving milk strains of indigenous cattle. He also emphasized that breeding policy must take into account the environment under which animal had to live and produce.

The Animal Husbandry Wing of the Board of Agriculture and Animal Husbandry of India at its fourth (1940) and sixth (1945) meetings discussed the mass improvement of inferior indigenous cattle and recommended that grading up of cattle should be taken up in a systematic way in selected areas. In these areas compulsory castration, proper feeding of the graded progeny and continuous supply of purebred should be ensured.

POST-INDEPENDENCE POLICIES

In 1949 the Goseva Sangh, Wardha advised the Government of India that the ultimate aim in the development of cattle should be the production of dual purpose animals and that the buffalo might also be treated as a dual purpose animal in those areas where male buffaloes were used for cultivation purposes. The ICAR considered the above suggestion of the Goseva Sangh and recommended adoption of the following course for the improvement of cattle in the country:

(i) In view of the fact that a large percentage of our cattle population comprises nondescript animals, it is essential in the interest of producing a general utility animal that it should combine in itself, draught and milking qualities to the optimum extent; in other words, if in nondescript cattle, these two qualities are combined to an average degree to start with, the purpose will be served.

(ii) In areas where specific types (as distinct from well-defined breeds) exist the policy should be to effect improvement by selective breeding with a view to improving both milk and work qualities.

(iii) In the case of well-defined breeds, the objective should be to put in as much milk in them as possible without materially impairing the work quality.

(iv) In the case of well-defined milch breeds, the number of animals which has considerably decreased after partition, the Committee was of the considered view that it would be in the larger interests of the country as a whole to develop their milking capacity to the maximum, by selective breeding and to utilize them principally for the development of cattle in underdeveloped areas.

National Policy on Agricultural Development, which ensures the welfare of rural people and stresses on social justice and equality of opportunity, is an important means in the development strategies. Within the confines of these basic objectives, the policy framework seeks to build a progressively modern and dynamic agricultural economy with continuously expanding production, maximum participation of weaker sections, increasing self-reliance, import substitution, diversification in crop production and dispersed development to reduce regional imbalances, ultimately leading to improved quality of life without disturbing the ecological balance.

So far India has not made any livestock policy statement as such. However, policy framework and strategies, as mentioned above, do find mention in the Five Year Plans. To begin with, in the First Five Year Plan, one of the goals in livestock development was increased milk production, improved milk supply to the large urban demand centres and to improve the quality and supply of the draught animals for agriculture. It also recognized the problem of feed and fodder and the huge livestock population, taking into consideration the carrying capacity of land under fodder. The problem of animal diseases also was identified as one of the limitations to productivity improvement. The launching of the Key Village Scheme, was one of the strategies adopted to increase milk production, removal of scrub bulls and to an extent supply of fodder. Another important project that was initiated was Gaushala Development Scheme for developing gaushalas into Centres of Economic Milk Production.

The first five year plan goals in livestock development were primarily to increase milk production, improve milk supply to the large urban demand centers and to improve the quality and supply of draught animals for agriculture. The strategies laid down were selective breeding of indigenous breeds for milk and work; and grading up of nondescript cattle and buffalo with selected Indian breeds.

The second and third plans followed the first plan policies and schemes without much of a change. By the end of the third plan the inadequacies of the key village scheme and government run city dairies became obvious, as also the need for greater rural orientation for milk production. There was virtually no growth in milk production during the first three plan periods.

Some of the most momentous policy initiatives in the livestock sector were taken during the interregnum between the third and fourth five year plans: milk production in rural areas through producer cooperatives and movement of processed milk to city dairies became the cornerstone of government dairy policy; key village schemes matured into the intensive cattle development projects, cross breeding of nondescript cattle with exotic dairy breeds became government policy for increasing milk production and a package of policies on animal coproducts and byproducts galvanized the leather industry.

The second comprehensive review of the livestock sector was by the National Commission on Agriculture in 1976. The NCA's review was during the fifth five year plan and therefore the NCA had the benefit of reviewing plan strategies and achievements under four five year plans between 1951-'74. the National Commission's Report, Part VII, deals with the problems and prospects of Animal Husbandry comprehensively.

Key village Scheme for increasing milk and fodder production, castration of scrub bulls for selectivity in cattle and buffalo population growth, government owned dairy plants for town milk supply and peri-urban cooperatives for city kept milch animals in metropolitan cities, were the major plan schemes under the first plan.

The government's dairy policy found institutionalization in the National Dairy Development Board and its translation into action in "Operation Flood Projects I to III". The country's milk production chart, stagnant over two decades, suddenly came alive: milk production grew rapidly from 22 mln mt in 1970 four times, to over 80 mln mt by 2002. Cross breeding of cattle gained momentum as the milk cooperatives under Operation Flood moved in to provide the much needed market stimulus.

Expert Committee on All India Key Village Scheme

An Expert Committee was set up by the Government of India in 1959 to review and evaluate work done under the All India Key Village Scheme. The Committee recommended that while draught quality in cattle was important, every effort should be made to increase milk production as quickly as possible. For achieving this objective, the Committee suggested that improvement of buffaloes should be undertaken wherever they have been found suitable and in the case of nondescript cattle even crossbreeding with exotic breeds might be resorted to where climatic and other conditions were favourable. In the case of well-defined breeds or specific types, it was considered essential that their milking quality should be improved through selective breeding. The Committee was of the view that in areas where specialized breeds already existed, no crossbreeding should be permitted.

ICDP and NDDB

Animal husbandry development plans suffered from several other limitations and great paucity of superior quality breeding bulls was one of them. Hence, the breeding policy during the first and the second plans was to develop dual purpose breeds which could provide good bullocks and increased quantities of milk. The need for registration of cattle conforming to certain preserved standards in the main breeding tracts was recognized as an important means for development of cattle breeds. Accordingly, a scheme to organize breeders' societies for registration of cattle milk recording and supply or breeding stock of Haryana, Gir and Ongole breeds of cattle and Murrah breed of buffalo was initiated. In the Third Plan, a scheme for progeny testing was started with Haryana cattle and Murrah buffalo at Hissar. During the later half of the Third Plan period it was realized that cattle development programmes started in the earlier plans could not make much impact on improvement of stock due to lack of sufficient inputs and absence of tie up of the production programmes with proper marketing systems. An area development approach for cattle development popularly known as Intensive Cattle Development Project (ICDP) was, therefore, formulated as a part of the special Development Programme. According to this policy cross breeding was undertaken in areas covered by ICDP and in Key Village blocks that lie in the milk sheds of existing and proposed dairies. The Key Village programme was merged into this programme. In fact, it was considered as a major shift to the livestock policy initiatives and the failure of Government run dairy development programme led to a change in the perception. This, in turn, led to the formation of the National Dairy Development Board in 1965. This policy initiative resulted in the launching of the Operation Flood programme through the National Dairy Development Board in 1970-1971, which continued till 1996 with spectacular results. The investment in the formation of dairy cooperative societies, and dairy processing plants in the rural areas helped to meet the rapidly increasing consumption demands of the urban centres and in turn gave the required stimulus to the milk producers to produce more. Thus, more than 10 million milk producers, 70% belonging to the landless labourers, small and marginal farmers, throughout the length and breadth of the country were benefited immensely. The policy regarding fodder development, disease control development of small ruminants, pack animals, continued without much change during the subsequent Plan periods.

Liberalisation and Delicensing

In the wake of the economic liberalization process set in motion by the Government of India in 1991, the government in the Ministry of Agriculture, Department of Animal Husbandry and dairying, constituted a Steering Group in 1994, to oversee and guide a comprehensive livestock sector review and to recommend to the government a new policy framework for the livestock sector, in keeping with the changing national and global economic environment.

The Report of the Steering group, comprising three sections: (i) the recommended policy approach; (ii) livestock sector perspectives 1995-2020; and (iii) Livestock Sector in India – Situation Analysis 1951-'95; was presented to the government of India in July 1996. The government is yet to act on the recommendations of the Steering Group.

Interest in what has been one of the world's largest development projects Operation Flood (OF) is now heightened by the challenge faced by the cooperative dairy, following delicensing of the industry in 1992. This has led to the influx of large private sector entrants, and more intense competition in the market. Cooperatives do not enjoy the same freedom as that by their competitors. Further, they remain committed to social as well as economic goals. Now, their viability seems seriously threatened. The immense infrastructure created under the OF Programme faces a daunting challenge. Should it not rise to the occasion, considerable economic and social loss is likely to take place.

Conservatively estimated, Operation Flood has reached more than 40 million rural Indians. Its achievements are well-documented. The programme strategies—creating infrastructure through monetization of commodity aid and investing in production enhancement while building processing facilities and developing markets—have also been well-researched and widely appreciated. In the 25 years from the launch of Operation Flood, milk production increased manifold and per capita consumption almost doubled. Most importantly, dairying emerged as an important income generating activity and source of rural employment.

In terms of infrastructure, rural processing capacity of 194 lakh litres per day (llpd) has been created and 67 llpd equivalent of chilling capacity set up to ensure better quality milk. For the urban consumers, milk marketing facilities of 72 llpd have also been commissioned. The project adopted novel and innovative measures to boost milk production, train professionals and workers alike to become more competent and educate members of the cooperatives about their rights and responsibilities so that a more informed and democratic cooperative structure emerge. The investments that have been made in all these activities, over the three phases of Operation Flood, are given in Table 9.2.

The investments made—which include substantial time, money and effort by milk producers themselves—are by no means small. It is necessary that no effort be spared to ensure that optimal returns are achieved in the future.

Challenges Ahead

A major factor affecting the future of the cooperatives is the liberlisation policy introduced in 1991. Before liberalisation, each cooperative union procured milk from a well-defined area and invested to increase milk production in the milk shed. It sold milk and milk products in its milk shed

Table 9.2: Investments in Infrastructure Under Operation Flood, 1970-95

(Rs. million)

Infrastructure	Investment
Rural processing facilities	8,742
Urban marketing facilities	3,727
Milk production enhancement	2,050
Training and Research	1,765
Cooperative education	776
Total	17,060

Source: Department of Animal Husbandry and Dairying, Government of India

and whatever surplus milk remained, it either sold to another union or converted into products for sale by a State-level federation. Delicensing of the dairy industry and the consequent mushrooming of private sector plants dramatically changed the competitive environment. At risk is the sustained investment in increasing milk production and the commitment to ensure maximum returns to producers while providing quality milk to consumers at affordable prices.

These have created the conditions for the orderly growth which has made India the world's largest milk producing country. What is clear, however, is that shackled as they are by the archaic laws and diktats of bureaucrats and politicians, cooperatives today are vulnerable to the challenges mounted by the private sector firms. While cooperatives are denied the right to make such basic business decisions as fixing their own purchase and sale prices and employing their own executives, at least some private sector dairy plants indulge in adulteration and tax evasion, practices antithetical to cooperative business.

While the new economic policies pose challenges to cooperatives, they are not without significant competitive advantages. As new entrants soon discover, it is one thing to build a plant while it is quite another to ensure that the plant is supplied with sufficient quantities of high quality milk. Cooperatives have invested in a milk procurement system that is unique and which would cost new firms levels of investment that they cannot afford if their products are to be competitive. Traditional powder plants, too, are facing significant problems in the new competitive environment. Relying on advances to secure milk supplies, they are increasingly at the mercy of brokers and contractors who demand increasing amounts of cash. No longer able to meet this demand from their own funds, powder plants owners are borrowing at high rates, squeezing profits on products which are already at the bottom niche of the market. Cooperatives, by contrast, have modern plants supplied with quality milk by a procurement structure that is already largely amortized.

Thus, while the long-term viability of cooperatives is challenged, the structure enjoys some important competitive advantage that offset some of the problems faced. The large investment that has already been made in developing these cooperatives makes it imperative that a fourth phase of Operation Flood focuses on helping cooperatives to capitalise on their strengths while dealing systematically with the challenges that they face, whether from competitors or the environment. The objective of this phase is to create a structure that can thrive in the new competitive environment, while at the same time strengthen its democratic values.

The future role of external financing will be an important factor in the pursuit of the fourth phase objectives. While discussions will continue with both EU and World Bank, it can be assumed that any future financing will carry different terms and conditions. This would imply that NDDB will both commit its own resources and secure funds commercially. This means a shift from the liberal lending terms that the NDDB enjoyed toward commercial terms more appropriate to the stage of development that has been reached by many OF-financed unions.

NINTH PLAN STRATEGY

Since the beginning of the Ninth Five Year Plan (1997/98 - 2002/2003), the government initiated steps to radically restructure the cattle and buffalo breeding operations in the country in consultation with major stakeholders involved. The novelties of the project are the attempts to integrate the artificial breeding programme with other sectoral programmes, emphasis on a long term breeding policy, institutional restructuring for autonomy of operations, recovery of cost of goods and services from the user and development of synergies of all involved players. This indicates a significant shift from the previous approaches of isolated scheme, and culminated in the launching of a new scheme "National Project for Cattle and Buffalo Breeding". This scheme was to be implemented throughout the country at a total cost of Rs. 4020 million, in two phases, each of five year duration, and necessary attention was to be paid towards the conservation of indigenous breeds, particularly, the draught ones and improve the quality of bulls used for natural mating in backward areas. There was emphasis on cost effectiveness of each of the components of the programme. It was also realized that rapid development of animal husbandry sector required establishment of appropriate linkages among various subsystem of animal husbandry sector viz. feed and fodder, draught animal power, livestock health and management, carcass utilization, etc. The scheme "Project on Animal System" seeks to facilitate proper linkages between various subsystems of livestock sector.

Basically the Government of India's Livestock Policy has been to promote livestock production through traditional production systems rather than based on modern/intensive livestock industries. Livestock forms an integral component of the Indian lifestyle. Agriculture and animal husbandry have been inseparable and this contributed to the sustainability of rural countryside. Livestock production practices in India are not only labour intensive but also labour distributive and rural in nature. The National Commission on Agriculture (1976) had therefore identified that promotion of livestock production through the weaker sections of farmers in the rural areas could be relied upon as a major instrument of social change, for supplementing the income of the poor and providing a large scope for employment for these sections of people in the rural areas. The exception has been development of poultry sector especially since the sixties, when the intensive poultry farming system was initiated as a commercial enterprise particularly for broiler production. Although currently major part of the eggs is produced in the commercial sector, the traditional backyard poultry system still prevails in tribal and rural areas in the country. However, it is losing its importance under the impact of the modernization and commercial intensive poultry production. Indigenous desi (local) fowl, which is poor in growth and productivity, still continues to be the mainstay of the traditional backyard poultry keeping. About 100,000 farms of varying flock sizes ranging from 5 to 250 birds are located in rural areas, which follow backyard or semi-backyard system of poultry farming.

Thrust Area

The major thrust of the Government Livestock policies has been scientific management and genetic upgradation of cattle and buffalo, expansion of existing infrastructure and delivery of breeding inputs and services to farmers, control animal diseases, creation of disease free zones, increased availability of nutritious feed and fodder, development of processing and marketing facilities and enhancement of production and profitability of livestock enterprises. Initially government used to take a very broad view of these programmes and project responsibilities in the livestock sector. However, during the last two decades there has been a considerable shift in these policies. Direct government intervention in the form of breeding and model farms that would supply "superior" cattle and buffalo to farmers

---

MAIN THRUST AREAS
- Animal diseases control.
- Livestock breed improvement and development.
- Fodder development.
- Dairy and Poultry development.
- Fisheries development.

STRATEGIES
- Expansion of infrastructure.
- Creation of seed stock of superior bulls and bull mothers.
- Develop adequate animal health services.
- Facilitate genetic improvement and conservation of indigenous breeds.
- Improve productivity of pasturelands through improved fodder seeds.
- Upgradation of fishing capabilities of existing vessels and Introduction of intermediate fishing crafts.
- Welfare programme for fisher folks.

have fallen out of favour after many costly failures. The Department of Animal Husbandry and Dairying has, however, been operating 38 Central Livestock Organizations and allied Institutions for production and distribution of superior germ plasms to the State Governments for cross breeding and genetic upgradation of the stocks.

Insemination Scheme for Dairy Farmers

The Punjab State Government has introduced a "mobile insemination" scheme in Amritsar, Nawanshehr, Kapurthala, Patiala, Ropar and Bhatinda districts in the State. The Scheme envisages creation of clusters all over the State where semen containers of 35 litres will be kept in store. These clusters will cater to a fixed number of dispensaries each of which will be equipped with a two-litre portable container. According to the scheme farmers will inform the nearest dispensary hospital about the end for artificial insemination following which it will deliver the service at their doorsteps. The service will be delivered to the dairy owners at the same rate being charged earlier which is Rs. 8 per injection. They will, however, have to pay a visiting fee of Rs. 3 per kilometre with a maximum fee of Rs. 20 to the visiting doctor. Under the programme, training would be imparted to veterinary practitioners. Optimum utilization of the semen of elite bulls would be ensured by bringing in modern methods to handle, process, preserve and utilize the semen.

Central Cattle Development Organizations

These organizations include the 7 Central Cattle Breeding Farms, the Central Frozen Semen Production and Training Institute, Hessarghatta and the 4 Central Herd Registration Units, which have been established by the Department in different regions of the country for production of genetically superior breed of bull calves, good quality frozen semen and identification of location of superior germplasms of cattle and buffaloes, to meet the requirement of bulls and frozen semen doses in different parts of the country.

Central Cattle Breeding Farms (CCBF)

The Central Cattle Breeding Farms located at Suratgrh (Rajasthan), Chiplima and Sunabeda (Orissa), Dhamrod (Gujarat), Hessaraghatta (Karnataka), Alamadhi (Tamil Nadu) and Andeshnagar (U.P.) are maintaining bull mothers of important cattle and buffalo breeds which include Tharparkar, Red Sindhi, Jersey, Holstein Friesian, Crossbred (HF × Tharparkar, Jersey × Red Sindhi), Surti and Murrah. The farms produce bull calves from these bull mothers and supply high pedigree bull calves and bulls to the State Governments and other breeding organizations for production of frozen semen. The farms located at Sunabeda, Suratgrh and Andeshnagar also have the facilities for production of frozen semen. The Central Cattle Breeding Farm, Alamadhi has been associated with Associated Herd Progeny Testing Programme of the Central Institute for

Research on Buffaloes, Hissar. The buffaloes available at the farm are used for test mating of Murrah bulls and semen of proven/high pedigree bulls is used for further genetic improvement. The Central Cattle Breeding farms follow the fodder cropping programme as recommended by Indian Grassland and Fodder Research Institute, Jhansi, and also produce fodder seeds for distribution under Central Minikit Testing Programme under which free fodder seed minikits are provided to farmers. The farms provide breeding facilities to the cows and buffaloes of the nearby villages free of cost and also conduct training of farmers in dairy farming under Animal Husbandry Extension Programme.

Central Frozen Semen Production and Training Institute, Hessarghatta

This premier Institute produces frozen semen doses of indigenous exotic and cross breed cattle bulls and Murrah buffalo bulls for use in artificial insemination. The institute also provides training in frozen semen technology to technical officers of the State Governments and acts as a center for testing the indigenously manufactured frozen semen and AI equipment. The institute has acquired proficiency in Embryo Transfer Technology sponsored by the Department of Biotechnology from 1987-88 to 1991-92.

Need for Appropriate Technology

The main conclusion of recent research in animal science suggests that the principal cause of poor performance and even failure in public and donor-funded livestock programmes and projects lies in the use of inappropriate technology. In India it was generally accepted that technological change would bring in higher productivity and lead the country to higher living standards. In the livestock sector this has largely meant a concentration on improved breeds of cattle and other animals. The country, through various development and research programmes, have imported and or bred improved breeds of cattle. To accelerate technological change in livestock, these animals were distributed to farmers without payment or at highly subsidized prices and gave the farmers loans to enable them to operate with this "new technology". Some of these projects failed. The banks, mainly publicly owned, which funded the farmers, were not repaid. There were usually subsidiary reasons, but the principal reason for failure was that the technology was inappropriate.

Livestock specialists, working without financial or economic constraints, designed projects which were capital intensive (imported or highly bred species) requiring costly inputs in the form of feed to enable these animals to produce to capacity, and were highly prone to disease. Financial returns were too low to allow repayment of bank loans.

The question of appropriate technology is more relevant in the context of biological parameters of livestock species in tropical environment, scale of operations and databases. It is a biological fact that tropical grasses and hot, humid climate make for higher costs of feed energy production in the tropics than in temperate zones, particularly.

A study by the National Centre for Agricultural Economics and Policy Research (NCAP) revealed that the livestock output grew at 2.59 per cent per annum over 1950-51 to 1995-96. The input index increased by 1.79 per cent per annum and Total Factor Productivity (TFP) grew at about 0.8 per cent, implying that technical change contributed about 30 per cent to overall output growth over the last 45 years (Table 9.3). Period-wise results are more revealing. There was no TFP growth in the first period (1950-51 to 1970-71) implying no technical change. Output growth proceeded along the traditional production function and was entirely driven by growth in measured inputs. Not surprisingly, the resulting growth in output was a modest 1.3 per cent per annum. There was sharp uptrend since then. Output as well as TFP growth picked up. The results show that the real upswing started in the eighties when sector's output growth touched nearly 4 per cent per annum and TFP growth jumped to nearly 1.3 per cent, contributing about 45 per cent to total output growth. Backed by an improved market and institutional environment, investments in livestock research have begun to pay off.

Table 9.3: Growth Rates of Output, Input and Total Factor Productivity Indices

Item	1950/51 to 1970/71	1970/71 to 1995/96	1950/51 to 1995/96
Output Index	1.28	3.59	2.59
Input Index	1.32	2.23	1.79
TFP Index	-0.04	1.36	0.81

Source: Birthal, P.S., Kumar, A, Ravishankar A., and Pandey, U.K., Sources of Growth in the Livestock Sector: Policy Paper 9, National Centre for Agricultural Economics Research, New Delhi, 1999.

Breeding Policy: Need for Appropriate Technology

Public Breeding Institution

Seven central and numerous state cattle breeding farms produce breeding bulls, rams and improved poultry stock for distribution to the various agencies involved in livestock development. These farms also supply bulls and elite donor females to the Central Frozen Semen Production and Training Institute. There are about 20,000 artificial insemination centres and about half of them are under the management of the NDDB.

Several schemes under different plan periods have been implemented both with Central and State Government funds to strengthen cattle and buffalo breeding activities in the States. Substantial infrastructure has been created leading to enhanced output from cattle and buffalo, particularly in terms of milk. Despite this, the low productivity level of Indian livestock is the major concern in the development of almost 290 million cattle and buffalo. Nearly 80 percent of Indian cattle and 60 percent of buffaloes are low yielding and do not belong to the defined breeds.

Crossbreeding of low yielding indigenous breeds with high-yielding exotic breeds has been widely acknowledged as a valuable strategy to improve animal productivity. Systematic crossbreeding research and development programmes in India were initiated during the 1950s. The focus of crossbreeding research has been mainly on cattle because of their dual role of milk production and use as draught animals in the crop sector. A number of crossbreeds with improved production potentials have been evolved. Some important crossbreeds include Haryana Friesian, Haryana Jersey, Haryana Brown Swiss, Rathi Jersey, Gir Jersey, Gir Friesian, and Sahiwal Jersey.

However, the impact of government breeding programmes has been limited. Artificial insemination programme covers only around 20 percent of all breedable bovines and conception rate of AI is about 20 percent. Adoption of crossbreeding technology has, however, been slow. Only 7.5 percent of the cattle population consists of crossbreeds. In other animal species too the status of crossbreeding is similar. Hardly about 5 percent of the sheep and 15 percent of pigs are crossbreeds. The reasons for the slow progress could be non-acclimatization and high incidence of morbidity and mortality in crossbred animals. Nevertheless, the success in the poultry sector is notable. Improved poultry constitute about 34 percent of the total poultry population. Crossbreeding is also practiced in other species, though statistical information is lacking.

Between 1982 and 1992, population of crossbred cattle increased at the rate of 5.6 percent a year. Female population increased at a faster rate than males. On the other hand indigenous stock seemed to be approaching stabilization. Annual growth rate of indigenous cattle stock was 0.52 percent, although the female population registered a higher growth. Low milk yield and decreasing demand for animal draught services are the main factors for the slow growth in indigenous stock. These trends indicate a gradual substitution of indigenous cattle by crossbred ones.

Breed improvement programmes for indigenous milch and draught breeds are not effectively organized. A systematic and focussed attention to provide pedigreed bulls for natural mating systems and revamp the AI network in terms of coverage as well as quality of resources and services is needed to realize full potential of the large bovine population. The existing artificial breeding infrastructure consisting of bull stations, semen banks, etc. suffers from several for inadequacies and has vast scope for improvement.

Moreover, despite being an important milch specie, the buffalo has not received much attention in breed improvement programme. Development efforts have focused on upgradation of low-yielding breeds through artificial insemination. The buffalo population increased at the rate of 1.9 percent a year between 1952 and 1982. The female population witnessed faster growth than the male population. Its adaptability to a wide range of climatic conditions, high milk yield compared to indigenous cattle, and price premium on milk due to its higher fat content have favoured faster growth in the buffalo population. Further, the salvage value of buffalo is higher; as unlike cattle there are fewer restrictions on buffalo slaughter.

Population of improved poultry grew at a rate of about 9 percent a year, more than double that of indigenous poultry. Technological transformation of the poultry sector seems to be market-driven as the demand for poultry meat and eggs is income elastic and has been rising continuously. The population of crossbred sheep and pigs also grew faster than their indigenous counterparts.

NPCBB AT A GLANCE*

Project launched in October 2000. Project envisages 100% grant-in aid for various cattle and buffalo breeding activities and to ensure sustainability of operations as well as quality in breeding inputs and services.

Project envisages
1. To arrange delivery of vastly improved artificial insemination at the farmers' door.
2. to progressively bring all the breedable females among the cattle and buffalo under organized breeding.
3. to undertake breed improvement programme through indigenous cattle and buffalo breed to improve genetic quality.
4. to provide quality breeding inputs in breeding tracts of important indigenous breeds so as to prevent breed from deterioration and extinction.

---

*National Project for Cattle and Buffalo Breeding.

Empirical evidence from the field studies proves the scientific claims of better economic performance of crossbred animals. Despite this, crossbreeding technology has not gained a foothold. One of the possible reasons could be non-acclimatization of crossbred animals to widely varying climatic conditions in the country. Indeed in India and even in much of the Asia, there appears to be a history of introducing breeds without proper evaluation and with little or no thought given to the breeding structure which will best use the available material. Non-acclimatization causes a number of health and physiology related problems.

Higher initial investment and maintenance costs could be other limitations to widespread adoption of crossbreeds. The first cross animals perform very well. However, the performance of animals from subsequent crosses declines significantly. Therefore, crossbred animals need to be replaced frequently in order to sustain the flow of benefits. Thus, frequent acquisition of first crossbreeds without realizing appropriate salvage value of the subsequent crossed animal renders crossbreeding technology capital intensive. In this connection it is observed that more than 50 percent of the farmers in Karnataka maintaining crossbreeds depend on the market for replacement of first cross animals[1]. This is to avoid the risk of getting unwanted male claves and the associated problems of breeding and feeding the calf.

Nevertheless crossbreeding strategy has been successful under certain environments and economic conditions such as in Kerala and Punjab. In Kerala, milk production system is cattle-based. Indigenous breeds are not good as milk yielder or draught power. Cropping system is largely plantation oriented, requiring less of draught power[2]. Further, unlike in may other states cattle slaughter is not prohibited by law in Kerala. This makes it easier to cull out the low yielding and unwanted animals. In Punjab on the other hand, increasing intensification of agriculture needed more power to perform agricultural operations on time, which indigenous cattle were not capable of. Moreover, feed and fodder have never been a problem in Punjab.

As mentioned above, the Government of India had initiated action at the beginning of 9th Five-Year Plan towards formulation of a comprehensive scheme for cattle and buffalo breeding in consultation with State Governments and other concerned agencies with an aim to consolidate the gains achieved till 8th Plan period, to maximize returns on investments, and to ensure sustainability of operations as well as quality in breeding inputs and services. These efforts culminated in merger of the ongoing centrally sponsored schemes on cattle and buffalo breeding, namely Extension of Frozen Semen Technology and Progeny Testing Programmes and National Bull Production Programmes into a new centrally sponsored scheme- the National Project for Cattle and Buffalo Breeding. This project aims at thorough reorganization and reorientation of the cattle and buffalo breeding operations in the country. The first phase of this National Project was launched with an allocation of Rs. 4020 million with effect from October 2000. The Project envisages inter-alia (i) radically improving coverage of bovine population under breeding programme: (ii); delivery of breeding inputs at the farmers' doorsteps; (iii) improvement of quality of bulls used for natural service; (iv) conservation of indigenous breeds; (v) imposing a levy on services and inputs to make the agencies providing the same self sustaining through recycling of receipts thus accrued; (vi) strict quality control of services and inputs; (vii) Optimum capacity utilization in institutional infrastructure; (viii) developing synergies among major players; (ix) putting in place field recording and progeny testing programmes through networking for indigenous cattle, crossbred cattle and buffaloes to identify and propagate superior germplasm for genetic improvement; and (x) making training and retraining of professionals and AI workers an integral part of the scheme.

---

[1]H. Alderman: Cooperative Dairy Development in Karnataka: India: an assessment. International Food Policy Research Institute, Washington, D.C.: 1987.

[2]A. R. Rajapurohit: Crossbreeding of Indian Cattle: An Evaluation: Economic and Political Weekly: 14(12/13): A9-24, 1979.

Private Breeding Services

Some private breeding farms are competing successfully with public breeding service in semen production. These farms charge Rs. 10-15 per dose of semen (Holstein Friesian and Jersey for cows and buffaloes). One private breeding operation in Haryana supplies semen to Uttar Pradesh (150, 000 doses a year), Rajasthan, and Punjab and exports semen and breeding animals to Nepal. The government breeding services in Uttar Pradesh and Rajasthan do not have the capacity to meet local demand for semen and thus must turn to private suppliers. In addition to providing AI services, the private firms also engage in milk recording.

Artificial insemination services in India are subsidized, including those provided by cooperatives and nongovernmental organizations. In addition to collection of milk and feed sales, the village cooperatives provide veterinary and AI services. Nongovernmental organizations such as the Bhratiya Agro-Industries Foundation (BAIF) also operate centres that provide AI and animal health services. Some states (such as Uttar Pradesh) contract BAIF to provide AI services in the state. Because of their limited profitability, privatization of AI services by themselves might not be feasible; a combination of private insemination and veterinary services would be more likely to provide an adequate income. An idea about the cost of production of frozen semen is as in table 9.4 below.

Table 9.4: Cost of Production of Frozen Semen

(In Rs.)

Items of Cost	Cost per straw	
	Cow	Buffalo
1. Maintenance of bull	8.16	8.82
	(49.31)	(51.34)
2. Collection of semen	0.71	0.74
	(4.29)	(4.31)
3. Processing of semen	2.41	2.35
	(14.56)	(13.68)
4. Freezing and storage	5.27	5.27
	(31.84)	(30.67)
Cost of Production	16.55	17.18

Figures in parentheses indicate percentage to total cost.

Source: Arun Pandit and D.C. Jain, Cost of Frozen Semen Production, Agricultural Economics Research Review, Jan-June 2002.

Strategy

Accordingly, the strategy and objectives pursued for development of animal husbandry and fisheries sectors can be summarized as follows:

(i) Expanding and strengthening the infrastructure for artificial insemination, improve its efficiency and effectiveness using frozen semen technology for crossbreeding purposes.

(ii) Creation of seed stock of qualitative superior bulls and bull mothers which would form the nucleus germplasm pool for rapidly building a national milch herd of high productivity cattle and buffaloes. For this purpose, modern technological tools such as embryo transfer will be deployed with increasing frequency.

(iii) Facilitating genetic improvement of important livestock breeds through selective breeding and cross breeding of low production nondescript stock, both for milk and draught purposes. Important indigenous breeds will be conserved.

(iv) Improving productivity of pasturelands by introducing improved fodder seeds and increased used of waste lands for fodder production.

(v) Developing adequate animal health services for protection of livestock, with special emphasis on eradication of rinderpest and control of foot and mouth disease.

(vi) Improving the database in respect of livestock products.

(vii) Enhancing the adoption of technological inventions for increasing productivity of livestock products.

(viii) Upgradation of fishing capabilities of existing mechanized vessels and introduction of intermediate range of fishing craft with capacity to fish in depth of 70-150 meters.

(ix) Development of large, medium and small reservoirs and floodplain lakes for fish yield optimization.

(x) Development of Freshwater aquaculture through Fish Farmers Development Agencies by providing assistance to fish farmers on various technologies packages of aquaculture.

(xi) Popularization of freshwater prawn farming including setting up small scale prawn hatcheries.

(xii) Development of environmentally sustainable aquaculture practices in coastal areas.

(xiii) Development of fisheries and aquaculture in hill areas for both food and sports fishing.

(xiv) Publication of extension material in print and electronic media on various topics for popularization of fisheries and aquaculture.

(xv) Welfare programmes for farmers and fisherman through insurance coverage, improvement of traditional habitats, etc.

The Government's Initiative and Assistance to States

As the Agriculture including Animal Husbandry, Dairying and Fisheries, is a state subject, the emphasis of the Department has been on supplementing the efforts of the State Governments in the development of these sectors. The Government's efforts are mainly concentrated on increasing the production of major livestock products, fish and fishery products. Accordingly the Department has been providing assistance to the State Governments for control of animal diseases, scientific management and upgradation of genetic resources, increasing availability of nutritious feed and fodder, sustainable development of processing and marketing facilities and enhancement of production and profitability of livestock and fisheries enterprises.

The Operation Flood Project: Impact and Lessons

During early seventies India was following a self-reliant macroeconomic development policy with heavy emphasis on import substitution. This policy remained essentially unchanged until 1991. In the dairy sector, a policy decision had been made to utilize farmer-controlled cooperatives to develop the dairy industry and to make import substitution as efficient as possible. The government also decided to withdraw from its own direct efforts to develop the dairy industry. Indirect efforts via extension, research, artificial breeding, etc., continued. Dairy commodity food aid was to be sold at commercial prices with the proceed being earmarked for support of Operation Flood.

It may be mentioned that Operation Flood programme was launched by the Government of India after it looked at the success of the Anand experiment. The farmer-owned Amul Cooperative at Anand, situated in Kheda District of Gujarat, has put the little known place on the dairy map of India and Amul has now become a household word. The Amul success was attributed to its integrated approach to production, procurement, processing and marketing of milk along cooperatives lines and the Centre decided that the pattern should be replicated throughout the country. Thus the Operation Flood programme was launched with the aim of setting up Amul like organizations in states to link rural milk procurement centers with urban demand centers with a view to stimulating milk production and marketing.

According to a progress report, the Operation Flood I aimed at creating 18 "Anands" with an investment of Rs. 1,160 million which were generated from gifted commodities received from the World Food Programme. The programme led to a "resurgence" in the dairy industry during the seventies and a much larger dairy development programme was launched through Operation Flood II in 1979 and funded by a soft loan of $ 150 million from the World Bank, money generated from the dairy commodities gifted by the European Community and by the internal resources of the erstwhile Indian Dairy Corporation. The Operation Flood III was funded by World Bank loan/credit of $ 365 million, money generated from the gifted dairy items and from the internal resources of the National Dairy Development Board (NDDB).

The number of milksheds covered had touched the target figure of 170 at the end of March 1995. The first phase of Operation Flood covered 18 milksheds which formed the catchment areas from which milk was drawn into the four metro cities of Delhi. Bombay, Calcutta and Madras. The organized marketing of milk now covers over six hundred towns which involves development of procurement, processing and transport facilities in 170 milksheds. The number of milkshed covered by the programme, it may be mentioned, was just five in 1970-71. Within a span of five years, the number had risen to 28 in 1975-76 and to 39 in the next five years to 1980-81. The next five years saw a phenomenal rise in the number of coverage and the number of milksheds more than quadrupled to stand at 164 in 1985-86. The farmers participation in the programme has also been constantly increasing. From about 278 thousand farmers in 1970-71, the number of farmers had already grown to nine million at the end of March 1995 exceeding the target of eight million till 1996. The target for cooperative societies also seemed to be nearing with already over 69,000 operational societies.

The inauguration of Operation Flood corresponded to a turnaround in per capita incomes. Rising per capita incomes, together with rising population and a high-income elasticity of demand for milk, resulted in a rapid growth in the demand for milk (technically, a rapid shift in the demand function for milk). In the absence of supply side adjustment this would have led to a rapid escalation in the price of milk or the need for extensive imports. But Operation Flood helped in meeting the rising demand and arresting sharp increase in real prices.

The overall expansion of the dairy industry from the early 1970s has been comparable to the more widely recognized Green Revolution crops of wheat and rice. Two key policy changes which accompanied the decision to provide direct financial assistance to the cooperatives to develop the dairy industry were the ending of direct efforts by the public sector to promote dairy production and the decision to sell dairy food aid at commercial prices within India. Both these changes reduced the price risks for farmers, small-scale milk traders and private processors. Crossbreeding of local cows with specialized dairy breeds provided the technology for rapid increases in the milk production, and Operation Flood provided the example of large scale modern milk processing fed by a well-organized milk shed procuring milk from a large number of producers in very small amounts (1 and 2 liters). The actual volume of milk handled by Operation Flood remains a small fraction of the increased supply. It is thus not possible to attribute increased production simply to the dairy processing, marketing infrastructure, and technical support provided by Operation Flood directly (important though these contributions have been). Rather, one has to look to the changed dairy policy environment that accompanied the decision supporting Operation Flood. The policy was promising because of its probable production impact, but even more because of its capacity to reach the poor. Present position and prospectus up to 2010 for Dairy Development is shown in Table 9.5.

NEEDED POLICY REFORMS

The livestock sector has been among the few growth sectors in rural India and the domestic demand for animal based food products is expected to increase rapidly with increase in income. Animal protein requirement, as discussed later in the study under the long term perspective, is expected to increase faster than from other sources. To meet these requirements, the

Table 9.5: Dairy Development

	2000	2010
A) *Operation Flood (of) Areas Key Action*		
Number of Village Level Dairy Cooperative Societies (DCS)	84,289	1,29,480
DCS Farmers Membership (Million)	10.63	15.63
Women Members (%)	21.19	50.00
DCS Milk Procurement (Million Kg. /Day)	15.78	48.80
B) *Non-operation Flood, (of), Hilly and Backward Areas*		
Milk Marketing (Million Liters/Day)	12.92	36.50
Additional DCS		10.00
Additional Farmer Members (Million)		0.6

Source: Government of India, Ministry of Agriculture, Department of Animal Husbandry and Dairying, Basic Animal Husbandry Statistics, 2002, New Delhi.

protein availability has to be more than doubled from the present 10 grams per day per person. For this to be achieved, the annual growth rate for milk, egg and meat production (which averaged 4.3 percent, 4.7 percent and 4.1 percent respectively) will have to be increased substantially.

Future strategies for development of livestock sector have to be based on a mixed approach of reduction in population number and vertical genetic improvement of livestock. One possible scenario could be that the livestock population growth will continue at the present level of 1-2 percent per annum in the large ruminants and around 7 percent in small ruminants (goats, etc.), with the resultant heavy feed burden leading to land degradation, loss of grass and environmental pollution. The present achievements cannot sustain the kind of growth rates achieved so far. The geotypes of cattle, sheep and other species will become Desi Mangaroles leading to significant drop in animal products, particularly milk, much to the distress of the large vegetarian population of over one billion in India. A significant change is needed in the policy frame and its mode of implementation if this situation is to be avoided.

Improvement is possible only with the people's participation, which needs direction. Without direction to the livestock production systems in the country, new technologies, which have been put in place during the last 40 years, will become self-defeating. Vertical genetic improvement will have to be linked with reduction in animal numbers. The reduction in animal number particularly of cattle and buffaloes is to be made mandatory by a policy frame otherwise all the feed resources will get exhausted sooner than later.

The growth in production in animal-based food will have to be brought through suitable programmes of government and by providing stimulus and creating an environment for increased private sector participation. The trend towards privatization will make it increasingly necessary for government to restrict its activities to policy formulation, creation of regulatory framework and development activities in areas where private sector participation does not exist or is minimal. Government will have to withdraw from production activities and from other areas, which should be best left to the private sector to operate.

The increased production of livestock products will have to be through higher productivity, which have to be brought about using sustainable production systems while maintaining environment and biodiversity. Environmental issues will play a major role in the years to come. The focus will have to be on sustainable development of livestock, keeping in view the need for maintaining the ecological balance between the needs of the human and animal in terms of pressure on land and other resources. Biodiversity and animal resources will have to be maintained in such a manner that the damage to the biosphere is kept at the minimum. Species should be reared and bred in regions whose agroclimatic conditions can meet needs of the animals for fodder and water. Towards this end, a livestock atlas should be prepared to identify the livestock species and breeds best suitable to a particular.

Under the new policy framework the number of cattle and buffaloes will be reduced, so as to achieve higher production targets of milk and meat through quality animals. Shortage of feeds and fodder, shrinkage of grazing land and environmental concerns specially methane emission from ruminants call for lower level of livestock population and improving productivity per animal to meet future animal food needs using new technologies. Extension network in animal husbandry, which is almost absent, will have to be put in place for better appreciation and acceptance of new technologies.

For Hygienic Meat Production an implementation of pragmatic slaughter policy is important. This should allow proper utilization of meat animals and economic consideration should play an important role in the disposal of unproductive animals. While the ethos of the country does not permit cow to be included in general slaughter policy, other animals should be governed by economic consideration alone.

Slaughter houses should be modernized to provide safe and wholesome meat, and utilize animal byproducts and prevent environmental pollution. A system of humane slaughter needs to be adopted. Private sector involvement in setting up of modern abattoirs should be encouraged.

The government long-term plan envisages policy measures *inter-alia* in the fields of: (i) Dairy Development, (ii) Cattle and Buffalo Breeding, (iii) Feed and Fodder, (iv) Animal Health, and (v) Risk Management. The last item envisages adoption of necessary measures for facilitating access to credit to small holders, together with forward and backward linkages. Moreover, a field study has been carried out to ascertain the reasons for poor capacity utilization, potential for development and technologies used in food processing industries, including milk and dairy products and meat and meat products. Based on the government's long-term plans for the development of the livestock sector and the findings of the field study on the Food Processing Industry (Chapter 20), the following further policy reforms for the livestock industries are considered necessary.

Promoting small farmer integration, through the cooperative marketing system is important both for livestock development and equity. One mechanism for achieving this objective is vertical integration or more specifically through backward integration of processors into production, by means of supply contracts. This approach is particularly relevant to the dairy and poultry industry and partially to the small ruminant sector, where international experience attests to the feasibility of such arrangements. For the producers, supply contracts and contract growing arrangements provide an assured market at assured prices and access to information on new production techniques. For entrepreneurs and processors, such arrangements help improve quality, reliability of supply, timeliness of delivery, which, in turn, improve cost efficiency, planning and utilization of capacity.

Transformation of the national and global market pull to the full advantage of sectoral growth enabling the small producers to participate in the process of globalization; ensuring ecological sustainability of livestock sector, growth and modernization, and the role of the Government only as a catalysts, in the growth of livestock sector are major policy changes expected to be followed gradually in the years to come.

The scenario emerging out of the preceding paragraphs underscores the need for cohesive and integrated planning taking into account specific needs of primary producers on an area/region basis on the basis of produces and their requirements for preliminary preservations, processing and value additions as well as vertical linkages with the industry so that the produce could be utilized fully without wastage and the specialized processing industry set up can work to its optimum capacity. In view of the fact that most of the primary produces from livestock enterprises, be it milk, meat or egg are highly perishable, area wise integrated planning is of paramount importance.

Food processing industry is a nascent sector in the country, which has enormous potential. The development of the sector so far is primarily because of the positive perception of its potential at Central Government level and not because of interest of domestic or overseas business community. Creation of the Ministry of Food Processing Industries is a result of these positive perceptions. Notwithstanding this, there is a need for preparation of an attractive case so far as livestock based food-processing industry is concerned. The case should ideally be strong both in terms of style and substance so that both domestic and international investors find it acceptable. This is of crucial importance since radical improvement in this sector could call for substantial investment and besides Central and State Governments, domestic and international investors must be convinced to put in their might.

Besides this, there is an absolute need on the part of the Government to formulate and announce proactive policy measures to dispel the general perceptions that livestock based food processing is a high risk – low return area, prone to poor capacity utilization and hence unviable as a business proposition in the long term. Needless to say, such policy measures must be framed with holistic approach and must involve all concerned Ministries and representatives of prospective investors to ensure that upstream and downstream linkages have sound basis. The existence of a large number of Panchayat Raj institutions and huge network of cottage, small and medium scale industries also points to the possibility of a bottom -up approach being more successful than a top- down approach in this matter.

The nodal concept that is being proposed is to eliminate/marginalize the role of middleman by providing a three tier structure wherein the primary producers have a preliminary storage/processing/packaging facility within twenty-five kilometers of his farm and such preliminary facilities are further linked as feeder to a modern processing plant. This will not only ensure better remuneration to the primary producers, but also improve availability of hygienic quality food for the domestic and overseas market, simultaneously reducing the risk perceptions of the investors. Since the entire process would involve integration on the basis of area wise planning of sectoral programmes, for which investments are normally being made, additional investment required will not be of a very high order but the spin-off of such a process could be enormously rewarding on many counts. There is also need to pursue the following set of strategies:

   (i) Identification of area/location with higher prospect for vertical integration of primary producers to industrial processing units.

  (ii) Creation of an interactive forum with select State Governments with higher prospects for processing industries in order to evolve a conducive policy environment for prospective entrepreneurs and to augment fund flow for the sector.

 (iii) Rationalization of tax structure on fresh and processed food as well as institutional investment in campaign for hygienic food, brand formation /market promotion, activities promoting producers' organization and industrial associations, etc.

 (iv) Sectoral programmes for improving raw material in target areas, creation of a dynamic database through studies and surveys at periodic intervals and dissemination of information to entrepreneurs.

  (v) Prioritizing infrastructural development like roads, power, communication, cold chain, etc., in prospective areas.

 (vi) Emphasis on quality control in production and processing in order to improve quality and acceptability of finished products. Adoption of Total Quality Management (TQM), Hazard Analysis and Critical Control Points (HACCP) in industrial units and extension campaign for primary producers to achieve this goal.

(vii) Adoption of appropriate technology both at the level of primary producers and at processing levels, incorporation of newer technology like remote sensing, information technology. biotechnology, etc. with concern for the environment.

(viii) Improving access to credit and transferable technology to the primary producers and promoting their own organizations should form integral part of the holistic approach.

(ix) The development of packaging technologies and harmonization of food laws to encourage reduction of high quality value added food.

(x) Assigning those roles and functions, which are necessary but cannot be performed in Government set up to non-Government organizations suited to take up the same is a prerequisite.

Evaluation of Government's Livestock Policy Perspective[1]

The Government of India and the Swiss Development Cooperation have prepared the Livestock Policy Perspective 1995-2020. This policy Perspective has been criticized in some quarters. For instance it is alleged that the indigenous approach to livestock is based on diversity, decentralization, sustainability and equity. Indian cattle are not just milk machines or meat machines. They are sentient beings that serve human communities through their multidimensional role in agriculture. On the other hand, extremely driven projects, programmes and policies emerging from industrial societies treat cattle as one-dimensional machines which are maintained with capital intensive and environmentally intensive inputs and which provide a single output - either milk or meat. Polices based on this approach are characterized by monocultures, concentration and centralization, non-sustainability and inequality.

It is felt that the new livestock policy framed in this paradigm of machines and monocultures is a serious attack on principles of diversity, decentralization, sustainability and equity in the livestock sector. The Livestock Policy Perspective is thus considered by some experts as a policy for the destruction of India's farm animal biodiversity and a threat to the survival of small farmers who depend on diversity based decentralized livestock economy. Detailed arguments against the New Policy Perspective are mentioned below.

The Cattle Economy: The Provider for the Poor

The policy document recognizes that the livestock economy is the economy of the poorest households in India. As stated in Section 2.3 of the policy perspective 1995-2020: About 630 million people reside in rural areas (74% of total population) of which 40% have incomes, which place them below the poverty line. Some 70 million households (73% of total rural households) keep and own livestock of one kind or another and derive on average 20% of their income from this source. Small and marginal farmers and landless

---

[1]This section is based mainly on Dr. Vandana Shiva's Paper: The New Livestock Policy: A Policy of Ecocide of Indigenous Cattle Breeds and a Policy of Genocide for Indian Small Farmers: January 1996: accessed through the Internet

labourers constitute almost two-thirds of these livestock-keeping households. The importance of the livestock sector can therefore not be measured purely in terms of its contribution to GDP but it plays a very crucial role in generating income and employment for the weaker sections of the economy. Rapid growth of the livestock sector can be a deciding factor in the efforts at improving nutrition and relieving poverty. Women provide nearly 90% of all labour for livestock management. However, all the analysis in the policy is totally insensitive to the systems, which allow cattle to serve the needs of the poorest. As a result the recommendations are a direct assault on this survival base of the poor.

The policy recommends government interventions to stimulate meat production even though this will totally undermine the basis of sustainable agriculture.

Undermining Sustainability of Agriculture

The economics of meat exports is totally flawed in a diversity-based culture of animal husbandry and farming. The 80 million work animals meet two thirds and more of the power requirements of Indian villages. Indian cattle excrete 700 million tons of recoverable manure. Half of which is used as fuel, saving 27 millions litres of kerosene, 35 million tons of coal or 68 million tons of wood. The remaining half is used as fertilizer.

As Maneka Gandhi has shown in the case of one export slaughterhouse, the value of nitrogen, phosphate and potassium provided annually by living cattle is fifty times more than the animal earnings from meat exports, which at current rates of slaughter will wipe out Indian farm animals in 10-15 years. If animals are allowed to live, we will get 1.92 million tonnes of farmyard manure with the help of their dung and urine.

The Livestock policy does not deal with the role of animals in the maintenance of sustainability in agriculture. In fact, the livestock policy if implemented would convert cow dung from a source of fertility into a major source of pollution since intensive factory farming of cattle for beef leads to concentration of organic waste from livestock in one place. Since such intensive production is not integrated and cannot be integrated with agriculture as in the case of small farms with decentralized livestock economies, the animal waste turns into a pollutant. Nitrogen from cattle waste is converted into Ammonia and Nitrates, which leach into and pollute the surface and ground water. A feedlot of 10,000 cattle produces as much waste as a city of 110,000 people. This is the reason the Netherlands has been able to export its toxic cow dung to India and is unable to reintegrate this animal waste into its own agricultural systems. Cow dung is a fertilizer only in small-scale integrated farm-dung systems. In large scale, concentrated and specialized factory farm-link systems, this wealth is converted into a hazardous waste. Further, since intensive factory farming of cattle goes hand in hand with intensive feeding and feed production, which in turn requires heavy use of fertilizers and pesticides, the cattle waste from factory farms is very heavily contaminated with chemicals.

Animal Energy

While in decentralized small-scale animal husbandry, cow dung is the most significant gift of the cow to sustainable agriculture, there is total neglect of the contribution of cattle to renewal of soil fertility in the livestock policy. Though reference is made to draught power, it is only with the objective of wiping out this source of sustainable energy production, without recognizing that if only tractors are to be used in India we would have to spend more than a thousand million US dollars annually on fossil fuels, worsening our debt crisis and our balance of payment. In total indifference to the huge economic costs to both farmers and the country generated by substituting animal energy by fossil fuel run mechanical energy, the livestock policy blindly proposes such a shift.

Section 2.4 deals with Draught Power: The number of work animals continued to increase through 1977 but had since fallen by about 10 million to a level of 70 million in 1987 of which 9% are buffaloes. To ensure replacement every sixth year one needs about 0.67 breedable cows per bullock. The bullocks have been largely replaced by mechanical means in transport and irrigation and are now almost exclusively used for land preparation. How much of the gross cropped area (180 m ha) that is cultivated by animal power is uncertain (an estimate of 60 m ha is given in a recent World Bank report) but it is clear that the bullocks may only be utilized for a short period of the year (at most 100 days). Since bullocks generally are not put out to grazing except possibly during the slack season, feeding them and the necessary replacement of stock imposes a major strain. Crossbreds are generally not appreciated as bullocks. Although there are opportunities to introduce improved bullock genes in F2 Second Filial Generation and subsequent crosses these are seldom utilized. In larger herds one may use some cows for crossbreeding while others are used for bullock (and marginal milk) production. In smaller herds one can however not separately pursue both the power and the dairy objective. The policy of upgrading bullocks and introducing improved implements has met with limited success (some implements like the seeder has been introduced). Where the field sizes, topography, etc. allow the farmer has the choice between keeping his own bullocks (and the stock needed for their replacement), disposing of the bullocks and either hire power for cultivation (animal or tractor) with the consequent risk that the timeliness of operations will suffer, or acquiring a tractor and offer its service for transport and cultivation. We have only limited material that illustrates the relative attractiveness of these options for different farm sizes with due consideration to the importance of timeliness of land preparation. The trend is obviously away from animal power.

Section 5.2 discusses Interventions: with respect of animal power further adds, if our aim, as suggested, is to accelerate the trend towards mechanization as well as to promote upgrading of bullock power and improvement of implements we will need to consider interventions for this purpose. In order to accelerate mechanization one may consider providing credit for tractor (incl. equipment) procurement and to make sure (through training programmes and subsidy) that the weaker sections get a fair chance to exploit this opportunity. At a time when as a result of the climate change crisis we should be moving away from fossil fuel use to sustainable sources of energy, the livestock policy recommends the reverse. It also neglects the fact that even in the affluent state of Punjab, farmers are shifting back from tractors to bullocks because the tractors have become too expensive to operate due to rise in fuel prices.

It is contended that the livestock policy is based on a flawed one dimensional linear and monoculture logic. One-dimensional thinking is based on perceiving cattle as linear and mechanical input-output systems with a single function, single output usually limited to milk or meat. Linearity is displayed in treating these inputs and outputs as linear flows. On this one dimensional and linear logic, it is that India's 70 million work animals have to be fed and managed over a "365 day feeding year" while they give a "100 day working year". On the basis of this flawed logic it is then stated that these "inefficient" work animals can become progressively redundant to the farming sector and cattle population can be reduced to one third of what it is.

This concept of efficiency applied to cattle is totally misplaced. Firstly, in India, farm animals are not single output, single function machines. They have many functions, only one of which is to provide work energy. Even when work animals are not pulling ploughs or bullock carts they are giving manure, the most significant contribution that cattle make to agriculture. Secondly, a comparative energy audit of inputs and useful outputs from US cattle and Indian cattle shows that Indian cattle are far more efficient than their counterparts in industrial economies in using energy. They use 29 per cent of organic matter provided to them, and 22 per cent of the energy and 3 per cent of the protein in contrast to 9, 7 and 5 per cent respectively in the intensive cattle industry in the US. Indian cattle provide food in the excess of the edible food consumed, in contrast to the US where 6 times as much edible food is fed to the cattle as is obtained from them. It is this wasteful and inefficient system of livestock management that the new livestock policy introduced in India in the name of improving "efficiency" of cattle.

Undermining Farm Animal Biodiversity

The Biodiversity Convention obliges all member states to protect bio-diversity. This includes farm animal biodiversity- India's indigenous livestock policy has been based on a wide diversity of cattle breeds. They are high milk yielders like the Gir, Sindhi, Sahiwal and Deoni. They are dual-purpose breeds such as the Haryana, Ongole, Gaolao, Krishna Valley, Ibarparkar, Kankrej. Finally there are specialized draught animals such as Nagori, Bachour, Kenkatha, Malvi, Kherigarh, Hallikar, Amritmohal, Kangayam, Khillari, etc.

The livestock policy document totally fails to address the issue of conservation of animal biodiversity even though it has been drafted after the Biodiversity Convention was signed. In fact, by recommending the wiping out of draught power, the policy is indirectly writing a death certificate for indigenous breeds, which have been evolved as dual purpose breeds for both dairy and draught power or a specialized draught animals. By a one-dimensional focus on dairy and meat alone, and a deliberate destruction of the animal energy economy, the policy clearly promotes the replacement of diverse indigenous breeds by uniform breeds from Europe. One-dimensional thinking thus leads to a monoculture of farm animals bred and maintained through external imported inputs for an export-oriented economy.

Aggravating the Fodder Crisis

It is contended that the primary reason for decline of cattle is the shortage of fodder. The fodder crisis has three roots - one lies in agriculture policy based on Green Revolution technologies, which undermined the sources of fodder from agricultural crops. High Yielding Varieties were bred for grain and led to decline in fodder. The second source of the fodder crisis lies in aid programmes such as "social forestry" and "farm forestry" projects, which promoted the planting of monocultures of non-fodder species such as Eucalyptus, thus aggravating the shortage of fodder.

Finally, the enclosure of the commons has also led to scarcity of grazing lands and pastures. In addition there has been a scarcity of cattle feed both because traditional sources of cattle feed such as oil cakes have declined as a result of the Green Revolution, which displaced oil seeds, and because new sources such as soybean cake are largely exported. The Agriculture Minister recently announced that he wanted a special port set up for the export of soyabean cake. Industrial countries such as Netherlands use seven times more land than in developing countries for fodder and feed to provide inputs to their intensive factory farming. The livestock policy does recognize the crisis of fodder and feed in India but fails to provide solutions. In fact, by promoting intensive factory farming, it is indirectly proposing a system that will intensify the pressure on land, divert land from food for people to food for animals and further erode the scarce environmental resources of the country.

As stated earlier, all livestock of course share the feed and fodder resources. However, lactating cows and bullocks receive preferential treatment while sheep and goats, dry and unproductive animals and backyard poultry to a large extent have to fend for themselves. Agricultural residues are currently estimated to provide 40%, grazing 31%, green fodder (cut and cultivated) 26%, and grain and concentrates (mainly for commercial poultry and high producing cows) 3% of total consumption. Over the last decade the straw grain ratio has deteriorated because of the large-scale adoption of high yielding varieties, which also produce poorer quality straw.

However, the amount of common property grazing land has deteriorated sharply from 78 m ha in 1950-51 to 55 m ha in 1988-89 (admittedly very crude estimates) together with the quality of grazing in the remaining areas. This has been at least partly compensated by encroachment into reserved forest areas (67 m ha) a large proportion of which (probably more than 50%) now exhibit serious degradation (other factors than grazing may have contributed to this state of affairs). Cultivated green fodder is estimated at 7 million ha and is gaining in importance (particularly in the NW Region). The nutritional constraints in dairy production are very real and the conditions under which stall-feeding, concentrate feeding and cultivated fodder become viable options are not very clear. There is no recommendation in the policy that would improve the natural resource and environmental base for ameliorating the fodder scarcity. Steps in this direction would include:

a. Shift to agricultural crops and crop varieties that produce food for both animals and humans. For example our seed conservation programme - Navdanya has shown that high fodder yielding varieties are the most popular among farmers.

b. Shift to fodder trees under agro-forestry and social forestry programmes

c. Recover and rejuvenate the commons

d. Stop export of cattle feed.

The policy perspective has no recommendations, with respect to (a, b and d) above. With respect to c, it recommends the opposite of what the environment movement has been saying. Section 3.4 states: "We are doubtful about the chances of success in relation to the village common (panchayat) lands and would not recommend any major effort to establish management for and to regenerate this resource."

The Government Livestock Policy developed in collaboration with the Swiss Development Corporation, the author alleges, is thus the opposite of what an ecologically sound animal husbandry policy should be; given the information we now have about the ecological and social externalities of intensive factory farming of animals. Instead of promoting the conservation of indigenous breeds of cattle, the policy prescribes the wiping out of local breeds. Instead of reducing dependence on fossil fuels, the policy recommends replacing ploughs and bullock carts with tractors. Instead of promoting reduction of meat eating it promotes increase of meat production. Instead of recovering the commons it suggests we should let the commons disappear.

This is a prescription for wiping out biodiversity and worsening the climate change crisis. Both the Indian government and the Swiss government are thus acting against their commitments made at the Earth Summit in Rio, in Agenda 21 as well as in the Biodiversity Convention and the Climate Change Convention.

The official policy needs to be totally revised to reflect people's concern, government obligations and full scientific and ecological knowledge that is available about the environmental and economic costs of large scale, centralized and intensive factory farming.

THE PEOPLE'S ECOLOGICAL AGENDA

For the livestock policy to be ecologically sound and socially just the following elements must be urgently addressed.

1. Protection of native breeds and conservation of animal biodiversity
2. Strengthening the role of farm animals in sustainable agriculture
3. Stopping the export of oil cake and cattle feed
4. Taking urgent steps to improve the fodder situation through planting appropriate crop
   species and trees and by rejuvenating the commons
5. Preventing the import of environmentally unsound methods of intensive factory farming of animals, which degrade and pollute the environment and cause health hazards to consumers.

Comments on the Above Section

Several comments mentioned above regarding the long term Livestock Policy Perspective seem to be valid in the present context. This specially relates to the introduction of exotic breeds while not improving and preserving the indigenous breeds. Nevertheless, it is too simplistic to assume that the government policy shall not take into account the preservation of the indigenous breeds. It is impossible to substitute whole of the local livestock population especially of cattle and buffalo, with the exotic breeds. Also the author seems to have raised issues such as an assault on the culture of conservation in connection with the promotion of meat, and also of undermining of sustainability of agriculture. However, there is urgent need to look after well the cows that are considered as holy and other cattle rather than continue to have a larger population of livestock year after year. It is essential to provide for adequate supplies of feed and fodder for the increasing stock, which is not feasible due to shortage of land and other resources. In fact the scarcity of feed and fodder has been one of the major limiting factors in improving livestock productivity. There is no doubt that currently India has too large cattle and bovine population compared to the feed and fodder supplies. The future policy, as discussed in the earlier section has to be based on reduction of number of cattle. This has to be made mandatory. The reduction of bovine population does not mean elimination of the whole stock. This will in no way undermining the sustainability of the agriculture sector in India. In fact, the lesser number of cattle and buffalo who are cared better both in terms of feed and health care, shall be able to perform more efficiently than in the past.

As regards the culling of holy cow, another view is expressed based on the Philosophy of Gita. It is suggested that dairy industry plays a vital role in the agro-based economics of India. Strengthening dairy industry is essential for removing poverty of the large majority of Indian population, which is living even today in rural areas. The three pillars of dairy farming economics – Milk, Meat and Use in Harness—need to be strengthened. It is suggested that just as National Dairy Development Board has done commendable work in the field of milk, there is an urgent need for similar work in the field of meat. For this the following has been suggested:

"Hindu religion takes a holistic view of the life and Hindu vision is free of any preconceived biases. Weakening society in the name of mercy, pity or nonviolence is ADHARMA and not DHARMA in the eyes of Hindu Philosophy. Cow is sacred and has an important place in Indian social and economic life. Yet, no one is above the overall interests of society and DHARMA. Lord Krishna asked Arjuna to kill his own brethren and beloved because that was the DHARMA at that time. Similarly in today's situation giving up the opposition to cow slaughter is indeed in accordance with DHARMA. Hindus must realize that enriching the life of bovine and other useful animals is DHARMA. Making efforts to build a healthy and large population of cattle in India is DHARMA, a wise man is not perturbed by death since he knows that soul is immortal - "Weapons cannot cut it nor can fire burn it; water cannot drench it nor can wind made it dry" (Verse 23, Chapter 2, Srimad Bhagavad-Gita)."[1]

Public Spending in the Livestock Sector

Central Government Public spending in the livestock sector (not including directed credit programme) comes from the central and state governments. The share of total agricultural spending going to animal husbandry and dairying activities ranged from 6-16 percent from the Fourth (1969-74) to the Ninth (1997-2002) Five Year Plan (Table 9.6). Until 1992, animal husbandry accounted for 65 percent of total spending on animal husbandry and dairying. Under the Eighth Plan, however, the share of animal husbandry fell to 31 percent and this share recovered to 43 percent during the last Plan.

Actual government spending (direct or through centrally sponsored schemes) on animal husbandry and dairying totaled Rs. 1.2 billion ($ 250 million) in 2000-01 (Table 9.7). An analysis of the 2000-01 expenditure indicates that:

- Activities that could be taken over by the private sector, such as poultry development, cattle breeding, and dairying (especially Operation Flood), received about 66 percent of total animal husbandry funds. Funding of such activities should be phased out.
- Feed and fodder development activities received very limited funding, Rs. 30 million or 2.4 percent of total spending on animal husbandry and dairying, although this does not include the support coming from

---

[1]Anil Chawla: Holy Cow: Philosophy of Gita and Economics of Cow and other Domestic Animals: 4 December,1999: Accessed through Internet. http://anilchawla.homestead.com/holycow.

Table 9.6: GOI Planned expenditure on Animal Husbandry and Dairying: 1969–2002

(Rs. million)

Five year plan	Agriculture and related activities	Animal Husbandry		Dairying		Total animal husbandry and dairying	
		Total	Share (%)	Total	Share (%)	Total	Share (%)
4th Plan; 1969-74	23,204	1,543	7	788	3	2,330	10
5th Plan: 1974-78	48,665	2,325	5	540	1	2,865	6
Annual Plan: 1979-80	19,997	2,088	10	1,158	6	3,246	16
6th Plan: 1980-85	136,203	8,025	6	4,363	3	12,388	7
7th Plan: 1985-90	276,611	12,805	5	6,034	2	18,839	7
8th Plan: 1992-97	111,050	4,000	4	9,000	8	13,000	12
9th Plan: 1997-02		4,483		5,890		10,373	

Source: Singh K, and Saxena R: " Some Macro Economic Aspects of India's Livestock Sector: A Situation Analysis," Institute of Rural Management, Anand: Department of Animal Husbandry: Annual Report: 2001-2002.

other departments (such as National Wasteland Development Board and the Departments of Crops and Seeds).[1] Given the significance of the feed and fodder problem and the magnitude of the deficit in their supply, more resources need to be channeled into this area.

• Spending on disease control is modest, only around 6 percent of total expenditure. Nevertheless it is balanced by a high level of state spending.

State Expenditure State governments are responsible for financing most animal husbandry and dairying activities. For example, in fiscal year 2000-01, the state total spending on these activities in Maharashtra, Tamil Nadu, Uttar Pradesh and Himachal Pradesh ranged from 89-98 percent. In several States (Punjab, Maharashtra, Tamil Nadu) animal health spending accounts for more than half of total state expenditure on livestock. Other major expenditure includes administration and cattle and buffalo development.

---

[1]In 2000-01, the budget allocation of the National Wasteland Development Board was Rs.285 million. The budget for the National Forestation and Eco-Development Board was Rs. 985 million.

Table 9.7: Actual GOI Expenditure on Animal Husbandry and Dairying: 2000-01

(Rs. million)

Sector	Budgeted		Actual	
	Total	*Share %*	*Total*	*Share %*
Animal Husbandry				
Cattle Development	530	30.1	377	30.2
Disease control and Rinderpest Eradication	280	15.9	195	15.6
Poultry Development	60	3.4	45	3.6
Feed and Fodder Development	40	2.3	30	2.4
Improvement of Slaughterhouse & Carcass Utilization Centres	25	1.4	22	1.8
Others	314	17.9	182	14.6
Subtotal	1,249	71.0	851	68.2
Dairying				
Integrated Dairy Development Programmes in Non-OF, Hilly and Backward Areas	200	11.4	203	16.3
Assistance to Cooperatives	250	14.2	170	13.6
Others	60	3.4	23	1.9
Subtotal	510	29.0	396	31.8
Total	1,759	100.0	1,247	100.0

Source: Department of Animal Husbandry and Dairying: Annual Report 2001-2002

Cattle Insurance Scheme

The General Insurance Company, a parastatal, provides insurance to livestock producers. The National Commission on Agriculture proposed livestock insurance in 1974 to encourage farmers to invest in higher-quality animals. For animals under government schemes such as IRDP, the government subsidizes the premium rate. While the premium rate is fixed at four percent of the value of animal, the beneficiary pays for only 2.5 percent of the value of the animal and the remainder 1.75 percent) is subsidized by the government.

Insurance schemes for poultry include comprehensive coverage for poultry farms, epidemic poultry insurance schemes for hatcheries, and poultry insurance schemes for parent stocks. The comprehensive programme for farmers covers broilers to the age of eight weeks and layers to the age of 72 weeks. The premium charged under the IRDP is Rs. 0.25 per bird as per batch or Re. 1 per bird a year. Non participants in the IRDP programme pay Rs. 1.20 per bird year. For layers, the premium charged under IRDP scheme is Rs. 0.80 per bird a year and 4.5 percent of the value of non-IRDP participants.

While livestock insurance helps address the risks associated with livestock production and might be required for the effective implementation of credit schemes, the government should not pay for the insurance of commercially viable enterprises–commercial enterprises should be graduated to full-cost insurance. The savings that result could be used to finance activities (such as research and extension for small farmers) that are more directly targeted at the poor. Insurance Statistics for cattle, other than cattle and for total livestock for the period 1988-89 to 1997-98 is given in Table 9.8.

The number of cattle insured increased from 7.2 million in 1988/89 to 9.1 million in 1997/98. Under the IRDP animal scheme the number insured had doubled to almost 6.1 million during this period, while in the Non-IRDP areas the number of cattle insured had declined by 25 percent to 3.1 million. However, the total premium amount had increased in both cases, resulting in 75 percent increase to Rs. 1,168 million. The insured claim amount has remained almost constant amount of Rs. 600 million. With increased premium amount and almost constant insured claim, the Insured-Claims ratio had declined from over 86 to 45 percent (Table 9.9).

As regards livestock other than cattle, the number insured declined by almost by one-third to 7.4 million in 1997/98. Though both the IRDP and the non-IRDP areas recorded decline in the number insured, the decline was rather sharp in the former area. Nevertheless, the Premium amount in the Non-IRDP area increased by almost 5 times despite 25 percent decline in the number of livestock insured. The increase in the premium in this area more than compensated the decline in the premium amount in the IRDP areas. The Insured Claim ratio, however, remained almost constant around 50 percent during the decade covered (Table 9.10).

Animal Health

Endemic diseases, such as rinderpest and contagious bovine pleuropneumonia, are still prevalent in India. In addition, the intensification of production and the introduction of exotic breeds have increased the incidence of other diseases, including foot and mouth disease, sheep, and Newcastle and infectious bursal disease (Gumboro) in poultry. Achieving sustainable output growth and maximizing the production potential of the livestock sector will require more effective disease control and better access to productive-enhancing technologies.

Both the central and state governments and the NDDB handle veterinary services. The central government develops the programmes and defines the policies through the Department of Animal Husbandry and Dairying's Animal Health Division and the Department of Agricultural Research and Education, which operates mainly through the Indian Council for Agricultural Research (ICAR) Institutes, such as the Indian Veterinary Research Institute, the species-oriented national research centres, and the ICAR Coordinated Projects (Surveillance of Animal Diseases, Foot and Mouth Disease and Haemoprotozoa Diseases).

The state animal husbandry and veterinary services departments provide animal health services down to the village level. They also work with the state agricultural universities on technology and extension services and overseas the Biological Products Division and research satiations.

Table 9.8: Cattle Insurance Statistics—I.R.D.P. and Non-I.R.D.P.—1988-89 to 1997-98

(Amount in Rs. lakhs, numbers in lakhs)

Year	I.R.D.P.				Non-I.R.D.P.				Total			
	No. insured	Premium amount	Insured claims amount	Insured claims ratio (%)	No. insured	Premium amount	Insured claims amount	Insured claims ratio (%)	No. insured	Premium amount	Insured claims amount	Insured claims ratio (%)
1988-89	31.09	2805.16	2149.52	76.60	40.46	3840.00	4119.97	107.29	71.55	6646.16	6269.49	94.33
1989-90	48.37	3665.46	2820.71	76.95	29.14	3283.62	3225.30	98.22	77.51	6949.08	6046.01	81.00
1990-91	34.40	3471.25	2401.55	69.18	26.80	3410.77	3294.05	96.58	61.20	6882.02	5695.60	82.76
1991-92	42.50	4070.11	2744.67	67.43	27.73	3241.78	2623.89	80.94	70.23	7311.89	5368.56	73.42
1992-93	48.34	4184.67	2909.91	69.54	40.01	3563.12	2589.51	72.68	88.35	7747.79	5499.42	10.98
1993-94	49.38	4764.63	3005.80	63.09	30.84	4052.91	2821.88	69.63	80.22	8817.54	5827.68	66.09
1994-95	65.03	4632.14	3170.35	68.44	26.18	4430.06	3333.11	75.24	91.21	9062.22	6503.46	71.76
1995-96	69.60	5278.48	3620.06	68.58	27.56	4514.13	3081.85	68.27	97.16	9792.61	6701.91	68.44
1996-97	52.26	5263.39	3152.64	59.90	32.81	5210.48	3440.35	66.03	85.07	10473.87	6592.99	62.95
1997-98	60.70	6423.35	2890.50	45.00	30.08	5255.50	2365.50	45.01	90.78	11678.85	5256.00	45.00

Source: General Insurance Corporation on India

Table 9.9: Livestock (Including Cattle) Insurance Statistics—I.R.D.P. and Non-I.R.D.P.—1988-89 to 1997-98

(Amount in Rs. lakhs, numbers in lakhs)

Year	I.R.D.P.				Non-I.R.D.P.				Total			
	No. insured	Premium amount	Insured claims amount	Insured claims ratio (%)	No. insured	Premium amount	Insured claims amount	Insured claims ratio (%)	No. insured	Premium amount	Insured claims amount	Insured claims ratio (%)
1988-89	106.29	4169.29	2849.96	68.36	80.45	4048.22	4217.11	104.17	186.74	8217.51	7067.07	86.00
1989-90	125.24	4590.25	3248.06	70.76	56.70	3908.01	3685.77	94.31	181.94	8498.26	6933.83	81.59
1990-91	95.24	4423.00	2656.62	60.06	77.40	4146.42	3479.08	83.91	172.64	8569.42	6135.70	71.60
1991-92	111.75	5109.88	3135.31	61.36	52.00	3851.42	3193.59	82.92	163.75	8961.30	6328.90	70.62
1992-93	93.94	5192.32	3215.43	61.93	44.25	4164.32	2763.02	66.35	138.19	9356.64	5978.45	63.90
1993-94	121.84	5892.98	3303.92	56.07	54.79	4493.66	3067.46	68.26	176.63	10386.64	6371.38	61.34
1994-95	96.43	5733.59	3599.78	62.78	46.27	4953.37	3550.50	71.68	142.70	10686.96	7150.28	66.91
1995-96	93.23	6040.81	4090.58	67.72	56.32	5297.54	3315.11	62.58	149.55	11338.35	7405.69	65.32
1996-97	91.55	6415.46	3655.91	56.99	55.53	5838.46	3826.85	66.55	147.08	12253.92	7482.76	61.06
1997-98	104.00	7419.55	3561.38	48.00	60.63	6320.24	2705.57	42.81	164.63	13739.89	6266.95	45.61

Source: General Insurance Corporation of India.

Table 9.10: Livestock (Other than Cattle) Insurance Statistics—I.R.D.P.—1988-89 to 1997-98

(Amount in Rs. lakhs, numbers in lakhs)

Year	I.R.D.P.				Non-I.R.D.P.				Total			
	No. Insured	Premium amount	Insured claims amount	Insured claims ratio (%)	No. insured	Premium amount	Insured claims amount	Insured claims ratio (%)	No. insured	Premium amount	Insured claims amount	Insured claims ratio (%)
1988-89	75.20	1363.13	700.44	51.38	39.99	208.22	97.14	46.65	115.19	1571.35	797.58	50.76
1989-90	76.87	924.79	427.35	46.21	27.56	624.39	460.47	73.75	104.43	1549.18	887.82	57.31
1990-91	60.84	951.75	255.07	26.80	50.60	735.65	185.03	25.15	111.44	1687.40	440.10	26.08
1991-92	69.25	1039.77	390.64	37.57	24.27	609.64	569.70	93.45	93.52	1649.41	960.34	58.32
1992-93	45.60	1007.66	305.52	30.32	4.24	601.20	173.51	28.86	49.84	1608.85	479.03	29.77
1993-94	72.46	1128.35	298.12	26.42	23.95	440.75	245.58	55.72	96.41	1569.10	543.70	34.65
1994-95	31.40	1101.45	429.43	38.99	20.09	523.29	217.39	41.54	51.49	1624.74	646.82	39.81
1995-96	23.63	762.32	470.52	61.72	28.76	783.41	233.26	29.77	52.39	1545.74	703.78	45.53
1996-97	39.29	1152.07	503.27	43.68	22.72	627.98	386.50	61.55	62.01	1780.05	889.78	49.99
1997-98	43.30	996.20	670.88	67.34	30.55	1064.84	340.07	31.93	73.85	2061.04	1010.95	49.05

Source: General Insurance Corporation of India

Animal Health and disease control programmes are discussed in detailed in the next chapter.

Livestock Research and Extension

Livestock research is undertaken by a multitude of institutions, often creating problems of duplication. At the central level, the Indian Council of Agricultural ·Research conducts livestock research through its six specialized national institutes, six research centres, and six coordinated livestock projects. The council serves as an apex organization for sponsoring, coordinating, and promoting research, education and extension services in agriculture and related fields. The Council oversees 43 central institutes, 4 national bureaus, 20 national research centres, 9 project directorates, 70 All India Coordinated Research/Improvement Projects, and 109 farm science centres.

Research is also carried out by the 28 state universities. The state agricultural university system supports 30 veterinary and animal science colleges. Most of the funding for the agricultural universities comes from state governments; some additional support comes from the ICAR. Private spending research is still negligible.

Expenditure on livestock research is in line with livestock sector's relative contribution to agricultural GDP, but the distribution of spending across livestock sub- sectors is not consistent with their relative importance. Under the Ninth Plan (1997-2002), ICAR spending on livestock research totalled Rs. 4710 million or 19 percent of ICAR's total expenditure. The breakdown of the research budget allocation is presented in Table 9.11, and a comparison of livestock research spending and total agricultural research spending, by states, appears in Table 9.12. This is in line with the sector's 30-33 percent contribution to agricultural GDP.

Livestock research, however, is skewed towards bovines and mainly focuses on cattle. The attention paid to buffalo, (which supply half of the national milk output) and small ruminants (which supply most of the national ruminant meat production) does not correspond to the importance of these sectors. Poultry, for which advanced technology is readily available and vibrant private sector exists, still receives seven percent of research resources. Spending breakdowns (breeding, health, nutrition and management and production system) are not available. However, the ICAR livestock research institutes tend to focus their efforts on genetic improvement, with considerable emphasis on the import of exotic breeds and biotechnology.

Key weaknesses of the livestock research sector include a shortage of trained personnel, poor staff and operating cost ratios and the lack of client orientation especially for smallholder production. An exception in dairy is NDDB research programme, whose success can be attributed to its client orientation. The programme covers the animal breeding, nutrition, and health problems of the mostly smallholder members.

Table 9.11: Share of Livestock Research in Total Research Outlay of ICAR

(Rs. million)

Plan	At current prices			At 1980-81 prices		
	Total outlay of ICAR	Research outlay of ICAR	Outlay for livestock research (ICAR)	Total outlay of ICAR	Research outlay of ICAR	Outlay for livestock research (ICAR)
IV Plan (1969-74)	914	579	152 (26.25)	1812	1111	318
V Plan (1974-78)	14535	932	259 (27.79)	2002	1215	338
VI Plan (1980-85)	3399	2497	356 (14.26)	3399	2497	356
VII plan (1985-90)	4250	3172	446 (14.06)	3094	2309	325
VIII Plan (1990-95)	13000	9682	1738 (17.95)	4874	3630	652
IX Plan (1997-2000)	33770	24556	4710 (19.18)	7650	5562	1067

Figures in parentheses are percent of total research outlay
IX Plan outlay also includes outlay on account of National Technology Project.
Source: ICAR Five Year Plans.

Table 9.12: Share of Livestock Research in Total Public

State	Share (%)	State	Share (%)
1. Andhra Pradesh	35.6	10. Madhya Pradesh	22.9
2. Assam	41.3	11. Maharashtra	22.9
3. Bihar	40.6	12. Orissa	25.7
4. Gujarat	36.5	13. Rajasthan	29.3
5. Haryana	54.7	14. Punjab	36.6
6. Himachal Pradesh	22.5	15. Tamil Nadu	27.6
7.Jammu andKashmir	31.1	16. Uttar Pradesh	40.4
8. Karnataka	27.5	17. West Bengal	
9. Kerala	20.7	18. Average	
		North and West	31.2
		East and South	31.5
		Uttar Pradesh	40.4

Source: M. Ruthyunjaya, P. Ranjitha, and S. Selvarajan: Congruency Analysis of Resources Allocation; In India Agricultural Research System," Division of Economics, Indian Agricultural Research Institute, New Delhi

Given the sector's technical and socioeconomic constraints and institutional weaknesses, the World Bank[1] had recommended that research efforts should be reoriented to focus on:

- Farming systems research, to identify key constraints at the smallholder level;

- Feed and fodder production, including:

    - Basic research, using modern biotechnology techniques, to improve the nutritive value of low quality high fibrous forages and crop residues. Research could include work on rumen ecology and manipulation, better *in vitro and in vivo* fermentation techniques, and improved utilization of scarce protein and carbohydrate resources using bypass techniques.

    - Applied research on feeds and fodder production, especially in the more arid zones, the use of multipurpose trees, the integration of the different feeds with the farming system, optimal supplementation of poor-quality crop residues, and considerably more emphasis on the economics of production. Priority should be given to buffalo and small ruminants and feeding systems. Reallocating the budget for research in cattle and poultry production could finance these systems. Research on intensive poultry production should be dramatically reduced.

    - Applied and multidisciplinary research, with a strong emphasis on the socioeconomic aspects of rehabilitating of the common property resource areas.

- Genetic improvement with a strategic shift from the current emphasis on introducing exotic breeds to one that identifies simple breeding schemes eventually using modern biotechnology techniques, to improve local breeds. More emphasis should be given to the evaluation, conservation, and use of local genetic resources in small ruminant and buffaloes;

- Epidemiological research, with an emphasis on gauging the relative importance of various diseases and developing cost-effective control strategies;

- Free range chicken production, with an emphasis on backyard poultry production systems. Specially attention should be given to specific free-range disease problems (of which Newcastle disease is the most important) and genetic improvement; and

- Socioeconomic evaluation of new and "on the shelf" (such as urea-molasses blocks) technologies.

---

[1] World Bank: India Livestock Sector Review: Enhancing Growth and Development: May 23, 1996, Report No.14522-IN, pp.79-79.

Livestock Extension

The government integrated agricultural extension service has not given enough emphasis to the dissemination of livestock technology. The World Bank, working with the central government, has provided financial assistance for the strengthening of extension services in the states of Madhya Pradesh, Rajasthan and Orissa under the Agricultural Extension Project (NAEP); in Haryana, Karnataka, Jammu and Kashmir, and Gujarat under NAEP II; and in Uttar Pradesh, Assam, Himachal Pradesh, and Bihar under NAEP III. Still the extension system continued to be heavily crop-oriented. The NDDB, however, has effectively incorporated livestock extension in its cooperative support activities.

In addition, nongovernmental organizations are conducting research and providing extension services. The Bhratiya Agro-Industries Foundation (BAIF) is one of the most efficient organizations. The BAIF operates in five states and has been active in developing artificial insemination services and in organizing livestock shows and training programmes. BAIF's spending on livestock research and extension totaled Rs. 160 million in 1998.

In the eighth and the ninth five-year plans livestock extension activities were given increased importance. The Central Government provide financial assistance under the Animal Husbandry Extension Scheme to State Governments, Agricultural and Veterinary Universities and Veterinary Colleges for establishment and development of information network to promote and propagate latest animal husbandry practices and technologies and to create awareness among farmers and breeders about the potential of the Livestock Sector. The Extension Scheme supports the following components/activities: (i) establishment of National Demonstration Unit on Animal Husbandry and Fodder Development; (ii) Organization of Seminar and Workshop and training for field staff on Animal Husbandry Extension; (iii) implements countrywide milk yield competitions; (iv) Organization of training programme for breeders and farmers including special programmes for women farmers; (v) organization of All India and Regional Livestock and Poultry shows; and (vi) participation in the National Exhibition and installation of pavilions on Animal Husbandry activities and related infrastructure. But while increased attention to livestock extension is needed and certainly justified, this should not lead to the creation of another bureaucracy. A flexible system involving non-governmental organizations and private veterinarians and companies (such as private agro-processors) through subcontracting or cost sharing arrangements would improve the delivery of extension services. International experience has shown that cost-sharing arrangements between the public sector and agro-processors (integrated into contract growing or supply scheme) can be effective means of delivering extension services to small farmers. Furthermore, better incentives need to be introduced for the extension agents, rewarding them on the basis of performance and impact in the field.

LIVESTOCK CREDIT PROGRAMMES

Integrated Rural Development Programmes

Poverty alleviation programmes, such as the Integrated Rural Development Programme (IRDP), now renamed as swarnajayanti from Swarozgar Yojana (SGSY), have been used to channel financial assistance to the poor to undertake productive activities such as livestock raising. The SGSY funds have also been channeled to the dairy cooperative sector. For families earning less than Rs. 6, 000 a year the SGSY provides a subsidy of up to Rs. 3,000 for projects with total cost of less than Rs. 10, 000. The funds, which are channeled through commercial banks, cooperative banks and regional rural banks, serve as margin money for getting loans (at subsidized interest rates) from commercial banks. Subsidized insurance coverage and training are also provided.

Livestock loans continue to account for a significant though declining proportion of SGSY loans. In 1998, livestock accounted for 60 percent of the SGSY-backed loans of commercial banks, 20 percent of the IRDP loans of cooperative banks, and 28 percent of the SGSY loans of regional rural banks. When the programme started (under the Sixth Five-Year Plan, 1981-86) dairy cattle loans accounted for 70 percent of total loans. This share had fallen to 22 percent by 1994. As noted in the Eighth Plan (1992-97), the SGSY programme was quite successful in terms of providing incremental income to poor families. However, the number of households able to cross the poverty line has been small. It may be partly due to the low levels of initial investment. On the other hand, it is also difficult to expect banks to raise the per capita loan assistance to beneficiaries, given the excessive overdues pending. In order to enhance the economic returns from an asset, it is necessary to integrate this scheme with the development plans of an area.[7]

Some factors contributing to the poor performance of SGSY beneficiaries include poor decision-making by local government officials, the diversion of funds for consumption purposes, and the poor availability of the projects. For example, the unavailability and low quality of dairy cattle and fodder, the high cost of concentrate feed, poor veterinary services, and poor linkages to the market critically affected the viability of diary activities. High maintenance cost during the dry season and cash constrains caused by delays in payments by cooperatives resulted in the disposal of the animals. Moreover, the government's 1990-91 debt relief scheme further affected loan recovery.

National Bank for Agriculture and Rural Development (NABARD)

Commercial banks provide 75-80 percent of the investment required for dairy ventures. For projects involving an outlay of more than Rs. 100, 000,

---

[7] Government of India: Planning Commission: Eighth Five Year Plan: p. 28, Para 2.2.4

refinance facilities are provided by the NABARD. The NABARD is the apex development institution for the rural credit system; its primary function is the refinancing of agricultural development loans of the cooperative, commercial and regional rural banks. Refinancing is available for veterinary clinic construction, livestock production activities (such as cattle and poultry raising), and small-scale food processing, feed mixing, and veterinary drug production. Investments are subject to NABARD standards on enterprise size and unit costs.[1]

National Credit Fund for Women

The national credit Fund for Women is another source of credit for livestock activities. The fund provides credit to poor women through voluntary associations and self-help groups (including women's credit cooperatives and women's development corporations) to support income-generating activities. The Department of Women and Child Development manages the fund. In 1994, the fund reached Rs. 310 million and had covered 34 voluntary associations in ten states since its December 1993 inception.

The fund targets families earning less than Rs. 11,000 in rural areas and Rs. 11,800 in urban areas. The ceiling for short term loans is Rs. 2,500 (US$ 52) to be paid within 15 months and Rs. 5, 000 (US$ 104) for medium term loans to be repaid within 3-5 years. The interest rate charged to the voluntary associations is 8 percent per annum, with a ceiling of 12 percent per annum for the ultimate borrowers.

APPROACH FOR 10th PLAN

The National Agriculture Policy announced by the Government in 2000 aims to attain a growth in excess of 4% per annum in the agriculture sector. Since the growth rate in crop production has stagnated to around 2% higher growth is feasible only through the growth of animal husbandry sector. The Agriculture Policy therefore lays stresses on animal husbandry and fishery sector. The Approach Paper to the Tenth Five Year Plan has also identified animal husbandry including dairying and poultry as an important component of agriculture diversification. The commitment of the Government in doubling of food production by the year 2007 also calls for rapid increase in the production of livestock, fish and fishery products. Keeping these in view, the emphasis of the Department will be on the all round development of these sectors.

In consonance with the overall strategy of the Tenth Plan, the major thrust of the policies and activities of the Department during 2002-03 was concentrated on rapid genetic upgradation of cattle and buffaloes, provision of health cover including creation of disease free zones, provision of nutritious feed and fodder, integrated approach to marine and inland fisheries, development of deep sea fishing, etc.

---

[1]The approved loan amount for the establishment of a veterinary clinic, for example is set at Rs. 350,000 plus a grant of Rs. 50,000.

The major thrust during the 10th Five year Plan is, hence, on the following critical areas;

- Rapid genetic up gradation of cattle and buffaloes and improvement in the delivery mechanism of breeding inputs and services to farmers.
- Extension of dairy development activities in non-Operation Flood, hilly and backward areas, including clean milk production.
- Promotion of fodder crops and fodder trees to improve animal nutrition.
- Provision of adequate animal health services with special emphasis on creation of disease free zones and control of foot and mouth disease.
- Improvement of small ruminants and pack animals.
- Development of backyard poultry in rural areas.

Cattle Development

Cattle are vital and integral part of our rural economy. To give a boost to the entire gamut of this economic activity, such as animal husbandry, dairying and sheep rearing, the Government will consider the setting up of a National Cattle Development Board with appropriate budgetary support.

International Cooperation and Interaction with States

Agreement with other countries

During the year 2002-03, no Agreements/Memorandum of Understanding have been signed by the/of Department of animal Husbandry Dairying : However, draft MOU/Agreement with following of Countries are at various stages, consideration for cooperation in the field of Animal Husbandry, Dairying, Fisheries Sector.

(i) MOU between Department of Animal Husbandry and Dairying of the Republic of India and Agriculture and Livestock Service, Ministry of Agriculture of the Republic Chile on Animal Health.

(ii) Agreement on cooperation in the sanitary veterinary field between the Government of Republic of India and the Government of Romania.

(iii) Agreement on Animal Health between the Ministry of Agriculture of the Republic of India and the Secretariat of Agriculture, Livestock and Rural Development of United Mexican States.

(iv) Agreement for cooperation in the Veterinary field between the Governments of the Socialist Republic of India and the Socialist Republic of Sri Lanka.

(v) MOU between the Government of Republic of India and the Government of Republic of Mauritius on cooperation in the field of Fisheries.

(vi) MOU between the Ministry of Agriculture, Department of Animal Husbandry and Dairying, Government of India and the Ministry of Fisheries and Aquatic Resources Development of the Democratic Socialist Republic of Sri Lanka for Fisheries Development and Technical Cooperation.

(vii) MOU between Ministry of Agriculture of the Federal Democratic Republic of Ethiopia and National Dairy Development Board (NDDB) of the Republic of India on the development of the Ethiopian Dairy Industry.

(viii) Agreement of cooperation in the field of Animal Health between the Government of Republic of India and the Government of Mongolia.

International Cooperation for Foreign Funded Projects

Many foreign funded projects are under implementation in the country. The agencies funding these projects are mainly Denmark (DANIDA), Switzerland (SDC) and the French Government. The Denmark Government (DANIDA) assisted projects are as under:

(i) Integrated Livestock Development Project in Puddokottai, Tamil Nadu;

(ii) Integrated Livestock Development Project in Koraput, Orissa;

(iii) Integrated Livestock Development Project in Bastar, Chhatishgarh;

(iv) Integrated Livestock Development Project in Andhra Pradesh.

The Switzerland Government assisted project (SDC) are as under:

(i) Cattle breeding and Fodder Development in Andhra Pradesh,

(ii) Animal Husbandry and Dairy Development in Orissa,

(iii) Animal Husbandry and Dairy Development in Sikkim.

Two projects for establishment of Fresh Water Prawn Hatchery are presently under implementation in the States of Gujarat and Maharashtra. These projects are being implemented with assistance from the French Government.

International Membership

This Department is also a regular member (paying annual membership contribution) of the following International Organisations related to animal health and fisheries:

(i) Office International des Epizooties (OIE), Paris, France

(ii) Indian Ocean Tuna Commission (IOTC), Sychelles – an organization under FAO

(iii) Animal Production and Health Commission for the Asia and the Pacific (APHCA), Bangkok, Thailand – an organization under FAO.

(iv) Bay of Bengal Project/Inter Governmental Organisation (IGO) on Fisheries – an organisation under FAO.

India is being permanent member of the Office International des Epizooties (I.O.E.), Paris, France an International Organisation responsible for setting Animal Health standards. India was so far making Annual contribution/Membership fee to OIE as 4th Category member country till-2002. However, OIE has upgraded the status of India from 4th category to 3rd category member country and Annual Payment of contribution paid of the enhanced rate, i.e. Euro 63150 since the calendar year 2003.

CONCLUDING REMARKS

Introducing high yielding varieties, newer technologies associated with their cultivation, improvement in the quality of livestock among all economically important species and the spread of irrigated crop production, were all areas clearly identified for extension support under the national extension programme launched during the first five year plan, in 1951. The national extension service blocks set up for this purpose country wide had well laid out plans and trained manpower for extension services in all sectors of rural development: crop production, animal husbandry, rural industry, development of women, farmers' organization, etc. The system worked extremely well during the first two plans and then petered out as it lost its momentum under the onslaught of programmes like "Grow More Food Campaign," shifting the focus entirely to crop production. Over the years, the agriculture departments in the country were able to structure an extension support system for crop production. The livestock sector was less fortunate: the animal husbandry department did not take any such initiative and therefore a national extension support system for the livestock sector does not exist.

However, the 5th, 6th and 7th five year plans for the dairy sector became the era of operation flood project: it dominated the policy environment during the 20 years 1970-'90. Another phenomenon which occurred during the same period is the stunning growth of the poultry industry in India: egg production grew from 5 mln in 1970 to over 32 bln in 2001, broiler production from 4 mln to 300 mln and poultry meat from 1 lakh mt to over 6 lakh mt.

Over the nine five year plan periods, there were however no achievements in improving draught animal quality, development of indigenous dairy breeds of cattle and buffalo, offsetting the ongoing genetic drain in Murrah buffalo population, improving feed and fodder supply; and above all in providing protection from animal epidemics to investment risks in livestock enterprises for the core livestock production sector in India, the small holder group.

Finally unlike in agriculture, subsidies are few in the livestock sector (some Rs. 300 crore in all, direct subsidies in 2000) as against some Rs. 16000 crore direct subsidy for agriculture from the central government alone. Credit to the livestock sector too is meager, Rs. 2500 crore as medium and long term loans: some 5 per cent of the total credit to the agricultural sector of over Rs. 50000 crore. Cash credit and micro credit is virtually unheard of in livestock production and Kisan Cards too do not cover livestock credit. Even at the turn of the century over 50 per cent of the farm level credit for livestock production comes from the traditional moneylenders.

Graph 9AI.1: Organisational Structure—Animal Husbandry Department

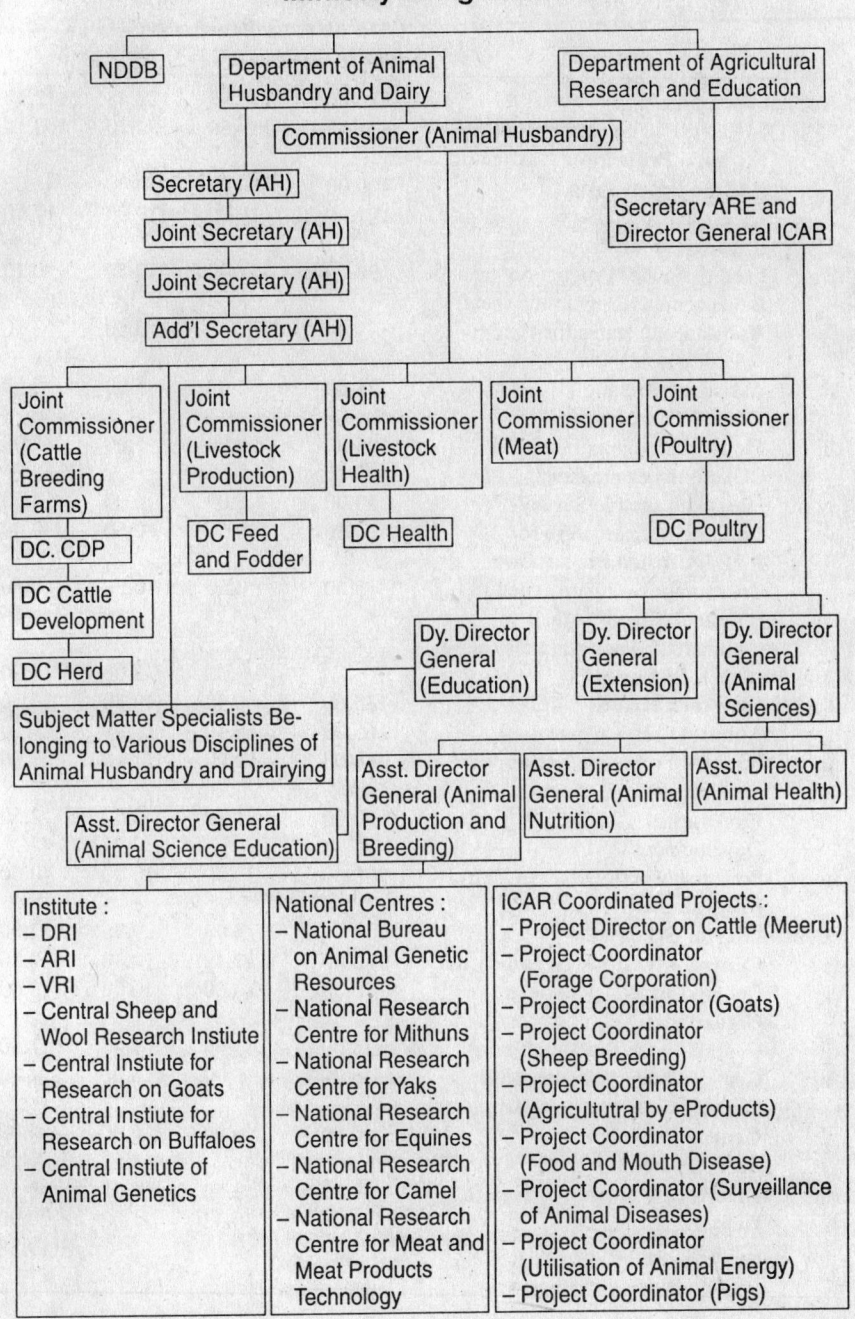

Table 9AII.1: Financial Allocation for Tenth Plan, BE 2002-03 and BE 2003-04

(Rs.in crores)

S.No.	Name of the Scheme	10th Plan (2002-07) Allocation	BE 2002-03	RE 2002-03	BE 2003-04
	Animal Husbandry	1380.00	156.98	122.48	172.10
	CENTRALLY SPONSORED SCHEMES		129.50	92.70	140.10
1.	**National Project for Cattle and Buffalo Breed Prog.**	400.00	50.00	30.00	48.00
2.	**Livestock & Poultry Improvement Prog.**	190.00	19.00	19.00	17.10
i	Feed & Fodder Production Enhancement Programme (new)	30.00	1.00	0.50	0.10
	Assistance to states for Feed 7 Fodder (old)*			3.50	3.50
ii	Assistance to State Poultry/Duck Farms	25.00	5.00	5.00	5.00
iii	Mod. Of Slaughter houses & CUC for hygienic meat	45.00	6.00	5.00	4.00
iv	Integrated sample Survey	50.00	6.00	4.00	4.50
v	Building infrastructure for A.H. Extension Prog. (new)	25.00	0.50	0.50	0.00
vi	Conservation of Threatened Livestock Breeds –small ruminants & Pack Animals (new)	15.00	0.50	0.50	0.50
3.	**Livestock Census $**			3.00	4.00
4.	**Livestock Health**	535.00	60.50	40.70	70.50
i	Animal Disease Control	265.00	15.30	15.85	21.00
ii	National Project on Rinderpest Eradication	40.00	12.00	11.50	7.00
iii	Professional Efficiency Development	30.00	3.20	3.50	2.50
iv	Foot and Mouth Disease Control **Programme (new)**	200.00	30.00	10.00	40.00
	Central Sector Schemes		26.98	29.76	32.00
1.	**Central Livestock Organisation**	140.00	17.48	17.48	18.50
i	Central Cattle Development Organisation	70.00	10.00	10.00	10.00
ii	Central Sheep Breeding Farm	25.00	1.48	1.48	1.50
iii	Central Fodder Development Organisation	45.00	6.00	6.00	7.00
2.	**Central Poultry Development Org.**	40.00	6.00	6.00	4.00
3.	**Directorate of Animal Health**	50.00	3.50	6.28	9.50
i	Dairy Development	355.00	36.52	31.02	29.90
ii	Centrally Sponsored Schemes				19.88

Table 9AII.1: *Financial Allocation for Tenth Plan, BE 2002-03 and BE 2003-04* (Contd.)

(Rs.in crores)

S.No.	Name of the Scheme	10th Plan (2002-07) Allocation	BE 2002-03	RE 2002-03	BE 2003-04
I	Integrated Dairy Development Project	184.00	20.50	17.00	18.88
II	Strengthening Infrastructure for Quality & clean milk prod. (new)	30.00	0.02	0.02	1.00
	Central Sector Schemes				10.02
i	**Assistance to Cooperatives**	140.00	15.00	13.00	9.00
ii	**Delhi Milk Scheme**	1.00	1.00	1.00	1.00
iii	**Dairy/Poultry Venture & Fisheries**	25.00	0.50	0.02	0.02
3.	**Fisheries**	750.00	102.00	82.00	95.00
	Centrally Sponsored Schemes				
I	**Dev. Of inland Aquaculture & Fisheries**	135.00	21.00	14.00	16.00
i.	Inland Aquaculture	120.00	19.00	14.00	15.00
ii	Inland Capture Fisheries	15.00	2.00	0.00	1.00
II	**Dev. Marine Fisheries, Infrastructure & post harvest**	260.00	15.00	9.10	13.00
i.	Development of Marine Fisheries	125.00	2.00	0.10	4.00
ii.	Dev. Of Infrastructure & post harvest operations	125.00	12.00	8.00	7.00
iii	Maintenance of Dredging Equipment	10.00	1.00	1.00	2.00
III	**Welfare Programmes/Human Res. Dev.**	135.00	20.00	20.00	21.00
	a) Welfare programme for Fishermen	120.00	19.00	19.00	20.00
	b) Training and Extension **including HRD**	15.00	1.00	1.00	1.00
	Central Sector Schemes				
I	**Assistance to Fisheries Institutes**	**175.00**	**45.00**	**38.40**	**43.00**
	a) Central Fishery Nautical Institute	38.85	2.00		0.61
	b) Central Fishery Coastal Engineering Institute	0.55	0.30		0.10
	c) Integrated Fishery Project	5.60	1.91		0.71
	d) Fishery Survey of India	130.00	40.73		41.58
II	**Strengthening of Database & Inf. Networking (new)**	**45.00**	**1.00**	**0.50**	**2.00**
	4. Secretariat and Economic Services	**15.00**	**4.50**	**4.50**	**3.00**
	Total	**2500.00**	**300.00**	**240.00**	**300.00**

10

Animal Health Services and Impact of Livestock Sector on Public Health

With the launching of extensive breeding programme, the quality of livestock has improved though to a limited extent. However, their susceptibility to various diseases has increased tremendously. In order to reduce morbidity and mortality in animals, efforts are being made by the State / Union Territory governments to provide better health care through a network of polyclinics, veterinary hospital, dispensaries, first-aid Centres and mobile veterinary dispensaries. Most livestock support services are in the public domain. These services are financed primarily by the State governments, although the Central government also plays some role.

Public spending in the livestock sector comes from the central and state governments. The share of the total agricultural spending allocated to animal husbandry, and dairying activities ranged from 5 percent in the First Plan (1951-56) to 6.6 percent in the Fourth Five Year Plan (1969-74) In the subsequent three plans the investment on animal husbandry and dairying declined. However, during the Ninth Five Year Plan (1997-2002) share of government funds allocated to this sector recovered to 6 percent. During the 9th Plan, a Budget outlay of Rs. 535 crore had been provided for animal health. This has been raised to Rs. 1,735 crore in the Xth Plan ('02-07). In the livestock sector increasing emphasis has been laid on the effective control of animal diseases and declaration of disease-free zones. Out of the total expenditure on animal husbandry, around 40 percent was spent on health services. A large proportion of the expenditure on animal health was accounted for by the National Rinderpest Eradication Programme and the rest for assistance to the states for controlling other diseases.

Livestock in India is ravaged by recurring epidemics, causing phenomenal production losses and lingering morbidity, costing the country dear in terms of money (Rs. 50 to 100 bln. annually, almost 10 per cent of the total annual output value of the livestock sector) and lost opportunities in global trade. As the smallholder group (marginal, small and landless) own over 75 per cent of all species of livestock in the country, they are the ones–the poorest of the poor in the country–who bear the brunt of these avoidable losses. Economic losses due to disease occur in the form of direct losses on account reduction of milk yield, quality and quantity of meat, work capacity and growth. There are eight major diseases afflicting livestock according to OIE (an international organisation for animal health) classification that are serious and fast spreading in India. These include foot and mouth disease (FMD), contagious bovine pleuropneumonia (CBPP) and Peste des petits ruminants (PPR), blue tongue (BT).

India as a country had never seriously attempted to control and eradicate animal diseases (with the single exception of NPRE in recent times); but had always spent the lion's share of the public funds available to the livestock sector on curative veterinary care, a private good, generating entirely private benefit to the livestock owners. Curative veterinary care does not influence the endemicity of diseases, whereas preventive veterinary care, a public good, generates enormous public benefit to the nation at large.

With the eradication of Rinderpest from India in the mid nineties, the only other diseases of concern to India are Foot and Mouth Disease and PPR. FMD is prevalent all over the country and strains O, Asia, and A were active throughout the country in 2001, while strain C has not been reported since 1996. No systematic control and vaccination programme against FMD exist even though massive, but sporadic vaccination (25 mln) are carried out every year. This, however, does not guarantee protection against the disease, as FMD protection is based on herd immunity: coverage of 85 per cent of the animals at risk in an area to establish herd immunity. As against a total of some 420 mln animals at risk, vaccinations cover only 25 mln, a mere 5 per cent.

PPR has become the most serious threat to small ruminants as susceptibility to the disease increased enormously after India introduced "no rinderpest vaccination" regimen. Vaccine for PPR though developed by the IVRI, is still in the testing stage and has not been released for mass protection. Another emerging threat for small ruminants is the spread of Blue Tongue in India. Cattle and buffalo too are infected and are carriers. A very large percentage of cattle and buffalo in the country are seropositive to the disease (short term: they are free of infection after three months, but can be reinfected). There is no vaccine available against Blue Tongue.

HEALTH AGENDA

On the Health Side

The focus throughout the past planning periods has been on enhancing the supply of veterinary services by strengthening the capabilities and coverage of the state animal husbandry departments. India has a large network of veterinary hospitals/dispensaries. In the year 2000-01, there were 7,749 veterinary hospitals/polyclinics, 15,554 veterinary dispensaries, 27,543 veterinary aid centres including mobile dispensaries, which were supported by about 250 disease diagnostic laboratories for quick and reliable diagnosis of diseases. In addition there are 43,782 AI centres.

Further, major livestock and poultry diseases are controlled by way of prophylactic vaccination. The vaccines are produced by 26 veterinary vaccine production units in the country. Of these, 19 are in the public sector and 7 in private sector. Import of vaccines is also permitted as and when required. Annexure 1 gives details of Poultry Vaccines

While efforts are made to ensure better livestock health in the country, simultaneous steps are also taken to prevent ingress of diseases from outside the country. For maintaining of standards of veterinary drugs and formulations, the Drugs Controller of India is responsible which regulates the quality of veterinary drugs and biological products in consultation with the Department of Animal Husbandry. Animal Quarantine and Certificate Services prevent ingress of livestock diseases by regulating the import and provide export certification of International Standards for livestock and livestock products. In order to implement the services, there are four quarantine stations located one each at New Delhi, Chennai, Mumbai and Kolkata. These stations are also providing export certificates of international standards for livestock and livestock products, which are exported from India. New quarantine stations are to be established at Bangalore and Hyderabad.

National Veterinary Biological Products Quality Control Centre

Currently there is no separate system for regulating manufacture, sale or distribution of veterinary drugs and formulations. Also there is no independent system for monitoring the quality of indigenously manufactured or imported vaccines and biological products. The Indian Veterinary Research Institute has been assisting in the task. This has necessitated the need to establish a National Veterinary Biological Products Quality Control Centre, which is to be set up at the existing building of Theileria Vaccine Libratory belonging to Punjab Agricultural University at Ludhiana.

Strengthening of Disease Diagnostic Referral Laboratories

Livestock owners in India are generally poor and own between one and three animals. Hence, it becomes necessary that facilities for diagnosis are made available close to the farmers' dwelling to provide timely health care. With this objective in view, a number of diagnostic labs have been set up in rural areas by the State Governments. In order to provide referral services for diagnosis of various livestock diseases prevalent in their respective regions, one Central and four Regional Disease Diagnostic Laboratories have been set up by strengthening the existing facilities of the state laboratories. The Indian Veterinary Research Institute, Izatnagar, is functioning as a Central Laboratory. The Disease Investigation Laboratory, Pune; Institute of Animal Health and Veterinary Biology, Kolkata; Institute of Animal Health and Biologicals, Bangalore, and Animal Health Institute, Jalandhar, are functioning as referral laboratories for Western, Eastern, Southern and Northern regions respectively.

A network of 26,717 Polyclinics / Hospitals / Dispensaries and 28.195 Veterinary aid centers supported by about 250 disease diagnostic laboratories functioning in the States and Union Territories.

Four Quarantine Stations one each at New Delhi, Chennai, Mumbai and Kolkata are operating in the country.

The Drugs Controller General of India regulates the quality of veterinary drugs and biologicals in consultation with this Department.

Chaudhary Charan Singh Institute of Veterinary Health at Baghpat, Uttar Pradesh is being established.

Control of Livestock Diseases

To supplement the efforts of the State Governments and Union Territories in health care programmes, the Government of India is implementing Centrally Sponsored Scheme, namely Assistance to States for Control of Animal Diseases. Under this scheme, grants-in-aid are provided to control certain important livestock diseases. This scheme has got three components, viz. Systematic Control of Livestock Diseases of national importance, Foot and Mouth Disease Control Programme and Animal Disease Surveillance.

Systematic Control of Livestock Diseases of National Importance

Under this programme assistance is provided to State/Union Territory governments for control of tuberculosis, brucellosis, swine fever, canine rabies, pulloram disease, control of infertility, sterility and abortions in bovines, control of emerging and exotic diseases, strengthening of poultry disease diagnostic laboratories and creation of disease free zones.

Foot and Mouth Disease Control Programme

The objective of this programme is to protect the valuable and high-yielding livestock belonging to weaker sections by proper vaccination against foot and mouth disease. For this purpose, vaccines are provided at subsidized price to the farmers i.e. sharing the cost between the Central and State Governments and the beneficiary in the ratio of 25:25:50.

Animal Disease Surveillance

Under this programme information is collected on the incidence of various livestock and poultry diseases from States and Union Territories and it is compiled for whole of the country. The information so compiled is disseminated in the form a Monthly Animal Disease Surveillance Bulletin to all States and Union Territories and also to organizations like Office International des Epizooties (OIE), Animal Production and Health Commission for Asia and Pacific (APHCAP), etc. The information system has been harmonized in accordance with the guidelines of OIE. The scheme indicates the disease situation in the country and also helps in working out the disease control programmes. Most of the State governments have started publishing their disease reports in local languages as well. These reports are disseminated to all concerned including livestock owners.

Creation of Disease Free Zones

The objective of this scheme is to create rinderpest, foot and mouth disease and contagious bovine pleuropneumonia free status in selected areas of potential growth of livestock products. The scheme seeks to improve export potential of livestock and livestock products. The scheme is yet to be approved and launched.

National Project on Rinderpest Eradication (NPRE)

Rinderpest is a highly infectious viral disease (Morbilli virus infection) of cloven-hoofed animals inflicting heavy mortality in bovine population as well as in small ruminants. Rinderpest Control Programme in India was initiated during 1957 as a part of the second Five Year Plan. Since then, the programme has been under execution adopting various strategies. The present National Project for Rinderpest Eradication (NPRE) was launched with effect from May 1992 as a part of Project ALA/89/04: "Strengthening of Veterinary Services for Livestock Disease Control with special emphasis on Rinderpest Eradication", for which the European Union had entered into a financing agreement with the Government of India to provide ECU 40.30 million grant. The total allocation of the project was Rs. 2,610 million of which Indian Government contribution was Rs. 330 million for six years. The financial agreement with EU expired on 31.7.1998. Since then the scheme is being implemented with the available domestic resources for continuing all the ongoing activities of the project. The Scheme was sanctioned with a total outlay of Rs. 480 million in January 1999 during 9th Five Year Plan.

The main objective of the project is to eradicate Rinderpest and Contagious Bovine Pleuropneumonia (CBPP) by strengthening the veterinary services across the country and to obtain freedom from rinderpest and CBPP infection following the pathway prescribed by Office International des Epizooties (OIE), Paris.

The Central Government's Department of Animal Husbandry and Dairying is implementing the project, with the participation of Departments

---

The whole country is at present provisionally free from rinderpest. Sero surveillance work initiated in randomly selected 1162 villages in country to generate information for preparing dossier for OIE to attain final stage Freedom form Rinderpest infection. Vaccine against PPR, a dreaded disease of sheep and goat developed at TANUVAS, Chennai. Rinderpest–C-Elisa kit developed by IVRI, Mukteshwar through NPRE funding Eradication programme for Contagious Bovine Pleuro Pneumonia (CBPP) initiated in 8 districts of Assam by NPRE in 2001-2002.

of Animal Husbandry of States and Union Territories, ICAR, and Research Institutes, etc. The technical programme of the project is as per the OIE pathway stipulation. Both Central Project Monitoring Unit and the State Monitoring Units do the implementation and monitoring of the Project by undertaking visits, discussions and regional meetings. The salient achievements of the project is as follows:

(i) Based on the past incidence of Rinderpest and the risk assessment, the country was divided into four zones, viz. (A Zone) North Eastern states, (B Zone) Indo-Gangetic Plains from Kashmir to Vindhas including Maharashtra and Goa, (C Zone) Southern Peninsular States and UTs, (D Zone) Island Territories of Andaman and Lakshadweep. The country declared "provisional freedom from Rinderpest" for A, B & D Zones in 1995 (effective June, 1994) and May 1996 (Maharashtra and Goa). The last provisional freedom declaration for the C Zone States was made with effect from 1st March 1998. Thus the whole country is currently provisionally free from rinderpest with effect from 1st March 1998.

(ii) To implement the NPRE Programme, the Project established 32 ELISA Laboratories, strengthened National Morbilli Virus Laboratory at Indian Veterinary Research Institute (IVRI), Mukteswar, Elisa Testing and Data Management Centre (ETDMC) at Institute of Animal Health and Veterinary Biologicals, Bangalore, to support the programme.

(iii) Veterinary services were strengthened by providing vehicles, sophisticated equipment, cold chain equipment and other support for infrastructure development of the veterinary services of the States and Union Territories.

(iv) Nine Biological Production Units were strengthened for production of Rinderpest and other vaccines.

(v) Rinderpest vaccination was undertaken in C Zone States up to 31 December 1997. The vaccination in the country was totally banned with effect from March 1998 excepting a 30 km wide immune belt maintained along the Indo-Pak border because of rinderpest in Pakistan. This was also stopped from October 2000.

(vi) Six strategic vaccine banks with a Rinderpest vaccine reserve of 2.5 million doses have been established to meet any eventuality due to reemergence of disease at any stage.

(vii) Dossier for attaining the second stage "Substantive freedom from Rinderpest disease" has since been submitted to OIE, Paris.

(viii) The programme for eradication of Contagious Bovine Pleuro Pneumonia has been initiated in Assam, which is to be taken up jointly by Department of Animal Husbandry, Assam, and Indian Veterinary Research Institute, Izatnagar under the supervision of NPRE.

(ix) With the stoppage of Rinderpest vaccination in the country, to control PPR, Rinderpest like disease in sheep and goats, steps have been taken for development of indigenous vaccine against PPR.

Government animal health programme however, seems to have limited impact. This is because despite large numbers there is only one veterinary institution per 10,000 animals. Tripura, Punjab, Haryana, Himachal Pradesh and Kerala has one unit for approximately 5,000 animals, whereas comparable figures for West Bengal and Rajasthan were 20,000-25,000 animals. The quality and accessibility of health services, barring some cooperatives and Non-Government Organizations (NGOs) generally remain poor. Moreover, the share of professional staff responsible for disease investigation and control has been meagre 3.5 percent, supplemented by a limited disease prevention role of the animal health services in the field. Thus, the primary emphasis is on clinical services, and, as a result, endemic diseases such as Foot and Mouth Disease (FMD) are still prevalent in India. During the three years period 1995-98, the incidence of FMD and Facioliasis has increased substantially. However in the year 2000 its incident as well as incidence of other diseases had declined sharply (Table 10.1). According to some estimates, India suffers a loss of Rs. 50 billion (US$ 1.2 billion) in annual production as a result of neglect of disease prevention and control. Indeed, the limited emphasis on preventive services contributes to India's inability to eradicate animal disease epidemics. This undercuts the country's competitive advantage in the global marketplace. Due to the prevalence of some diseases, the sanitary and phytosanitary regulations of many OECD countries deny entry to Indian livestock products, despite the 'minimum access clause' of the World Trade Order, which is open to all countries.

Curative veterinary services, delivered to the farmers with heavy subsidies, have expanded considerably over the last few decades. But they continue to be characterized by poor quality. Among over 51,000 veterinary institutions in the country–employing over 10,000 of professionals and para-professionals–very few are equipped with clinical diagnosis facilities and those that do exist are very old. Lack of facilities for clinical diagnosis is at least in part responsible for indiscriminate use of antibiotics and anti-infectives, leading to high cost of drugs and medicines and presenting a threat to human because of the risk of inducing drug resistance.[1]

As mentioned earlier, on the health side, the focus throughout the planning period has been enhancing the supply of veterinary services by expanding the capabilities and coverage of the State Departments of Animal Husbandry. Over 75 percent of the total staff either provided curative health services or implemented other livestock development schemes. The share of professional staff responsible for disease investigation and control was a meagre 3.5 percent. As a result, endemic disease such as Foot and Mouth Disease (FMD) continues to prevail in India. As a result of neglect of disease

---

[1]Vinod Ahuja et al: Agricultural Services and the Poor: Case of Livestock Health and Breeding Services in India: Indian Institute of Management, Ahmedabad: The World Bank and Swiss Agency for Development and Cooperation

Table 10.1: Disease-wise Incidence of Livestock Disease in India During the Calendar Year 1997-2001

Sl. No.	Disease name	Species name	Outbreaks (in Nos.)					Attack (in Nos.)					Death (in Nos.)				
			1997	1998	1999	2000	2001	1997	1998	1999	2000	2001	1997	1998	1999	2000	2001
1.	Foot and Mouth Disease	Bovine	6343	572	940	900	2638	46022	64240	35574	18532	62499	589	2472	697	119	1274
		Ovine/Caprine	54	15	31	4	21	2214	3479	420	67	12542	200	45	72	4	208
		Swine	4		3	6	28	14		11	16	163	5		0	2	29
		NS	54	43	44	8	789	2046	2070	2228	106	11757	148	74	64	0	28
		Cattle				11					306					1	
		Buffalo				3	14				74	6781				0	105
	TOTAL		6455	630	1018	932	3490	50296	69789	38233	19101	93742	942	2591	833	126	1644
2.	Haemorrhagic Septicaemia	Bovine	1251	994	409	299	1150	6751	7833	4521	1724	6177	3594	2910	1847	774	2867
		Ovine/Caprine	22	7	18	11	11	559	40	150	224	1439	142	7	66	54	149
		NS	179	72		1	32	1049	1666		160	505	644	113		10	39
		Cattle				6					84					14	
		Sheep and Goat					0					21					10
		Buffalo				6	410				58	2399				18	894
		Swine		1					17					7			
	TOTAL		1452	1074	427	323	1603	8359	9556	4671	2250	10541	4380	3037	1913	870	3959
3.	Black Quarter	Bovine	615	457	273	318	840	2592	1715	1389	1105	2905	1351	950	513	517	1273
		NS	96	68	1	1		383	232	4	401		179	124	3	10	
		Cattle				2					15					10	
		Ovine/Caprine			14		0			111		45			19		41
		Avian			1					4					4		
		Buffalo					11					106					44
	TOTAL		711	525	289	321	851	2795	1947	1508	1521	3056	1530	1074	539	537	1358

Table 10.1: Disease-wise Incidence of Livestock Disease in India During the Calendar Year 1997-2001 (Contd.)

Sl. No.	Disease name	Species name	Outbreaks (in Nos.)					Attack (in Nos.)					Death (in Nos.)				
			1997	1998	1999	2000	2001	1997	1998	1999	2000	2001	1997	1998	1999	2000	2001
4.	Anthrax	Bovine	75	41	43	31	157	230	154	117	166	690	153	110	80	144	417
		Ovine/Caprine	58	43	41	3	128	756	233	229	23	456	646	183	146	21	388
		Buffalo					3					15					13
		NS	9	3	1	5	5	27	34	4	5	10	24	9	0	0	7
		Ovine	8					13					13				
	TOTAL		150	87	85	39	293	1026	421	350	194	1171	836	302	226	165	825
5.	Fascioliasis	Bovine	113	121	96	125	625	9341	17594	3135	2790	5165	105	866	99	4	4
		Ovine/Caprine	35	20	30	9	52	2125	2553	1523	660	1385	14	79	145	3	59
		NS	1			3	83	4			7249	9273	0				368
		Carpine	8			10		583			136		5			1	
		Ovine	9			2		205			131		0			0	
		Cattle				18					1050					0	
		Swine										2					
		Buffalo		1	4	1	9		12	4	36			2	0		0
		Camel					2					24					0
	TOTAL		166	142	130	168	771	12258	20159	4662	12052	15849	124	947	244	8	431
6.	Enterotoxaemia	Ovine/Caprine	94	93	166	34	421	1965	1136	1472	476	4340	702	552	1034	105	1694
		Ovine				1					200					0	
		Carpine				2					5					1	
		Buffalo				1					4					0	
		Avian			0					0					0		
		Bovine	6	19				59	87				51	71			
		NS	58	3				670	24				622	14			
	TOTAL		158	115	166	38	421	2694	1247	1472	685	4340	1375	637	1034	106	1694

Table 10.1: Disease-wise Incidence of Livestock Disease in India During the Calendar Year 1997-2001 (Contd.)

Sl. No.	Disease name	Species name	Outbreaks (in Nos.)					Attack (in Nos.)					Death (in Nos.)				
			1997	1998	1999	2000	2001	1997	1998	1999	2000	2001	1997	1998	1999	2000	2001
7.	Sheep and Goat Pox	Ovine/Caprine	93	55	48	63	434	3831	5685	861	2930	7434	438	558	193	216	1907
		Carpine				6					22					0	
		Ovine				5					848					9	
	TOTAL		**93**	**55**	**48**	**74**	**434**	**3831**	**5685**	**861**	**3800**	**7434**	**438**	**558**	**193**	**225**	**1907**
8.	Blue Tongue	Ovine/Caprine	29	9	75	5	710	1018	8999	960	114	17983	250	188	176	11	1884
		NS						5									
		Ovine	2			1					20		0			0	
	TOTAL		**31**	**9**	**75**	**6**	**710**	**1023**	**8999**	**960**	**134**	**17983**	**250**	**188**	**176**	**11**	**1884**
9.	Contagious Caprine Pleuro-Pneumonia	Ovine/Caprine	10	5	6	1	16	1075	306	624	100	964	55	63	155	0	197
		NS				1					5					0	
		Carpine				3					28					0	
		Ovine				2					38					11	
	TOTAL		**10**	**5**	**6**	**7**	**16**	**1075**	**306**	**624**	**171**	**964**	**55**	**63**	**155**	**11**	**197**
10.	Amphistomiasis	Bovine	6	14	15	23	231	852	341	47	435	3993	9	30	1	0	14
		Ovine/Caprine	12		6	1		1169		23	17		0		0	0	
		NS	2				8	30				190	0				0
		Carpine				7	25				20	311					2
		Cattle				7					34						
		Buffalo				5	3				20	9					0
	TOTAL		**20**	**14**	**21**	**43**	**267**	**2051**	**341**	**70**	**526**	**4503**	**9**	**30**	**1**	**0**	**16**

Table 10.1: Disease-wise Incidence of Livestock Disease in India During the Calendar Year 1997-2001 (Contd.)

Sl. No.	Disease Name	Species name	Outbreaks (in Nos.)					Attack (in Nos.)					Death (in Nos.)				
			1997	1998	1999	2000	2001	1997	1998	1999	2000	2001	1997	1998	1999	2000	2001
11.	Schistosomiasis	Bovine	6		1	1	37	32	1	1	8	257	0	0	0	0	0
12.	Swine Fever	Swine	60	34	66	47	236	2669	818	4560	1217	13224	552	354	921	43	1195
		NS		56	45				2673	2530				681	436		
		Bovine		1					6					1			
	TOTAL		60	91	111	47	236	2669	3497	7090	1217	13224	552	1036	1357	43	1195
13.	Ranikhet (New Castle) Disease	Avian	766	148	324	330	1387	125531	22692	24418	23653	71478	27823	2732	7802	10953	27994
		NS		5		26			370		4156			15		1357	
	TOTAL		766	153	324	356	1387	125531	23062	24418	27809	71478	27823	2747	7802	12310	27994
14.	Coccidiosis	Bovine	2	18	5	14	104	74	448	5	141	17840	0	69	0	1	373
		Ovine/Caprine	2	10	3	2	62	1488	1448	44	5	3745	158	52	17	0	0
		Swine				1	32				3	569					47
		Avian	95	107	133	118	962	43340	47401	35880	57629	134449	3179	4618	5419	2767	7690
		Carpine				3					38					0	
		Cattle				2					7					0	
		Buffalo					31					202					0
		NS		1	12		129		10	700		1053		10	40		194
	TOTAL		99	107	153	140	1320	44902	49307	36629	57823	157858	3179	4809	5476	2768	8304
15.	Fowl-Pox	Avian	105	88	48	38	429	18519	1954	7918	1780	15256	657	78	2149	224	1194
16.	Fowl Cholera	Avian	21	24	8	7	80	790	606	119	223	1494	162	125	2	81	373
		Swine				4					13					0	
	TOTAL		21	24	8	11	80	790	606	119	236	1494	162	125	2	81	373

Table 10.1: Disease-wise Incidence of Livestock Disease in India During the Calendar Year 1997-2001 (Contd.)

Sl. No.	Disease name	Species name	Outbreaks (in Nos.)					Attack (in Nos.)					Death (in Nos.)				
			1997	1998	1999	2000	2001	1997	1998	1999	2000	2001	1997	1998	1999	2000	2001
17.	Infectious Bursal Disease	Avian	1320	98	211	42	472	111913	36298	8912	8279	34565	14066	3190	1442	1389	7584
		NS	10	4				5970	8340				506	2190			
	TOTAL		1330	102	211	42	472	117883	44638	8912	8279	34565	14572	5380	1442	1389	7584
18.	Marek's Disease	Avian	1	3		1	3	21	90			138	21	90		301	0
19.	Salmonellosis	Avian	59	9	17	26		40714	23465	34729	70157		3753	647	5117	2911	
		Bovine				3	1				50	100				0	23
		Swine				7	24				57	336				1	6
	TOTAL		59	9	17	36	25	40714	23465	34729	70264	436	3753	647	5117	2912	29
20.	Duck Plague	Avian	4	2	4	3	24	424	10	1150	141	1434	17	10	1099	85	400
21.	Canine Distemper	Canine	20	5	72	126	436	597	11	1504	1146	2984	88	2	212	118	571
22.	Rabies	Bovine	12	10	11	14	83	113	140	65	34	384	70	137	35	34	297
		Canine	24	24	8	9	20	76	181	9	10	71	34	166	9	5	70
		Equine	2					18					0				
		NS	1	16		5	11	1	34		21	91	1	33		21	75
		Ovine/Caprine	1			1	10	1				65	1				65
		Cattle				1					2					2	
		Buffalo					6					43					41
	TOTAL		40	50	19	29	130	209	355	74	67	654	106	336	44	62	548
23.	Brucellosis	Ovine/Carpine	5	1	1	1	1	131	198		41	26		0			0
		Swine				1					1						
		Ovine				2					108						
		Bovine		2	1		2		44	1		34		7	0		1
	TOTAL		5	3	1	4	3	131	242	1	150	60	0	7	0	0	1

Table 10.1: Disease-wise Incidence of Livestock Disease in India During the Calendar Year 1997-2001 (Contd.)

Sl. No.	Disease Name	Species name	Outbreaks (in Nos.)					Attack (in Nos.)					Death (in Nos.)				
			1997	1998	1999	2000	2001	1997	1998	1999	2000	2001	1997	1998	1999	2000	2001
24.	Chronic Respiratory Disease	Avian	54	57	43	13	123	6258	57849	274	3180	19338	1119	3795	239	96	563
25.	Babesiosis	Bovine	31	17	15	124	447	1458	83	145	1872	9454	4	19	4	11	26
		NS	9	1		1	2	42			37	56	0			0	1
		Avian				2	27				251	196				15	0
		Caprine															
		Cattle				9					13					0	
		Camel					1					1					0
		Buffalo				3	15				6	33				0	0
	TOTAL		40	17	15	139	492	1500	83	145	2179	9740	4	19	4	26	27
26.	Anaplasmosis	Bovine	12	1	3		16	56	2		3	251	0	0			0
		Caprine	1					4					0				
	TOTAL		13	1	3		16	60	2		3	251	0	0			0
27.	Mastitis	Bovine	59	34	88	102	155	8027	887	1443	1649	25624	3	24	0	0	9
		NS	1			2		7			24		0			0	
		Ovine/Caprine	16				26	1810				3940	0				0
		Cattle				13					51						
		Buffalo					20					162					0
	TOTAL		76	34	88	117	201	9844	887	1443	1724	29726	3	24	0	0	9

Table 10.1: Disease-wise Incidence of Livestock Disease in India During the Calendar Year 1997-2001 (Contd.)

Sl. No.	Disease name	Species name	Outbreaks (in Nos.)					Attack (in Nos.)					Death (in Nos.)				
			1997	1998	1999	2000	2001	1997	1998	1999	2000	2001	1997	1998	1999	2000	2001
28.	Theileriasis	Bovine	7	11	2	2		52	1360	6	10		3	116	1	4	
		Cattle				2					2					0	
		Ovine/Caprine	1		1			30		1			4				
	TOTAL		**8**	**11**	**3**	**4**		**82**	**1360**	**7**	**12**		**7**	**116**	**1**	**4**	
29.	Trypanosmiasis	Bovine	11	36	44	11	49	56	478	386	184	529	5	35	27	9	62
		Camel	1		2	3	1	3		6	15	1	0		0	0	0
		Buffalo				1					58					0	
		NS	1		12			4		13			0		2		
	TOTAL		**13**	**36**	**58**	**15**	**50**	**63**	**478**	**405**	**257**	**530**	**5**	**35**	**29**	**9**	**62**
30.	Mange	Bovine	15	10	77	24	88	384	627	603	687	3990	0	6	0	0	4
		Ovine/Caprine		54	3	5	3		4876	444	26	18		85	0	0	0
		Canine		4	3	94	280		34	42	868	1303		0	0	5	5
		Avian				1	1				60	150				0	0
		Carpine	2			16		203			199		0			0	
		Ovine				1					54					0	
		Camel					3					15					1
		Swine				144	494				2081	5917				0	0
		NS			83					430					0		
		Buffalo					1					58					0
	TOTAL		**17**	**68**	**166**	**285**	**870**	**587**	**5537**	**1519**	**3975**	**11451**	**0**	**91**	**0**	**5**	**10**
31.	Pests Des petitis Ruminants	Ovine/Caprine	82	164	180	2	320	3456	7411	13568	101	35115	852	2037	3260	32	5477
		Ovine				2					401					65	
	TOTAL		**82**	**164**	**180**	**4**	**320**	**3456**	**7411**	**13568**	**502**	**35115**	**852**	**2037**	**3260**	**97**	**5477**

Table 10.1: Disease-wise Incidence of Livestock Disease in India During the Calendar Year 1997-2001 (Contd.)

Sl. No.	Disease Name	Species name	Outbreaks (in Nos.)					Attack (in Nos.)					Death (in Nos.)				
			1997	1998	1999	2000	2001	1997	1998	1999	2000	2001	1997	1998	1999	2000	2001
32.	Sheep Pox	Ovine	103			2					192					0	
	TOTAL	Ovine/Caprine	**103**			**2**	**2**	**1457**			**192**	**56**	**895**			**0**	**3**
33.	Goat Pox	Caprine	13			24	2	347			379	56				9	3
	TOTAL	Ovine/Caprine	**13**			**24**	**2**	**347**			**379**	**56**	**88**			**9**	**3**
34.	Cow Pox	Bovine	1			1	5	600			15	24	10			0	0
35.	Surra	Bovine	6					115					9				
36.	Pullorum Disease	Ovine/Caprine		11					2787					266			
		Avian		1	1				1	1				1	1		
	TOTAL			**12**	**1**				**2788**	**1**				**267**	**1**		
37.	E.Coli/ Collibacillosis	Avian		4					7					7			
	TOTAL			**4**					**7**					**7**			
38.	Lencosis	Bovine		6					2073					155			
	TOTAL			**6**					**2073**					**155**			

Source: Basic Animal Husbandry Statistics, Ministry of Agriculture.

prevention and control India continues to suffer a colossal loss in production each year and it is the poorest section of the society who bears the brunt of these avoidable losses.

AN EVALUATION

In this connection, findings of a field study in three sates: Gujarat, Rajasthan and Kerala, where the Animal Husbandry Departments have already introduced fees for providing some services, would be of interest. The study covered two major components: (i) an evaluation of the efficiency and effectiveness of the primary animal health and breeding services delivery systems in the three states, and (ii) a survey of livestock owners to determine the factors influencing their demand for these services, their willingness to pay and the impact of cost recovery and/or privatization on the welfare of the poor. In terms of livestock and service type, the focus of the survey was on curative veterinary and AI services for cattle and buffalo.[1]

The result of the field survey indicated that the cost of delivering curative veterinary and AI services were significantly higher in the government system compared to the private and other nongovernment veterinarians/inseminators. A major share of these costs were due to the salaries and benefits of veterinarians and para–veterinarians, employed by the government on full time basis, opportunity cost of land and building and other overhead costs. Although the government veterinary services were only available at the centre, the household survey showed that a large number of cases were attended to at homes of the farmers. In Gujarat, for instance, less than 10 percent of total cases in the survey were attended to at the center. It was quite common for the government veterinarians to attend even the ordinary sickness cases at farmers' homes and a majority of these cases were attended in private capacity. The extent of in-centre service appeared to be somewhat higher in Rajasthan although even here over 70 percent of all cases were attended at home. Comparable figure for Kerala was 60 percent.

However, the service users rarely received the service at the prescribed price. Indeed, to receive the government services the users paid prices several times higher than the legally mandated. Moreover only a small proportion of those who received services at the official prices belonged to the 'poor' category. For instance in Rajasthan only about 10 percent of these free services belonged to the poorest 20 percent category. In Kerala, the comparable figure was about 30 percent. In both these states about 40 percent of those receiving free service belonged to the richest households. It was clear from this survey that there was no targeting of free services towards the poor.

As regards the AI, the private providers charged the highest fee in both Gujarat and Kerala. Nonetheless, the rate of conception was also higher for the inseminations done by the private providers. In Kerala, for example,

[1]Ahuja, Vinod et al., op. cit.

for the total 393 sample cases for which results were known, only 142 resulted in pregnancies. This gives a conception rate of about 43 percent. A comparable figure for private providers was 58 percent. At these conception rates, services of private inseminators turn to be cheaper than those of government providers.

Based on these findings, the study recommends a redefinition of the role of governmental sector by moving the curative veterinary and AI services into the realm of the private sector. The fear that such a policy could lead to a drastic decline in the use of services is unfounded. Farmers, including the poor farmers and landless households, value these services tremendously and are not seeking free or subsidized services. Indeed they are already paying prices that are not significantly lower than those charged by private veterinarians.

LIVESTOCK HEALTH SERVICES

All livestock services in India are provided by the state governments with the minor exception of services provided by the milk cooperatives to their members and some marginal activity by nongovernmental organizations. Curative veterinary care and artificial insemination are the two most important services that the governments provide. The state department of animal husbandry is the governments implementing arm for services delivery. All services are free or are heavily subsidized; and are provided at the institutions of the department.

When the planned era of development started in 1951 with the launch of the first five year plan, India had only some 2000 veterinary institutions. By the turn of the century and after 9 five year plans, this has grown to 51000 veterinary institutions, manned by 36000 professional veterinarians and 70000 para vets. These institutions are all for delivery of free veterinary services and some 30000 of them also provide AI services. This growth, the institution based delivery of services and the free services together have made the network unwieldy and financially unsustainable. Fiscal constraints have now forced the state governments to restrict financial support to these institutions to barely cover the establishment costs: animal husbandry departments spend 90 per cent of their annual budgets on salaries, travel and transport; and leave less than 5 per cent for medicines and consumable for treatment of animal diseases. The livestock owners therefore receive in these centers only a prescription and he has to procure all medicines and consumable for treatment, from the local trade at his cost. The combined share of all states in the pharmaceutical trade of over Rs. 500 crore (1997) annually, all India, is less than 5 per cent or Rs. 25 crore for veterinary drugs and pharmaceuticals. The governments believe that the services are free, but there is now empirical evidence to show that livestock owners incur substantial expenses for availing of the services and that the subsidies built into them seldom reach the poor.

Almost all veterinary drugs, pharmaceuticals and vaccines required for livestock health care are manufactured. In India: drugs and pharmaceuticals predominantly by the privates sector, while vaccines and biological both by the public and private sector. Special drugs and vaccines, not made in India are imported on need basis. In spite of the very large animal and poultry populations and an annual output value of over Rs. 1,23,000 crore, the veterinary pharmaceutical industry in India is small and circumscribed, with a turn over of around Rs. 500 crore per annum.

AI Services

Artificial insemination services for cattle and buffalo too are provided in the AI Centres of the department. Livestock owners have to take the animals in heat to the centre for receiving AI. India has a very large AI infrastructure, perhaps the single largest in the world: 63 frozen semen production stations, production of some 36 mln doses of frozen semen per year, some 42,000 AI Centres nation wide. Annually this services carries out some 25 mln artificial inseminations in the country 90 percent of it in cattle and some 10 per cent in buffalo.

Nevertheless the service covers only some 20 per cent of the breeding female among cattle and not even 5 per cent of the buffalo, the conception rate to AI is less than 20 per cent and AI does not result in successive generations of superior progenies as the bulls used for AI are unselected. The centre based delivery of the service limits its scope and coverage. In short, the quality of AI services in India is very poor.

Use Pattern of Government Services

According to a study (Vinod Ahuja) the government is the primary provider for veterinary services, and the services are to be delivered at government veterinary centers, except in case of emergencies. The household survey data, however, revealed that, in reality, a large number of veterinary cases are attended at home (Table 10.2). In Gujarat, for example, the in-center veterinary service was practically nil. Of a total of 140 sample visits by government veterinarians in Gujarat, only 7 per cent were attended at the centers. The comparable figures for Rajasthan and Kerala were 30 and 43 per cent. It was quite common for the government veterinarians to attend even ordinary sickness cases at the farmers homes and a majority of such visits were undertaken in a private capacity.

Table 10.2: Number of Sample Veterinary Visits Disaggregated by Provider Type

District	Number of visits by				
	Government veterinarian		*Home services by private veterinarian*	*Home services by Co-operative veterinarian*	*Total*
	At home	*At the centre*			
Gujarat	130	10	98	69	307
Rajasthan	178	79	55	9	321
Kerala	304	230	22	2	558

For veterinary services at the center, the prices prescribed by the government were either zero or very nominal (Rs. 5 per visit in Gujarat and free in Rajasthan and Kerala). However, the services users often paid much higher prices. To understand the structure of the price paid by the users, data were collected on three components – (i) fee paid to the veterinarian (comprising service charge, transportation charge in the case of home service and any drugs and medicines supplied by the veterinarian); (ii) price of additional medicines purchased from the private medical stores; and (iii) additional transportation and communication expenditures incurred by the user. The average fee paid to the veterinarian for in-centre service was about Rs. 41 in Rajasthan and Rs. 18 in Kerala (Table 10.3). The average price paid per visit including the price of drugs and medicines was Rs. 128 in Rajasthan and Rs. 55 in Kerala. It may be recalled that the treatment received in both these centers were supposed to be provided for free.

Table 10.3: Average Expenditure for Veterinary Service at the Government Vetrinary Centre

(Rs)

State	Doctor's fee	Total visit cost*
Rajasthan	41.3	128.1
Kerala	18.4	54.9

*Including the cost of additional medicines

This is not to say, however, that no one received free services at the veterinary centers. Indeed, over 60 per cent of the cases attended at the veterinary centers in Rajasthan and about 58 per cent in Kerala were provided free services (excluding the cost of medicines purchased at the stores). However, as only about 30 per cent of the total cases attended by government veterinarians in Rajasthan were at the veterinary centers, free services actually only accounted for about 18 per cent of total cases attended by government veterinarians in Rajasthan and 25 per cent in Kerala. The prescribed fee for emergency home visits was equivalent to that for in-centre service except that the government veterinarians were allowed to charge a nominal amount to cover transportation cost. In reality, however, the charges were significantly higher than what could be justified as the transportation cost.

The projected livestock population growth and the increased emphasis on more productive crossbreeds, coupled with other sector's competing demands for financial resources will increase budgetary and administrative pressures on the central and state level animal husbandry and dairy departments. Indeed, ensuring an adequate supply of quality livestock services in the face of declining real spending on animal husbandry and dairy activities poses a serious challenge for the future. A more efficient allocation of resources is critical. Achieving needed objectives will require: (i) Redefining public and private roles in the livestock sector; (ii) creating a level playing field; and (iii) establishing appropriate incentives.

Public and Private Sector Roles

The appropriate roles of the two sectors in providing livestock services should be determined by the economic characteristics of each service. Public involvement is required when market failures prevail. This applies three categories of services which are as follows:

- *Delivery of public goods.* The benefits from these types of services, which include sanitary controls and basic research, are available to the entire community, and it is impossible to restrict use to the individual or group who paid for the service. Because of the free-rider problem, the private sector has no incentive to provide these services. They must, therefore, remain a public sector responsibility.
- *Products or services whose quality cannot be immediately assessed.* Also called hazard problems, incentives exist to pass on substandard products such as veterinary drugs, vaccines and semen, since quality cannot be judged at the time of purchase. Public sector regulation is necessary to ensure that products meet established quality and safety standards.
- *When externalities or spillover occur because the services are used.* Services such as vaccinating for infectious diseases protect an individual farmer's animals from diseases (private benefits), and at the same time reduce the risk of a disease transferring to other farmers' animals (extra social benefits). Since farmers purchasing the service do not consider these extra social benefits, they tend to use the service less often than is socially optimal. Consequently, the government needs to control or subsidize these services to increase their use by the farmers.

A New Perspective

The role of public and private sector in the Indian livestock services sector must be adapted to market realities. Economic classification of types of economic services for the public, private and toll goods services is presented in Table 10.4. The private sector can efficiently and effectively, as discussed above, provide those services classified as private goods or toll goods. In the case of private goods, the user can exclusively appropriate the benefits and is thus willing to pay the private fees. Consequently, private suppliers can appropriate the returns for the delivery of these services. Examples include clinical services, artificial insemination, and the production and distribution of veterinary pharmaceuticals. The private sector can also efficiently deliver toll goods. Toll goods are products and services whose supply does not diminish as a result of one person's use, but access to them can be restricted

Table 10.4: Economic Classification of the Type of Livestock Services

Service	Type of economic good			Measures to correct for		Public sector		Private sector
	Public	Private	Total	Externality	Moral hazard	Funding	Provision	Provision
Clinical Interventions								
Diagnosis	X**							YY
Treatment	X**							YY
Preventing services								
Vaccination	X*					Y*	Y*, S	YY
Vector (tick) control	X*					Y*	Y*, S	YY
Veterinary Surveillance								
Epidemiology	X					YY	YY, S	Y*
Diagnostic Support		X*				Y*	Y8, S	YY
Quarantine				X		YY	YY	
Drug Quality Control					X	YY	YY, S	
Food Hygiene/ Inspection					X	YY	YY, S	
Provision of Veterinary Supplies (including vaccines)								
Production		X						YY
Distribution		X						YY
Production services								
Semen Production		X						YY
Artificial Insemination		X						YY
Veterinary Research								
Basic Research	X					YY	YY, S	Y*
Applied Research		X*				Y*	Y*, S	YY
Agriculture Extension	X	X*				Y*	Y*, S	Y*
Milk Recording			X					YY
Herdbook Registration			X					YY
Livestock Insurance		X						YY

X* – private good, with consumption externalities;
X** – private good, with consumption externalities only in case of infectious diseases;
YY – economically justified;
Y* – economically justified only in special circumstances;
S – delivery can be subcontracted out.

Source: Adapted from D. Umali, G.Feder, and C de Hann: "Animal Health Services: Finding the Balance Between Public and Private Delivery: World Bank Research Observer, Vol. 9, No. 1, pp 71-96, 1994.

so that only those who pay for the product or services can enjoy their benefits. Toll goods include milk recording or herdbook registration.

Future policies should strengthen the capacity of central and state agencies to manage tasks that remain in the public sector, such as basic research and most agricultural extension activities. Policies should limit public sector involvement to these tasks as the private sector becomes more established. In addition, the public responsibility does not necessarily imply public implementation. Some services, such as vaccination, food inspection, and veterinary research, can be subcontracted by the state governments for delivery by private sector. The government's role in these activities will be reduced to monitoring and regulation. In some countries vaccinations (Argentina, Brazil, the US, the EU, and West Africa) and food inspections (the US and EU) are being subcontracted to private veterinarians, and delivery is regulated through the inspection of vaccination and inspection certificates. Such an approach will require some modifications of India's regulation.

Creating a Level Playing Field

Public sector domination of delivery of livestock services also constrains private initiative in commercial functions. To remove these barriers, establishing a level playing field between state governments and private veterinarians will be critical. Specifically, clinical care, veterinary drugs, improved genetic stock and semen, and artificial insemination services should be provided with full cost recovery.

For example, semen banking is set to turn professional in Punjab, with the government preparing a business and marketing plan to sell quality semen. This has been done to provide high quality semen of proven and elite bulls to dairy farmers. Under the new scheme which would be taken up by the semen banks of Patiala, Ropar, Kapurthala and Nabha, sire profile directories would be published where in all technical data of bulls would be published along with photographs. While the department publications were likely to encourage farmers to go in for artificial insemination, the department would also market its semen by going down to the grassroot level to convince dairy farmers to go in for the facility.

A study was also conducted by Vinod Ahuja to have estimates of Willingness To Pay (WTP) for curative veterinary services in three states of India, and an analysis of its determinants. It was found that most farmers were willing to pay for receiving veterinary services. Since a larger proportion of households are opting for home service, it suggests that the farmers have a preference for home service. For home service, a significant positive relationship is found between income and WTP in Gujarat. This suggests that the WTP for home service by Government veterinarians is lower for poor households in this state. In the other two states, such a relationship could not be established. For in-centre service, on the other hand, the WTP for government service is lower for poorer households in both Gujarat and Rajasthan.

Constraints in Artificial Insemination System

1. Poor quality of semen, mainly due to inadequate care during its preservation and transportation limited the conception rate.
2. High cost of insemination inhibited many farmers from availing the services of artificial insemination, particularly when the farmers had to take the Artificial Inseminations to their villages.
3. Due to distant location of the Government Veterinary Centers (AI Centers), farmers who resided even 2-3 km away from the center could not avail its services as it was difficult to bring their livestock to the A.I. Center for insemination.
4. Insemination services were available only during the office hours and high temperatures during this time did not favour conception. This resulted in the AI process becoming ineffective. Moreover, the services were not available on holidays.
5. Poor transport facilities to tribal and interior areas restricted the mobility of the government staff.
6. Promoting awareness on the post-insemination care and management aspects was neglected.

One direct message from this analysis is that there is significant demand for these services. The service users, including the poor, are willing to pay, and are paying, to receive these services. There is significant potential for private sector participation and for cost recovery. Adjusting official rates towards full cost recovery can enable the government to raise the necessary resources to improve the availability and private providers, attract greater private participation that could improve the availability of livestock services for all the farmers. As area-specific characteristics, such as income level, size and composition of livestock of herds, do influence the WTP significantly, these factors will need to be considered in formulating an appropriate pricing policy for livestock services.

Establishing Appropriate Incentives

Incentives to encourage public sector vaccinations to enter private practice should be introduced. Such incentives could include granting a one year leave of absence, assuring that the government will cease all interventions in areas where private veterinarians operate, assuring that the government will subcontract services at remunerative rates, leasing out existing public sector facilities to prospective veterinarians, and allowing private importation of veterinary drugs.

It is argued that full cost recovery will lead to a drastic decline in the use of services such as clinical case, vaccination, and artificial insemination, especially by the poor. India's long tradition of livestock raising and management and its considerable experience with veterinary services have made farmers appreciate the value of these services - a fact that should not be underestimated. Given the importance of livestock in many families (as a source of protein and income, draught power, insurance substitute, and store of wealth), the preservation of this asset is highly valued. Indeed cooperatives already explicitly (through direct charges) and implicitly (through lower milk procurement prices) charge their 8 million (most poor) members for veterinary services. Full cost recovery would only improve the market transparency of these fee structures.

Experience in India, as mentioned above, and other countries, shows that farmers are willing to pay for services that are reliable and effective. In Kenya the total availability of services improved markedly and the poor gained greater access to the services when cost recovery was introduced.[1] When veterinary services became commercially oriented in the 1980s, with staff charging for their curative visits, the work output increased significantly and inequality in distribution was reduced by at least half, and more fully commercialized veterinary staff graduated their charges according to the consumer's ability to pay.

For a full cost recovery programme to succeed, the delivery of quality and consistent services must be guaranteed. Moreover, a promotional campaign must accompany the programme to bolster farmer appreciation of the returns from investing in livestock services.

Expanding the extension service under the Tenth Five Year Plan offers good possibilities for absorbing the public sector staff that will be displaced by privatization. Their extensive veterinary training and familiarity with local conditions provide strong foundation for effective extension provision. The continual training of public sector staff in extension techniques, technologies and approaches, will be necessary to ensure the effectiveness of these measures.

NGOs ROLE IN LIVESTOCK IMPROVEMENT—A CASE OF ANTHRAX

Anthrax is an organization based in India, working towards the development of livelihoods of marginalized communities including pastoralists, dalits and tribal groups. Anthrax's approach for improving the livelihoods of the farming communities dependant largely on livestock rearing, is being discussed.

The various activities and interventions carried out by anthrax are largely community led action research projects. While working with diverse livestock rearing and farming communities, problems are defined, different strategies and approaches are identified and implemented and the experiences are documented which serves as an input for enriching the organization's activities, strategies and policies. Some of the interventions carried out by anthrax are:

---

[1]Leonard, D.K., "African Practice and the Theory of User D=Fees: International Livestock Centre for Africa, Addis Ababa, Ethiopia, 1984.

Strengthening Rural Veterinary Health Care Delivery Systems Through Training of Animal Health Workers

In most parts of India, veterinary services are very poor. There is an estimated one veterinarian per 7000 animals. The services are concentrated in the urban and more affluent parts of the country. To make veterinary services available in rural areas, especially in the more remote and inaccessible parts of the country, it has been necessary to look for alternatives. Local healers and trained Animal Health Workers (AHW) do provide an important interface between rural communities and formal veterinary care systems. Healers and AHWs do provide primary health services and valuable preventive solutions such as deworming and vaccinators. They act as change agents by educating and training rural communities on improved health and management practices.

Healers and Animal Health Workers from the local communities are trained in the use of different systems of medicines. As women are the primary caretakers of the livestock in many households, a large number of women have been trained. These Animal Health Workers have been responsible in bringing down the mortality and morbidity rates of livestock in their villages. In addition, they have formed state level networks through which they are able to deal with varied issues related to resources, finances, medicines, etc.

Community Efforts in Conserving Livestock Diversity

Most poor rural communities are dependent on local species of livestock. However, government programmes in the past have given scant attention to these breeds. Programmes for preserving the gene pools of the traditional breeds like *Kanchu Mekha* (dwarf variety of goat), *Dangi* breed of cattle and, *Decanni* sheep, are being taken up by the local communities. For instance, conservation of the *A seel* breed of poultry is being carried out in the East Godavari district of Andhra Pradesh, along with Girijan Deepika, a tribal people's group, and Yakshi, a resource group.

Community Biodiversity Parks: Herbal and Fodder Nurseries

A number of small bio diversity parks and nurseries have been initiated by involving local communities. Here, local varieties of medicinal, fodder and food crops and local breeds of livestock are being grown and reared, thus promoting preservation.

Documentation and Dissemination

Anthrax adopts different methods to reach out to a larger group of farmers. Newsletter and journals are brought out regularly in local Indian languages. Books, posters and other educational materials are also being published in different Indian languages on various aspects pertaining to livestock health management as well as Natural Resource Management. Anthrax had documented details of over 300 traditional species used as fodder.

In one of its projects, the documentation, validation and dissemination of traditional livestock rearing practices has been done by bare foot field researchers trained by anthrax. This has ensured local communities involvement and participation in the process. As a part of the project, anthrax has documented over 700 different traditional remedies used for treating approximately 70 different conditions affecting domestic farm animals and 14 conditions affecting poultry. Extensive directories of the plants and their properties, herbaria and directories of well-known local traditional healers of livestock have been created. The information is shared with the communities in the form of books, newsletters, and other educational materials.

Village outreach programmes are important means of spreading information. Village yatras (campaigns) are held every year in different villages. The topics include livestock health and productivity, natural resource management, social issues and human health. Stalls are also set up at prominent Animal Bazaars. These have become extremely popular among the farmers from different villages. The Animal Health Workers also visit different villages and hold meetings and training programmes and extend their knowledge to other farmers with the help of educational materials designed and produced by the organization.

Policy, Research and Advocacy

Livelihoods of livestock farmers are greatly affected by the policies at the State, Central and global levels. Anthrax attempts to analyze different policy documents and analyse their implications on livestock rearing, especially those practiced by poor rural households.

PARA TECHNICIANS AS ALTERNATIVE VETERINARY SERVICE FOR LIVESTOCK MANAGEMENT

Artificial Insemination (AI) with improved semen has contributed significantly towards upgradation of local cattle and maintaining the genetic superiority of crossbred cows. The artificial insemination has also been instrumental in reducing the calving interval through timely servicing and better conception. Together with the good marketing network, this practice has played a pivotal role in making the Operation Flood, a reality.

However, Artificial Insemination system itself had many constraints (see box), which created a need for looking at alternatives.

The Krishi Vigyan Kendras (KVK), initiated efforts in enabling farmers to access the services of Artificial Insemination for their livestock. The KVKs in collaboration with local NGOs, promoted alternative veterinary services to unreached areas. The experiences are described below.

Case 1: KVK - Mitraniketan NGO, Trivandrum District, Kerala

The Indian Council of Agricultural Research (ICAR) established a Krishi Vigyan Kendra (KVK) under the management of Mitraniketan NGO in

1979-80. Mitraniketan, located in Vellanad village of Trivandrum District, was already working towards alternative livestock services, by providing artificial insemination service by collecting liquid semen from the bulls maintained in its farm. From 1979-80 onwards, the artificial insemination services were brought under the fold of KVK. One of the mandates of the KVK was to provide self-employment oriented vocational training programmes. The idea of promoting para-technicians, served the dual purpose of helping the unemployed youth to be gainfully employed and also in providing service at the farmers' doorstep.

The Animal Husbandry Department in Trivandrum district, has 222 artificial inseminators in its network. The ratio of cows to artificial inseminator was about 1135.1. With about 80% of the cows being breedable, each artificial inseminator has to work with and monitor at least 980 cows in a year. The distribution density of cows in this district is 68 per sq. km Thus, each artificial inseminator was required to cover at least an area of 15 sq. km. But, in reality, the coverage was less than 10 sq. km and the service remained, less than required.

Rural Extension Sub Centers (RESC)/Cattle Improvement Centres

The RESCs are sponsored by the local institutions like panchayat, youth club, village library, milk cooperative society, sports club or some NGOs. There are 22 RESCs in Trivandrum district established during the last two decades. Each serves 2-3 panchayats over an area ranging from 15-25 sq. km. Each RESC is managed by an Artificial Inseminator and is normally located in tribal and interior areas. Few of them has one helper as an additional staff.

Constraints in Artificial Insemination System

1. Poor quality of semen, mainly due to inadequate care during its preservation and transportation limited the conception rate.
2. High cost of insemination inhibited many farmers from availing the services of artificial insemination, particularly when the farmers from availing the services of artificial insemination, particularly when the farmers had to take the Artificial Inseminations to their villages.
3. Due to distant location of the Government Veterinary Centres (AI Centres), farmers who resided even 2-3 km away from the centre could not avail its services as it was difficult to bring their livestock to the AI Center for insemination.
4. Insemination services were available only during the office hours and high temperatures during this time did not favour conception. This resulted in AI process becoming ineffective. Moreover, the services were not available on holidays.
5. Poor transport facilities to tribal and interior areas restricted the mobility of the government staff.
6. Promoting awareness on the post-insemination care and management aspects was neglected.

The youth sponsored by local institutions are trained for 2 months at the KVK. The local institutions provide the necessary infrastructure. The para technician purchases the minimum equipment required like cryocan. KVK provides the technical support and also the liquid semen at a subsidized rate. The para technicians exchange information among themselves, discuss problems and help each other when needed. In addition to the scheduled fortnightly meetings at KVK premises, they often have unscheduled meetings to plan for contingencies and to tide over the difficulties. The para technicians provide the insemination service at the rate of Rs. 75, thus generating income.

The para technicians use several approaches to keep in regular contact with their clients. Farmers located in far-off and interior villages are contacted through contact telephones available in the village, petty shops, medical shops, milk societies, etc. A register is maintained in the RESC to enable the visiting farmers to leave information on the services required, while the para technicians are away on village visits. On return, the para technicians check the register and ensure timely services. Record on every insemination is maintained which helps in monitoring the conception.

Impact on the Project Area

The alternative extension service provided to the dairy farmers by the RESCs and the KVK has several significant features. It has succeeded in filling the gap in the public extension service and thereby meeting the information and service requirements of the dairy farmers. There is a significant impact on various aspects of livestock development since RESCs have started functioning. As compared to 1980, when the RESCs started functioning, currently, the percentage of breedable cows has increased from 54% to 68%, the age at first conception has been reduced from 28 months to 20 months owing to regular contacts and technical support, the conception rate has improved from about 24% to more than 40% due to timely provision of good quality semen, the inter-calving period has been reduced from 20 months to 12 months, simultaneously reducing the dry period from 8 months to 4 months, thereby enabling farmers to get one calving every year.

There has been a substantial improvement in the average daily milk yield from 1.82 litres to 7.5 litres, thus enabling farmers to reap higher returns from dairy.

The para technicians, with the help of veterinary expert from KVK, provide the information on nutrient and disease management. Various camps on livestock health, vaccination, deworming, infertility identification and its treatment are organized at appropriate times. As a result, most of the diseases and problems related to parasites and nutrient deficiencies, have been brought down. This was accomplished by mobilizing communities on a large scale to get desired results.

Case 2: KVK-Myrada NGO, Erode District, Tamil Nadu

The Tallavadi block of Erode district is largely inhabited by tribal population. Owing to geographic remoteness, poor transport and communication facilities, these areas do not have access to, even minimum veterinary services. Demand for an alternative veterinary service was expressed by the tribal people during the participatory processes. The KVK along with MYRADA, initiated the concept of Animal Health Promoters, where a batch of youth selected from remote villages are trained for six months on various aspects. These include livestock upgradation, forecasting and prevention of seasonal diseases and other simple practices like first aid, vaccination, pregnancy test etc. The six-month training is a collaborative effort of the KVK, EDCMPUL (Erode District Cooperative Milk Producers Union Limited), Government Veterinary Hospitals, Milk Producers Cooperative Societies (MPCS), Commercial Dairy Units and Self Employment Training Institutes located in the area. The first batch of training was completed in April 2002. The trainees are attached to an MPCS for better rapport with the customers. Considering the fact that the average education being 10th standard, these youth have been doing a tremendous job with the guidance and support of veterinary doctors and constant monitoring and supervision of the KVK personnel.

Health Implications of Livestock Product Production and Consumption

A discussion of health implications should start with the animals themselves, and the matter of animal welfare should not be dismissed as overwrought outbursts of vegetarian activists. All domesticated species reared for meat are social animals, and their well-developed group organisations are drastically disrupted or altogether eliminated by modern farming methods that force these animals to live either in extreme overcrowding or in complete isolation. These unnatural conditions result inevitably in heightened stress and lead to a higher incidence of density-promoted diseases. Excessive crowding is most obvious in poultry production. Broilers reared in groups of many thousands in tightly packed cages can have as little space as 450-500 cm^2 per bird. That is a square with a side as small as 21 cm, providing just enough room to stand. In contrast, free-range birds may have as much as 25 m^2 of grass per bird, or 500 times as much space— but because of their higher metabolism they will consume up to 20 percent more feed than their caged counterparts.

Pathological demonstrations of crowding include cannibalistic attacks among poultry and pigs. Other common practices that prompt ethical questions about the treatment of domestic animals range from inflicting pain by castration, branding, dehorning, beak trimming, and inadequate stunning before slaughter. No less disturbing are the stress induced through extreme confinement of calves and deep muscle myopathy (atrophy of the inferior pectoralis muscle caused by an inadequate blood supply to the tissue) and skeletal disorders, particularly in the bones of the pelvic limb, associated with the accelerated growth of muscle that is not commensurate with skeletal development in chicken and turkeys. These abnormalities are further exacerbated by the denial of free movement. Moreover, lack of synchronous growth among body components in broilers can contribute to pulmonary hypertension causing excess accumulation of fluids.

These quotidian inhumanities were recently overshadowed by concerns about epizootics that swept through western Europe and parts of East Asia. By far the most dangerous is BSE, commonly known as mad cow disease. Its cause is another unfortunate and still widely used practice of modern animal husbandry, namely the feeding of processed animal tissues (meat and bone meal) to herbivorous species: in the case of BSE it was the meal prepared from sheep infected with scarpie, and encephalopathy-related disease, fed to calves. Between 1980 and 1996 some 750,000 head of cattle infected with BSE were slaughtered for human consumption in Britain, and edible products from these animals could have exposed up to 500,000 people to the risk of VCJD, an aggressively fatal disease. In contrast, foot-and-mouth disease epizootics had taken place in most of the world's countries during the twentieth century, but the British outbreak of this highly transmissible viral infection in 2001 was both serious and spectacular because of the total number of animals involved—8.65 million pigs, sheep, lambs and cattle were killed—and the gruesome manner of their disposal by burning the carcass on giant pyres.

Recent epizootics have not been limited to mammals: H5NI virus spread avian influenza from chickens to 18 people in Hong Kong in 1997 (six of them died). The episode necessitated the destruction of all of the territory's 1.6 million chickens beginning in December 1997. Because the infections coincided with the onset of the usual influenza season, health experts were concerned that human strains might co-circulate with the avian influenza and create new avian reassortant viruses that could be readily spread person-to-person, a development that would raise fears of a new pandemic. Less widespread and less virulent returns of the virus in 2001 and 2002 led to further preventive killings of chickens (nearly 900,000 in February 2002).

Another health concern has been with us since the beginning of massive animal slaughter in America's sprawling Midwestern abattoirs, memorably portrayed by Upton Sinclair (1906). Few people realize that, nearly a century later, meat-packing remains the country's most dangerous occupation. In the year 2000 some 25 percent of all employees in meat-packing plants, or exactly four times the private-industry average, has a nonfatal occupational injury or a job-related illness. In addition, serious injuries and illness (compared in terms of lost workdays) are nearly five times the national average found in private industry (average incidence of 14.3 percent vs. 3.0 percent in 2000), and the frequency of disorders associated with repeated traumas (mainly back problems and tendinitis) is 30 times higher than the private industry mean (812 versus 26.3 cases per 10,000 full-time workers in 2000). These statistics are less surprising when one realizes that some modern slaughterhouses process as many as 400 cattle per hour and some workers make up to 10,000 repetitive knife cuts every day.

Effects of meat-rich Western diets cannot be seen in separation from other nutritional practices and, indeed, from prevailing lifestyles. The traditional Inuit demonstrated that humans can adapt to a diet consisting of little else but a mixture of meat and animal fat. But particulars of that existence—ranging from a basal metabolic rate higher than in non-Arctic populations to active lives energized by a diet rich in polyunsaturated fatty acids typical of marine mammals — have nothing in common with modern urbanites sheltered from temperature extremes by heat and air conditioning, rarely engaged in prolonged strenuous activity, and consuming both food energy and saturated fatty acids far in excess of actual requirements.

Plotting the average meat supply (carcass weight) in the 30 countries with the highest ranking according to the Human Development Index against the average life expectancy of their populations shows a slightly negative slope (lower life expectancy with higher meat intakes), but the correlation between the two variables is practically insignificant (Graph 10.1) On the other hand, there is little doubt that high consumption of animal products in general, and of fatty meat in particulars, is responsible, particularly when combined with high intakes of sugar and low levels of everyday activity, for highly obese populations and elevated incidence of several chronic diseases. It has been observed in the United States that lower food prices brought by agricultural innovation have been responsible for about 40 percent of the recent rise in weight, while the remainder is due to declining physical activity and other factors.

Prevalence of obesity, defined as having at least a 35 percent excess over ideal body weight, was stable in the United States between 1960 and 1980 at about 25 percent of the adult population and it increased by 8 percentage points during the 1980s. By the early 1990s the mean weight gain of 3.6 kg had made every third US adult overweight, with the highest increases among men over age 50 and women between ages 30–39 and 50–59 years.

In Canada, where obesity rates are very similar to those in the United States, it is estimated that the total direct cost of obesity accounts for as much as 4.6 percent of the country's health care expenditure for all diseases . A higher incidence of obesity is now also seen in Europe and in such lower-income countries as Mexico, Egypt, and South Africa. Even in China the nationwide proportion of the overweight urban adults rose from 9.7 percent in 1982 to 14.9 percent in the early 1990s; Beijing's rate of over 30 percent approaches the North American incidence.

Epidemiological studies have linked obesity with generally reduced longevity and specifically with type 2 (non-insulin dependent) diabetes, hyperglycemia, hypercholesterolemia, hypertension, and coronary heart disease (CHD), stroke, and certain malignancies (colon, rectum, prostate, breast, ovary). Obesity's most common structural impacts are orthopedic impairment, pulmonary difficulties, and surgical risk. Among nonsmokers up to 90 percent of type 2 diabetes, between a quarter and a third of CHD and cancers, and nearly a quarter of total premature mortality can be attributed to obesity. For the United States it is estimated that CHD incidence could be cut by 25 percent and congestive heart failure and brain infarction by 35 percent if the country's entire population were at optimal body weight.

In spite of a growing demand for low-fat cuts of meat, most of the iconic meaty meals consumed by millions of Americans every day are very fatty, either naturally or because of fat added during the cooking process. Burger King's Whopper has 55 percent of its 640 kcal of food energy in saturated fat, and fat shares are 54 percent for McDonald's Chicken McNuggets, 53 percent for Sausage McMuffin, 50 percent for Big Mac (560 keal), and 47 percent for KFC's Tender Roast Thigh as well as for Pizza Hut's Meatlover's Pizza. Increasingly popular Mexican fast food, particularly beef (or even more so beef-and-cheese) enchiladas and ehimichangas, also contains 40–50 percent fat. Compare all of that with less than 5 percent fat in wild meat, less than 20 percent food energy as fat in traditional diets, and with no more than 30 percent of food energy as fat recommended by the American Heart Association.

There has been some moderation of fat intake, with the overall share of lipids in the average American diet declining from the peak of about 42 percent during the mid- 1980s to about 37 percent during the late 1990s; but the total amount of saturated fats available in the average US per capita food supply fell by less than 10 percent from the high of 54 g/day to 50 g. Two circumstances explain the extraordinarily high fattiness of popular US meals: beef's high lipid content and the preference for deep-fried foods. While modern breeding has produced some very lean pigs, beef animals remain such more fatty. As a result, prime-grade, boneless cuts of pork have between 25 and 35 percent less fat than similar cuts of beef.

Carcasses of US feedlot-fed beef contain about 57 percent water, 24 percent fat, and 18 percent protein, which means that lipids account for 75 percent of the edible portion, and even what the industry calls "lean trim product" has 50 percent fat. This fact leads to a peculiar situation in which the country that is the world's largest beef producer (and exporter) has become also the world's largest beef importer, purchasing recently nearly one Mt/year of lean trim in order to mix it with its 50 percent-fat trim and lower the share of fat in ground beef, the product whose sales now represent nearly half of the country's beef production and whose appeal is enhanced by making it leaner.

Mass addiction to deep-fried foods changes even the leanest meat into a concentrated package of fat. Raw chicken breast is converted from an extremely lean foodstuff with only 110 kcal per 100 g and less than 3 percent fat to McNuggets of 314 kcal per 100 g with 54 percent of food energy in fat. The increasing popularity of processed meat is another source of concentrated fat. The annual US consumption of all types of sausages now surpasses 11 kg/capita, of which nearly 500 g are pepperoni used on pizza. These processed meats commonly contain 40–50 percent of their food energy in fat.

Cholesterol, a major well-known risk factor in the etiology of coronary heart disease, is an integral part of the cell membrane of animal tissues, hence its presence in meat does not correlate with the fat content of the muscle. Fatty pork and beef have about 70 mg of cholesterol per 100 g, extremely lean white-tailed deer and pronghorn antelope about 110 mg, and even chicken and turkey have about 60 mg. This means that frequent consumption of any kind of meat, and particularly so when such organs meats as heart (275 mg/100 g) or liver (450 mg/100 g) are also eaten frequently, is associated with higher intakes of cholesterol. Classic studies of the dietary cholesterol–CHD link have been recently augmented by a unique set of 100 years of dietary data from Norway (Johansson et al. 1996). They show that a doubling of fat's contribution to total food energy (from just 20 percent in 1890 to 40 percent in 1975) was paralleled by an increase in serum cholesterol corresponding to a 60 percent rise in risk for coronary heart disease. A subsequent fall in fat's contribution to 34 percent of all food energy by 1992 resulted in a 30 percent reduction in CHD.

A health impact of an entirely different kind arises from the massive use of antibodies in all forms of animal husbandry. The Union of Concerned Scientists estimates that more than 11,000 t of antibodies, eight times as much as used in treating humans, are now fed every year to US domestic animals for nontherapeutic reasons in order to prevent outbreaks of infectious diseases in crowded conditions. Pigs and poultry each receive about 40 percent of the total and cattle get the rest. What is most worrisome about these practices is that several antimicrobials that are important as human medicines, including tetracycline, penicillin, and erythromycin, are used extensively for these extensively for these prophylactic treatments. These massive dispensations promote bacterial resistance to essential antibiotics.

The most widely debated recent example is food poisoning (gastroenteritis) caused by the bacterium *Campylobacter jejuni* that acquired resistance to fluoroquinolones (ciprofloxacin and related compounds) when these were used to treat chickens for bacterial infections . Every year an estimated 8,000–10,000 people in the United States contract fluoroquinone-resistant *Campylobacter* by eating chicken. The spread of vancomycin-resistant enterococci in humans is a development of particular concern among hospitalized patients. Thus it has been argued that we should not wait for incontrovertible evidence of harm before acting to preserve the usefulness of many antibiotics in human medicine.

Finally, a relatively widespread acute medical problem is caused by enterovirulent *Escherichia coli* serotype O 157:H7 that causes gastroenteritis and, particularly in children under age five years and in the elderly, a hemolytic uremic syndrome that destroys red blood cells and can lead to kidney failure. Most of this illness, estimated to reach 73,000 cases of infection and about 60 deaths in the United States every year, has been associated with eating undercooked, contaminated ground beef. Meat usually becomes contaminated during slaughter by bacteria living in cattle intestines, and the pathogens can then be thoroughly mixed into large production facilities, infections from a single batch of contaminated meat can occur in many locations simultaneously.

LIVESTOCK AND ENVIRONMENT

Relentless increases in livestock numbers and indiscriminate use of natural resources for livestock production have, over the centuries, rendered all animal agriculture in India unsustainable. It is often argued that large animal numbers are the result of burgeoning demand for animal products. But this argument doesn't hold good in the Indian context, as a substantial portion of the cattle population, the species most responsible for this sorry state of affairs, are unproductive and so dispensable.

Mixed crop-livestock farming is the preponderant farming system and accounts for over 90 per cent of all farming in India. Anthropogenic influences in recent times have upset the crop-livestock and the land-livestock interactions in the most irrigated areas of the country; Trans-gangetic and upper-gangetic plains. The rice-wheat crop crop rotation system in these areas has brought with it many practices that have started to threaten the sustainability of the farming system itself: Livestock production in Punjab for example no longer uses rice or wheat straw as ruminant fodder: over 70 per cent of the straw is burnt in situ. Farm yard manure is no longer used for enriching soils in Punjab. Use of chemical fertilizers and irrigation has crossed ceiling levels, all leading to increasing salinity, deteriorating soil textures and increasing soil toxicity.

Nearly a third of the dry matter intake of large ruminants and almost 100 per cent in the case of the small ruminants come from grazing the common property resources and their numbers are increasing without restraint: cattle population by over 50 per cent, buffalo 100 per cent, sheep 50 per cent, goat 300 per cent over the past five decades. Over grazing by animal populations far higher than its carrying capacity have degraded the CPRs, leaving them with scanty biomass cover, reduction in water points and heavy wind erosion, almost to the point of no return. Forests too are part of the CPRs in India and deforestation in India is one of the highest in the world. Processing animal products is another source environmental damage: untreated effluents from slaughter houses, dairy and other food processing plants. Tanneries and leather processing units are all leading to serious levels of urban soil and water pollution and toxicity. Added to this are the gaseous emissions from ruminants, contributing to global warming.

Impact of Livestock Sector on Public Health

Livestock production is a source of risk to human health in both traditional low-and high-intensity production systems. Risks exist not only from the endemic diseases that prevail in developing countries including India, but also from those that prevail in the highly developed production system when animal concentrations are high, feeds contain contaminants, or milk and meat are improperly handled. Human are exposed to these risks through several pathways. Zoonotic diseases those shared by human and animals, can mutate and spread in animal hosts before passing to humans. Animal waste can carry disease or chemical toxins into the environment. Similarly, milk and meat can expose humans to disease and toxins contained in the animals or produced by improper handling and processing.

In India livestock poses a particular risk to human health, as animal concentrations are located near or around the human habitation including in the cities, because of limited transportation facilities and infrastructure. The risks are compounded by inadequate or nonexistence of health infrastructure (particularly in rural areas), regulations, monitoring or enforcements. Zoonotic diseases such as tuberculosis, which has been nearly or entirely controlled in the developed countries, continue to pose a major problem in India. In fact incidence of this disease that was controlled some time ago, is on the rise again both in the urban and rural areas. Apart from livestock, the increase in the incidence of tuberculosis and other contagious diseases among the human population in India is also due to unhygienic living conditions, malnutrition due to poverty and lack of basic health facilities especially in rural areas.

The drive in India to satisfy the increasing demand for animal protein has resulted in many changes to common agricultural practices. The intensification of the some of the animal production industries, combined with urbanization, global changes and the increasing ease of travel/transport, has produced environments that may lead to an increase in impact of formerly uncommon diseases or even the emergence of new diseases. These changes challenge the normal control methods and indicate that new ways need to be found if these emerging diseases are to be controlled. Measures have already been taken to relocate animal production systems away from where they have developed in peri-urban to an area-wide integrated approach. These man-made relocations will significantly affect the disease determinants and can, if well understood, be used to significantly reduce the occurrence of disease in both animals and man.

Health status of cattle and buffalo has a direct bearing on the health of consumer's milk, meat and their products. There are a few major sources of pathogens in cattle and buffaloes; the animal itself, the environment of the farm where the milk is collected and stored, transport system and hygiene of milk processing. Milk (milk product) borne diseases are classified into two major groups; those that lead to classical gastroenteritis and those, which cause systemic manifestations (brucellosis, tuberculosis and Q fever). One of the major sources of milk borne diseases is the mastitic animal. Mastitis in farm buffaloes is a common aliment in India. Also brucellosis, tuberculosis and Q fever continue to remain endemic in many parts of the country and pose a direct threat to public health. Many diseases are transmitted through contaminated milk viz salmonellosis, Bacillus cereus infection and anthrax.

There are also human health hazards due to environmental pollutants from cattle and buffalo products. Studies conducted in India on toxic metal content in blood and milk of cattle and buffalo reared in urban and various industrial localities, showed a presence of high level of toxic heavy metal as well as toxic levels of chemical residues like insecticides, herbicides, drugs and steroidal hormones. Translocation of these pollutants to consumers not only induces acute health hazards but also cause subtle health hazards. Most alarming effects are: hypertension, neuronal deficits, immunotoxicity, chromonal aberrations and cancer. In view of the serious situation, it is essential that buffalo and other livestock should be reared in pollution free environment far away from highways and industrial location. Drugs and hormonal preparations, when used, statutory caution for withholding of milk and slaughter needs strictly to be followed. National level surveillance and monitoring of environment pollutants in livestock milk, meat and their product are therefore, considered essential.

Biotechnology and Poultry Vaccines: Present Status and Future Possibilities

Poultry industry all over the world has made significant progress in production efficiency due to innovative management practices and the regular use of vaccines to reduce disease related losses. But, the diseases (bacterial and viral) still remains one of the most important hurdle in development of poultry sector not only in India but throughout the world. Annual losses due to various diseases in poultry industry in India are to the tune of Rs. 300 crores. In the International scenario, for instance, the losses due to latest outbreaks of Newcastle diseases (NDV) in California (US) have been estimated to the tune of US $ 300 million. Yet, it is quite reasonable to acknowledge that the incidence of many poultry diseases has been lowered through the use of currently available vaccines consisting of either attenuated (live) or inactivated (killed) vaccines. Today the annual market for poultry vaccines in India is to the tune of about Rs. 140 crores and looking at the growth rate (@ 8%) in the industry, it is expected to rise to the tune of Rs. 240 crores by yr. 2010. However, most of the present day vaccines are produced using age old technologies and therefore have their own pros and cons. Some of the most important drawbacks associated with these vaccines include the following.

1. Laborious and highly expensive production processes.
2. Conventional live vaccines: require maintenance of cold chain up to the point of vaccination, has a possibility of contamination with adventitious agents or other cells, chances of reversion to virulent state, need for refrigeration temperature for storage and limited shelf life. Apart from these, there is a potential hazard to personnel working with large amounts of live micro-organisms like *Salmonella spp.*

3. Killed vaccines also has its own drawbacks like need to ensure complete inactivation, presence of cellular debris, repeated injections and the period of immunity offered by most of these vaccines at the field level are still questionable.
4. Most important factor contributing to the reducing of efficacy of conventional vaccine is the difficulty in differentiating between vaccinated and infected birds or animals.
5. Methods used for quality control of vaccines are time consuming and laborious. For instance, detection of mycoplasma spp. As a contaminant in vaccine product requires weeks to months for isolation and identification.
6. The standards fixed by the international bodies such as OIE, FAO, WHO also limit the use of the number of vaccines. Since poultry and poultry products finally enters human food chain, the residual effects of chemicals used in vaccine production, excretion of virus in case of live vaccines, effect of vaccine strains or ingredients on meat and egg quality are some of the burning issues of the hour linked with conventional vaccines.

During the last two decades, a new subject called biotechnology has emerged as a possible remedy to such problems. Biotechnology is an amalgamation of subjects like microbiology, biochemistry and molecular biology. The use of advanced molecular biology, techniques, identification of immunogenic component of organisms, better understanding of avian immune system and pathogenesis of diseases has mandated that introduction of a number of new approaches to develop and deliver vaccines. Therefore, poultry industry is in favour of developing new generation vaccines that will partly if not completely replace the conventional vaccines.

To attest to that statement, the first genetically engineered fowl pox virus vectored vaccine against Newcastle disease (NDV) virus infection in chicken has been licensed for use in the US. A recombinant avian influenza (AI) – fowl pox (FP) vaccine has been approved for use in Mexico following an outbreak of a highly pathogenic avian influenza (HPAI) virus in 1995. Recently, a live gene deletion mutant Salmonella enteritidis vaccine has also been approved for use in poultry. Various biotechnological approaches have been used for development of poultry vaccines. For better understanding, these modern biotechnologically designed vaccines can be classified into two major categories.

a. Killed/inactivated vaccines
    1. Sub unit vaccines
    2. Recombinant DNA (rDNA) vaccines
    3. Synthetic peptide vaccines
    4. Anti-idiotype vaccines
b. Live vaccines
    1. Gene deletion/mutant vaccines
    2. Live vectored vaccines

Applications of Biotechnology in Quality Control of Poultry Vaccines

Quality Control (QC) of biologicals for poultry use include certification of freedom from extraneous agents. Contamination of vaccines may originate from various materials used for production and during manufacturing process. To date the methods to detect contaminating agents in biologicals consists of either isolation or cultivation in embryonated eggs or demonstration of antibody induction in chicken after immunization. These methods are time consuming and laborious. Therefore, certain biotechnological tools such as polymeraze chain reaction (PCR) is recently being looked as a promising tool since the method is highly specific, sensitive and rapid in yielding results. PCR has been used for detection of mycoplasma, infectious laryngotracheitis, chicken anaemia virus and many other contaminant of poultry vaccines. It may not be surprising if we see this method finding place in European Pharmacoepoiea (EP) in near future.

Applications of Biotechnology in Research and Development of Poultry Vaccines

Strains of infective agents used for production of vaccines are generally antigenically well characterised. Some of the micro-organisms like infectious bronchitis virus (IBV), avian influenza (AI) are highly susceptible to changes like frequent antigenic shift and drift. Due to this, variant strains of such viruses may emerge from time to time and pose problems in control of such diseases by vaccination with standard strains. Under such circumstances some of the recent biotechnological tools like PCR, restriction fragment length polymorphism (RFLP), restriction endonuclease analysis (REA) and gene sequencing are of great value in determining newly emerged variant strains. Such variant strains can be incorporated in a vaccine formulations so as to produce autogenous vaccines. This strategy has helped to a great extent for the control of diseases like infectious bronchitis, fowl cholera and infectious coryza.

Conclusions

The intensive poultry industries rely heavily upon the use of vaccines for disease control. The use of biotechnology to create recombinant DNA vaccines, viral vector based vaccines and gene deletion vaccines offer new avenues for the development of modern vaccines for effective control in poultry. ND, AI, ISD and MD antigens expressed recombinant fowl pox virus have been shown to be effective vaccines for poultry. Although, only few products have seen market place, we may see many more in near future since biotech vaccines are novel, safer, more efficacious and less expensive to produce in order for them to gain a niche in the market place. It may not be an exaggeration if we say that biotechnology promises revolution in poultry industry.

11

Environmental Impact of Livestock Industry

In India, research in economics of livestock production has hardly paid any attention to environment's determining influence on the livestock production system, or for that matter on the reproductive characteristics of the livestock. Nor has any attention been paid to livestock production systems feedback to environment. As regards the feedback from livestock production system to environment, the environmentalists and scientists concerned with global climatic change took the lead in 1980s, and carried it through the 1990s. They focused, however, only on the negative feedbacks, i.e., on the environment damaging effects of the livestock production system. The main focus was on the small ruminants as culprits causing environmental damage in the fragile zones of the country.

In addition to the negative feedbacks, there are a number of positive feedback from Indian livestock production system to the environment, which are either not recognized or if recognized, are not brought up at national or international discussions. The proverbial 'cow dung' used either as manure or as domestic fuel by millions of rural households in India has, for instance, pretty high environmental value. Similarly, India's livestock function as a gigantic recycling machine of agricultural byproducts, and thereby contribute to saving of land, a scarce natural resource. The positive feedbacks are discussed further in this chapter. However, it will be useful to deal with the environments' determining influence on Indian livestock resources.

Livestock Diversity due to Environmental Diversity

India is of subcontinental size and its geographical spread extends from near equator to sub-temperate latitudes (about 8° to 37° N) and from 67° to 98° E longitude. The vast landmass, her physiography and the diverse climatic conditions have made India a home for biodiversity of livestock. That is incomparable to any other country in the world. Let us consider only cattle, for example. Some of the lightweights black cows of the trans-Himalayan Spiti region are reported to have lactation length up to 5-6 years;

so also their crossbreds with yak males called *dzomo*. At the other end, there is Kerala's "dwarf cow", the Vechur, about to be extinct, now revived, which is high milk yielder. A cow in Brahamputra valley is a very different animal than a cow in Haryana. It is quite common to say that the country has 25 well-defined breeds of cattle, but most of the cattle population is 'nondescript". But this common view is based upon lack of complete knowledge. Only recently the National Bureau of Animal Genetic Resources at Karnal has started genetic mapping of our livestock resources. A complete mapping will give the true picture of the country's livestock biodiversity, i.e. not just the number of livestock species, and types of breed within a species but also the genetic difference among the latter including so called 'nondescript'. Given the vast environmental diversity of the country, mentioned above, the complete mapping of livestock is likely to yield a high degree of livestock biodiversity. This is a natural endowment that needs to be preserved. With revolutionary changes taking place in biotechnology of breeding and genetic engineering, it has tremendous potential for generating economic wealth in the future.

Positive Environmental Feedback from the Livestock Production System

The livestock sector requires a balance between animal and man to maintain the ecological biosphere and to enable economic exploitation of the resources without causing irreversible damage to the environment. In India, the livestock sector has played a critical role in the process of agricultural intensification. Cropping systems in the country, based as they are on different agroclimatic and bio-economic pattern, enable farm animals to provide valuable inputs at reasonable costs: e.g. draught potential for cultivating the soils, transporting the produce as well as manure to improve the structure and life of the soil and enrich the soil with plant nutrients. Using farm animals on the field keeps the damage to physical soil parameters within justifiable limits, while growing fodder crops improves the rotation system and helps to reduce soil erosion. Livestock stocks recycled nutrients on the farm, produce valuable output from land that is not suitable for sustained crop production and provide energy and capital for successful farm operations. Livestock helps to maintain soil fertility in soils lacking adequate organic content or nutrients. At the same time they subsist for a major part of their feed on the waste and bye-products of agriculture

By recycling of agricultural byproducts as animal feed, major land saving occurs because the alternative is to produce equivalent amount of green fodder (in terms of DCP and TDN) by allocating required land area. Similarly, the use of dung as manure which substitutes for chemical fertilizers, besides providing plant nutrients (NPK), it protects soil-born micro organisms, and prevents greenhouse gases emission that would otherwise occur in the manufacture, transport and distribution of the equivalent amounts of chemical fertilizers. Further, the use of dry dung-cake as domestic fuel results in land savings because the alternative is to plant and harvest firewood trees, and supply equivalent amount of dry firewood (in terms of thermal energy). Since there is a gestation lag between planting and harvesting of firewood, it requires much more land than the area required to be harvested each year.

The use of working animals in agricultural operations and also for rural transport serves as substitute for tractors and other agricultural machinery run on fossil fuel. The working animals stock thus prevents greenhouse gases emission, in particular CO_2 emission that would otherwise occur due to burning of fossil fuel in running the substitute number of tractors. Incidentally, whereas as fossil fuel is a nonrenewable resource, the working animal stock is renewable.

To quantify the above-mentioned positive environmental contributions to Indian livestock production system is not easy. The Society for Economic and Social Research, (SERS), Delhi, is conducting a major study on this subject with the financial support of the National Dairy Development Board (NDDB). The major difficulty being faced is the lack of reliable, up-to-date data on a large number of parameters that are involved in the estimation. Livestock statistics of the country even otherwise are in a poor state. For instance, the representative up-to-date feeds consumption rates for different age-groups and functional categories of animals, so very crucial for estimation of land saving due to recycling of agricultural byproducts, are just not available.[1]

Negative Environmental Effects

Nevertheless, in India livestock has been one of the causes of environmental degradation. The growth in livestock populations, coupled with shrinking areas, has put intense pressure on existing pastures, encouraged encroachment into forestlands, and contributed to the degradation of land resources. Moreover, livestock processing, particularly leather processing also has been a major cause of industrial pollution. Hence, while livestock development activities generate significant benefits, it must be balanced with environmental conservation measures. A large increase in livestock population in the country seems to be out of balance with feed supply capacity of available land and the waste absorption. While there has been almost 50 percent increase in the livestock population during the last three decades (1970 to 2000), area under fodder crops has shrunk to less than 4 percent of the total cropped area. This is hardly sufficient to support a fraction of livestock. The increased demand for cattle fodder has resulted in overgrazing in some areas. This has led to the degradation of grazing

---

[1]Mishra, S. N: A Note of Environment and Livestock in India: in Conference Proceedings of Livestock in Different Farming Systems in India: Editors: Birthal, Pratap S., Kumar, Anjani and Tiwari, L., Published by Agricultural Economics Research Association (India); 2002, p.81.

land, soil compaction and erosion and decreased soil fertility. Overgrazing in hilly environment has accelerated erosion. There is no doubt that overstocking and overgrazing is damaging to environment. However, if area under permanent pastures in the country is declining, animals are not to be blamed for this. Given the increasing human population pressure on land, the decline in pastures could be due to slicing away of land for other uses.

Overload of livestock population in the country has been responsible for the following environmental problems: (i) Emission from animal husbandry waste load, e.g. microbial or gaseous: and (ii) disposal of carcasses. Excess concentration of livestock produces gases. Some, such as ammonia, remain. Others, such as carbon dioxide (CO_2), methane (CH_4) and nitrous oxide (N_2O) affect the atmosphere by trapping the sun's energy and contribute to the global warming.

The major negative effect of the livestock production system is the methane emission, a greenhouse gas, which has many time more global warming potential than the ubiquitous carbon dioxide. There are two ways in which methane emission occurs: (i) through enteric fermentation of feed in the animals' rumen, and (2) the way dung-manure is managed. Ruminants – cows, buffaloes, sheep and goat, contribute to global warming. India's contribution to global warming from the source is considered high because it has large cattle population. Methane is one of the products generated by the ruminants through chemical reaction of feed by bacteria present in the animal's gut. The other products are volatile fatty acids, microbial cells and carbon dioxide. An international team of scientists in Hyderabad has suggested that India can help reduce global warming by changing the diet of its cows and buffaloes. Micheal Blummel, Chief Scientists of the Team, has suggested that it is possible to select feeds with high degradability in the rumen. The current research using sheep is aimed at finding the ideal feed for Indian cattle that will lead to less methane production[1].

Since in India manure is stored in solid form in the open aerobic conditions, emission on this account is expected to be very small. This is because when managed this way it provides little opportunity to methanogenic bacteria to grow and form methane. Quite in contrast, when dung is stored in covered lagoons and slurry pits, as it happens to be the case in the developed countries, it provides ample opportunity for growth of methanogenic bacteria and methane formation. Methane emission from enteric fermentation depends upon a host of factors, the chief among them being the quantity and quality of feed fed to animals, and of course the number of animals. Experimental research in some of the developed countries has shown that methane emission as a percentage of gross energy intake (GEI) varies from 3 percent to 8 percent as feedgrains are reduced

---

[1] The Economics Times: Feed the Cows Properly to Prevent Global Warming: 18 October 2002.

and forage is increased in the diet. In most normal feeding situations methane emission in the case of bovines works out to be about 6 percent of the gross energy intake (GEI).[1] However, no such measurements in Indian field conditions are yet available. One could nevertheless, apply 6 percent of GEI to Indian bovine stock, and make an estimate of total methane emission form enteric fermentation. But it all depends upon the availability of the data on GE intake of animals in different age-group and functional categories. The GE intake can be derived from the reliable and up-to-date data on feed consumption rates. So the data on the latter is crucial not only for estimating the positive environmental contribution of livestock arising out of recycling of agricultural byproducts as animal feed, but also for estimating methane emission from enteric fermentation. A large number of studies on feed availability and requirement have been done in the country since 1950s. But studies on actual consumption are few and far between.[2] The two studies on feed and fodder availability were carried out based on IASRI pilot surveys in different livestock tracts of the country. However, both these studies are outdated since IASRI stopped conducting such survey way back in 1980s. If the environmental dimension of the country's livestock production system is to be properly studied, it is necessary to take up feed-fodder consumption studies in right earnest.

Escalating demand for dairy products especially in urban areas had resulted in the setting up of a large number of dairy units close to urban centres in India, because of weak infrastructure, high transportation costs and weak regulations. Large-scale poultry operations are also now found in periurban areas in some of the metropolis in the country. These systems have led to severe environment problems. To overcome the pollution and human health problems resulting from concentration of livestock production units amidst residential areas in the cities, some of the state governments, such as Delhi, have established dairy colonies on the periphery of these cities. Most of these units have been relocated to these areas. However, the rapid urbanization has led to the extension of boundaries of the cities. Consequently, residential areas have sprung up around these dairy units, thus nullifying the benefit of the relocation programme. For this, the technology on waste utilization can offer solution to growing environmental and health hazard. Most of the slaughterhouses are old, unhygienic, overcrowded and lack essential services like water, light, drainage, waste disposal and effluent treatment. It is high time that the Government of India should formulate policies and regulatory measures to address the problems of pollution of land, water and air associated with the livestock production.

---

[1]Johnson, K.A. and Johnson, D.E., Methane Emissions from Cattle: Journal of Animal Science, 73: 1995, pp. 2483-2492.

[2]Mishra, S.N. and Sharma, R.K.: Livestock Development in India; An Appraisal. Institute of Economic Growth, Vikas Publishing House, Delhi. 1990.

A production system oriented policy will promote measures needed to gradually reduce animal production and processing in areas with high animal concentrations and waste loads, as well as to attract specialized livestock production into rural areas. Policies that can help correct the negative effects of livestock production include pricing regulations and institutional development. The collective purpose of these instruments is to establish feedback mechanisms that ensure the impact of livestock production is consistent with overall social objectives.

Environmental concerns related to livestock production have focused on such issues as overgrazing leading to the degradation of grasslands and desertification, the grazing of steep slopes causing greater soil erosion, deforestation to create more pastures for cattle ranching, and water pollution arising from intensive livestock enterprises. There is, however, a growing consensus that the importance of overgrazing has been misjudged in the past. This is in part caused by the poor understanding of rangeland ecology, and in part by the lack of appreciation of traditional range management practices in arid and semirigid areas. Similarly periodic overstocking which does occur is often the consequences of institutional and infrastructural problems which form constraints for the marketing of livestock products. These constraints are likely to be overcome as growing urbanization and income growth stimulate expansion of markets for livestock products. Lack of opportunities to raise the productivity of extensive livestock systems and the possible advent of alternative income sources are causing livestock producers to either shift to more intensive systems or to migrate out of agriculture altogether.

Looking ahead, it can be expected that the structure of livestock production in a country like India will converge towards that prevalent in the industrial countries. The dominant proportion of cattle and dairy production will be feedlot, stallfed or other restricted grazing systems, albeit at scales going from simple pens with five or more head to industrial scale enterprises with 100 or more heads. We may assume that by 2030 the bulk of at least poultry production will be from largely landless. This expansion will entail a major increase in the area used for feed and fodder production so that a considerable share of the environmental damage arising from these crops could be attributed to the livestock sector.

This perception has several implications for future environmental pressures arising from livestock production, most of which are not readily quantifiable. The main ones are: overgrazing, soil acidification, compaction and erosion, emission of ammonia eutrophication because of leaching of nitrates in to the soil and water systems, and discharge or runoff of nitrogen and other nutrients from intensive livestock production units into surface waters because of bad waste management; environmental impacts of feed and fodder production. There are two other pressures of global importance, namely emissions of the powerful greenhouse gases-methane and nitrous oxide, and threats to wildlife biodiversity.

Agriculture, particularly livestock production is the dominant source of ammonia, cattle is the main causative factor. The environmental importance of ammonia emissions is that they are potentially more acidifying than the emissions of sulphur dioxide and nitrogen oxides. Moreover, with the past and ongoing efforts to reduce industrial and domestic emissions of sulphur dioxide and to improve energy use efficiency, future emissions of sulphur dioxide are likely to be lower whereas there is little action on reducing cattle emissions of ammonia. The release of ammonia from intensive livestock systems contributes to both local and longer-distance downward deposition of nitrogen causing tree damage and the acidification and eutrophication of terrestrial and aquatic ecosystems leading to declining species richness. Based on projected livestock numbers, ammonia emission in India is estimated at 5.73 million tonnes by the year 2030. (Table 11.1)

Table 11.1: Ammonia Emissions Implied by the Livestock Projection – India

Items	Animal numbers (million)		N excretion (kg/animal/year)		NH3- N class (percent)	Emissions NH3-N/year (million tonnes)	
	1992	2030	1992	2030		1992	2030
Cattle Buffalo	288	160	40	56	20	2.30	1.79
Dairy	64	50	60	84	29	1.11	1.22
Sheep & Goats	232	232	12	16	10	0.28	0.37
Pigs	13	50	16	22	36	0.08	0.40
Poultry	507	6780	0.6	0.8	36	0.11	1.95

Source: F.A.O Asia Study Perspectives

Poultry Industry

According to the report from the National Chicken Council (NCC), two thirds of the country's chicken farms are actively participating in a voluntary programme intended to manage environmental impact of chicken litter used as fertilizers. Offensive odours from animal farming may one day be a thing of the past with the use of essential oils, according to an Agricultural Research Service report. In a recent study, microbiologist Vincent Varel used the essential oils carvacrol and thymol in quantities as low as one gram in one-half-liter slurries of cattle faeces and urine to completely block formation of foul-smelling volatile fatty acids using the oils in combination. Studies were conducted at the Roman L., Hruska U.S. Meat Animal Research Center (MARC), in Clay Center, Neb., to find ways to preserve manure's value as a fertilizer, reduce emission of global warming gases and decrease the prevalence of foodborne pathogens on livestock headed to processing plants. Varel's studies also showed that the essential oils might reduce fecal bacteria such as *E. coli* in slurries. The scientists are now taking their research to manure in the feedlot to test the essential oils against *E. coli* and other pathogens.

Rendering Industry

Almost one-fourth of broilers go waste. Slaughters wastes consist of inedible offals, feathers, blood and condemned birds. Rendering is an excellent way of profiting from waste and thinking 'green' by recycling what would otherwise contaminate the environment. Processed material contains up to 65% protein and a good protein supplement for poultry feed. Dead birds and hatchery wastes (dead-in-shell chicks, unhatched eggs) can all be collected together for valuable poultry manure. However, the cost of setting up a rendering plant is as much as the poultry processing plant itself. A rendering plant would only be justified, if volumes exceed 8,000 birds per day. For setting up of such a plant, sufficient number of broilers should be available within the radius of 100 km and there should be market for 7–8 tonnes of poultry meat per day.

Disposal of slaughter waste is always a problem for the processing plant as these are high nitrogen–and water-containing perishables. Most of the plants which have the byproduct plants, run them when sufficient quantity of waste is accumulated. The main aim is rather the disposal of the waste then profit making. Slaughter waste originating from thousands of retailers spread throughout the length and breadth of the country goes unutilized. This also causes public nuisance when thrown in the municipal waste bins or pits.

In India, considerable work has been done for making fertilizer from unprocessed poultry waste. This method is popularly called the 'Bangalore Method'. However, there is a long way to go for popularizing rendering industry since it is still not cost effective.

By-Products

By-products of poultry industry may be defined as everything from farm or processing that may be used directly as human food. The byproducts may be edible and inedible. Edible byproducts are mainly tissue and bones from the carcasses. Inedible byproducts include manure, feathers, offal, blood, egg shell and hatchery waste. Many of these inedible byproducts from the poultry-processing plant are wasted or dumped in open areas giving a possibility of environmental pollution. Nowadays, environmental pollution laws are becoming stringent and the old practice of dumping waste in open land is no longer acceptable to the environmentalists. The wastes may be salvaged by suitably processing them in byproducts processing plant utilizing wet-or dry-rendering process. The main problem faced in utilization of poultry byproducts is collection of enough material for processing it economically. Insufficient raw material can be utilized along with other animal byproducts. Yield of byproducts from broilers, fowl and turkey of inedible nature is estimated to be immense in future (Table 11.2).

Classification of Byproducts

Byproduct from poultry industry are classified into 3 categories, viz. byproducts from production phase which include litter and manure from the farm; byproducts emanating from the hatchery which represent shells of hatched eggs, dead embryos and dead chicken; and byproducts of the poultry processing plant which include blood, feathers, offals, condemned birds etc. All these 3 categories of byproducts are suitable for converting them into value added products.

With the fast growing poultry industry, the availability of byproducts will be a great menace to the environment if they are not used properly. Conversion of feathers to feather meal will be beneficial, as it has a great potential in the feed industry. Conversion of these byproducts into either feather meal or poultry byproducts meal is more economical than to convert them into manure.

Table 11.2: Byproducts from Broilers, Fowl and Turkey

Material	Live weight (%)		
	Broiler	*Fowl*	*Turkey*
Offals	18.5	18.0	12.5
Blood	3.5	3.0	3.5
Feathers	7.0	7.0	7.0
Mixed byproducts (total byproducts obtained)	28.0	28.0	24.0
Dry products (8% moisture)			
Offals	5.8	7.4	5.0
Blood meal	0.8	0.7	0.8
Feather meal	5.5	5.5	5.9
Mixed poultry byproduct meal	12.8		11.7
Pressed products (1% fat)			
Byproducts meal	5.2	4.3	4.2
Grease	0.6	3.2	0.8

LEATHER INDUSTRY

It is one of the most polluting industries in the country. Its unorganized nature had made it very difficult to implement pollution control norms. Further, the players do not have the money to erect pollution control equipment. The maximum amount of pollution is generated at the time of tanning of leather. This activity is being completely handled by the unorganized sector. After much criticism for its ignorance regarding pollution and being under pressure, the industry has begun to take initiatives for controlling this plague.

With a view to complying with the pollution control standards, the tanning industry in India has started setting up the emission treatment plants and Common Effluent Treatment Plants (CETPs) for cluster of tanneries. There are about 120 individual ETPs and 18 CETPs in Tamil Nadu covering about 80 per cent tanneries.

For controlling the pollution from the tanneries in West Bengal, the state government is trying to relocate the tanneries in the Integrated Leather Complex to be developed as per the directives of the Supreme Court. Tanneries in Kanpur (UP) have already implemented the Common Effluent Treatment Plant in Jaimau under Ganga Action Plan with support from the Dutch government. These measures adopted by the industry are expected to place it at par with environmental standards complied with by units in China and the South Asian Countries.

The industry has attracted a lot of criticism on environmental grounds. First, it has become a major pollutant of ground water and second, it causes a malodorous atmosphere around such locations. This is due to the fact that there is continuous discharge of untreated effluent by tanneries into open drain and rivulets. Western countries also object to increasing use of synthetic chemicals such as pesticides, solvents, dyes, finishing agents and processing chemicals. Environmentally clean processes cost between five and ten per cent of the cost of capital investment for the tanneries.

This problem first surfaced in the early 1970s, when the government of India, realizing that value-added products could fetch more foreign exchange, banned the export of raw hides, skins, and semi-finished leather. The Seetharamaiah Committee set up by the Union Commerce Ministry to study the export potential of value added products which submitted its report in September, 1992, made three major recommendations and pushed for the export of finished leather products. However, the Government implemented the report in part, conveniently forgetting the effluent treatment systems, which the committee insisted upon. At the same time many European countries and the United States banned export of finished leather, preferring to send out raw hides and skins and semi-finished leather for processing, essentially in the third world countries.

PROBLEMS OF DEVELOPING COUNTRIES

As with so many other realities, environmental consequences of animal husbandry are different in rich and poor countries. Expansion of livestock production in the poor world brings further degradation of natural ecosystems and loss of biodiversity arising from deforestation (although the expansion of pastures is not, as in sometimes claimed, the primary reason for the loss of forest cover in most tropical countries) and regular grassland burning. Overgrazing, trampling and excessive soil erosion are common environmental degradations on improperly managed pastures. In contrast, the rich world's carnivorousness, based on high quality concentrates, requires large areas of feed crops. Its most obvious environmental impacts result from concomitant increases in applications of fertilizers and pesticides and from greater soil erosion under corn and soybeans, the leading row crops. How much additional plant food could be produced if we were not growing all those feed crops for our animals?

A great variety of concentrate feed mixtures, crop yields, and feed shares supplied by byproducts and ruminant means that actual land requirements of animal feeding can range two-or even threefold for the same species. The representative North American means have been calculated by using a weighted average for typical yields of concentrate feed crops, assuming a common share of 20 percent of the feed coming from byproducts (as well as the minimum 15 percent share of ruminant roughage) and applying these factors to the previously derived typical feeding efficiencies. Chickens and pigs have similar land requirements in terms of overall food energy, but broilers need the least amount of land to produce a unit of protein, less than one-tenth the need of beef cattle.

But the farmland needed to grow feed for animals is not simply proportional to specific conversion efficiencies. A significant share of feed comes from byproducts generated by processing of food crops, mainly by grain milling and oil extraction. In addition, even when raised in feedlots, ruminants need a minimum share of roughages (straw, hay) whose production does not compete with the growing of food crops. Perhaps a more revealing approach is to compare the overall land claims between largely vegetarian and highly carnivorous societies. An overwhelmingly vegetarian diet produced by modern high-intensity cropping needs no more than 800 m^2 of arable land per capita; the typical Western diet now claims up to 4,000 m^2/capita. Implications of the last rate are clear: today's world's population eating the Western diet whose meat would be produced with feeding efficiencies prevailing during the late 1990s would need about 2.5 billion hectares of agricultural land, that is, 67 percent more than the existing total.

Extension of the affluent world's carnivorousness to the rest of the global population is thus impossible with current crop yields and feeding practices, and many as yet unavailable bioengineering advances could bring it to the realm of conceivable achievement. Quantification of current impacts of competition between food and feed crops is not simple. The more than 700 Mt of cereals and leguminous grains now consumed annually by the world's animals are equal to roughly one-third to the global harvest of these crops, and they contain enough energy to feed more than 3 billion people—but only if those people were willing to eat a largely vegetarian diet dominated by corn, barley, sorghum, and soybeans, today's leading feed crops. A more realistic approach is to assume that the area now devoted to feed crops would be planted, to the extent possible, in a mixture preferred food crops dominated by wheat and rice and that only their milling and processing residues would be used for feeding.

These assumptions would lower the estimate of the additional number of people who could be accommodated on predominantly vegetarian diets to about one billion. The actual number of people who would freely choose such a diet would obviously be much lower. Moreover, because nearly 90 percent of arable land that could be converted from feed to food crops is in affluent countries, additional food produced in that way would only add to the already vast food surpluses to the rich world and would not be readily available to some 800 million of the world's undernourished people who do not have incomes to buy it. A recent report by a leading agricultural organisation goes so far as to conclude that diverting grains from animal production to direct human consumption would result in little increase in total food protein.

Adequate water supply is now widely seen as one of the key concerns of the twenty-first century. Few economic endeavors are as water-intensive as meat production in general and cattle feeding in particular. Broilers have by far the lowest direct (drinking) water requirement, no more than one-third of pigs' need per unit of protein, and less than one-tenth the rate needed by cattle. Naturally, as with the land, the indirect water needs for growing feed far surpass the direct requirements because the production of common feed crops needs at least 1,000 times their mass in water. Consequently, one could think about international meat trade, even more so than about the grain trade, as one of the most effective ways to avoid huge water consumption by importing nations with scarce water resources, or to exercise comparative advantage by water-rich producers.

The lower the feeding efficiency, the higher the production of wastes. In relative terms (per kg of live weight), beef cattle are the largest producer of feces and urine among meat animals, followed by poultry and pigs. Animals are also particularly inefficient users of nitrogen: even such good protein converters as young pigs will excrete 70 percent of all ingested nitrogen. Not surprisingly, Bleken and Bakken calculated average nitrogen retention in animal foods in Norway at just about 20 percent. Annual global production of animal manures (including considerable output by dairy animals) now amounts to more than 2 billion tons of dry matter, and with average nitrogen content of about 5 percent it contains about 100 mt of nitrogen, more than we apply annually in synthetic fertilizers. However, less than half of that total is produced in confinement where it would be available for collection and later recycling to fields. The relative nutrient content of fresh wastes is very low, mostly between 0.5 and 1.5 percent nitrogen and 0.1-02 percent phosphorus, compared to 46 percent nitrogen in urea and 8-9 percent phosphorus in superphosphate.

Even so, animal manures were a valuable resources in all pre-industrial agriculture, and they were regularly applied to fields to renew soil fertility. This recycling kept a substantial share of nutrients excreted by animals circulating within agroecosystems. Modern research confirms that adequate manure applications produce crop and pasture yields indistinguishable from those obtained through the use of inorganic fertilizers. But while traditional farmers often had too little manure to produce the best possible yields, the modern separation of large-scale livestock production from field agriculture makes it impossible to recycle the large volume of wastes produced by thousands of animals concentrated in huge feedlots or sties: for example, four-fifths of all US pigs are now fed on farms selling 1,000 or more animals a year.

Moreover, these large feeding units are increasingly concentrated in particular areas: in the United States six Midwestern States produce about two-thirds of the country's pork, and Iowa has about 1.6 pigs for every hectare of farmland, a low rate compared to about 3.6 animals/ha in Nordrhein-Westfalen and 21.5 animals/ha in Zuid-Nederland. Obviously, cropland in these regions becomes rapidly saturated with manure. Since fresh waters are mostly wasted, the radius of their economic distribution is limited to a few km and they cannot be exported to distant nutrient-deficit areas. Consequently, it is not the provision of feeds but the disposal of wastes that is now putting limits on the size and density of animal production. Some countries have already legislated the limits on the density of farm animals based on their waste output.

Nitrogen volatilized and leached from animals wastes has become a major source of both local and regional environmental pollution. Volatilization of ammonia is the source of objectionable odours from large-scale operations. After their removal from the atmosphere and subsequent bacterial conversion to nitrates, these emissions also contribute to eutrophication and acidification of terrestrial ecosystem. Most of the eutrophication—enrichment of waters with plant nutrients—is caused by leaching of nitrates from fertilizers and animal manures. Intensive fertilization of feed crops is the single most important source of these losses. US corn receives about 40 percent of the country's nitrogen fertilizer, and, to the great surprise of most people who think that leguminous crops secure their own nitrogen through symbiosis with rhizobia, about one-fifth of US soybeans now receive supplementary nitrogen in order to guarantee consistently high yields.

Aquatic eutrophication causes excessive algal growth in streams, lakes, estuaries, and coastal waters. These blooms sometimes contain species producing human toxins. One of the most dangerous is *Pfiesteria piscicida*, an estuarine dinoflagellate that kills fish and can cause temporary loss of memory and gastrointestinal problems in humans. Algal blooms increase water's turbidity, and their eventual decay leads to oxygen deficiency, disruption of entire aquatic ecosystems, and loss of biodiversity. Their effects are now found above all in coastal waters heavily affected by nutrient runoff such as the northern gulf of Mexico, the Chesapeake Bay, the northwestern shelf of the Black Sea, and Japan's Seto Inland Sea. Terrestrial eutrophication may lead to temporary increases in productivity of forests and grasslands as well as to changes in the composition of dominant species and to a loss of biodiversity as nitrophilic plants thrive.

Meat production is also a significant source of greenhouse gases. Enteric fermentation in bovines is a major source of methane (CH_4), a greenhouse gas whose global warming potential (GWP, over a period of 100 years) is 23 times that of carbon dioxide (CO_2) during the first 20 years of its atmospheric residence. And denitrification of nitrates in synthetic fertilizers and in animal manures releases nitrous oxide (N_2O), a greenhouse gas with a GWP nearly 300 times that of CO_2. But because meat production requires heavy inputs of agrochemicals and inputs of fuel and electricity for manufacturing and operating field and barn machinery, its most important impact on global warming is, nevertheless, due to CO_2 generated from the combustion of fossil fuels used to make these additional inputs. CO_2 is also released from the burning of tropical forests that are being converted to pastures.

THE ENVIORNMENT — DEVELOPMENT LINK

The 'Asian Brown Cloud' — the three km-deep cocktail of deadly pollutants that hovered in July-August, 2003, over Asia and much of India— should illustrate the connection between environment and development. The latest report on the Asian Brown Cloud reveals that the concentration of ash, acids and aerosols in the atmosphere above vast areas in Asia and most of India is changing monsoon patterns, reducing harvests, causing droughts and leading to premature deaths and respiratory illness.

The interlinkages of and the concept of "sustainable development" have been emphasised repeatedly since the UN Conference on Environment and Development in Rio de Janeiro. Why did it not make a difference? Mr. Nitin Desai, Secretary–General of the World Summit on Sustainable Development (WSSD), acknowledged that more needed to be done to get government to integrate different sectors in environmental planning. But on specific sectors, he held that progress had been made. For instance, in the area of energy he said that the addition of wind power in the last few years was comparable to the additional energy being generated through hydropower. Similarly, energy savings through the introduction of compact fluorescent lamps, for instance, was considerable given the scale of use in countries such as China. The energy focus at the conference would bring in the top seven international energy utilities to discuss issues of not just sustainable energy but also programmes for universal rural electrification. Essentially, Johannesburg will be an action-oriented summit. We will not try and redefine issues but instead try spell them out in more concrete terms.

The WSSD is expected to bring together an estimated 60,000 people, including over 100 heads of Government. Given that India played an important role at Rio de Janeiro in articulating the views of developing countries, India would make a useful contribution in Johannesburg too. India can make it clear that there is a strong commitment in developing countries for sustainability. But it can also get the world to recognise that there is a global dimension to this. It is not enough to get the policy right at the national level.

Global summits such as the WSSD usually sort out most contentious issues in preparatory meetings held over a year. In this instance, too, three-fourths of the issues to be discussed have been already agreed upon. But the contentious 25 percent include perennials such as the commitment to additional resources by industrialised countries and the impact of globalisation. Mr. Desai acknowledged that the latter would be an important issue. "This is going to be one of the major conceptual issues — in way we can make globalisation and sustainable development compatible." He did not think it would be "insuperable" but hoped that any agreement that emerged out of the conference would address the "genuine concerns of people about the impact of globalisation on social development and environmental management at every level.

In the same context, nongovernmental organisations have proposed a treaty on corporate accountability. Mr. Desai said that the text of the document to be adopted at the summit already had hoped that it would be passed. There were also other programmes under consideration such as a global reporting initiative, comprising corporations, NGO's and international bodies, that would strive to set standards of environment and social reporting for large corporations. It is expected that over a thousand chief executives of large private corporations would participate in the summit.

Every UN conference, whether on environment or women or population, usually stumbles on getting industrialised countries to commit additional financial resources to implement programmes. The Rio conference led to the setting up of the Global Environment Facility (GEF). Until a few days ago, its future was in a question. Mr. Desai said that the commitment of $ 2.9 billion for the GEF and an additional $ 13 billion agreed upon at the Moneterrey conference on financial commitments earlier this year was a "positive signal". He emphasised, however, that in addition to these commitments and bilateral and multilateral flows to developing countries, domestic budgets also needed to be taken into account. "We have to remember that as great a challenge is to make sure that sustainability guides private flows and domestic budgets, especially in areas like energy.

Asian Brown Haze Clouds

A woman burning cow dung to cook her meal in her slum tenement could be engaging in slow suicide and also taking a small step towards killing her environment and people around her. The report by the United Nations Environmental Programme (UNEP) on the 3-km brown cloud hanging over Asia, zeroes in on this kind of fuel burning as the source of the cloud that is disrupting monsoons, lowering agricultural output and creating air pollution leading to respiratory diseases. The big problem here could be cooking at home. The haze is the result of forest fires, burning of agricultural wastes, dramatic increases in burning of fossil fuels in vehicles, industries and power stations and emissions from millions of inefficient cookers burning wood, cow dung and other bio fuels. Acids in the haze may, by falling as acid rain, have the potential to damage crops and trees. Ash falling on leaves can aggravate the impact of reduced sunlight on earth's surface. The pollution that is forming the haze could be leading to several hundreds of thousands of premature deaths as a result of higher levels of respiratory diseases. It is a problem that will now have to be addressed by governments in India and in other countries in South Asia. The silver lining in this cloud is that it can be tackled relatively soon if the correct policy decisions are taken.

Scientists indicate that a revolution of lifestyles will be needed across India, Pakistan and China acting together. This will mean common policies against burning of fossil fuels and agricultural wastes, against emissions from industries and power stations, and above all, against emissions from the millions of inefficient cookers in homes using fuels like wood and cow dung. The brown clouds these fuels have created over Asia have already led to a 20-40 percent disruption in the monsoon. That has meant more rain in the east and south, and relative drought over northwest India and Pakistan.

India and the rest of south Asia are covered by this deadly blanket of pollution, which is radically changing monsoon patterns, causing drought, reducing India's winter rice harvest by 10 per cent and literally killing hundreds of thousands of people by respiratory disease. A study on the Asian Brown Haze was recently released by scientists working with the United Nations Environment Programme (UNEP). It said that the vast "pollution parcel" could endanger the economic success of South Asian countries, particularly India.

Already, higher levels of respiratory diseases are leading to a large number of premature deaths, as revealed by data from seven Indian cities, including Ahmedabad, Kolkata, Delhi and Mumbai. The Indian data suggested some kind of air pollution was responsible for 24,000 annual premature deaths in the early 1990s, said the report. A few years later, the number rose to an estimated 37,000 per year. In India they are expecting more than two million people to die because of the incomplete burning of biomass. The scientists, who are calling for an action plan to address the threats across Asia as a whole, have also frightened much of Europe by the suggestion that the Asian haze has "global implications". It was pointed out to a shocked Europe that "a pollution parcel like this, which stretches three kilometers high, can travel half way round the globe in a week".

Brown Cloud Hampers Monsoon

The global models used in the report suggest the haze may reduce precipitation over northwest India, Pakistan, Afghanistan, Western China and neighbouring western central Asian region by between 20 and 40 per cent. There have been two consecutive droughts in 1999 and 2000 in Pakistan and the northwestern parts of India while increased flooding in the high rainfall areas of Bangladesh, Nepal and northeastern states of India. Air pollution caused by the cloud is leading to at least half a million deaths a year and agricultural production has begun to decline.

According to Prof. V. Ramamurthy of the University of California, who is associated with the project, this haze, is not just dust and gases, but manmade particles "made up of sulphates, sulphuric acid, black carbon, fly ash, nitrates, aerosols and the like." The haze was "reducing the amount of direct sunlight reaching the earth surface in these areas by 10 to 15 per cent," This has radical consequences. It is reducing evaporation and cloud formation and rainfall. The reduced sunlight is also reducing photosynthesis and therefore agricultural productivity. Asian Brown cloud is "modifying rainfall patterns including those of the mighty monsoon" and also "triggering droughts in western parts of the Asian continent". The report says research in India indicates the haze may reduce the winter harvests by as much as 10 per cent. If the drought persists for about four to five years, then we should start suspecting that it may be (because of the haze). India, China and Indonesia are the worst affected owing to their population density, economic growth and depleting forest cover. The concern is that the regional and global impacts of the haze are set to intensify over the next 30 years as the population of the Asian region rises to an estimated five billion people.

WHAT DOES EMISSIONS TRADING CONVEY?

What is Emissions Trading or Carbon Trading?

The idea is to reduce the level of the six so-called greenhouse gases, such as carbon dioxide, methane and oxides of nitrogen, which prevent heat from escaping from the earth and gradually raise global temperatures and induce climate change with disastrous consequences. Under the Kyoto Protocol to the UN Framework Convention on Climate Change, (UNFCCC), 36 developed countries, called the Annex 1 countries have to reduce their emission of greenhouse gases below their 1990 levels over the five-year commitment period of 2008-12. Under Article 17 of the Kyoto Protocol, approved in 1997, an international emissions trading scheme (IET) has been established to enable Annex I parties to meet some part of their targets in a flexible and cost-effective manner. IET is, however, limited, in that Article 17 also makes it clear that emission trading 'shall be supplemental to the domestic actions' of Annex I countries.

Countries that can reduce emissions in excess of their commitments can sell them to countries that are unable to meet their targets. Since reduction commitments are assigned at a sub-national level to individual enterprises, such international trading of emission reductions will translate into the trading of emission reductions among firms.

What is traded is certified units of emission reduction. Emissions can be abated (a programme to increase energy efficiency would reduce emissions), avoided (instead of a conventional coal-based thermal plant, one could have cogeneration in a sugar plant or a gas-based plant) or removed (a man-made forest or a plantation would act as a sink, absorbing carbon dioxide from the atmosphere). A number of auditing agencies duly authorized by the UNFCCC would have to certify that a particular project has generated so many emission reduction units.

What is the Clean Development Mechanism?

The Kyoto Protocol has a strong market orientation in its approach and recognizes that it may be more cost-effective for Annex I parties to reduce emissions in non-Annex I countries. Consequently, Article 12 of the Kyoto Protocol grants Annex I parties the right to generate or purchase emission reduction credits from projects undertaken by them within non-Annex I countries.

In exchange, developing countries parties will have access to resources and technology to assist in development of their economies in a sustainable manner. This is called the Clean Development Mechanism (CDM). The CDM is supervised by an 'Executive Board' (Article 12.4) and the credit earned from CDM projects are known as 'certified emission reduction' (CERs). CDM projects will be externally verified and certified by 'operational entities' (Article 12.5).

These are third party organizations that will be designated by the parties to the Protocol. Projects initiated after January 1,2002 qualify for consideration under CDM.

Can the Kyoto Protocol come into force without ratification by the US?

Article 25 of the Protocol outlines a complex procedure for the Protocol's entry into force as a multilateral agreement. It specifies that it will enter into force " ...on the ninetieth day after the date on which not less than 55 Parties to the Convention have ratified it.

Although the US is the largest producer of greenhouse gases and the Bush administration has decided to keep out of Kyoto, the protocol can come into force even without US ratification, provided other major greenhouse gas producers such as the European Union members, Russia and Japan join in. The progress in ratification has been such that now only Russia and a minor polluter alone need to ratify the Protocol for it to come into force. It is in Russia's interest to ratify it as economic decline over the 1990s has reduced its emission levels below the 1990 levels even without major technological changes and the country is in a position to cash in on a huge quantity of reduction units in excess of its own commitment.

12

Foreign Trade In Livestock Products

India has been described as a "slumbering giant of the international dairy trade". The General Agreement on Tariffs and Trade (GATT) offers exciting trade prospects. With the reduction in the heavy subsidies that support livestock producers in the developed countries, India's livestock products may improve competitiveness in the international market (Kumar and Singh, 1999). The market-oriented economic policies of the country have brought into focus new issues, which were not very important or relevant in the past. These issues can be broadly classified into two groups: (i) those arising out of the opening of the economy to trade, investment and technology flow, and (ii) those arising out of deregulation or market freedom. Livestock trade has emerged as an important area of economic enquiry as a result of opening of the economy. The concern is how the livestock sector will respond to a free market economy and liberal trade regime. With this background, the study examines (i) the temporal change in the composition of exports and imports of livestock products, (ii) the magnitude of growth in exports and imports of livestock products, (iii) the performance of livestock sector trade and (iv) the price competitiveness of livestock products in the international market.

WORLD TRADE AND INDIA

World trade in livestock products especially meat and dairy products takes place in a relatively small residual market and the volume traded accounts for a small proportion of world production. For instance less than 8 percent of the world meat production and 5 percent of global dairy products were traded internationally in the year 2001. The position regarding various categories of meat was as follows: poultry meat 11 percent, beef and veal 9 percent, sheep and goat meat 7 percent and pork 4 percent. Over 70 percent of international trade in dairy products is through EU, New Zealand and the United States. The EU is the largest beef exporter, accounting for about 26 percent of world exports in 2001, with Australia contributing another 17 percent. Some of these countries are also major importers, the USA taking 17 percent of the world beef imports, the EU 12 percent and Japan 13 percent. In an environment dominated by a few market participants, market price movements and expectations are largely determined by the domestic meat and diary policies of the key producing countries.

Concerns with food security and the secular trend of declining importance of agriculture in national output in developed countries have caused agricultural producer support policies to flourish. These are enforced by import controls as well as direct market interventions to maintain high prices for domestic farmers. These policies impose high and increasingly transparent costs on consumers and taxpayers. In the context of global trade relations they have also come to have important spill over effects on efficient producers in other countries, including developed countries. The agriculture price raising policies of the major developed countries succeeded in inducing·over production in many EU countries and the USA. This has weakened world prices of meat, poultry products (and other agricultural commodities) indirectly via the effects of import controls and directly by dumping of excess government commodity stocks and officially subsidized exports—butter exported from EU in 2001 needed a subsidy of almost US$ 3000/tonne and non-fat dried milk a subsidy of almost US$ 520 per tonne. The US raised its export subsidies for skimmed milk powder tom US$ 864 tonne in March 2002-3.

The world fresh meat trade is also faced with non-tariff barriers based on health restrictions. The EU bans meat produced with growth hormones but the most important restrictions are those of meat imports from countries where there is foot and mouth disease (FMD). Combined with domestic farm and livestock support policies the restrictions promote segmentation of world markets for livestock and lead to exclusion of most developing countries exporters from the lucrative markets of developed countries.

Most of the livestock products in India are consumed domestically. Export trade in edible livestock products is tiny and accounts for less than 1 percent of the global trade in livestock products. The external trade includes value added milk products, meat and meat preparations, leather, leather products and inedible offal. Table 12.1 shows India's exports of livestock products during the years 1997-98 to 2000-01

Table 12.1: The Export of Livestock Products from India (Value in Rs. Crores) 1997-98 to 2000-2001

Items	1997-98	1998-99	1999-2000	2000-01
Buffalo meat	729.30	691.29	706.43	1375.04
Sheep meat	62.66	78.47	80.90	78.16
Processed meat	2.22	2.90	4.58	1.59
Poultry products	88.84	51.72	54.25	86.18
Dairy products	13.39	13.65	37.22	83.90
Animal Casings	11.96	1356	11.70	12.29
Total exports	908.37	851.73	905.08	1637.16

Source: APEDA

India's share in the world exports/imports of selected livestock products in different years is presented in Table 12.2. The share of live animals from India in the world exports of live animals increased from 0.03 percent in TE 1976 to 0.31 percent in TE 1985 and it dropped afterwards and reached to 0.03 percent again in TE 1998. An increase in the share in world exports was observed in the case of meat and meat preparations and dairy products and eggs. There was a quantum jump in the share of meat and meat products in TE 1998 taking its share in the world export of this item to 0.70 percent. The share of eggs in the world export of eggs remained very less till TE 1994 but increased to about 2 percent in TE 1998. The share of dairy products remained negligible throughout (0.01-0.02 percent). India's share in the world import of live animals, meat and meat preparations and eggs remained negligible. A sharp decline in the share of world import of dairy products

Table 12.2: India's share in World Trade of Selected Livestock Products

(Percent)

Period/commodity	Export				
	Live animals	Meat and meat preparations	Milk and milk products	Butter	Eggs
(1)	*(2)*	*(3)*	*(4)*	*(5)*	*(6)*
1974-76	0.03	0.12	#	0.01	0.02
1977-79	0.22	0.19	0.01	0.02	0.03
1980-82	0.16	0.35	0.01	0.02	0.04
1983-85	0.31	0.36	0.02	0.05	0.05
1986-88	0.25	0.25	0.02	0.05	0.02
1989-91	0.11	0.24	0.01	0.03	0.02
1992-94	0.09	0.28	0.02	0.05	0.30
1996-98	0.03	0.70	0.02	0.04	1.71

Period/ commodity	Import					
	Live animals	Meat and meat preparations	Milk	Butter	Milk and milk products	Eggs
(1)	*(8)*	*(9)*	*(10)*	*(11)*	*(12)*	*(13)*
1974-76	0.01	#	1.00	0.48	0.54	0.02
1977-79	#	#	0.97	0.89	0.61	0.01
1980-82	0.01	#	1.59	1.28	1.02	#
1983-85	0.06	#	0.97	0.71	0.58	#
1986-88	0.12	#	0.51	0.48	0.32	#
1989-91	0.05	#	0.14	0.19	1.14	0.01
1992-94	0.03	#	0.08	0.08	0.05	#
1996-98	0.01	#	0.01	0.07	0.01	#

Source: FAO Trade Year Book, various issues.
Note: Indicates negligible share.

was observed, its share declined from 0.54 percent in TE 1976 to almost negligible level (0.01 percent) in TE 1998. It is thus evident that India has only a marginal presence in the world trade of livestock products. Thus India is not in a position to significantly influence the world market situation either in prices or supplies. However, it may be argued that though trade in livestock products is small in relation to world trade, India's output is large in relation to the latter, and opening up of India's large livestock sector to world trade may have large effect on the nature of the world equilibrium in terms of prices, and, subsequently, outputs.

International Competitiveness

Nominal Protection Coefficients (NPCs) have been worked out by Anjani Kumar, et al. to measure the export competitiveness of selected livestock products in the global market (Table 12.3). An examination of NPCs for different livestock commodities indicates that butter has not been competitive internationally after TE 1982 (Table 12.1). Although producer milk prices in India are significantly lower than in the United States and Western Europe, dairy product prices are considerably higher than international market prices. This may be attributed to the domestic processing inefficiency in India (World Bank, 1999). India also lacks international competitiveness in poultry products though it was price competitive in TE 1991. There has been an increase in NPCs after reforms and at present domestic poultry meat is over 50 percent costlier than world prices. India exhibited international price advantage in beef, pork and mutton. Beef was highly export competitive in all the reference years and it NPCs varied from 0.162 in TE 1994 to 0.414 in TE 1985. Though NPCs for mutton and pork were more than unity (not competitive) in the initial years of reference, NPCs became price competitive in the later years.

Some studies have assessed the impact of the GATT on dairy and meat products and projected that world dairy product prices increase by about 2.3 per cent in real terms by the year 2002, while world meat products increase by 1.4 percent. However, despite the expected increase in world

Table 12.3: Nominal Protection Coefficients (NPCs) of Selected Livestock Commodities in the Global Market

Year	Butter	Beef	Mutton	Pork	Poultry meat
(1)	(2)	(3)	(4)	(5)	(6)
1980-82	0.856	0.367	1.192	1.253	-
1983-85	1.262	0.414	1.012	1.162	-
1986-88	1.473	0.402	0.991	0.975	-
1989-91	1.532	1.176	0.825	0.314	0.988
1992-94	1.850	0.162	0.627	0.211	1.045
1996-98	1.978	0.258	0.795	0.259	1.531

Source: Anjani Kumar, et al, Trade in Livestock Products

market prices, domestic product prices remained higher (excluding mutton, pork and beef) than world market prices. Thus increasing production and processing efficiency in the livestock sector was critical. The sector is to remain competitive with imports.

Indian Scenario

In India exports of live animals and livestock products make a valuable contribution to the foreign exchange earnings. Livestock products include meat and edible meat offals, dairy and poultry products, animal fodder and feed, leather and raw wool and animal hair. The value of export of these products more than doubled during the decade, from Rs. 9,570 million in 1990/91 to Rs. 21,134 million in 1999/2000. (Table 12.3). The increase was mainly due to growth in exports of meat and met products, which accounted for two-third of the increase. Dairy products contributed around 5 percent to the increased foreign exchange earnings. Export of meat and preparations provides valuable foreign exchange, which was to the tune of Rs. 8,014 million in 1992/2000, almost 6 times higher than in 1990/91. The main meat-producing animals in India include cattle, buffalo, sheep, goat, pig and chicken. Amongst these, 10 million buffaloes slaughtered during 1999 contributed 31 percent of the total meat production by providing 1.41 million tonnes of meat, as compared to 31%, 5%, 10%, 11% and 12% meat contributed by cattle, sheep, goat, pig and chicken with slaughtered statistics of 13.8 million (cattle), 17 million (sheep) and 13.4 million (pigs), respectively.

ACTUAL EXPORT AND IMPORT SCENARIO

Live Animals

Import and export of live bovine animals and live swine are negligible to and from the country. However, a sizable quantity of poultry fowls of the species Gallous is exported from India. The export of live poultry birds that shot up from more than 2 million birds valued at around Rs. 18 million in 1993-94 to more than 9 million birds valued at Rs. 81 million in 1995/ 96 declined to only 3 million birds worth Rs. 35 million in 1999/2000. India also exports a small number of live sheep and goats. Exports of such animals declined from 29.4 thousand in 1993/94 valued at Rs. 26.02 million, to only 4.6 thousand valued at Rs. 3.3 million in 1999/2000. On the other hand, India imported quite a sizable number of live sheep and goats varying between 30.6 thousand heads valued at Rs. 10.3 million in 1995-96 and 22.3 thousand, worth Rs. 6.8 million in 1999/2000.

Meat and Meat Products

Bovine Meat Fresh or Chilled

There is practically no import of bovine meat fresh or chilled in the country. However, there has been a steady increase in export of fresh or chilled bovine meat. It increased from 8.4 thousand tonnes (valued at Rs. 140.6 million) in 1990/91 to 68.6 thousand tonnes (valued at Rs. 2793 million) in 1999-00.[1] India's export of frozen bovine meat is however much larger than the fresh bovine meat. Export of frozen meat was to the tune of 54.9 thousand tonnes valued at Rs. 925.6 million in 1990/91. But by 1996-97 these exports peaked at about 140.7 thousand tonnes valued at Rs. 5525.7 million. However, in recent years exports have declined and totaled 100.8 thousand tonnes worth Rs. 4237 million in 1999/00.

Total export of bovine meat is considered to be only about ten percent of the domestic production. Some private slaughterhouses and processing plants have established footholds in foreign markets for bovine meat.

There has been a continuous increase in export of buffalo meat. The exports have increased from 63.5 thousand tonnes in 1990/91 to 153.9 thousand tonnes in 1998/99. Despite the rapid increase, India's share in the total world buffalo meat trade remains meager (1.3 percent) South East Asia and Middle East Countries are the major destinations for export of buffalo meat. Malaysia is the largest importer accounting for 32% of buffalo meat exports, followed by the UAE (22%) and Philippines (20%). Saudi Arabia, Turkey, Eastern Europe, CIS countries and African countries are the new markets, which could be developed for Indian buffalo meat (Table 12.4).

Although buffalo meat exports have increased in recent years, there is a need to expand the trade further. There is no religious taboo on slaughtering buffaloes for meat. About 86 percent of the world buffalo meat comes from Asia, mostly from old and culled animals. According to an estimate about 10 million male buffalo calves are born annually, but mortality rate is high due to poor nutrition and care. It is of utmost importance to save male calves from early death for conserving germ plasm. There is also a need for systematic nutrition studies on fattening of buffalo calves.

The reason for tardiness in recognizing the buffalo's economic potential goes back to the 1960s and 70s when the frenzied era of development and modernization first hit the developing countries. Everything new, especially foreign, was in and everything old, especially if it was indigenous, was out. Water buffalo – the mainstay of Asian agriculture for millennia became an embarrassment and an all too-visible symbol of low-tech, even no-tech, present backwardness, apathy and rural poverty. There would be no progress, ran the arguments, until farmers replaced the offending beast with modern machinery.

Farmers and officials have now discovered that the water buffalo is not merely a work animal, but a dependable producer of milk and meat needed

---

[1]The FAO's estimate for export of bovine meat from India varies considerably from government data. FAO's figures for export of fresh bovine meat is around 0.3 million tonnes valued at around 0.4 million US$ during 1997 and 1998. There is an urgent need to reconcile these two estimates.

Table 12.4: India's Share in World Export of Buffalo Meat – 1998-99

(Qty. in tonnes and value in US$ million)

Countries	Total import of product		Imports from India		% Share		Major competitors
	Qty.	Value	Qty.	Value	Qty.	Value	
World	5,005,538	13684	153956	174.90	3.08	1.28	
Malaysia	63481	81.60	40054	46.84	76.30	57.40	Australia, New Zealand, Argentina, Brazil
UAE	42011	66.29	37469	41.90	89.19	63.21	EU, Australia, New Zealand
Philippines	52495	70.89	26383	30.01	50.26	42.33	Australia, New Zealand, Argentina, Brazil
Iran	61400	131.00	13524	14.57	22.03	11.13	EU, Argentina, Australia, New Zealand, USA
Jordan	8718	16.46	6576	8.25	75.43	50.12	EU, Argentina, Australia, New Zealand, USA

Source: FAO Trade Year and Centre for Monitoring Indian Economy: July 2000

for an expanding international market. A recent report by the US Department of Agriculture (USDA), written with American tastes in mind demolishes much of the negative buffalo dogma. The USDA compared the nutritional value of water buffalo meat with beef and chicken. This shows that Asian buffalo meat has 41 percent less cholesterol, 92 percent less fat and 56 percent fewer calories than traditional meat, the report says. It also has a good flavour and texture, can be substitute for beef in practically any American recipe, and stores well. Overall, the report says buffalo can be regarded as a delicacy for health conscious Americans.

In India buffalo meat generally sells for 40-50 percent less than cow beef, because it comes from animals worked until old age. Their meat is, therefore, tough and stringy. But when the buffalo is raised as a meat producer it gives a completely different quality. The meat becomes succulent and tender, at least as tasty as beef and many would say more so. Pakistan, with about 20 million buffalo, has built a flourishing industry on the slaughter of male calves for high quality veal. Non-vegetarian Hindus in India and Nepal have no qualms about eating buffalo meat, though cow meat remains taboo.

Prevalence of various livestock diseases and inadequate modern and integrated facilities are the two major constraints for promoting the export of meat. India has achieved the Rinderpest free status. India is also free from BSE, and scrapie. However, certain other livestock diseases like FMD etc., are still prevalent in the country. The exporters are willing to set up modern and integrated meat production facilities. However, they are finding it difficult to get necessary approval of the Government for setting up of these facilities because of the socio-political problems. India also has the advantage of being price competitive particularly for the buffalo meat. In view of the above, India has huge potential for export of meat and meat products.

Domestic beef prices in EU and some selected countries in US$ per tonne are as under EU internal price: US$ 3000. Iran: US$ 2200. Middle East countries: US$ 1700-1750 Wet Africa: US$ 800 (compensated beef). New Zealand and Australia have access to developed countries like Japan and export prime cuts at a very high price. Low-grade cuts and trimmings are exported to Malaysia and Philippines at price lower or equal to prevailing Indian buffalo meat prices (Table 12.5).

Table 12.5: Cost of Buffalo Meat Production in India: (Rs./KG)

(i)	Cost of Indian raw material/production	30-35
(ii)	Cost of processing	6
(iii)	Cost of Inland transportation	2.50
(iv)	Cost of freight	3.60
(v)	Import duty at destination	NIL
(vi)	Any other costs (handling)	1.50
Sub Total (excluding freight)		40-45
Realization of Exporters		45

Meat Sheep Fresh, Chilled or Frozen

Mutton (sheep and Goat meat) exports increased from 8.33 thousand tonnes (valued at Rs. 312 million) in 1990/91 to 11 thousand tonnes, (valued at Rs. 622 million) in 1993/94. However, during the next three years it declined to 8-9 thousand tonnes, but recovered to 12.4 thousand tonnes.[1] Export earnings from mutton increased from Rs. 312.5 million in 1990/91 to Rs. 909 million in 1999/00. The increase in quantities comes to 49 percent, while the value of exports increased by more than 129 percent. This implies higher unit price earned from mutton exports. Mutton is exported mainly to Middle-Eastern countries (Bahrain, Oman, Saudi Arabia, UAE). Unlike beef, high domestic demand and prices limit larger exports of mutton, which accounts for only 4-5 percent of domestic production. The Government of India has withdrawn the export quota and minimum export price restrictions as export incentives for mutton. There is practically no import of mutton in the country.

Swine Meat

A small quantity of pork is exported from the country. As per the statistics compiled by the DGCIS, there was an erratic trend in the volume of export

---

[1]*Source:* Directorate General of Commercial Intelligence and Statistics: Monthly Statistics of Foreign Trade of India: Various issues.

of swine meat during the period from 19910/91 to 1999-00. While in 1993/94 the export was around 56 tonnes valued at Rs. 1.25 million, in 1994-95, the export shot up to 741 tonnes valued at Rs. 25.2 million, and then further went up to about 934 tonnes valued at Rs. 26.2 million in the following year. However, since 1996-97 the quantity and value of export of swine meat declined sharply. As per the government official record, in the earlier years there was no import of swine meat, and only in 1996-97 there was some import, valued around Rs. 0.6 million. The pork eating population in the country is very limited and is mainly confined to the tribal population of the North-Eastern Region. Expansion of swine meat is of considerable importance for increasing its exports and to meet the rising domestic demand. Piggery development in the country is of considerable importance, particularly in the North East. The pig is one of the most efficient food converting animals among domesticated livestock, and can play an important role in improving the socioeconomic status of the weaker sections of the society. A major constraint in piggery development is the lack of adequate high quality breeding stock. Exotic breeds, which are being maintained in the 158 State Pig Farms, are prone to inbreeding and require a fresh input for genetic upgradation. The Central Department of Animal Husbandry and Dairying is providing assistance to States under its Integrated Piggery Development Scheme to strengthen state pig farms and to assist them in genetic upgradation of their breeding stock.

Poultry Meat Fresh

Despite tremendous growth in its production, the export of poultry meat has been very limited. This is largely due to lack of price competitiveness. In fact, there was a sharp decline in the export of meat and edible offal of the poultry from 102.5 tonnes in 1993/94 valued at Rs. 3.25 million to 13.7 tonnes valued at only Rs. 0.54 million in 1995-96. Since then exports of poultry meat and offal recorded a further precipitous fall and was worth only Rs. 1.7 million in 1999/00. There is however, scope for expansion of export of poultry meat if the phyto-sanitary restrictions of the importing countries are strictly followed and packaging requirements are met properly. For example, in most countries in Europe, and primarily America, breast meat of chicken is sold at a premium, whereas, the leg meat is virtually considered as waste matter, to be dumped at throwaway prices in developing countries. Breast meat in USA is sold at a price of US $3 -3.5 per pound while leg meat is sold at 45 cents per pound. Hence, India may avail of the golden opportunity of exporting breast meat that fetches a better price at the markets of Europe and USA. But it is also feared that the US may try to dump leg meat at cheaper prices in India. However, if the bound rate of import of most poultry products is enforced, dumping of leg meat may be difficult.

Eggs in Shell

Export of eggs in shell has registered a mixed trend. The foreign exchange earning from their exports increased Rs. 0.53 million in 1993/94 to Rs.

105.3 million in 1998/99, but declined to only Rs. 2.3 million in 1999/00. A sharp increase up to 1998/99 was due to demand from the neighbouring countries like Bangladesh, Maldives, and Middle East countries, which slackened in the next year.

Eggs not in Shell

Export of eggs, not in shell and egg yolk fresh has been significant in recent years. Export earnings rose from Rs. 0.38 million in 1990-91 to Rs. 555.7 million in 1999-00. According to the industry sources India is the cheapest egg producers in the world and if proper incentives are given to the processing industry, India may be able to further improve its export performance.

A new avenue for poultry exports is opening up a result of the growing worldwide trend towards the consumption of eggs and meat from birds reared under free-range conditions. Essentially backyard farming, which is unlike the factory-farming methods, birds are not subjected to stress or fed with specially-formulated rations for higher production. The demand for these products is largely in the developed countries. In addition, growing segments of health and fitness conscious young people are cutting down on red mat consumption and so prefer poultry meat.

One indication of the changing trend is the ninefold increased consumption in Britain of free-range and organically raised meat increasing in value from £ 1 million to £ 9 million between 1988 and 1992. Further, the knowledge that the sale proceeds from free-range poultry products would benefit the rural poor in the developing countries is by itself an incentive enough for the socially–conscious section of people in the developed countries to patronize such purchases.

Free-rage poultry rearing is common in India and other developing countries among the weaker sections, including tribal folks and scheduled castes. Normally, *desi* eggs and chickens attract premier prices.

Since April 1, 2001, all Quantitative Restrictions on imports of livestock productions have been removed, as per the WTO agreement, thus opening up the Indian market to imported livestock products including poultry meat and egg products. While players in the industry maintain that they are not scared of competitions, the farmer fear that this will lead to dumping of cheaper imported products in the country and lead to loss of livelihood. The Indian poultry industry maintains that it can complete with foreign players at all levels, except price. In a bid to provide some protection to the Indian poultry industry, the Government of India had earlier enhanced the import duty on certain products from 35% to 100%. The poultry industry has suggested to the government that the current rate of duty of 100% be retained for another two years, i.e. till March, 2003, when the ongoing Review of Agreement on Agriculture will be completed. In fact, India's poultry industry is not asking for protection, but only a level playing field. The industry is not inefficient. Its productivity levels are among the best in the world.

Dairy Products

The strength of the dairy economy lies in a livestock of 272 million. The country occupies the first position in the world in livestock holding. It has 51 per cent of the Asian bovine population of 530 million and 19 per cent of the world population of 1,420 million. Cattle population comprises 198 million which is 50 per cent of Asian and 15.4 per cent of the world population.

As the country has now started looking at overseas markets, it may be mentioned, that it has an added advantage in buffalo milk. It has 53.3 per cent of the world and 55.0 per cent of the Asian buffalo population, the ratio of cattle to buffalo approximates 100 to 11 in the world and 100 to 38 in India. Nearly 55 per cent of the milk in the country is produced by buffaloes. The IDA paper says buffaloes are better convertors of feeds into milk. Buffalo milk has superior fat and calcium contents and buffalo milk has fat less cholesterol and more tocopherol, which is a natural non-oxidant. Buffalo milk has a special advantage for production of several products such as dairy whiteners, various cheese such as Mozzerella, Ricotta, Domiati, concentrated milk products, including condensed milk and malted milk foods.

The dairy sector is closely integrated to agriculture and can be considered as a subsystem of agriculture. Most milk production, according to IDA, is based on utilisation of agricultural byproducts and crop residues. In other words, cattle convert wastes into wealth, adding to food production. Because of this advantage, the cost of milk production in the country is much lower than many developed countries. The farm gate milk price in India is Rs. 7.26 (one dollar equivalent to Rs. 49) per litre as compared to Rs. 33.53 in Japan, Rs. 19.60 in Canada, Rs. 18.41 European Community, Rs. 13.86 in the US, Rs. 11.17 in Australia. Only New Zealand with a farm gate milk price of Rs. 7.64 per litre comes close to India.

As for the milk productivity per animal, it is one of the lowest when compared to the developed countries. Despite being the second largest milk producers, the density of milk production per square kilometre is substantially low. According to Bulletin to New Zealand Board, quoted by IDA, the average milk productivity per year per animal in India in 1994 was 522 kilograms as compared to 6,874 kilograms in the US, 6,223 in Denmark, 5,751 in Holland, 5,590 in Canada, 5,054 in the UK, 4,096 in France, 4,758 in Germany, 4,500 in Australia, 4,176 in Ireland, 4,121 in Japan and 1,327 in CIS (excluding USSR). Milk production in the country is widely scattered and millions of farmers are involved in the subsidiary occupation. Majority of the milk production possess one or two milch animals. Milk production is not homogeneous and not all areas have the potential or the resources to produce milk efficiently. Due to low density and widely spread milk production areas, the cost of milk transportation is very high as compared to the advanced dairying countries.

There is a broad consensus among analysts that world markets for dairy products are likely to expand. Production growth is expected to be concentrated in those countries where production is not subject to quota system and more so in countries with a low level of support for this sector, and where farmers can respond rapidly to new market opportunities. Production in the European Union, Canada and in some of the Former Socialist is projected to decline. A marked increase in production is expected in Latin America and Asia. Global consumption is likely to follow the same trend.

Improved market balance for dairy products combined with a decline in subsidized exports resulting from WTO agreement and relatively small demand in a number of countries was forecast to lead to higher international prices for dairy products compared to the first half of 1990s. However, contrary to earlier forecast, international prices of dairy products have dropped substantially since mid 2001. In fact by mid year 2002, the prices of most dairy products were, at levels rarely seen over the past decade. The FAO price index for dairy products was 85 in April 2002, compared to 121 for the same month in 2001. The price for all commodities, however, milk powder was most affected. In April 2002 prices of skimmed powder and whole milk powder were around 30 percent below those of 2001. Butter price was 22 percent less, while price of chandler cheese dropped by 7 percent. The sharp decline in prices was due to reduced import demand in some key markets in South East Asia and Latin America and a build up of uncommitted stocks in the main dairy exporting centres including New Zealand, Australia, Argentina, The United States and the EU. By April 2002, the international prices for dairy products have stabilized, albeit at extremely low levels. This was a result of supply and demand becoming more evenly balanced, in particular a reduction in unsold products in Oceania. The difference between domestic prices and world market prices in many developed countries is likely to make market prices of some dairy products like cheese, skimmed milk powder and whole milk powder more sensitive to changes in supply and demand in the international market. With the presence of a specialized organisation like National Dairy Development Board, India has the potential to gain a share of the new market opportunities from the most likely beneficiaries, namely, Australia and New Zealand.

Milk-Condensed, Dry and Fresh

India has a good scope for exports of dairy products as it enjoys several comparative advantages vis-a-vis other countries. While milk market in the developed world is getting saturated, the demand in the developing countries is expanding manifold. The demand for milk and milk products in the developing world is also high because of greater population density. For instance, in the Asian region, the population of China and India alone could demonstrate the market potential of Asia. Similar niche market of ASEAN and petro-dollar Afro-Asian countries are to be reckoned.

India's geographical location, being in the midst of these markets, is definitely a comparative advantage over other advanced dairying countries, viz.Scandavia, the US, Australia and New Zealand. Apart from these, he says India has the largest cattle population, strong procurement infrastructure, a large number of processing and allied facilities and highly skilled manpower pool. However, in spite of these advantages, the country is yet to create a proper dent in the export market. We have been adopting an easier path by going in for occasional milk exports instead of sustainable branded product exports.

Wherever we have seasonal surpluses resulting out of extra production, instead of maintaining a buffer stock, we have resorted of export. Whenever we have got into shortages particularly in the summer months, we have gone for imports to maintain liquid milk supply to the urban consumers. Stressing the necessity of prioritising branded product exports instead of occasional bulk exports. However branded products export can not be just commenced. A lot of campaign is required to support such exports and the policy-makers will have to give incentives for the purposes. The country should also look for other value added live sweetmeats and desserts. India has to convert its comparative advantages into competitive advantage in the global market, the first and foremost step would be to impose self-regulation. The problem of quality, should be dealt with stringently by all concerned including regulatory authorities such as the Prevention of Food Adulteration Act (PFA), Milk and Milk Products Order (MMPO), etc.

However, regulatory mechanisms alone would not yield any positive results until and unless milk producers, processors and marketers also take a positive attitude in discarding inferior quality milk. Equal attention would have to be given to quality packaging. One of the important aspects which is considered a serious impendiment is our packaging quality. Hence, Research and Development incentives should be given for developing quality food packaging at reasonable price.

Export of milk & cream concentrated/containing sugar/sweetening matter from India exhibited an erratic trend during the period from 1990/91 to 1999/00. In fact, during 1995-96 and 1996-97, there was a declining trend in the export of these commodities both in quantitative and value terms. Nevertheless in 1999/00 India exported over 2 thousand tonnes of these products earning Rs. 160 million. Due to remarkable increase in milk production in the country following successful implementation of Operation Flood, very little quantity of liquid milk is imported from other countries. However, India imports a sizable quantity of milk powder. Imports of milk powder and cream increased sharply in 1999/00 following the lifting of the QRs on their imports, but have declined during the next two years. Value of imports of these product totaled Rs. 1980 million in 1999/00, but only Rs. 75.6 million in 2000/01 and Rs. 81 million in 2001/02. It is observed that despite Operation Flood and consequent phenomenal increase in domestic milk production, India's export of milk and milk products is trifling mainly due to unfavourable international prices of the products.

Butter and other Facts and Oils derived from Milk

Export of these commodities also fluctuated quite abruptly from year to year. India's export of these commodities suffers mainly due to higher prices as other major producing countries in Europe offer those at a much lesser price due to the heavy subsidies given to livestock farming sector by the EU and the USA. In fact, India import quite a sizable quantity of butter and fats oil derived from milk to meet the domestic demand.

With $75,000 sales in three weeks, 'Amul Milk Powder', a product of an Indian mega-cooperative has been well-received in the Dubai market dominated so far by multinational brands. The Gujarat Cooperative Milk Marketing Federation (GCMMF), Asia's biggest, already enjoys 10 per cent of Gulf Cooperation Council (GCC) market share for purified butter with annual sales of 400 tonnes. They are also launching Amul Butter in the Gulf shortly and hope to sell 15 tonnes every month. The $400-million cooperative, the largest dairy product exporter from India recorded overseas sales of Rs. 183 million ($5.4 million) in 1995-96 up from Rs. 165 million ($4.6 million) the previous year, marking an increase of 11 per cent. In the Dubai market, Dutch 'Nido' has 60 per cent share followed by Coast (10 per cent) and Anchor of New Zealand at 8 per cent. Though no figures are available for the GCC, the entire market is believed to be as large as 80,000 tonnes a year.

HIDES AND SKINS

Hides and skins are the principal raw materials for the tanning industry. The body cover of big animals is called 'hide' and the body cover of small animals is called 'skin'. Hides and skins differ in size, thickness, and weight. Hides are larger, thicker, and heavier than skins. Normally, the skins of domestic livestock (cows and buffaloes), sheep, and goats are used in the tanning industry. The country is fortunate to have an old established tanning industry which can be classified into household and cottage, small-scale, and finally medium/ large-scale segments. The total number of tanneries in India is estimated to be 2091. Out of these, only 15000 to 16000 are functional. The tanning industry at Erode is a century or even more old. Vegetable tanning of cow hides for making leather buckets, locally known as Kavalai, was popular here. Vegetable-tanned cowhides, popularly known as East Indian Leather, were famous all over the world. While there is no export of hides and skins from India, quite a sizeable quantity of both bovine/equine animals and sheep/lambs are imported for manufacture of leather and leather goods. Import of bovine/equine hides and skins recorded a steady growth in the country following increase in demand from leather manufacturers (Table 12.6). Imports of raw skins of sheep/lambs rose from 3.6 thousand tonnes in 1993/94 to 5.2 thousand tonnes in 1999/00. Value of imports increased from Rs. 85 million to Rs. 139 million. India also imports large quantities of other raw hides and skin. These ranging between 1000 tonnes and 2000 tonnes during the last four years. India has 10 per cent of world's hides and skins but it has only 4 per cent share in leather and leather product trade worldwide.

Table 12.6: Indian Imports of Leather Products

(US $ million)

Item	1996-97	1997-98	1998-99	1999-2000	2000-2001	2001-2002
Finished Leather	298.43	287.80	428	450	472	496
Footwear	340.29	287.08	644	806	1007	1259
Components	222.99	230.51	338	372	409	450
Garments	420.91	418.22	631	726	835	960
Goods	324.81	343.69	691	864	1080	1350
Saddlery &Harness	25.73	28.68	—	—	—	—
	1633.16	1595.98	2732	3218	3803	4515

Source: Council of leather exports

Leather

Leather links rural farmers to the fashion world. It is used in leather goods, garments, and footwear. Leather is one of the few commodities where demand is independent of supply. India has emerged as a reliable source of leather and leather products in the last 50 years. During the eighteenth century the East India Company established a vibrant trade in raw hides and skins in India and the country became a large supplier of raw hides and skins to U.K. However, it was only in 1947 that the economic employment, and export potential of the leather sector was recognised. Then onwards, the focus was directed on the conversion of raw hides and skins into finished leather and value-added products.

The leather industry in India now has a record of exporting nearly 70 percent of the total production. It boasts of nearly 10 percent of the global raw material availability, exports of leather shoes from India to Italy have jumped more than 100 percent. Major market for footwear are the US, Australia, Belgium, the Netherlands, Germany, and the U.K.

The leather industry has made a commendable progress during the decade ending in 2000-01. Besides meeting all the domestic needs, this industry continues to increase its export earnings year after year. In 2000-01, India's exporters of leather and leather products increased by 22.7 per cent. In the eleven years ending in 2000-01, this industry's export earnings were of the order of US$ 16.9 billion or US$ 1.54 billion every year, on an average. In the latest Exim Policy, duty-free import of trimmings and embellishment up to 3 per cent of FOB. value hitherto alone, has been extended to all leather products.

The credit for the expansion of the leather industry also goes to the Central Research Institute at Chennai which has played a useful role in strengthening this industry, It may be recalled that in 1995, the government of India announced the appointment of the Leather Technology Mission with an outlay of $6.3 million for a period of four years to provide guidance in various fields such as improvement in the quality of raw hides and skins and cleaner production with reduced wastage.

Since the quality of leather goods produced in our country is of the international class, the domestic market has also expanded. The industry has certainly expanded its exports without starving the domestic market, which is creditable. As was expected, we have now skilled, semiskilled and unskilled workmen whose relentless efforts are helping to win over new pastures. It may be recorded that China is a leading exporters of leather goods followed by Italy. Both these countries hold about half the world market of leather products. We have a long way to go in carving out a bigger share of world trade in leather goods.

India imports and exports substantial quantities of leather derived both from bovine and sheep or lambskins. With the increase in per capita income, the domestic demand for leather goods has recorded a steady growth. Also India exports footwear to many developed countries. In fact, footwear exports constitute 19.6 % of the exports of leather and leather products. Exports of leather footwear increased by 1.43 per cent during April to September, 2001, as compared with the corresponding period of 2000. The total value of leather and leather manufactures also increased from Rs. 44.89 billion to Rs. 47.15 billion during the same period. Most of the leather products are exported to developed countries like Germany, France, USA, U.K., Italy, Japan and CIS countries.

Leather industry occupies a place of prominence in the Indian economy in view of its massive potential for employment, growth and exports. Apart from a significant foreign exchange earner, leather industry has tremendous potential for employment generation. Direct and indirect employment of the industry is around two million. The skilled and semi skilled workers constitute nearly 50 per cent of the workforce. Around 2.5 million people are employed in the leather sector in India. Out of these, 85 percent with primary skills are in the small and rural areas. Sixty to 65 percent of production comes from the small-scale and cottage sector. Major production centers are located in Chennai, Ambur, Ranipet, Trichy, Dindigul Vaniyambadi, and Erode. There has been an increasing emphasis on its planned development, aimed at optimum utilization of available raw materials for maximizing the returns, particularly from exports. Policy initiatives taken by the Government since 1973 have been instrumental to such a transformation. In the wake of globalization of Indian economy supported with liberalized economic and trade policies since 1991, the industry is poised for further growth to achieve greater share in the global trade. There is also going to take place a revolution in footwear consumption pattern within the country, the signs of which are clear from various developments in the last five years. Launching of various brand names, including foreign brands, is one such example. With the increase in middle class population. the consumption patterns are likely to change rather dramatically.

The exports of leather and leather products gained momentum during the past decades. There has been a phenomenal growth in exports from Rs. 320 million 1965-66 to Rs. 89,140 million in 2000-2001. Indian leather industry today has attained well-merited recognition in the international market besides occupying a pride of place among the top export earners of the country. The exports from leather sector constituted four per cent in the country's export basket in 2000-01.

Thanks to the persistent rise in exports of leather products, the industry is achieving new heights year after year as is evident from Table 12.7. It is encouraging to note that steady expansion in this industry is accompanied by handsome rise in export of finished products. Export of leather and leather products recorded an improvement of the order of 22.7 per cent in 2000-01 in relation to the preceding year. Finished leather had the highest rate of growth in exports at 59.23 per cent in 2000-01 followed by leather garments at 32.62 per cent and saddlery and harness at 25.24 per cent (Tables 12.8).

Table 12.7: India's Leather and Leather Goods Exports

(Rs million)

Category	1997-98	1998-99	1999-2000	2000-01	2001-02
Finished leather	10,944.44	11,293.45	10,392.25	17,428.15	21,813.08
Leather footwear	10,467.76	13,665.26	16,353.35	17,422.75	18,799.82
Footwear components	8,937.27	10,143.86	9,320.62	10,877.10	11,128.27
Leather garments	15,802.77	16,072.22	15,048.63	21,035.59	18,057.34
Leather goods	11,212.94	13,276.77	12,077.80	15,704.40	15,301.00
Saddlery and harness	964.67	1,394.82	1,478.00	1,948.73	1,692.91
Leather gloves	3,181.76	4,020.92	4,238.01	4,413.79	4,086.79
Non-leather footwear	565.20	747.80	611.95	873.16	1,244.12
Total	62,135.81	70,615.10	69,520.61	89,703.67	92,123.33

Source: Council of Leather Exports.

Five decades ago, India was an exporter of raw hides and skins and an importer of finished leather. Today, our capacity to convert raw hides and skins into finished leather has multiplied manifold with the result that we are importing raw hides as well as skins. The manufacturing of leather goods has expanded sharply with the result that the country is obliged to import special quality leather from abroad. Consequently, India's total imports of raw hides and skins, and leather rose by 25 per cent from $ 149 million in 1999-2000 to $ 190 million in 2000-01.

Table 12.8: Export of Leather Manufactures

Year	Rs. Crore	$ Million
1990-91	2,600	1,449
1991-92	3,128	1,269
1992-93	3,700	1,227
1993-94	4,077	1,300
1994-95	5,057	1,611
1995-96	5,790	1,731
1996-97	5,609	1,580
1997-98	6,061	1,631
1998-99	6,847	1,580
1999-00	6,890	1,590
2000-01	8,914	1,951

The export effort of leather and leather products has been accelerated by the leather industry fairs which are organized regularly every year at three centers- Chennai, Delhi and Kolkata. These fairs offer an opportunity to the international community to pick and choose from a vast variety of products on display. Besides the Indian enterprises, foreign companies also participate because these fairs provide an opportunity to display finished leather, machinery and equipment, accessories, dyes and chemicals. In a way, the participation of foreign companies in these fairs has helped Indian manufacturers to improve the quality of their products. At the 17th India International Fair held at Chennai from January 31,2002 to February 7, 2002, exhibitors from 26 countries had participated.

The credit for the expansion of the leather industry also goes to the Central Research Institute at Chennai which has played a useful role in strengthening this industry. It may be recalled that in 1995, the government of India announced the appointment of the Leather Technology Mission with an outlay of $ 6.3 million for a period of four years to provide guidance in various fields such as improvement in the quality of raw hides and skins and cleaner production with reduced wastage[1].

---

[1] Leather goods and wool products were classified as manufactured products as per the classification of products given by the Directorate General of Commercial Intelligence and Statistics (DGCI&S). Therefore, these products were not included in the composition of the trade of livestock products.

Since the quality of leather goods produced in our country is of the international class, the domestic market has also expanded. The industry has certainly expanded its exports without starving the domestic market, which is creditable. As was expected, we have now skilled, semiskilled and unskilled workmen whose relentless efforts are helping to win over new pastures. It may be recorded that China is a leading exporter of leather goods followed by Italy. Both these countries hold about half the world market of leather products. We have a long way to go in carving out a bigger share of world trade in leather goods.

The industry has made a commendable progress during the decade ending in 2000-01. Besides meeting all the domestic needs, this industry continues to increase its export earnings year after year. In 2000-01, India's exports of leather and leather products increased by 22.7 per cent. In the eleven years ending in 2000-01, this industry's export earnings were of the order of US$ 1.54 billion every year, on an average. In the latest Exim Policy, duty-free import of trimmings and embellishments up to 3 per cent of the FOB value hitherto limited to leather garments alone, has been extended to all leather products.

COMPETITION WITH CHINA

China has taken the leather off Indian leather garment business. By wrapping up key markets like the US and Japan with competitively-priced leather garments, the Chinese have managed to effectively choke up Indian exports in this segment. This has resulted in a staggering 35.6% decline in India's leather garment exports during the first five months of the 2002-03 financial year, apart from steady decline in market share. With the American and Japanese market under their domination, the Chinese are now planning a big invasion of the European market and this is likely to turn into a major blow for the Indian leather garment industry. China is setting up huge capacities to supply leather garments to Europe.

Exporters feel the slide in leather garments exports due to diversion of orders to China. A study commissioned by Council for Leather Exports (CLE) and Indian Leather Garment Association (ILGA) also points out that China has walked away with a dominating share in the world market, leaving Indian rivals gasping. A decade of planned export development by China has taken wind out of Indian leather garment industry's sails. From almost identical level of exports in 1990, China now commands 42% share in the global market while India is left behind at 10% at a time when demand is also shrinking.

Exports from India during the first five months of 2000-3 fiscal stood at $121 million as compared to $189 million during the corresponding months in fiscal year 2001-02, according to ILGA president M L Sethi. All other segments of the leather business, leaving footwear components alone, have shown increase in exports during this period. The decline in leather garment exports is attributed to loss of business to China and decline in global demand. Other players like Indonesia, Turkey and Pakistan are also catching up, according to the study commissioned by CLE and ILGA. China is very strong in pig skin varieties and their huge manufacturing capacities make their leather garments globally competitive. A large portion of the global market is limited to garments priced at $100 to $200 and China is the main source of supply in this price range. Sadly, India has not been able to match up to Chinese competition despite being home to 10% of world's cattle population. Exporters now want to emulate the China example by going in for larger production capacities which can result in cheaper prices. They also want the government to intervene in encouraging large tanning capacities, a simpler tax structure and a liberal import regime.

ILGA is now planning to set up a design centre with Indian Institute of Fashion Technology (IIFT) to lay emphasis on this key aspect, better fore casting and technical support are also needed. China enjoys 70% market share in the US, the largest market for leather garments while India lags far behind at 7%. In the case of Japan, leather garments from India are nowhere to be seen while China has captured half of this market. India trails in the German and British markets too, though the margin of lead in favour of China is narrower. Similar is the case with Spain and France. The only market where India is leading is Italy which is known to consume leather garments of higher value as compared to other key markets.

Export of leather and leather products from China was about $ 1 billion per annum, double that of India's, in the late 1980s. In 2000, China's export had surged to $ 12 billion, more than six times that of India's (less than $ 2 billion). Two trade delegations from India visited China recently to understand the drivers of such stupendous development. Both are greatly impressed, but consider that given the right environment, Indian industry can perform far better. The distinguishing features of today's China are the world-class infrastructure, substantial foreign investment in this sector and a disciplined workforce at competitive wage levels.

Specifically, province compete fiercely among themselves for promoting Greenfield Special Economic Zones (SEZ). The SEZs in Zhejiang, Guangdong, Hangzhou, Donguang, Shenzhen and Fujian host a large number of leather-related industries. Water and power at competitive rates and excellent telecommunication facilities in SEZs are the other attractions. FDI in export-oriented industries is actively encouraged. More than 2000 foreign enterprises, accounting for 24% of companies, owned 53% of total assets and 57% of total sales of the leather sector in 2000. Labour regulations facilitate achieving higher productivity. Workers work longer hours when pressure of export orders is high. Average wage levels at $ 60-100 per month are competitive, given the comparatively higher productivity.

When the leather industry declined in Taiwan and South Korea due to rising wage levels in late 1980s, attracted by the open door policy of mainland China, they shifted their manufacturing base there. Despite initial hiccups, these enterprises are doing well at present. On top of its sizeable raw material base (100 million pig skins, 200 million sheep and goat skins and 30 million cattle hides annually), China's annual import of about

$ 3 billion worth of raw material sustains its spectacular export growth. China's export today meets about 22% of global import of leather and leather products. According to strategic plans of China for this sector, 5% per annum growth in output and 7% p.a. growth in foreign exchange earning are envisaged until 2005; from 2005 to 2015, 3% p.a. growth in output and 5% p.a. growth in foreign exchange earnings are expected. Judging by the pace of investments currently being made, achieving these targets would appear quite likely.

In terms of production systems or technology, India is not behind. Though labour productivity is higher in China, with some efforts and labour reforms, India can match it. In terms of prices, Indian products can compete well. With regard to banking systems and language, India scores positive points. However, the enormous capacity available in China in different product segments—at least five time India's–being expanded dramatically, and its ability to secure and execute large volume orders have been major attractions for buyers in China. Quality consistency and timely delivery are its major strengths. China's ability to accept and execute orders for smaller volumes and short delivery schedules too has improved. China no longer is a lower end market supplier : its target now is the higher end and branded product segment. With an overwhelming presence in the USA, Canada and Japan, China's current efforts are to expand its already growing presence in the EU.

What Can India Do?

First, let us look at the support expected of the government. Unless basic infrastructure improves, the overall productivity of Indian industry will be lower. Even as India's SEZ scheme takes shape, infrastructure such as water, power and road connectivity in existing export clusters could be vastly improved. The major leather clusters are the Ranipet-Ambur Vaniyambadi belt of Tamil Nadu, Kanpur and Agra in Uttar Pradesh and Jalandhar in Punjab. Activity in Kolkata Leather Complex must be speed up. Equally important is the need to improve port efficiency. In today's competitive environment, the export product must reach the destinations in the USA or Europe within 15 to 20 days. Labour regulations for a seasonal industry like this must be flexible. Reportedly, for the canning industry in the UK, the total working hours per year is prescribed, with an absolute maximum per day, with flexibility to work longer when required. Next, imported consignments of inputs must not languish in air or sea ports but cleared within a maximum of 48 hours. For star export performers, an express channel of clearance may be provided.

Now, let us turn to the industry-with a meagre production base, India cannot hope to remain competitive and attract buyers. There is an urgent need to augment domestic and foreign investments, particularly in the tanning and footwear sectors. Managerial improvements, targeting higher productivity, cost reduction and overall efficiency at the enterprise level are a must. Material development, design and product development must get adequate importance. India has to be proactive, developing new materials and products each season. Services provided by Indian exporters to the buyers must be comprehensive and more attractive than China's Aggressive marketing is an other urgent necessity. Taking advantage of China's strengths, Indian enterprises.may open offices in China to procure various inputs and production. Strategic alliances with India's traditional export markets in the EU must be urgently established. The question today is how India can retain its current share in the global market and possibly increase it. Procrastination will result in Indian exporters being inundated by competitive forces.

The Indian leather industry has a share of 7 per cent in total exports. It experienced the highest export growth of 23 per cent in the year 2000-01, and the value exports was $ 1.93 billion in 2001-02 due to certain unfavourable international developments. During the first seven months, from April to October 2002, exports touched $ 1.1 billion (Rs. 56 billion). Exports are estimated at around $ 2 billion (Rs. 100 billion) during 2002-03. A clear indication that the threat from organizations like people for Ethical Treatment of Animals (PETA) is on the wane. While some big leather brands in the US and Europe like Reebok, Kenneth Cole and Wolverine Worldwide, are still desisting from buying Indian leather products, most importers are now of the view that Indian producers have started taking adequate measures to improve animal transportation and handling, the crucial issues of Peta resistance against Indian products.

The Council of Leather Exports, under the Union Commerce Ministry, has started addressing these problems in the right earnest. It has taken up a pilot project to reform one market/transport/slaughter unit in Tamil Nadu. For this CLE has raised more than a crore of rupees half of which has come from the central government. According to leather industry sources, Peta has not been able to influence some of the key European market for Indian leather products. As a result leather garment exports and other personal products have continued to show signs of improvement over the past few months. But the biggest irony seems to be the huge success in the exports of finished leather from India. Even as a number of importers have refused to buy Indian products, India has managed to export finished leather worth about Rs. 2,000 crore to Italy. Buyers there use Indian leather to manufacture products and sell them as 'Made in Italy' None of the raw material is used for domestic consumption there. Now, if one looks at the value addition, the same leather would have been used for manufacturing goods worth not less than Rs. 8,000-10,000 crore, which is nothing less than a couple of billion US dollars.

The leather industry has set an ambitious export target of $ 3 billion by the year 2005, as against $ 2 billion projected for the year 2002-03. Intensive efforts are being made to enter into the leather export markets of Russia and South East Asia. Of course, India should make its presence felt in the upcoming second line overseas market like South Africa, Australia, New Zealand, Canada, Japan, Spain, Portugal Saudi Arabia, etc. While the US accounts for about 19 percent of the total Indian leather exports, Germany, Italy, the UK and France together absorb over 40 per cent of the exports. Leather exports rose from Rs. 7790 million in 1985 to Rs. 92, 123 million in 2001. In 2000-01, India exported $ 1970.98 million worth of finished leather and leather goods, translating into 22.85 per cent growth in dollar terms. The lions share was from the South which contributed 42.58 per cent, as against the North's 18.78 per cent and the East 15.70 per cent. The impact of Chinese competition could be severe if that country progressively restructures its exports form labour-intensive to skill-and knowledge-intensive goods. The inconsistent duty policy of the government and competition from China are the main hindrances to India's leather industry. Some state governments, like UP government, impose taxes which are great deterrents. The imposition of an entry tax on leather goods is a case in point. The leather entrepreneurs have a key role to play. As far as marketing is concerned, strategies will have to be appropriately oriented, both at macro and micro levels, to meet the challenges. Market credibility will have to be established as a long-term measure. Also, the industry must invest on brand promotion, and, at the same time, support the national effort of image building through innovations in marketing, backed by quality of production and development of supply-line suited to the specific demand situations. However, Indian leather industry planners, researchers, and forecasters are now talking of brand building, fashion designing, and coining plans to enter top-end fashion markets of the world. The current stress is on product designing and development of leather parks.

There is a need to improve port efficiency. Because of competitive environment, the export product must reach the destinations (in the US or Europe) within 15 days. The industry is no doubt prepared to invest on all environmental measures, whatever be the cost, but needs proven technologies to undertake such investment. The industry must change its

---

The Chinese Factor

Indian exporters will feel the heat of increased competition from China and Europe and other markets where exports were subjected to quota restrictions till recently. Of course, India can take advantage of the progressive opening up of the huge Chinese market for footwear and other leather goods. There is also the likelihood of increased import of raw material by China from India. In 1999, the total leather exports from China were valued at $ 11,321.81 million, while it was $1970.98 million from India. Of course, India will ride the wave and come out stronger. China's annual import of about $3 billion worth of raw materials sustains its spectacular export growth. China's export today meets about 22 per cent of global import of leather and leather products. According to the strategic plans of China for this sector 5 per cent per annum growth in output and 7 per cent growth in foreign exchange earnings are envisaged until 2005.

attitude and should have global view of the opportunities, both in terms of availability of inputs for the industry and for marketing its products. Of course, measures should be initiated to curb dumping by China. The industry will be in trouble unless it lays emphasis on planned development aimed at optimum utilization of available raw materials for maximizing the returns, particularly from exports.

Outsourcing Attraction

The leather sector holds the promise of turning out to be yet another big outsourcing story for India. Last year, small-scale industry reservation for leather products was withdrawn, opening up the way for foreign direct investment (FDI) sector. Several European countries are preparing to relocate their manufacturing facilities to low-cost centres in Asia, which already supply most of the finished leather for the world market. India thus has a chance to attract some of this investment directly, and also to supply components to other manufacturing units being set up in Asia. India's leather product exports crossed $ 2 bn for the first time in 2003-04, a sharp recovery after successive years of decline. Footwear, the biggest item, registered a 27 per cent increase, accounting for almost half of the export earnings. Policy initiatives have also been announced, though in fits and starts. Allocation for the leather sector has been sharply hiked in the 10th Plan. The Plan proposals include employment-oriented policy promotion, integrating environmental protection with development, and offsetting the effects of dereservation and tariff reduction through gains in efficiency and higher investments. The Planning Commission has approved a Rs 400 crore modernisation and infrastructure fund. The foreign trade policy, among other incentives for export production in the sector, has given customs duty exemption for import of equipment for effluent treatment plants.

However, dereservation and policy support will not suddenly bring in a flood of FDI. India's leather industry faces several challenges. Foremost among these is scale efficiency. Although an integrated leather goods park in Kolkata is inching its way towards completion, and other facilities such as a tannery complex in Andhra Pradesh and a footwear park in Tamil Nadu are coming up, the scale of operations is nowhere near the gigantic proportions of China's leather industry. China turned out almost 500 mn sq m of leather and over 6 bn pairs of shoes in 2003. Its leather industry comprises over 16,000 large enterprises, with an output valued at over $ 25 bn last year, against India's $ 4 bn. India has only a 2 per cent share in the global footwear market; China has 20 per cent. China's leather exports accounted for about 5 per cent of its total exports in 2003, and almost a quarter of the $ 80 bn global market. China continues to register strong growth, both in its volume and range of operations. And it is certain that a significant chunk of the leather manufacturing facilities moving towards Asia will find their way into China.

India will, therefore, need to significantly ramp up capacities, and do it fast, if it is not to be overwhelmed by the competition. Besides, numerous obstacles, especially in infrastucture, still need to be overcome. Modernisation of existing units and effluent treatment at tanneries, an important environmental issue, should be taken up more actively. Manufacturing costs must be reduced through optimal use of raw material, which accounts for 60 per cent of total costs, to cut wastage and improve efficiencies. Infusion of technology is essential for productivity gains. In India, the industry average of shoe manufacture is 10-12 pairs per worker per day, only half that of China. And not withstanding the excitement over the prospective inflow of FDI, it is important to remember that two-thirds of the industry's output is from the small and cottage sector, which employ's a large workforce. A lack of credit for operations has been the small sector's bane, a shortcoming that has affected competitiveness and the quality of output. But the phenomenal success of the Tirupur textile cluster shows that the resources and output of a large number of small production units can be synergised, using the cluster approach to facilitate the flow of credit, technology and inputs. Another example is that of Italy, whose success in leather in leather exports is largely attributed to the cluster model. Leather processing clusters pattern should be taken up more aggressively in other parts of the country, especially in the south, where the industry is concentrated. With the largest livestock population in the world, India has a strong resource base, and it is also an important tanning centre. The leather industry can capitalise on these advantages to make India an important production base for the world market.

Growth Trends in the Trade of Livestock Products

The estimated annual compound growth rates are given in Table 12.9. While the growth rate in the exports of agricultural products was 5 percent, the exports from the livestock sector increased at an impressive growth rate of more than 11 percent during 1974 to 1998. Exports of eggs registered the highest annual growth rate (26 percent), followed by dairy products (21 percent) and meat and meat preparations (12 percent). Remaining products did not witness significant growth. The growth of exports of livestock products has accentuated and eggs witnessed higher growth in post-liberalisation period. The trade reforms initiated in the 1990s might have resulted in a significant improvement in the export of these livestock products. For instance, the minimum export prices for buffalo meat and mutton were removed in April 1993, which should have encouraged exports of these commodities. Export quotas were also recently removed.

The total imports of livestock products registered a negative growth rate. Among various items of imports, hides and skins presented most striking growth; their imports showed an annual growth of 25 percent. It is followed by imports of live animals (10 percent) during the period 1974-78. Imports of dairy products and animals fats showed a negative rate of growth. Imports of hides and skins slowed in the nineties (12 percent) as compared to the earlier period (24 percent). This may be attributed to the various measures taken to enhance the domestic availability of raw hides and skins.

Table 12.9: Commodity Wise Growth Rates of Indian Exports and Imports of Livestock Sector

Commodities	Exports			Imports		
	Annual compound growth rate (per cent)			Annual compound growth rate (per cent)		
	1974-90	1991-98	1974-98	1974-90	1991-98	1974-98
(1)	(2)	(3)	(4)	(5)	(6)	(7)
1. Total merchandise exports	8.02*	9.73*	8.85*	9.09*	11.67*	8.01*
2. Total agricultural products	3.27*	12.32*	4.86*	-0.07	22.09*	2.01**
3. Total livestock products	11.77*	21.60*	11.15*	0.69	3.75	-2.66**
4. Live animals	19.94*	18.60**	4.06	26.49*	-23.35*	9.91*
5. Meat and meat preparations	11.82*	22.49*	11.65*	4.31	21.88	3.30
6. Dairy products	23.12*	7.11	20.99*	-2.74	-1.94	-4.06
7. Eggs	15.48*	37.64*	25.76*	3.32	-28.19	0.68
8. Hides and skins	-13.72	-12.93**	1.45	24.36*	12.23*	24.90*
9. Animal fats	-10.55	40.25	0.58	-34.31*	4.94	-22.18*

Note: * and ** Significant at 1 and 5 percent level respectively.

Performance of Livestock Sector Trade

The data on net trade (exports minus imports) of livestock sector are presented in Table 12.10. A close perusal of the table revealed that we were net importers in livestock products till 1988. This scenario changed drastically during the nineties. This sector now holds good export potential as its exports exceed total imports significantly. A comparison of these figures in total agricultural and total merchandise trade brings out the fact that while the agricultural sector provided surplus foreign exchange, the trade deficit in the nonagricultural sector was the main cause for the problem of balance of payments. It is interesting to note that the share of exports from livestock sector in the total agricultural exports increased continuously from 1974-76 to 1983-85 (Table 12.11). Though the share of exports declined slightly for the triennium ending 1988 and 1991, it has again registered an increasing trend in the recent years. At the same time the share of total livestock exports in the total merchandise trade increased till 1982 and declined afterwards. However, again the trend reversed after 1994 and reached its peak in TE 1998. Thus the growth in export earnings from livestock products were better than those from other agricultural products. The share of imports of livestock sector in total agricultural and total merchandise imports in recent years has been declining (see Table 12.11). The ratio of livestock exports to livestock GDP has improved from 0.6 percent in TE 1982 to a little over one per cent in TE 1998. A reverse situation obtained in the case of livestock imports.

Table 12.10: Average Annual Imports, Exports and Trade Deficit of Livestock Sector, Agricultural Sector and Total Merchandise Trade in India

(10,000 US. dollars)

Item	1974-76	1977-79	1980-82	1983-85	1986-88	1989-91	1992-94	1996-98
(1)	(2)	(3)	(4)	(5)	(6)	(7)	(8)	(9)
1. Livestock sector								
(i) Imports	5,668	8,691	20,609	9,090	8,943	4,620	4,289	4,912
(ii) Exports	1,409	4,042	8,604	8,333	7,795	9,295	12,502	35,336
(iii) Trade surplus/deficit	-4,259	-4,649	-12,005	-757	-1,148	4,675	8,213	30,424
(iv) Exports as percent of imports	24.86	46.50	41.75	92	87.16	201.22	291.51	719.38
2. Agricultural sector								
(i) Imports	1,52,477	1,26,132	1,44,418	1,73,243	1,63,321	96,368	1,44,036	33,23.163
(ii) Exports	1,59,487	1,89,711	2,45,547	2,30,760	2,28,208	2,84,267	3,17,913	5,68.271
(iii) Trade surplus/deficit	7,010	63,579	1,01,129	57,517	64,887	1,87,899	1,73,877	2,45.108
(iv) Exports as percent of imports	104.59	150.41	170	133	140	294.98	220.72	175.85
3. Total merchandise trade								
(i) Imports	5,76,670	8,06,486	14,61,686	14,80,190	17,50,386	21,68,466	25,28,664	48,51.443
(ii) Exports	4,63,704	6,71,400	8,39,017	9,12,211	11,72,825	17,62,711	23,02,324	33,34.333
(iii) Trade surplus/deficit	-1,12,966	-1,35,086	-6,22,669	-5,67,979	-5,77,561	-4,05,755	-2,26,340	-15,17.110
(iv) Exports as percent of imports	80.41	83.25	57.40	61.63	67.00	81.28	91.05	68.73

Source: FAO Trade Year Book, various issues # indicates negligible share.

Table 12.11: Percent Share of Exports and Imports of Total Livestock Products in the Exports and Imports of Total Agricultural, Merchandise Trade and Livestock GDP

Triennium	Exports			Imports		
	Total agricultural exports	Total merchandise exports	Livestock GDP	Total agricultural imports	Total merchandise imports	Livestock GDP
(1)	(2)	(3)	(4)	(5)	(6)	(7)
1974-76	0.88	0.30	-	3.72	0.98	-
1977-79	2.13	0.60	-	6.89	1.08	-
1980-82	3.50	1.02	0.60	14.27	1.41	1.44
1983-85	3.61	0.91	0.50	5.25	0.61	0.55
1986-88	3.42	0.66	0.37	5.48	0.51	0.42
1989-91	3.27	0.53	0.42	4.79	0.21	0.21
1992-94	3.93	0.54	0.57	2.98	0.17	0.20
1996-98	6.22	1.05	1.01	1.52	0.10	0.22

Source: FAO Trade Year Book, various issues # indicates negligible share.

Destination of Trade

As regards India's trading patterns for export of both meat and preparation and poultry and dairy products, there are two or three major routes and a large number of countries are importing only small quantities. Each of the later countries contributes between 1-2 percent to the total foreign exchange earnings from these commodities. Data on the value of exports of these commodities and the relative share of different countries in the total exports are shown in Tables 12.12 and 12.13. Data on relative share of different countries in exports of eggs, raw hide and skins are shown in Tables in 12.14 and 12.15.

Table 12.12: Destination of Exports: Meat & Preparations

(US $ million)

Country	1993-94	1994-95	1995-96	1996-97	1997-98	1998-99	1999-00
World	109.72	128.30	187.73	199.86	217.77	187.29	180.44
Malaysia	37.35	47.83	54.54	68.85	62.80	44.04	50.81
UAE	26.16	25.46	45.80	41.76	49.62	46.86	50.26
Philippines	1.32	14.66	20.72	30.75	40.80	28.19	24.32
Saudi Arabia	9.33	9.75	7.29	8.98	8.06	9.19	7.83
Iran	1.40	0.06	2.45	7.88	10.31	13.69	7.10
Kuwait	4.65	3.29	5.88	4.69	5.56	5.88	5.29
Jordan	7.82	0.90	8.02	2.68	6.64	7.7	5.26
Oman	6.55	7.81	10.49	9.26	5.62	2.6	4.35
Mauritius	3.07	3.81	4.67	4.53	4.68	4.2	3.39
Gabon	-	0.29	0.10	0.59	2.63	1.87	2.49
Yemen	4.45	2.10	2.36	2.03	2.02	2.1	2.37

Table 12.12: Destination of Exports: Meat & Preparations (Contd.)

(US $ million)

Country	1993-94	1994-95	1995-96	1996-97	1997-98	1998-99	1999-00
Lebanon		0.04	1..95	0.99	2.71	2.64	2.31
Bahrain	2.64	2.06	2.93	2.88	2.91	2.35	1.79
Portugal		1.00	0.82	1.10	1.63	1.60	1.53
Angola		0.03	0.04	0.04	0.92	1.38	1.44
Egypt	0.20	0.13		0.05		0.03	1.25
Germany	0.04	0.13	0.36	0.24	0.19	0.34	0.72
Qatar	0.44	0.65	0.67	0.75	1.23	1.17	0.69
Turkey			2.45	1.56	0.79	1.76	0.66
Netherlands		0.35	0.99	0.44	0.25	1.22	0.51
Brazil						0.04	0.47
Greece	0.10	1.20	4.86	1.92	0.04	0.06	0.43
USA	0.06	0.31	2.90	2.94	0.67	0.33	0.41
France		0.55	1.30	0.78	1.24	1.13	0.41
Italy		0.10	0.10	0.15	0.13	0.21	0.39
Congo					0.14	0.13	0.37
Belgium				0.13		0.62	0.36
Japan	0.35	0.13	0.80	0.26	0.25	0.39	0.30
Singapore	3.24	2.83	0.47	0.19	0.51	0.34	0.28

(% share in total exports)

Country	1993-94	1994-95	1995-96	1996-97	1997-98	1998-99	1999-00
World	100.00	100.00	100.00	100.00	100.00	100.00	100.00
Malaysia	34.05	37.28	29.05	34.45	28.84	23.51	28.16
UAE	23.84	19.84	24.39	20.89	22.79	25.02	27.85
Philippines	1.20	11.43	11.04	15.30	18.74	15.02	13.48
Saudi Arabia	8.50	7.60	3.88	4.49	3.70	4.91	4.34
Iran	1.27	0.05	3.31	3.94	4.74	7.31	3.93
Kuwait	4.23	2.56	3.13	2.35	2.55	3.14	2.93
Jordan	7.12	0.70	4.27	1.34	3.05	4.14	2.92
Oman	5.97	6.09	5.59	4.63	2.58	1.41	2.41
Mauritius	2.80	2.97	2.49	2.26	2.15	2.24	1.88
Gabon		0.22	0.06	0.30	1.21	1.00	1.38
Yemen	4.05	1.63	1.26	1.01	0.93	1.45	1.32
Lebanon		0.03	1.04	0.50	1.24	1.41	1.28
Bahrain	2.41	1.60	1.56	1.44	1.34	1.26	0.99
Portugal		0.78	0.44	0.55	0.75	0.85	0.85
Angola		0.03	0.02	0.22	0.42	0.74	0.80
Egypt	0.18	0.10		0.22		0.01	0.69
Germany	0.04	0.10	0.19	0.12	0.09	0.18	0.40
Qatar	0.40	0.51	0.36	0.37	0.56	0.62	0.38
Turkey			1.31	0.78	0.38	0.94	0.37

Source: Centre for Monitoring Indian Economy, July 2000, P. 34.

Table 12.13: Destination of Exports: Poultry and Dairy Products

(US $ million)

Country	1994-95	1995-96	1996-97	1997-98	1998-99	1999-00
World	15.56	17.59	34.90	31.80	23.04	22.76
UAE	3.01	4.30	6.76	5.92	6.38	5.46
Bangladesh	3.10	3.89	2.28	3.32	3.37	5.20
Germany		0.67	6.53	3.29	1.55	1.66
USA	0.31	1.04	1.46	0.68	0.87	1.15
Oman	0.93	1.27	3.94	2.82	2.69	1.00
Belgium	0.02	0.45	2.44	0.35	0.06	0.85
Japan	0.01	0.21	1.90	2.29	1.00	0.83
Philippines	1.32	0.88	0.30	0.41	0.24	0.74
Kuwait	0.20	0.23	0.63	0.68	0.79	0.62
Saudi Arabia	0.70	0.46	1.47	2.53	0.75	0.55
Norway			0.05	0.13		0.51
Singapore	0.44	0.11	0.04	0.06	0.39	0.32
Poland		0.07	0.31	0.10	0.66	0.32
Australia		-	0.32	0.28	0.09	0.22
Morocco						0.21
Myanmar (Burma)				-	-	0.20
Korea Republic		0.10	0.37	0.59	0.24	0.19
Thailand		0.24	0.33	0.47	0.25	0.19
Bahrain	0.20	0.08	0.26	0.18	0.10	0.19
Indonesia		0.20	-	0.15	0.07	0.15
Sri Lanka	0.89	0.15	0.06	0.28	0.60	0.15
Canada		-	0.14	-	0.03	0.15
France			0.10	-	0.02	0.14
Hong Kong		-	0.26	0.07	0.16	0.14
Nepal	0.28	0.25	0.06	0.30	0.75	0.13
Taiwan (Taipei)				0.06		0.11
Austria			1.93	1.92	0.06	0.11
Mexico				-	0.16	0.11
South Africa	0.02	0.13	0.05	0.07	0.06	0.10

(% share in total exports)

Country	1994-95	1995-96	1996-97	1997-98	1998-99	1999-00
World	100.00	100.00	100.00	100.00	100.00	100.00
UAE	19.33	24.42	19.38	18.62	27.69	23.98
Bangladesh	19.92	22.11	6.54	10.45	14.62	22.86
Germany		3.78	18.70	10.35	6.71	7.30
USA	1.97	5.89	4.17	2.14	3.78	5.04
Oman	5.98	7.22	11.28	8.86	11.68	4.41
Belgium	0.14	2.58	6.98	1.12	0.27	3.72
Japan	0.08	1.20	5.46	7.19	4.34	3.66
Philippines	8.67	4.99	0.87	1.29	1.04	3.27

Table 12.13: Destination of Exports: Poultry and Dairy Products (Contd.)

(% share in total exports)

Country	1994-95	1995-96	1996-97	1997-98	1998-99	1999-00
Kuwait	1.32	1.31	1.80	2.14	3.45	2.72
Saudi Arabia	4.50	2.62	4.22	7.94	3.24	2.42
Norway			0.14	0.41		2.23
Singapore	2.82	0.61	0.11	0.20	1.68	1.42
Poland		0.40	0.88	0.30	2.85	1.39
Australia			0.19	0.89	0.39	0.96
Morocco						0.90
Myanmar (Burma)					0.02	0.90
Korea Republic		0.57	1.06	1.84	1.04	0.85
Thailand		1.35	0.95	1.47	1.07	0.84
Bahrain	1.29	0.46	0.76	0.57	0.42	0.83

Source: Centre for Monitoring Indian Economy, July 2000, P. 34.

Table 12.14: Countrywise Shares of Eggs Exported from India

(Per cent)

Country	1993-94	1994-95	1995-96	1996-97	1997-98	1998-99
(1)	(2)	(3)	(4)	(5)	(6)	(7)
UAE	11.03	13.65	29.04	20.02	19.14	28.51
Bangladesh	39.61	2.80	1.82	1.02	7.20	16.69
Oman	20.22	28.40	17.45	13.03	10.41	16.04
Japan	-	-	3.22	6.44	8.60	6.15
Kuwait	0.16	0.02	1.25	2.08	2.55	4.87
Saudi Arabia	23.58	32.82	6.61	4.81	9.25	4.35
Poland	-	-	1.07	1.04	0.29	4.02
Netherlands	-	-	-	3.37	6.14	2.90
Singapore	-	-	-	-	0.06	2.15
U.S.A.	0.39	0.83	-	0.36	0.28	1.44
Korea	-	-	1.54	1.78	2.11	1.23
Thailand	-	-	0.97	1.12	1.75	1.22
Germany	-	-	9.72	21.13	10.87	1.22
Philippines	-	-	-	0.06	0.76	0.70
Qatar	0.49	0.65	0.06	0.08	0.26	0.62
Australia	-	-	-	1.08	1.07	0.55
Belgium	-	-	0.58	7.90	1.34	0.38
South Africa	0.16	1.16	0.09	0.16	0.28	0.36
Maldives	1.95	12.82	3.88	0.57	0.47	0.35
Austria	-	-	-	6.51	7.22	0.35
Iran	2.04	6.58	1.08	0.54	0.21	0.22
Italy	-	0.14	-	3.05	-	0.10
Sri Lanka	-	0.12	0.19	-	0.06	-
Russia	0.16	-	21.38	0.81	3.70	-

Table 12.15: *Country wise Shares of Raw Hides and Skins Imported to India*

(Per cent)

Country	1992-93	1993-94	1994-95	1995-96	1996-97	1997-98	1998-99
(1)	(2)	(3)	(4)	(5)	(6)	(7)	(8)
Germany	5.44	7.32	8.42	9.61	9.76	12.95	12.71
Italy	0.53	0.48	0.75	0.53	2.09	3.94	12.65
New Zealand	33.44	25.03	21.56	26.33	15.11	10.72	9.43
U.K.	19.33	15.73	14.43	11.23	7.39	6.47	6.86
Indonesia	0.02	0.15	-	0.06	0.13	0.43	5.98
Netherlands	0.70	1.27	8.60	6.30	3.52	2.47	4.14
France	5.48	0.32	0.74	0.86	0.32	1.59	3.38
Saudi Arabia	2.30	8.74	4.40	4.65	6.27	4.56	3.14
China	0.90	0.80	1.62	0.94	5.04	4.09	3.04
U.S.A.	0.18	1.38	0.97	1.83	5.04	4.09	2.90
UAE	0.39	1.08	2.03	2.11	1.71	5.98	2.89
Sudan	1.11	1.75	1.69	1.61	1.65	0.93	2.61
Nepal	3.48	5.21	3.33	2.57	3.64	3.70	2.32
Sweden	-	0.35	5.67	5.82	2.67	0.98	2.24
Yemen	-	0.53	0.87	-	0.64	2.13	2.04
Ukraine	-	0.60	0.03	1.38	1.12	2.16	1.99
Russia	2.02	2.88	0.92	1.80	2.13	1.76	1.85
Kenya	4.77	2.47	3.32	1.21	5.18	4.69	1.73
Brazil	1.48	0.29	0.53	3.90	7.03	5.04	1.62

1. Leather goods and wool products were classified as manufactured products as per the classification of products given by the Directorate General of Commercial Intelligence and Statistics (DGCI&S). Therefore, these products were not included in the composition of the trade of livestock products. However, the inclusion of these products would substantially enhance the share of livestock exports in total agricultural exports.
2. Other benefits include concessional rents, exemption from sales tax, excise duty on capital goods, components and raw materials, income tax for a block of five years, etc.

Although, the concept of organic livestock production is very attractive, so far not much has been done to promote organic farming system in India. While a few NGOs and other agencies like Apeda have taken lead in organic agricultural production, by and large, the livestock component of the system is virtually untapped. For ensuring organic livestock production, organic agriculture is a must. To capitalize on this niche market, a National Programme for Organic Production has been launched and the road map includes preparation of documents like national standards, accreditation criteria and procedures for a crediting, inspection and certification agencies has been prepared.

Export Market Opportunities for Livestock Products

India's international trade in livestock and poultry (live and products) is small despite the country having a very large livestock population. The major factors which impede exports of livestock and their products are, inter alia, high prices of the products making those uncompetitive in the international market, rigid phytosanitary restrictions in the importing countries and absence of adequate export promotional drives for livestock and poultry products along with virtual nonexistent market intelligence collection system. Exports of major livestock products - including live animals, meat, meat and dairy products, eggs and hides and skins - account for only 7 per cent of total agricultural exports estimated at US $ 5.8 billion. This ratio was 4 per cent in 1992.

An examination of international competitiveness of livestock products, indicate that India enjoys international price advantage in buffalo meat and mutton. However, the Indian dairy product prices relative to other countries have not so far been competitive internationally. Although producer milk prices in India are significantly lower than those in the United States and Western Europe, dairy product prices (butter and whole and skim milk powder) are substantially higher than international market prices. This is due to domestic processing inefficiencies (Table 12.16). Only during 90's, with the devaluation of the Rupee and the sharp rise in world dairy product prices, did the gap between Indian dairy prices and world market prices narrowed. In addition, fluid milk marketing margins are high in India– for example, it is about 67 percent higher than in the United Kingdom. India also lacks international competitiveness in poultry products.[1]

With the removal of all QRs. on the imports of agricultural product since 1 April 2001, the Indian Authorities would have to address urgently the issue of increasing efficiency in the production and processing of livestock products as well as improving their quality. With the relatively low cost of labour and the introduction of modern technology, it is expected that in due course India may become internationally competitive in most of the livestock products mentioned above.

Currently India exports only a fraction of most of the livestock products out of its total output. Similarly, India's share in the total imports of each of the products by its major partners is not significant. There seems to be considerable scope in increasing export of some of the major livestock products during the next three decades. Prospects for exports of some of these items are discussed below.

Two binding agreements relevant for food regulations under WTO regime which are of major concern to India are the agreements on Sanitary and Phytosanitary measures (SPS) and Technical Barriers on Trade (TBT) which stipulate quality assurance such as hazard analysis critical control point

---

[1] World Bank: India: Livestock Sector Review: Enhancing Growth and Development, May 23, 1996, p.62

Table 12.16: Comparison of Indian and World Market Prices for Selected Dairy and Meat Products: 1995-2000

(US $ per ton)

Item	1995	1996	1997	1998	1999	2000
Milk Producer Prices						
India: Cows (40% fat)	210	214	218	237		
Buffalo (70% fat)	280	286	291	305		
Germany	360	383	360	328	321	
U.K.	371	364	328	294	283	
U.S.	281	321	294	340	317	
Butter						
India: Wholesale	2868	3011	3086	3163		
Export Price European Port (FOB)	2246	1877	1911	1907	1445	1384
Skim Milk Powder						
India: Wholesale	2186	2326	2420	2450		
Export Price European port (FOB)	2077	1838	1675	1414	1295	1797
Beef						
India: Wholesale price	850	925	1036	1087		
US Domestic wholesale	2352	2273	2277	2202	2449	2591
Australia (CIF)	1947	1741	1880	1754	1894	1957
Argentina (FOB)	1935	1788	1869	2229	1910	1986
EU Export Price (FOB)	1627	1556	1540	1677	1356	1297
Mutton						
India: Wholesale Price	1590	1795	1970	2150		
New Zealand (CIF London)	2621	3295	3393	2750	2610	2619

Source: NDDB: Ministry of Agriculture: Prices in India; Statistical Office of the European Community Eurostat Agriculture Statistical Yearbook: Australia: Meat Exporters News; New Zealand: World Bank's Monthly Commodity Prices- Pink Sheet. Argentina: Analysis de Mercados Internationales de la Carne – SAGYP. FAO's Commodities & Trade Division supplied to the authors the International prices quoted above.

(HACCP) based system, code of practices on good animal food, good hygienic practices (GHPs) and cold chain system. To accomplish quality, modern processing and infrastructural facilities should be developed to achieve the goals. Prospects of exports of some of these items are discussed below.

Meat Trade: FAO's Projection to the Year 2015 and 2030

indicate a lower growth in world meat consumption. This is due to lower population growth compare with the past and the natural deceleration of growth accompanying the attainment of fairly high consumption levels in the few major developed countries that dominated past increases. The total world meat demand is projected to grow at 1.9 percent per annum in the next 20 years, down from 2.8 percent in the preceding 20 years. For developing countries the growth in demand is projected at 2.8 percent per annum against 5.5 percent during the previous two decades. However, for South East Asian countries as well as for the Near East and North Africa due to the better prospects for income growth during the next ten years, higher growth in meat consumption is anticipated. Fortunately, India's main partners for meat and meat products belong to these two regions.

Despite Projected Low Growth Rates for Meat Consumption, Buoyancy in World

meat trade of the recent past is likely to continue. This is due to the changes in the trade policy regimes due to WTO Agreement and rebound of the economies in the South East Asian region. The FAO projections for meat production and consumption in the different regions imply a significant increase in the volume of trade in meat during the period 2015/2030. Total meat trade is projected to increase from 7.1 million tonnes during 1995/97 to about 12 million tonnes by the year 2015 and 17.4 million tonnes by the year 2030. The volume of net imports mainly by the developing and transition countries is projected to increase from 2.5 million tonnes in 1995/97 to about 5 million tonnes in 2015 and 7.6 million tonnes by the year 2030.[1] Overall, the trend for the developing countries to become growing net importers of meat is set to continue. Imports of poultry meat will likely dominate the picture of growing dependence on imported meat. Salient features of the latest FAO import projections for meat and milk and dairy products are summarized below:

MEAT Import: World Imports of Total Meat

are projected to increase at the rate of 4 percent per annum during 1995-97 to 2015 and 4.5 percent per annum during 2015 to 2030. Total imports will increase from 2.35 million tonnes in 1995-97 to 5.16 million tonnes by 2015 and 8 million tonnes by the year 2030. **Imports of bovine meat** are projected to rise from 0.56 to 1 million tonnes during the first period and to 1.45 million tonnes during the second period. Bulk of imports of the bovine meat would be in the developing countries. Their imports will total 0.8 and 1.3 million tonnes respectively in 2015 and 2030.

Among Different Regions

import requirements for total meat for **the Near East/North Africa** are projected to increase annually by 4.5 percent during 1995-97 to 2015 and by 5 percent per annum during 2015 to 2030. Their total imports of all meat are anticipated to increase from 1.21 million tonnes to 2.9 million tonnes during the first period and to 4.72 million tonnes by the year 2030. Imports by the South East Asia are projected to recover dramatically by

---

[1]FAO: Agriculture: Towards 2015/30, Technical Interim Report: April 2000.

almost 13 percent per annum during the first period. It will also rise during the second period but by only 4.5 percent per annum. Their total meat imports would rise from 2.55 million tonnes by 2015 and 3.94 million tonnes by the year 2030.

Growth in Poultry Meat Trade

is likely to continue. World imports of poultry meat are projected to more than double (from 1.52 million tonnes to 3.20 million tonnes) during 1995-'97 to 2015 and increase further by 46 percent to 4.78 million tonnes by 2030. The growth rate would accelerate from 3.8 percent per annum to 4.1 percent. Among the total, poultry meat, imports into developing countries are projected at 2.4 million tonnes (i.e. 75 percent of the total) and 3.95 million tonnes (i.e. 82 percent) respectively.

India can and must take advantage of the expanding world trade in meat and meat products as well as for milk and diary products. As discussed above, most of the increased import requirements for meat and meat products are projected to be in the Near East/North Africa and South East Asian countries, which are the major trading partners of India.

The export of meat from India began in the early 1970s. The bulk of its meat exports consists of buffalo meat. With the boom in the price of the Persian petroleum products, meat exports to the Persian Gulf and the Middle East registered rapid growth during the 1970s. The major importing countries include United Arab Emirates (UEA), Kuwait, Saudi Arabia, Oman, Bahrain, Qatar, Iran and Yemen. Meat exports from India suffered a setback on account of a ban imposed by Saudi Arabia in 1982 because of the presence of Rinderpest and Foot and Mouth disease. This has been partly compensated by developing new markets in Malaysia and Philippines. During 1994/95-1996/97 out of India's total annual average exports 154.5 thousand tonnes, around 86 percent were shipped to the above-mentioned ten countries. The remaining 14 percent were exported to twenty countries.

For the ten major importing countries, out of their total meat imports of 1.27 million tonnes Indian supplies accounted for only 7 percent. The import requirements of these countries are likely to increase in accordance with the projected rate of growth for the Near East/North Africa and for the South East Asia. Based on the projected rate of growth of these two regions, total meat import requirements in these ten countries are forecast to increase from 1.27 million tonnes in 1995-97 to 4.25 million tonnes by the year 2010 and to 6.72 million tonnes by the year 2030. India has the potential in the medium and long terms to expand its meat exports to these as well as to some other countries.

VERMIN-COMPOST EXPORTS

There's always a first time for everything – exports included. After sending everything from cycle-rickshaws to khadi jeans to the Big Apple, Delhi has literally tied up all the 'loose ends' in the export book. An MCD brainwave will see the civic agency exporting to the US the dung and urine produced by the thousands of stray cattle on Delhi's roads. Going by the black and white of the MCD's blueprints, while the dung will be processed into vermin-compost, the urine will be converted into a bio-pesticide, Productivity- wise, an estimated 1.6 lakh kg of vermin-compost and 70,000 litres of bio-pesticide are expected to be churned out on a daily basis.

'Dung-ho' over its ambitious plan, the MCD maintains that its initiative will not only milk foreign resources from the US, but also take a local problem by the horns. "Delhi has approximately 35,000 shelterless cows," There has been attempt to solve this problem by working with the Morarka Foundation, an NGO engaged in eco-projects. To put its plan on track, the process of purchasing hydraulic trucks which will help it catch stray cattle and transport them to shelters in and around Delhi. With dearth of cows in the US, the demand for Indian cow-dung there is quite high. In fact, chemical analysis reveals that the dung of the Indian cow scores over the US version by way of organic content.

Products from dung and urine are new becoming very popular the world over. Having its network in Rajasthan, Punjab, Haryana, Gujarat, Delhi, Maharashtra, Tamil Nadu, Andhra Pradesh and North-Eastern Region, the Morarka Foundation has been given consultative status for developing value added products from cow dung by several State Governments and international development organizations like UNICEF, Help Age India and Care India. Right now the MCD has launched a massive drive to catch stray cattle in the Capital and shift them to gaushalas, even though it is facing tough resistance from the local people running unauthorized dairies in residential areas. The Delhi High Court has directed the Delhi police to provide protection to the MCD team engaged for such a purpose after reports appeared in the media that civic body officials were being beaten by those running illegal dairies. Given the large number of stray cattle on Delhi road whose dung is mostly thrown into a drain and finally ends up in the Yamuna, it was a good proposition to utilize hundreds of tonnes of cow dung for such a purpose which would ultimately be exported to the developed world.

MILK AND DAIRY PRODUCTS — WORLD TRADE

The FAO's projection of demand and production suggest that developing countries will continue to face a growing trade deficit in diary products. World trade in dairy products is likely to recover with the net imports of the developing countries resuming growth after a period of stagnation from the mid-1980s onwards. This would reflect essentially continuation (after the recovery from the recent economic crisis) of the growth of imports of East Asia as well as the resumption of import growth into the major deficit regions, (the Near East/North Africa), following recovery in the growth in demand. All developing regions would continue to be large net importers of milk and dairy products during the three projection sub-periods viz. to the year 2010, 2020 and 2030. Of the total increase in their import requirements of 24.7 million tonnes during the period 1995-97 to 2030,

South East Asia will account for over 50 percent followed by Near East/ North Africa, accounting for 32 percent.[1] The petroleum exporting countries in the Near East will remain the largest importing countries with Saudi Arabia, Iran, Kuwait, Malaysia and Indonesia being the principal customers. Other important buyers will be Thailand, the Philippines, Sri Lanka and Pakistan. The Republic of Korea with its protected young diary industry by restrictive import policy until the late 1980s, will allow foreign supplier to satisfy a greater share of its growing demand. The world biggest net importer is expected to be Japan whose total market for dairy products continues to expand with its degree of self-reliance tending to decline. Much of the Japan's import requirements will come from New Zealand and Australia.

With the rapid expansion of the dairy sector particularly since 1980s, India began to export dairy products. However, India still exports only limited quantities of milk and cream concentrated/containing sugar/ sweetening milk and butter. It seems to have good potential for further growth in exports of these products. The major importers include Bangladesh, Kuwait, Saudi Arabia, and Oman. India can strengthen its position in these markets and try to develop a few new markets, especially for milk products such as milk based sweat-meat, which are quite popular among the expatriates as well as ethnic Asian community abroad. The bulk of the future expansion of milk imports is projected to originate in the two regions, which India can take advantage of.

Based on the FAO projected rates of growth in trade for different meats and for milk and dairy products, total as well as of different regional groups, and India's production and export potential an attempt has been made below (Table 12.17) to project Indian exports of different categories of meat, milk and diary products by the years 2010, 2020 and 2030.

India also exports live animals, eggs, wool and hair. However, it is not practical to prepare a medium and long-term projections for these items. Nevertheless, there is no doubt that trade in these products will also increase substantially during the next three decades. Indian exports of these products will also increase further. The existing egg powder plants are primarily for exports. There is every possibility that more plants may also come up and exports pick up further.

Indian exports of livestock and dairy products have to be competitive price wise and qualitatively equal if not superior to those of the developed countries. Export oriented meat and poultry dressing plants require to be enlarged with strict enforcement of quality control programme. As regards meat exports, the requirements in the Middle East are not just regulatory in nature. These also involve the requirements imposed by the importers, i.e. those relating to quality, prices, punctuality of delivery, etc. The basic regulatory requirements for meat imports in the Near Eastern countries are

---

[1] FAO: Agriculture Towards 2015/2030. op.cit.

Table 12.17: Actual and Projected Exports of Meat, Milk and Dairy Products from India

(Tonnes)

Category	Actual exports Average 1994/95- 1996/97	2010	2020	2030
MEAT				
Buffalo Meat	144,461	193,580 (2.0)	259,400 (3.0)	365,750 (3.5)
Sheep and Goat Meat	9,374	16,680 (4.0)	29,860 (6.0)	64,500 (8.0)
Pig Meat	676	1,670 (3.5)	2,470 (4.0)	4,420 (6.0)
Poultry Meat	19	50 (7.0)	130 (10.0)	410 (12.0)
Total	154,530	211,980 (2.1)	291,7860 (3.2)	453,080 (4.0)
Milk & Milk Products				
Milk and Cream	5,127	9,230 (4.0)	15,050 (5.0)	26,940 (6.0)
Butter	581	1,040 (4.0)	1,685 (5.0)	3,020 (6.0)
Total	5,708	10,270 (4.0)	16,735 (5.0)	29,960 (6.0)

N.B: Figures in brackets are compound rate of growth percent per annum over previous period.

Source: Actual 1994/95 – 1996/97: Directorate General of Commercial Intelligence and Statistics, Calcutta: Foreign Trade Statistics: various issues.

Projections made by Professional Team of Techno-Economic Research Institute, Saket, New Delhi

the "Halal" slaughter and the fitness for human consumption certificate. Zoo-sanitary requirements are the primary regulatory consideration and these are the main bottlenecks in expanding Indian exports. To minimize the possibility of disease transmission through the animals and meat exports, it is essential that the veterinary services be brought up to a standard where they would be fully effective. The requirements for effective disease control in trade animals (vaccination and certification, quarantines and veterinary control of animal and meat movement) should be efficiently and effectively implemented.

The competitiveness in the world market dictates the requirements of modern export marketing infrastructure as well as for business efficiency. In India the exporters face a number of obstacles in developing a sustained export trade. The structural factors include: cumbersome bureaucratic procedures, lack of market information, export financing and payment problems. Urgent attention is needed to tackle these problems for taking advantage of the growing world livestock product market for which India has good potential.

Livestock Trade Policy Reform

Agricultural exports and imports (which encompass livestock products also) were regulated through quantitative restrictions such as quotas and licenses or channelled through a state trading organisation or some combination of both until recently (Nayyar and Sen, 1994; Chand, 1997). In April 1995, the Government of India (GOI) introduced major trade policy reforms that encompassed livestock products. Most of the quantitative restrictions (QRs) for livestock trade flows have been dismantled. Import tariffs for most livestock products were significantly reduced. Tariffs for skimmed milk powder (SMP) and pureline poultry stocks were completely eliminated.

Trade reforms have relaxed most of the restrictions on the export of livestock products, as well as some export promotional schemes are also operational. Exports of non-breedable or culled buffaloes, sheep and goats were subjected to quantitative restrictions and minimum export prices. These restrictions continued during the initial phase of liberalisation and were removed only in 1994 (NCAER, 1996). The export of buffalo meat was free from any restrictions since the 1980s. Sheep and goat meat exports were restricted by quotas and minimum export prices (MEPs). Now, the export of these items is allowed without a license and the associated terms and conditions were also deleted. By and large, exports of hides and skins are prohibited. The only exceptions are skins of stray dogs and lambs. Exports of milk and milk products were prohibited earlier. However, exports of milk, baby milk and sterilised milk are now permitted subject to licensing requirements. The export of powdered milk was prohibited earlier and later canalised through the NDDB. Subsequently, decanalisation has taken place. Restrictions in butter exports have been similar to those for powdered milk. However, the export of ghee was subjected to quantitative restriction in the 1980s, followed by canalisation with NDDB. Finally, exports were decanalised. The quantitative restrictions on the above items have already been removed with effect from April 1, 2000. Some export promotional schemes are also operational. For instance, firms classified as export-oriented units (EOUs) and those within export processing zones (EPZs) may import, duty free, any goods including capital goods required for manufacturing, production of processing activities, provided that the goods are not prohibited under the negative lists of imports. In the case of animal husbandry and poultry, the EPZ unit or EOU may sell up to 50 percent of production domestically (World Bank, 1999). EPZs have been established in Delhi, Mumbai, Calcutta, Madras, Vishakhapatnam, Kandla and Cochin. These firms also enjoy tax breaks and other benefits. Establishment of Special Establishment of Special Economic Zones (SEZs) was proposed in the different parts of the country on the lines of highly successful Chinese experiments, in the Exim Policy announced on March 31, 2000.

The idea behind the establishment of SEZs is that in these areas export production can take place free from the plethora of rules and regulations governing import and export. The government is willing to permit 100 per cent fully foreign-owned units in these zones, provided that the entire output is exported. Moreover, the existing EPZs would be converted into SEZs.

There are some other financial incentive schemes sponsored by the Agricultural and Processed Food Products Export Development Authority

(APEDA). The authority provides subsidies to exporters, growers, trade associations and government agencies to pursue export promotion and market development activities, strengthen market intelligence and information channels, improve export quality, develop infrastructure and human resource capacity, modernise meat processing facilities and perform research and development (World Bank, 1999).

The policy of trade liberalisation seems to have provided impetus to livestock exports, which have registered remarkable growth during the 1990s. Liberalisation offers both opportunities and challenges to the policy makers. For instance, the recent lifting of most import restrictions on dairy and poultry meat may adversely affect producers if it is not coupled with structural changes in the processing and marketing sectors to reduce marketing costs and margin (World Bank, 1999). Diversity of livestock farming systems in India and the existing differentials in actual and potential yields augur well for export of livestock commodities. However, India has to be cautions with regard to sanitary and phytosanitary measures and intellectual property rights issues.

CONCLUSIONS

It can be concluded that export of meat and meat preparations showed most stable and promising performance. To give a further boost to it, the various sanitary and phytosanitary measures should be taken up vigorously to ensure the international hygienic standards of our livestock exports particularly to developed countries which are lacking now. Within meat and meat preparations, India is very competitive in buffalo and cow meat and reasonably competitive in mutton. However, the sociocultural factors may hinder export of cattle meat. Mutton exports may be constrained by domestic demand. Despite impressive growth of exports of dairy products and eggs (especially in the 1990s), their exports may be limited by their lack of international competitiveness. To make dairy products internationally competitive, domestic processing efficiency has to be improved substantially. The exports of leather goods are consistently increasing and the earnings thereof can pay for the imports of raw hides and skins, although China is taking a big chunk of share in leather garments.

Appendix I

Table 12AI.1: *Countrywise Shares of Meat and Meat Preparations exported from India*

(Per cent)

Country	1992-93	1993-94	1994-95	1995-96	1996-97	1997-98	1998-99
(1)	(2)	(3)	(4)	(5)	(6)	(7)	(8)
UAE	24.81	23.84	19.84	24.39	20.89	22.79	25.20
Malaysia	36.47	34.05	37.28	29.05	34.45	28.84	23.10
Philippines	-	1.20	11.43	11.04	15.30	18.74	14.85
Iran	-	1.27	0.05	1.31	3.94	4.74	7.46
Saudi Arabia	7.27	8.50	7.60	3.88	4.49	3.70	5.03
Jordan	9.66	7.12	0.70	4.27	1.34	3.05	4.19
Kuwait	3.76	4.23	2.56	3.13	2.35	2.55	3.04
Mauritius	2.26	2.80	2.97	2.49	2.26	2.15	2.28
Lebanon	-	-	0.03	1.04	0.50	1.24	1.50
Yemen	4.92	4.05	1.63	1.26	1.01	0.93	1.41
Oman	6.45	5.97	6.09	5.59	4.63	2.58	1.27
Bahrain	2.20	2.41	1.60	1.56	1.44	1.34	1.23
Turkey	-	-	-	1.31	0.78	0.36	1.12

Appendix II

Table 11AII.1: Countrywise Shares of Dairy and Dairy Products Exported from India

(Per cent)

Country	1993-94	1994-95	1995-96	1996-97	1997-98	1998-99
(1)	(2)	(3)	(4)	(5)	(6)	(7)
UAE	23.40	20.77	27.96	22.98	-	40.95
Nepal	4.47	2.02	2.64	1.15	7.21	17.12
USA	0.76	1.39 ·	7.71	19.22	8.62	13.88
Bangladesh	35.62	19.83	20.81	8.14	30.82	9.96
Mexico	0.13	-	-	-	-	4.07
Hong Kong	0.15	-	0.01	4.62	0.77	2.26
Sri Lanka	8.69	6.87	0.68	1.27	4.54	2.09
Oman	-	2.78	1.50	1.87	1.20	1.45
Thailand	-	-	2.21	-	-	1.18
Philippines	0.18	11.00	11.16	8.25	5.37	1.15
Singapore	0.18	2.65	1.36	0.32	1.14	0.90
Saudi Arabia	-	0.14	-	-	0.84	0.62
Bahrain	5.17	1.64	1.01	2.83	-	0.58
Netherlands	0.39	21.53	9.89	0.85	0.06	0.51
Bhutan	-	0.04	-	1.86	-	0.28
Russia	11.34	-	-	-	-	0.05
Germany	0.33	-	0.34	6.42	0.42	0.03
Belgium	-	0.17	5.28	2.86	-	-
Indonesia	-	-	2.57		0.02	-
Kuwait	4.29	1.67	1.90	1.17	-	-
South Africa	-	-	1.55	-	-	-
U.K.	-	-	0.80	13.45	-	-
Mauritius	1.19	0.18	0.01	-	-	-
Ghana	-	-		1.70	15.36	-
Yemen	-	5.59	-	-	-	-

13

Economics of Livestock Enterprises

The livestock farming in general and the dairy industry in particular have undergone great changes both in its structure and in its methods of production. For instance in the dairy farming, more and more small farmers, marginal farmers and landless agricultural labourers are being brought into the fold of the schemes in these sectors. Dairy farming is practiced mainly as a subsidiary rural occupation. However, for the weaker sections and landless agricultural labourers, dairying, goat and sheep rearing offer promising returns especially daily returns. For dairy farming initial capital requirements are high. But milk production has the important advantage of being less dependent upon seasonal working capital than arable stock rearing or fattening enterprises due to the regular nature of its sales in the form of weekly or monthly milk cheque.

When judged on the basis of gross margin produced per forage hectare, dairying would seem to be one of the most efficient ways of converting grass and forage crops into cash. The profitability of the enterprise will depend upon the levels of fixed costs and capital investment. Under Indian farming systems and conditions, dairying offers ample job opportunities especially for the rural women, unable to get regular employment due to seasonality in agriculture. Further, women cannot travel that long to get employment also, especially in the rural areas.

A wide range of factors are involved in determining the ultimate profitability of milk production and consequently much confused thinking persists on the relative importance of each. The significance of one factor will vary from farm to farm and each case needs to be judged upon its own merits and farming conditions. The most useful measure of profitability within an enterprise is the return on farmers' capital, since this single factor involves and is influenced by just about every other possible factor of production. However, profitability is more frequently expressed for comparative purposes as gross or net margin per cow or per buffalo, or net margin per hectare. Interpretation of profitability expressed in this way will depend largely upon the farm in question.

In general, a high overall return on capital is the aim. In order to achieve this, it will be necessary to obtain the maximum possible margin within the limits that are imposed. Thus, if physical factors like buildings, labour, etc., limit the number of cows or buffaloes to be kept, then it is necessary to achieve a higher margin per cow or buffalo in order to achieve a good return on capital for the enterprise.

However, if land is the only factor imposing a limit on the enterprise, then it may be possible to achieve the same or even better return on capital from a lower margin per cow or per buffalo, but with a lot more cows or buffaloes on the same hectarage, provided that the stocking rate is increased sufficiently to result in an increased margin per hectare.

Final profitability or "net margin" will be the difference between (a) gross margin, (b) fixed costs, whether expressed per cow or buffalo or per hectare. Factors affecting "gross margin" include gross output per cow or per buffalo. Gross margin represents the quantity of milk sold multiplied by price realized. The value of milk sold per cow or buffalo per year is the result of several factors. Quantity of milk sold per cow or per buffalo per year is a function of (i) Yield per cow or per buffalo per lactation; (ii) Calving index i.e. the interval in days between calvings: (iii) Hygienic quality of milk produced and (iv) Seasonality of production. Factors affecting the profitability of production are depicted in Graph 13.1.

Enterprise gross output per forage hectare: This measure is simply a function of gross output per cow or per buffalo and stocking density. Gross output per hectare will increase as stocking density increases since it is not affected by extra feed costs, which usually accompany a heavier stock density.

Enterprise net output per forage hectare: This is a far more valuable measure upon which to compare output per hectare since it relates to the margin achieved per hectare after deducting the cost of purchased and homegrown feeds from the gross output. It is easy enough to increase gross output per hectare, simply by buying in large quantity of feeds and thereby increasing stock density. Any ultimate profit will come from the net output, i.e., the difference between gross output and feeding-stuff cost.

VARIABLE COSTS

Concentrates whether purchased or home grown, are usually the principal items of variable cost incurred in milk production and represent one section of expenditure, over which the farmer has some degree of immediate control. The rate of feeding concentrates will depend upon the availability of quality fodder as well the price at which milk is sold. The feeding of concentrates is, therefore, practiced in order to sustain or increase the level of milk yield. The most economic level of concentrate feeding will depend upon the response of the animal to concentrates, which in turn will depend upon the quality of their diet, upon their genetic potential and upon the level of yield already being achieved.

The important concentrates feed economy measures include (i) Kilogram of concentrate fed per litre of milk and (ii) Cost of the concentrate per litre of milk. The ratio of milk produced to concentrates fed can only be a valid

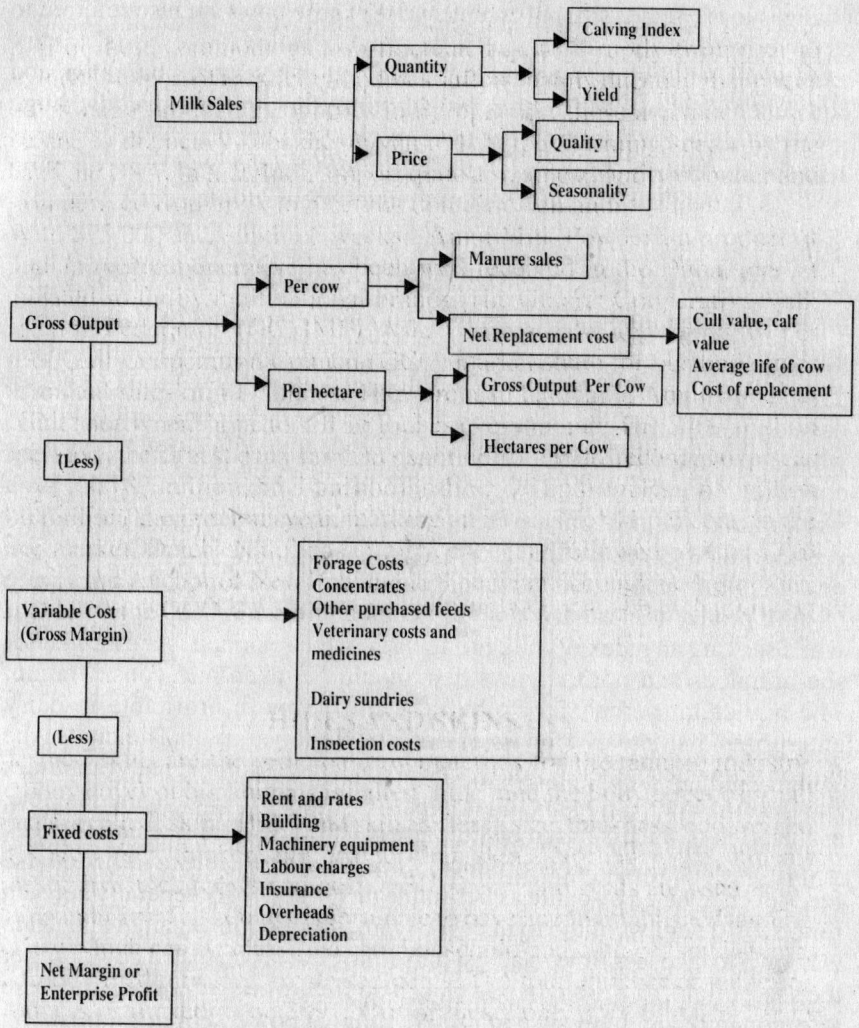

Graph 13.1: Factors affecting the profitability of production

measure of comparing the efficiency of feed used between herds when their levels of yield are the same.

However, caution has to be exercised regarding the quality of concentrates obtained from the market. Other variable costs include cost of feed and fodders, cost of veterinary medicines, service fees, cost of minerals etc. and labour charges.

FIXED COSTS

These are defined as those farm cost items which are not easily allocated to particular farm enterprise and which do not vary very much with small changes in the scale (size) of an enterprise. These costs are also referred to as 'overhead costs', 'common costs', and 'unallocatable costs'. Dairy enterprises require high capital cost involved in livestock, buildings and equipments. However, under Indian rural farming conditions, huge investments in building and equipments are not necessary. The labour is also family labour. Thus, as compared to developed countries' farming systems, Indian system requires lower investment in fixed costs.

BUFFALO AND SMALL RUMINANT ENTERPRISES

Dairy Buffalo Enterprise

Similar economic analysis for buffalo and small ruminants has been attempted in this chapter. Buffalo makes a value contribution to rural development in India. Buffaloes are valuable for the triple purpose of milk, work and meat. The relative importance of these purposes differs between countries. In India the bulk of milk produced comes from buffalo. As a work animal, it is next only to the bullock. The meat potential of the buffalo is unexploited as yet. Buffalo is also a pack animal. The Royal Commission on Agriculture recognized the superiority of buffaloes over cows as a source of milk production as early as 1928. The Commission had suggested that while seeking an index of milk production in the region, it is the number of she-buffaloes and not the cows that should be taken into consideration. The higher fat percentage in buffalo milk is more profitable in dairy enterprises, particularly for toned and double toned milk. The higher the fat content which generally ranges between 7 and 8 percent and sometimes shoots up to even 12-15 percent, enables the farmers to get a higher income, as the price of milk is based on fat content. It is also held that buffalo milk is comparatively cheaper to produce, since a buffalo is able to utilize coarse feeds even rejected by cattle as her stable diet. Feed costs generally account for 60 to 70 percent of the total cost of milk production. Again, the buffalo is known to take less time to adjust herself to new ration than a cow. Further the she-buffalo, as a draught power, can do field work without any adverse affect on milk yield, because of its high draught power. For this it is rightly called living tractors. In fact, especially in Southeast Asian countries buffaloes are affectionately labeled as Asian mini tractor and mobile fertilizer factories.

The importance of buffalo as a source of milk and as work animal has been duly recognized since prehistorical times. The contribution of draught power by buffalo is unparalleled. Harnessing of buffalo is simple. Their body build, enormous strength, docile temperament, amenability for easy training, capacity for long sustained work, adjustability in a variety of coarse feeds make it an excellent animal for haulage and a variety of agricultural work. Especially for the cultivation of paddy under swamp conditions with small and marginal farmers the buffalo works with efficiency. Large hooves and great flexibility of the pastern and fetlock joints facilitate this. Their proclivity for water also makes them very well adapted to this kind of work in slush and mud. Although possessing a massive body frame and large hooves, buffaloes are quite nimble-footed and work with ease in very small plots without damaging the bunds. Besides their contribution to ploughing and harrowing, they are also used for threshing, lifting water for irrigation, extracting oil through local crushers, crushing sugarcane, treading clay for preparing bricks, logging and haulage of loads on sledges or carts. Buffaloes are slow as compared to oxen for traction, but can draw much heavier loads and have greater staying power. On good roads, a pair of buffaloes can draw a load of 2 tonnes at a pace of 3.2 km an hour. However, buffaloes are incapable of working long hours on hot days when they are exposed to direct sunlight during the hot summer. Nevertheless, unlike cattle, they can perform their duties even if there is heavy rain.

Dairy Young Stock Enterprise

Each crossbred cow generally has five lactations and each lactation period is 305 days, followed by a dry period of 60 days. Thus, one production cycle takes 365 days. At the end of the productive period, the animal will be sold on the basis of a certain price per kg of live weight. At the time of purchase of the animal, she should be in the first lactation and either in the advanced stage of gestation or in colostrums stage.

The financing agencies should be depending on the feed and fodder availability, finance one or two animals at a time, so that the farmer will have sufficient surplus to repay the loan as well derive reasonable income to maintain his family. The second loan for additional one or two crossbred cows should be advanced after six months from the purchase of the first lot. This will help the farmer to repay the installments and provide more or less uniform returns, throughout the year. This is important, since after six months of lactation, sufficient surplus will be generated due to declining phase of lactation, advanced stage of pregnancy and dry period.

The daily feed and fodder requirements will have to be met either by (a) high roughage—complete green, silage and hay ration, (b) medium roughage and concentrate ration, (c) straw and concentrate ration. If green feeds and fodders are available, the cost of milk production will be lower. This should be the aim. If the animals are maintained on straws and concentrates, the cost of milk production will be high. Usually feeds and fodders account for 60 to 70 percent of the cost of milk production. Poor quality straw rations will have to be supplemented with minerals also. Good quality leguminous fodders like barseem, lucerne, can support 6-8 litres of milk per day, without any concentrate. Proper feeding during pregnancy and dry period is of paramount importance. Actually the nutrient requirements are more during pregnancy and in first lactation of animals. The concentrate ration is usually fed at the rate of 1 kg for every 2.5 litres of milk production. Crossbred cows, if properly fed during lactation, pregnancy and dry periods, will definitely produce a minimum of 300 litres of extra milk in the subsequent lactation.

Cost of veterinary aid, medicines etc. per animal is assumed at Rs. 200 per year. Cost of minerals is taken as Rs. 300 per animal per year. Insurance premium is 5.3 percent of the value the animal. Family labour charges are imputed at Rs. 1000 per year. The average milk production is assumed at 3000 litres per first lactation and it is increased by 10 percent during the subsequent two lactations. Ten percent of the total milk production is assumed to be fed to calf. The average price of milk is taken as Rs. 10 per litre, fat content being 4 percent. The net sale proceeds of one calf, net of expenses on its rearing, is assumed as Rs. 300, and the income from sale of manure is estimated at Rs. 500/animal/year. The farmers belonging to the "weaker section" can reduce their loan burden due to the availability of various levels of subsidies.

At present only scanty data on the economics of livestock enterprises in India are available. Based on the available data and current costs of various inputs and the assumptions described above, the economics of one cow dairy unit has been worked out in Table 13.1 The Gross return per cow comes to Rs. 27,800. The enterprise can recover its initial investment in three years. The input-output ratio is favourable l: l.46. The family income per year increases from Rs. 7,271 in the first year to around Rs. l4, 510 in the fourth year.

A major expenditure more than 50 percent in dairy farming is on feeding the milch animals. In scientific terms, milch animals have to be provided maintenance and production rations. The crude protein requirement, which is the costliest component, is 500 gm as maintenance ration and 70 gm per

*Table 13.1: **Economics of Livestock Enterprises for Rural Development***

Dairy Unit – One Cow

One dairy cow: Semi-stalled-fed system. High Roughage ration

Capital Investment	Rs.
(a) Cost of one buffalo in the first lactation, expected yield 3,000 litres/lactation	15,000.00
(b) cost of housing (two buffaloessemi-permanent construction 50 sq. ft. @ Rs. 70 sq. ft.	3,500.00
(c) Equipment- milking pail buckets. Measuring jar, etc.	1,000.00
Total Capital Investment	19,500.00
Total Capital Investment	19,500.00
Term Loan for 4 years	15,000.00
@ 15% percent interest	
Subsidy 25 percent	3,750.00
Effective Loan	11,250.00
Repayment per year	2,813.00
Repayment Schedule	

Months	1st year Rs.	2nd year Rs.	3rd year Rs	4th year Rs.
1.	600	600	600	600
2.	600	600	600	600
3.	600	600	600	600
4.	400	400	400	400
5.	400	400	400	400
6.	213	213	213	213
Total	2,813	2,813	2,813	2.813

Fixed Costs
	Rs.

I. Interest @ 15% on	
(a) Investment	2,925.00
(b) working capital of Rs. 6,000 (for 6 months)	450.00
II. Insurance	800.00
III. Miscellaneous expenses	500.00
IV. Depreciation	
(a) Livestock @20%	3,000.00
(b) Equipment @10%	100.00
(c) Shed @10%	350.00
Total	8,125.00

Variable Costs
	Rs.

I. Feed & Fodders		
(a) Roughage . about 9 tonnes @ Rs. 700/tonnes		6,300.00
(b) Concentrates- Supplemented with roughages @ Rs 3.5/ Kg.		3.089.00
2 kg/day for 305 days =	762.5 kg.	
2 kg/day for last two months of pregnancy = 120.0 kg.		
Total	882.5 kg.	
II. Labour-family labour- imputed		1,000.00
III. Veterinary aid/year		200.00
IV. Minerals, slat, etc. 10 kg/year		500.00
Total		10,889.00

Income
	Rs.

I. By sale of milk: out of 3,000 litres, 300 litres fed to calf Sale of 2,700 litres @ Rs. 10/litre	27,000.00
II. By sale of calf	300.00
III. By sale of manure	500.00
Total	27,800.00

Table 13.1: Economics of Livestock Enterprises for Rural Development (Contd.)

Net Surplus

Net Surplus = Total income – (FC+VC)

= Rs. 27,800 – (8,125+ 10,889) = 8,786

$$\text{Viability of the Enterprise} = \frac{\text{Initial Investment}}{\text{Net Surplus}} = \frac{19,500}{8,786} = 2.2$$

The enterprise can pay back in three years.

1. Input-Output ratio = 1: 1.46
2. Fixed Cost-Output ratio = 1: 3.42
3. Variable Costs-Output ratio = 1: 2.55

Annual Surplus and income Statement

Items	1st Year Rs.	2nd Year Rs.	3rd Year Rs.	4th Year Rs.
1. Installment	2,813	2,813	2,813	2,813
2. Interest on Term Loan	1,687	1,265	843	421
3. Interest on Working Capital	450	450	450	450
4. Insurance	800	800	800	800
5. Depreciation	3,450	3,100	2,760	2,420
6. Miscellaneous expenses	500	500	500	500
Sub total	9,700	8,828	8,166	7,404
Variable Costs	10,889	10,889	10,889	10,889
Total	20,589	19,717	19,055	18,293

Net Surplus = Gross Income-Total Expenses

	1st year Rs.	2nd year Rs.	3rd year Rs.	4th year Rs.
Sale of Milk	2,700 litres	3,000 litres	3,200 litres:	3,200 litres
	27,00,000	30,000	32,000	32,000
Sale of manure	300	300	300	300
Sale of 1 calf	500	500	500	500
Sub total	27,800	30,800	32,800	32,800
Income per Year (Rs.)	7,271	11,083	13,745	14,507
Income per Month (Rs.)	600	924	1145	1209
Income per Day (Rs.)	20	30	38	40

milk as typical production ration. For example, if we have one milch animal yielding 18 litres of milk, its ration would be 500 gm crude protein plus production requirement of 1,260 gm (18 × 70) – a total of 1,760 gm.

Let us compare it with three milch animals yielding 6 litres each. They would require 1,500 gm (3 × 500) crude protein as maintenance ration and 1,260 gm (18 × 70) as production ration, making a total of 2,760 gm as against 1,760 gm of the single animal giving 18 litres. Thus, there is a saving of 1,000 gm, which can become maintenance ration of two milch animals, in the first alternative. Accordingly, it is economical to have one high-productivity animal than three low-productivity ones. In addition, in sizeable herds there would be saving in space, sheds, labour and management.

A buffalo, with lactation yield of 1,300 kg, with average 7 percent fat and 9 percent solids-non fat (SNF), would give 91 kg fat and 117 kg SNF. As opposed to that, a crossbred cow, in its 3,000 litres of lactational yield, would give 105 kg fat and 255 kg SNF on a 3.5 percent fat and 8.5 percent SNF basis. In the case of improved crossbred cows with 7,500 kg, lactational yield there would be 252 kg fat and 637 kg SNF.

Meat Purpose

The meat production potential of buffalo has not been fully explored. So far, it has remained by and large, only as an incidental although important by-product from the buffalo when this animal ceases to be economical in any other manner.

Studies carried out at the IVRI on meat production characteristics of weaned male Murrah buffalo calves have shown interesting results. Groups of 9-month-old calves weighing 75 kg were divided into two groups, one lot being fed *ad lib* a high grain ration and the other *ad lib*, roughage type, leguminous hay and wheat straw ration. On attainment of 300 kg body weight, the animals were slaughtered for evaluation of carcass quality. Animals fed the high grain ration demonstrated growth rates ranging between 0.555 kg and 0.625 kg per day and attained a slaughter weight of 300 kg at 16 to 18 months of age. Those on the roughage type ration gained at the rate of 0.410 kg and 0.450 kg per day and reached slaughter weight at 20 to 22 months. The dressing percentage of the high grain-fed animals ranged from 56.8 to 59.6 (mean 57.3 percent), while in the animals fed roughage type rations it varied from 50.8 to 53.5 (mean 50.9).[1]

These results indicate that if buffalo is properly managed and fed as a meat producing animal and slaughtered at around 16 to 20 months of age, it can produce meat that would equal choice as that of beef obtained from cattle, both in quality and quantity. India is having great potential to tap this enterprise. Farmers can take up these schemes in a big way with green and dry fodder available in the sugarcane growing areas, mulberry growing areas, besides other regions. Supplementation of urea and molasses to these rations will definitely help reach better body weight. Further, organized slaughter houses can augment the income of these farmers. In slaughter houses the byproducts obtained from buffalo slaughter include skins, bone, blood and horns. The value of the skin is generally affected by inexpert and improper handling. When meat industry develops, the hide can be spilt to make thin strong sheets, which after processing and dyeing make as good leather as that obtained from other animals.

---

[1]Gopalakrishnan, C.A., and Lal, G.M.M.: Livestock and Poultry Enterprises for Rural Development. Vikas Publishing House Pvt. Ltd., 1986 Edition: p. 324.

Comparative study of carcass characteristics of bulls of different cattle breeds and a group of water buffaloes showed that in spite of having lower slaughter weight; the buffaloes had higher proportion of meat than cattle. By virtue of possessing the absolute amount of meat more than cattle (i.e. the ratio of bone to meat is more favourable), the buffaloes are preferred by butchers. Another characteristic feature of water buffalo meat is the presence of little fat, which is seen around kidney and in the mesentery and not deposited in the muscle fibre. Buffalo meat consists of large muscle fibers and more cell nuclei than beef. Taste panel after organoleptic examination of buffalo meat (cara beef) and beef have certified that buffalo meat is more tender and palatable than beef. The general opinion that the buffalo meat is poorer in quality than beef can be attributed to the fact that in most cases only older animals enter the slaughterhouse. Italian and Bulgarian research workers reiterate that the meat of young buffaloes in caloric value, nutrient and taste is equal to those of the meat of young cattle.

Economics of Buffalo Production

The production parameters of buffalo and other inputs are generally similar to those described earlier in the Section on Cow. Each buffalo cow has five lactations and each lactation is 270 days, followed by a dry period of 125 days. Thus one production cycle takes 395 days (13 months, against 12 months for cow). As in the case of cow, at the end of productive period, buffalo will be sold for meat purposes on the basis of price per unit of live weight. Other conditions are assumed to be generally similar to those discussed under the Cow enterprises. The economics of one buffalo dairy unit has been worked out in Table 13.2. The returns in the case of buffalo are higher, mainly because of the higher price of milk per kg.

Based on the ratio of initial investment to net return, the buffalo enterprise can recover its initial investment in two year times, compared to three years required in the case of cow dairy unit. The input : output ratio is also favourable as is the family income per year. For instance in the fourth year the annual family income from buffalo diary unit is estimated at Rs. 19,000 against Rs. 14,500 for the cow diary unit. (Table 13.2)

Table 13.2: Economics of Livestock Enterprises for Rural Development

Dairy Unit – One Buffalo

One dairy buffalo: Semi-stalled-fed system. High Roughage ration

Capital Investment	Rs.
(a) Cost of one buffalo in the first lactation, expected yield 2,400 litres/lactation	20,000.00
(b) cost of housing (two buffaloessemi-permanent construction 50 sq. ft. @ Rs. 70 sq. ft.	3,500.00
(c) Equipment- milking pail buckets. measuring jar, etc.	1,000.00
Total Capital Investment	24,500.00

Capital Investment	*Rs.*
Total Capital Investment	24,500.00
Term Loan for 4 years	20,000.00
@ 15% percent interest	
Subsidy 25 percent	5,000.00
Effective Loan	15,000.00
Repayment per year	3,750.00
Repayment Schedule	

Months	1st year Rs.	2nd year Rs.	3rd year Rs	4th year Rs.
1.	700	700	700	700
2.	700	700	700	700
3.	700	700	700	7 00
4.	650	650	650	650
5.	650	650	650	650
6.	350	350	350	350
Total	3,750	3,750	3,750	3,750

Fixed Costs	*Rs.*
I. Interest @ 15% on	
(a) Investment	3,900.00
(b) working capital of Rs. 6,000 (for 6 months)	450.00
II. Insurance 6	00.00
III. Miscellaneous expenses	500.00
IV. Depreciation	
(a) Livestock @20%	4,000.00
(b) Equipment @10%	100.00
(c) Shed @10%	350.00
Total	9,900.00

Variable Costs	*Rs.*
I. Feed & Fodders	
(c) Roughage i.e. about 12 tonnes @ Rs. 700/tonnes	7,800.00
(d) Concentrates- Supplemented with roughages @ Rs.3.5 Kg.	1,592.00
1 kg/day for 270 days = 270 kg.	
1 kg/day for 75 days = 65 kg.	
2 kg/day for Last two months of pregnancy = <u>120</u> kg.	
Total	455 kg.
II. Labour-family labour- imputed	1,000.00
III. Veterinary aid/year	200.00
Total	11,092.00

Table 13.2: Economics of Livestock Enterprises for Rural Development (Contd.)

Income	Rs.
I. By sale of milk: out of 2,400 litres, 130 litres fed to calf	
Sale of 2,270 litres @ Rs. 14/litre	31,780.00
II. By sale of calf	300.00
III. By sale of manure	500.00
Total	32,580.00

Net Surplus

Net Surplus = Total income – (FC+VC)

= Rs. 32,580 – (9,900+ 11,092) = 11,588

$$\text{Viability of the Enterprise} = \frac{\textbf{Initial Investment}}{\textbf{Net Surplus}} = \frac{\textbf{19,500}}{\textbf{11,588}} = 1.68$$

The enterprise can pay back in two years.

1. Input-Output ratio = 1: 1.55
2. Fixed Cost-Output ratio = 1: 3.29
3. Variable Costs-Output ratio = 1: 2.94

Annual Surplus and income Statement

Items	1st year Rs.	2nd year Rs.	3rd year Rs.	4th year Rs.
1. Installment	3,750	3,750	3,750	3,750
2. Interest on Term Loan	2,250	1,688	1,125	562
3. Interest on Working Capital	450	450	450	450
4. Insurance	600	600	600	600
5. Depreciation	4,600	3,740	2,880	2,020
6. Miscellaneous expenses	500	500	500	500
Sub total	12,150	10,728	9,305	7,882
Variable Costs	11,092	11,092	11,092	11,092
Total	23,242	21,820	20,397	18,974

Net Surplus = Gross Income-Total Expenses

	1st year Rs.	2nd year Rs.	3rd year Rs.	4th year Rs.
Sale of Milk	2,270 litres	2470 litres	2660 litres:	2660 litre
	31,800	34,500	37,240	37,240
Sale of manure	300	300	300	300
Sale of 1 calf	500	500	500	500
Sub total	32,600	35,300	38,040	38,040
Income per Year (Rs.)	9,358	13,480	17,643	19,066
Income per Month (Rs.)	780	1,123	1,470	1,589
Income per Day (Rs.)	26	37	48	52

Small Ruminant Enterprise

Goatary, because of some misconception, is still in a primitive stage in India. The small ruminant – goat – has remained the most underrated and perhaps the least appreciated of farm animals in India, even though archaeologists and historians have established that the goat was perhaps the very first animal species domesticated by man.

The depiction of the goat on Mohenjodaro seal (4,000 BC) is proof of its status and popularity in the evolution of agriculture since ancient times. Actually, the domestication and spread of the animal is believed to have occurred about 7,500 to 7,000 B.C. in what is today the Turkey, Palestine and Jordan region and almost immediately the species spread all around in Asia and then into other parts of the globe. The goat is rated to be one of the most adaptable domesticated species of animals next only to the dog.

When, however, the National Commission on Agriculture (1976) decided to treat goat and sheep as "indiscriminate grazers" and thus a "hazard to the ecology and environment" it paved the way for a grave neglect or rather elimination of these hardy and useful animals from any kind of development work in India. However, their survival and growth in nature, despite their condemned status, has proved that if anything, these animals cannot be blamed for bringing about any more damage to the environment than man himself.

It has now generally come to be recognized that the goat is not necessarily a degrader of the environment. In fact it helps eliminate some of the obnoxious weeds, which are difficult to get rid of in farming practices. Also their ability to survive on the scant vegetation in wasteland makes them a favorite for reclamation of these tracts as various State governments have provided incentives to corporate houses for this purpose. Goatary today is in a primitive stage in India like poultry farming was in 1950 While poultry has found patrons in the industry, goat keeping is still looked down upon, partly due to social taboos and partly due to a glaring lack of understanding of the adaptation and the physiological or reproductive behaviour of this hardy animal especially when it is stall fed like the dairy cattle.

Goats constitute only a small part of farmer's agricultural wherewithal primarily with the underprivileged farmers and often the landless rural poor. Traditional goat keepers are more likely to be tribals leading nomadic life, grazing their herds on the natural pasturelands or even freshly harvested fields having crop residues and sometimes (stealthily) the reserved/ unreserved forest areas. These herd keepers pride themselves on being goat keepers/sheep breeders, even though in most of today's herds, the characteristic breed features are missing and there are more likely to be" mixed" genetic stocks. Also, some of the well-known breeds of Indian origin are now threatened due to indiscriminate genetic introgression of the nondescript breeding stocks coupled with a poor effort at replenishment of pure stocks.

Together, goat and sheep annually produce 450 million kilograms of chevon (goat meat), 230 million kilograms of mutton (sheep) meat, 63 million pieces of skin for leather making and 3 million tonnes of milk (from goat only). The foreign exchange earnings from small ruminant meat export were Rs. 890 million in 1999-2000, or 25 percent of the total meat export (including carcass), and are rising at the rate of over 4 percent per annum. Besides, live animals are often exported especially to Near East at the time of Haj. The Pashmina of the Indian goat breeds is certainly one of the finest in the world, though its production is low. In order not to overlook the comprehensive contribution of these animals to the agricultural scenario, an evaluation of their excreta could be placed at more than Rs. 3000 million per annum. Their contribution to the agricultural GDP of the country amounts to 5.4 percent. Thus the status of small ruminants in the agricultural economy of India is substantial.

Studies on the economic viability of animal farming with various species of farm animals vis-à-vis goat keeping show that the best benefit: cost ratio is provided by goat to all the three classes of farmers (marginal, small and others) and that too at an investment level of less than one-half of cattle.[1] It is therefore, quite clear that goat farming even in the traditional small-scale system renders adequate income and deserves to be supported as an enterprise in the interest of reducing underemployment and even to provide employment to less educated rural and semi-urban entrepreneurs.

The settled *vs.* nomadic types of systems are regarded as having a relative share of about 75-25 in terms of farmer numbers but only 40-60 percent in terms of goat/sheep populations. The land under forest and pasture cover is fast shrinking in almost all the states. All these factors pose a serious constraint to the future growth and survival of small ruminants. Perhaps it is no longer feasible to expect the continued growth rates of goats registered in the past. The best way to reconcile the recombine the factors for a judicious growth of goat as a commodity with economic force is to support goat farming on a reasonably large scale by adopting integrated farming system namely adequate backup of agriculture, forestry or other green activity for mutual support enabling synergy and efficiency to production systems for added outputs with zero wastages.

In this direction, encouragement has to be provided for greening (energy-efficient management) of wastelands by afforestation/crop raising, coupled with controlled grazing by goats. The fact that the goat can accept as food the hard and fibrous green or dry fodder, not normally acceptable to other domesticated animals, as well as their amenability to easy handling management (due to small size) makes the goat an ideal foil for integrated farming systems under diverse agroclimatic zones. The goat has the ability to multiply at a fast rate and could provide meat animals at a reasonably quick pace for cash purpose to the farmer and at the same time, provide reasonable degree of risk cover in the event of failure of regular crop, especially in marginal low-capability farming conditions.

---

[1]Chandra, S: Goat Rearing: Unmerited Low Status: in The Hindu Survey of Indian Agriculture 1999; p.134.

The small ruminants form a small part of the total farming establishment of a majority of cultivators. In China, however, 50 percent of the total returns of farming units have small ruminants as a component of its set up. Generally, it is known to vary between 10 to 25 percent in most of the mixed farming establishments, including in India. But small ruminant farming as a distinct enterprise has taken a new shape in Europe, especially in countries like Greece, Spain and France, where new uses have been found for goat milk. Moreover, the goat farming technology has been developed to such a level that mortality rates are now down to an unbelievable level of three percent. It is a challenge to goat farmers in tropical and subtropical countries to emulate the success story of European goat keepers. Incidentally, attempts to harness European technology have begun in India, one such unit has been set up in Maharashtra with an initial export tie up for goat milk products.

Farmers are not aware of the scientific methods of management of goats, which are now penned in open fields. Extreme weather and wet ground conditions take a heavy toll of goat herd and mortalities are high especially due to soil borne ecto and endo – parasites and respiratory diseases. On the other hand, efforts made to rear goats on an in-house or intensive stall-fed regime (to the exclusion of grazing) have generally met with negative results in flock size.

It has been found and demonstrated that the best course for sustaining the growth of small ruminants and achieving quick gains in lactation cycles, milk yields and body weight gains for meat production, is to adopt a more controlled semi-intensive system of maintenance which will entail grazing during light hours followed by in-house stall feeding of the herd. This system removes over-dependence on pen-care and gears the animals to combat the natural incidence of diseases. For this purpose, it is necessary to adopt a scientific approach to the style and the design of animal sheds providing for sufficient space, favourable microclimate, disinfecting the housing quarters, proper vaccination of the animals against major diseases and pests and last but not the least, a proper balanced diet (green, dry and concentrate feed mixture) including major nutrients with minerals and vitamins.

Despite indiscriminate slaughter of goats, the total goat population of India accounted for 17 percent of world total in 1999. The number of goat in India had increased from 47 million in 1951 to almost 123 million in 1999. Perceptible increase in goat population is because of its prolificacy in producing more than one young at one time of kidding and of short generation interval. Being a prolific breeder, the unique ability of the goat, kidding twice in 14 months and of producing several female kids in eight years cannot be achieved either by cow or buffalo in their life period.

The importance of goat in the rural economy is evidenced by its unparalleled economic traits; ability to get acclimatized under diversified agro climatic conditions, high fertility and short generation interval; practically no religious restrictions for goat and its products among the diversified religious people in rural area. Economically goat is ideally suited for poorer rural folk especially for marginal and landless labourers by its low cost maintenance, short-term return on capital with low risk capital investment. No involvement of extraneous labour, as such the entire rural family members especially women folk and children are brought into the gamut of activity; thereby the health status is bound to improve with availability of cheap and good quality protein through goat milk and mutton. Goats thrive and add to the rural economy even in areas where it is difficult to raise cows or buffaloes. The multivarious methods of utility of goat render the animal to be labeled as a "Poor Man's Cow".

Some studies indicated that crossbred cow are not economically feasible proposition for the rural poor, because of their high cost maintenance and the poor animal health cover available in rural India. The goat is found to be an ideal milk and meat animal for these people because of its lower money inputs and relatively better returns. It is also found that goats can be stall-fed with farm wastes, thereby preventing their wanderings and damage to the vegetation around. In addition, goat rearing has several advantages over cow keeping in rural areas, especially drought prone area, tribal areas, and remote villages, where transportation is a problem.

The best-known representative breed of the tropical milch group is Jamnapari of India. The average live weight of Jamnapari goat is 54 kg and buck 80 kg. The average lactation period under good management practices in India was found to be 205 days. The average milk yield is 250 kg. in 274 days, the highest daily yield was 3.8 kg. and the highest lactation yield was 561 kg. The butter fat content averages 5.1 percent, with a maximum of 7.4 percent. Another good goat breed in India is Surti. The Surti is estimated to produce, in a lactation period of about the same length as that of the Jamnapari, 1.4 kg to 2.3 kg. of milk a day. The average daily milk yield of Indian goats is estimated to be 0.2 kg. to 0.45 kg in a lactation of 150 days.

A Dairy Goat Unit for Domestic Purposes

Majority of the farmers in India maintain 2 to 3 goats to meet their domestic demands for milk and they would sell the surplus male stock for meat. There is considerable scope for breeding and improvement in goat. Native breeds can be improved to double their milk production by crossbreeding. Improved feeding and management practices will definitely sustain milk production. The goat breeding has been undertaken to produce crossbred goats capable of yielding 300 kg milk in 120 days under stall feeding management. The breeding programmes for making native goat (Beetal, Jamnapari, Babbari, Malabari) with exotic bucks (Sannen and Alpine) have been undertaken to produce the progeny of ½ and ¾ exotic germ plasm with two or three breed combination. Pure breeding on selective mating has been done on a small member progeny for contemporary comparison as well as to produce good bucks from nucleus stock of exotic goats.

Weight at Slaughter Stage

This varies considerably because of wide variation among the breeds. However, 20, 25 and 30 kg live weight may be achieved in small, medium and large breeds of goat in 10 to 12 months period provided they are properly fed. Castration of male kids improved the carcass quality. Usually fattening males are castrated at 2 to 3 months age. Gaddi and Chamba breeds are considered to produce meat of every low fat content.

The economics of goat unit enterprises, like for diary cow and buffalo, has been attempted in Table 13.3. Most of the economic indicators for goat unit husbandry are quite favourable.

Table 13.3: Economics of Livestock Enterprises for Rural Development

GOAT UNIT 25 +1

(For milk and meat purposes)

Capital Investment	Rs.
Livestock	
(a) Cost of she goats	
- 25 goats @ Rs. 1000/goat	25,000.00
- One Buck @ Rs. 1,200	1,200.00
Building: Low cost Sheds	
- Cost of penning 26 goats	3,500.00
- Cost of penning 50 kids	5,000.00
Equipment	
- Equipment	3,000.00
Total Capital Investment	37,700.00
Total Capital Investment	37,700.00
Term Loan for 5 years	35,000.00
@ 15% percent interest	
Subsidy 33 percent	11,667.00
Effective Loan	33,833.00
Annual Repayment	6,767.00

Fixed Costs	Rs.
I. Interest @ 15% on	
(a) Investment	5,655.00
(b) working capital of Rs. 15,000 (for 6 months)	1,125.00
Insurance of 26 goats 3.3 percent of value	1,389.00
III. Miscellaneous expenses	500.00
IV. Depreciation	
(a) Livestock @10%	2,620.00
(b) Equipment @10%	300.00
(c) Pens @10%	850.00
Total	12,439.00

Table 13.3: Economics of Livestock Enterprises for Rural Development (Contd.)

Variable Costs		Rs.
I. Feed & Fodders		
Roughages by grazing		
Concentrate—Supplemented with grazing @ Rs 3.5/kg.		
for does-25: @300g/day/doe		
i.e. 109.5 kg/doe/year	= 2,737 kg.	
(b) for buck @ 500 g/day	= 182 kg.	
©for kids-fattening kids 50 for		
90 days of age to 300 days i.e.		
210 days @300 g/kid/day		
to 210 days i.e. 63 kg/kid	= 3,150 kg	
Total	6,069 kg	21,242.00
II. Labour- Family Labour-imputed grazing charges		1,000.00
III. Veterinary aid Rs. 15/goat/year		390.00
Rs. 8/kid/year		400.00
IV. Minerals, slat, etc. 10 kg/year		500.00
Total		23,532.00

Income	Rs.
I By sale of young stock 50 kids Expected to service at the end of 10th month: Average body weight 20-25 kg. @ Rs. 800/head	40,000.00
II. By sale of milk Expected production/doe/ kidding- 180 litres: 80 litres utilized for kids. Total milk available for sale 100 × 25 = 2,500 litres @ Rs. 10/litre	25,000.00
III. Value of manure (not taken into calculations) @ Rs, 10/month	
(i) Goats 26x10x12 = Rs. 3,125.00	
(ii) Kids 25x10x10 = Rs. 2,500.00	
Total s.	5,625.00
Total	65,000.00

Net Surplus

Net Surplus = Total income – (FC+VC)
= Rs. 65,000– (12,439+ 23,532 = 29,029

$$\text{Viability of the Enterprise} = \frac{\textbf{Initial Investment}}{\textbf{Net Surplus}} = \frac{37,700}{29029} = 1.30$$

The enterprise can pay back in two years.

1. Input-Output ratio = 1: 1.81
2. Fixed Cost-Output ratio = 1: 5.23
3. Variable Costs-Output ratio = 1: 2.76

Annual Surplus and income Statement

Items	1st year Rs.	2nd year Rs.	3rd year Rs.	4th year Rs.	5th year Rs.
1. Instalment	6,767	6,767	6,767	6,767	6,767
2. Interest on Term Loan	5, 075	4,060	3,045	2,030	1,015
3. Interest on Working Capital	1,125	1,125	1,125	1,125	1,125
4. Insurance	2,514	2,514	2,514	2,514	2,514
5. Depreciation @ 10%	3,770	3,393	3,000	2,700	2,430
6. Miscellaneous expenses	500	500	500	500	500
Sub total	19,751	18,359	16,951	15,636	14,351
Variable Costs	23,532	23,532	23,532	23,532	23,532
Total	43,283	41,891	40,483	38,988	37,883

Net Surplus =	1st year Rs.	2nd year Rs.	3rd year Rs.	4th year Rs.	5th year Rs.
Net Surplus = Gross Income-Total Expenses					
i.e. Income per Year (Rs.)	21,717	23,109	24,517	26,012	27,117
Income per Month (Rs.)	1,810	1,926	2,043	2,168	2,260
Income per day (Rs.)	59	63	67	72	74

ECONOMICS OF SHEEP UNIT ENTERPRISE

Sheep like goat is a small ruminant with a high adaptability to extreme climate. Sheep by nature is gregarious animal and it is generally uniparous unlike goat, which produces more than one young at the time of one kidding. Sheep plays an important role in the animal production and rural economy in arid and semiarid regions and largely in marginal and submarginal holdings. Of the 1069 million sheep in the world in 1999, India accounted for only 5 percent of the total, against 17 percent of the world goat population. The production potential of sheep in India is estimated to be around Rs. 5100 million per annum. This is based on yearly production of 50 million kg of wool, 220 kg of mutton, 17 million of skin and 30 million tons of manure.

Role of sheep rearing in improving the rural economy is well established. In the event of failure of seasonal rains, the rearing of sheep gives a helping hand to the farmers at the time of crisis arising from crop failure. Sheep rearing can be recommended as an occupation to the rural people especially to the weaker sections in hilly, drought prone and desert areas. In the north and northeastern hilly regions comprising Jammu and Kashmir, Himachal Pradesh, Uttar Pradesh, Assam, Meghalaya, Nagaland, orchards and cereals are raised in combination with sheep rearing. Sheep farming through small and marginal farmers and landless agricultural labourers will provide employment opportunities for most of the unemployed and underemployed in rural areas.

Sheep can thrive well in all agroclimatic conditions excepting in rainfall areas. Sheep can subsist on lowest and sparse vegetation whereas other species of farm livestock may have to struggle to thrive. This is possible because of their inherent capacity to browse very close to the roots of herbage. Sheep manure excels cattle manure and penning of sheep in harvested fields enhances the fertility of the soil by the richness of nutrients in the faecal materials voided. Penning of sheep in the fields brings in additional income to the flock owners. Since sheep rearing does not warrant any large investment in building and equipment, it opens scope for exploitation by the small, marginal farmers and landless agricultural labourers. In the drought prone and desert areas shepherds are compelled to lead nomadic life for the welfare of their sheep. Studies on economics of sheep rearing indicate that the sheep population was subject to considerable fluctuations on account of drought, diseases, wild animals, fluctuation of prices of mutton and wool and uneconomic holdings and soil erosion over which the Indian sheep farmer had little control.

Compared with an average annual production of 3.5 to 5.5 kg of quality wool per sheep in Australia, New Zealand and USA, the yield is 1.4 kg in India. Poor management, feeding and health care mean that only about 20 percent of the possible meat yield per ewe is obtained. The maximum concentration of the wool yielding sheep remains in the arid regions of northern Indian plains and Joria region, comprising the area of Rajputana, Kutch, Saurshtra and North Gujarat. The Deccan plateau extending from Vindya mountains possesses the largest number of flocks in India and this is especially on the eastern sides of Hyderabad, Andhra Pradesh and Tamil Nadu. The majority of sheep in these areas are hairy and produce little wool. Kashmir and adjacent districts of Himachal Pradesh are specially suited to raising superior wool types of sheep. The Lohi breed of the Punjab is well known for its large size and milk and meat producing traits. The hairy type of southern Deccan is mainly for meat production.

Sheep has carved a niche in the agricultural economy of the country by effective utilization of the uncultivable wastelands and unwanted shrubs and weeds from the fields. Due to the great adaptability of sheep to widely varying biological and socioeconomic environmental conditions, there are varying methods of sheep farming. These include nomadic or partial nomadic or permanent rearing systems, which in their turn, can have a subsistence or a commercial character to their production aim.

Sheep Development Programmes

From time to time sheep development programmes have been carried out in India. The East India Company initiated programmes for crossbreeding indigenous sheep stock with exotic fine wool breeds to improve the quality and quantity of wool to meet demands of the woolen mills in United Kingdom. Perhaps these were the pioneering attempts to improve the indigenous stock for increased wool production. Records indicate that some progress was achieved in crossbreeding work, particularly with Cape

Merino, around Pune. During the first decade of the twentieth century crossbreeding programmes of indigenous and Bikaneri breeds with Merino and Ramney Mash breeds were initiated in number of places in the then United Provinces both in plain and hilly regions. No definite results were achieved in the crossbreeding programme since the experimental work was discontinued after obtaining second generation of crossbred progeny for want of financial support and lack of organization.

With the formation of the Imperial (now Indian) Council of Agricultural Research (ICAR), several projects for breeding superior sheep were initiated in 1938 and later the ICAR started development projects in sheep on regional basis. In 1952, a detailed plan for sheep development on regional basis to identify the several problems of evolving superior breeds and for studying different aspects of sheep husbandry was formulated by the ICAR. The first two plans however, saw very little development of sheep other than the activities carried out by the ICAR and the establishment of a full-fledged centre for conducting research on sheep and wool in each of the three regions, viz., the temperate Himalayan region, the dry northern plains and the southern region. Sheep breeding farms were established at Banihal Riasi in Kashmir, Gwaldun in Uttar Pradesh, Sarhan in Himachal Pradesh, Darjeeling in West Bengal, Jorbir (Bikaner) in Rajasthan, Pattan in Gujarat, Poona in Maharashtra, Nilgiris (Ootacammund) in Tamil Nadu and Gaya in Bihar.

Sheep development programmes for improved mutton production and for wool, continued during various plan periods. Food and Agriculture Organization and the World Bank have also provided assistance for development of goat and sheep in India.

To obtain best possible combination of the existing—the mostly extensive—natural and economic influence factors, utilization of alternatives have developed for particular locations, to which special production results can be attributed. While the production of purely wool and fur, can be developed into a profitable system in India, because of low fodder requirements and relative intensity of climate, meat and milk production very quickly come up against the natural limitation of poor feed supplies and the low performance potential of native breeds. Only favourable market conditions can justify the increased cost of pasture management, providing feed, breeding and marketing. Adoption of modern techniques of breeding, improvement in the feed and fodder resources, better management practices and provision of health cover, will promote the sheep development and in turn improve the rural economy.

Meat Production

The best way to increase meat production in sheep is to improve fertility and breeding performance. Economical lamb production depends more on ewe's breeding performance than growth rate and carcass. In farms of wool production, lambs are reared only to replace herd. As the production of lams over and above those required to replace the herd become profitable, interest shifted from exclusive pure wool production to overall productivity per sheep, per hectare and per head.

Wool Production

Wool growth depends on annual cycle and more so in summer than in winter. Photoperiodicity, temperature, intake of feed, body weight and general condition of the animal are the factors that influence the annual cycle. The amount of precipitation also has an indirect effect on fineness of wool. A good nutritional support with a high rainfall leads to coarser fleeces. Feeding is a deciding factor, which is connected with seasons and temperature. The wool growth cycle may disappear if food supplies are better in winter than in summer. However, the cycle remains as long as food supplies are kept constant. The nutritional condition of the ewe can influence the subsequent wool growth of the lamb even before its birth in as much as poor intake of nutrients in prenatal condition lowers the number of follicles. They are fully formed in Merinos within six months of birth. Wool production can be 20 percent lower if the nutrition condition is poor in the first month of a lamb's life. Sheep reared for wool production require additional nutrients to meet the demand for wool growth. Most of the wool-producing breeds mature slowly and make smaller daily live weight gain than the mutton breeds.

Requirement of building units are more or less the same for sheep and goat. Generally they do not need elaborate buildings. However, the shelter provided should be dry and clean. They should give protection from severe hot and cold climatic conditions as well as from heavy rains. Usually loose housing system is practiced. Only half-walled sheds are provided for sheep with open paddocks. Sheep are folded in the sheds during the night after grazing and taken out for grazing during day time. Under Indian rural farming conditions, costly investments are not practicable, since sheep are moved from place to place in search of suitable grazing lands.

Production Parameters

Sheep

1. Lambing rate—80 percent lambing is common and 2 lambings are obtained in a period of one-and-half year. **2. Lambing Ratio**—50 percent male – 50 percent female. **3. Mortality Rate: (a) Adult sheep**—5 percent: **(b) Lambs**—10 to 15 percent. **(4) Culling rate: (a) Ewes**—4th year onwards—20 percent of the total livestock will be culled. **(b) Lambs**—All the surviving male lambs will be disposed off after they attain the age of 6 months. **5. Wool Yield. (a)** 1 ½ kg per year from local breeds. **(B)** 3 kg per year from crossed breed sheep. **(c)** ½ kg per year from lambs over 6 months.

Financial Parameters

1. Sale of Lamb @ Rs. 475 per lamb.
2. Sale of adult sheep @ Rs. 750 per sheep.

3. Sale of wool
   (a) Wool from local breed sheep: @ Rs. 30 per kg.
   (b) Wool from cross/exotic breed of sheep and lambs @ Rs. 45 per kg.
4. Sale of manure @ Rs. 30 per sheep per year.

Expenditure Per Year

1. Cost of supplementary feeding during rainy days @ Rs. 20/ day/ sheep.
2. Cost of medicine and sheering charges Rs. 20/ sheep/year

Useful age	7 years
Weight of Lamb	2-2.5 kg
Maturity	8-9 months
Breeding age	15-18 months
Weight of ewe	25 kg
Lambing	80 percent.

Based on the production and technical parameters mentioned above, economics of a sheep unit enterprise consisting of 25 ewes and one ram, is worked out in Table 13.4.

Table 13.4: Economics of Livestock Enterprises for Rural Development

SHEEP UNIT 25 + 1

Capital Investment	Rs.
I. Livestock	
Cost of 25 ewes @ 570 each	14, 250.00
Cost of One Buck @ Rs. 950	950.00
II. Building: Cost of Katcha pen	1,500.00
- Equipment	1,500.00
Total Capital Investment	18,200.00
Total Capital Investment	18,200.00
Term Loan for 3 years	35,000.00
@ 15% percent interest Subsidy 33 percent	-6,000.00
Effective Loan	12,200.00
Annual Repayment	4,067.00

Fixed Costs	Rs.
I. Interest @ 15% on	
(a) on Investment	2,730.00
(b) working capital of Rs. 5,000 (for 6 months)	375.00
Insurance of 26 sheep 3.3 percent of value	730.00
III. Miscellaneous expenses	200.00

Table 13.4: Economics of Livestock Enterprises for Rural Development

Fixed Costs	Rs.
IV. Depreciation on	
(a) ewes and rams @10%	1,520.00
(b) Equipment @10%	150.00
(c) Pens @10%	150.00
Total	5,855.00

Variable Costs	Rs.
Feed & Fodders	
Roughages by grazing Feed cost during lean season as a lump sum	1,500.00
II. Labour- Family Labour-imputed,grazing charges	1,000.00
III. Veterinary aid Rs. 15/sheep/year	390.00
Rs. 8/kid/year	400.00
Total	3,290.00

Income	Rs.
I. By sale of 25 lambs (yearlings)	
@ Rs. Rs. 475 each (475 × 25	11,875.00
3. By sale of wool l 1/2 kg/adult	
4. 39 Kg. @ Rs. 30/kg.	1,170.00
III. Value of manure	
Adult 26 × 30	780.00
Young 8 × 15	64.00
Total	13,889.00

Net Surplus

Net Surplus = Total income − (FC+VC) = Rs. 13,889− (5,855+ 3,290) = 4,744

Viability of the Enterprise = $\dfrac{\textbf{Initial Investment}}{\textbf{Net Surplus}}$ = $\dfrac{\textbf{18,200}}{\textbf{4,744}}$ **= 3.84**

The enterprise can pay back in four years.

1. Input-Output ratio = 1: 1.31
2. Fixed Cost-Output ratio = 1: 2.37
3. Variable Costs-Output ratio = 1: 4.22

Cash Flow and Net income for Sheep unit 25+1

Items	1st year Rs.	2nd year Rs.	3rd year Rs.	4th year Rs.	5th year Rs.
1. Investment	6,767	6,767	6,767	6,767	6,767
2. Interest on Term Loan	5,075	4,060	3,045	2,030	1,015
3. Interest on Working Capital	1,125	1,125	1,125	1,125	1,125
4. Insurance	2,514	2,514	2,514	2,514	2,514

Items	1st year Rs.	2nd year Rs.	3rd year Rs.	4th year Rs.	5th year Rs.
5. Depreciation @ 10%	3,770	3,393	3,000	2,700	2,430
6. Miscellaneous expenses	500	500	500	500	500
Sub total	19,751	18,359	16,951	15,636	14,351
Variable costs	38,704	38,704	38,704	38,704	38,704
Total	58,455	57,063	55,655	54,340	53,055

Net Surplus =	1st year Rs.	2nd year Rs.	3rd year Rs.	4th year Rs.	5th year Rs.
Net Surplus = Gross Income-Total Expenses i.e. Income per Year (Rs.)	6,545	7,937	9,345	10,570	11,945
Income per month (Rs.)	545	662	778	880	995
Income per day (Rs.)	18	22	26	29	33

Annual Surplus and income Statement (Rs.)

Items	15 Months	23rd Month	31st Month
1. Instalment	3,500	4,350	4,350
2. Interest on Term Loan	2,250	979	489
3. Interest on Working Capital	375	375	375
4. Insurance	805	805	805
5. Depreciation @ 10%	1,820	1,638	1,456
6. Miscellaneous expenses	200	200	200
7. Sub total	8,950	8,347	7,675
8. Variable Costs	3,290	3,290	3,290
Total	12,240	11,637	10,965

Net Surplus

Income	I. 15 Months	II. 8 Months	III. 8 Months
I. By sale of 25 lambs (yearlings) @ Rs. Rs. 475 each (475 × 25)	11,875	I. 11,875	I. 11,875
II. By sale of wool 1 1/2 kg/adult 39 kg. @ Rs. 30/kg	1,170	II. One kg/adult 26 kg. 780	II. 780
III. Value of manure		III. Sale of manure	III.
Adult 26 × 30	780	Adult 26 × 15 390	390
Young 8 × 15	64	Young 8 × 15 120	120
Total Income	13,889	13,165	13,165
Net Surplus	13,889 - 12,240 1,134	13,165 - 11,637 1,528	13,165 - 10,965 2,200

i.e. 94.50 per month   i.e. Rs. 131.67 per month   i.e. Rs. 183.33

Comparative Economics of different Livestock Enterprises

The result of economics of different enterprises discussed above is summarized in Table 13.5. Economics of poultry layer and broiler farm is presented in Table 13.6 and 13.7 respectively.

Table 13.5: Economics of Different Livestock Enterprises

Item	Dairy cow Unit	Dairy buffalo Unit	Goat unit	Sheep Unit
1. Capital Investment (Rs.)	19,500	24,500	37,000	18,200
2. Fixed Costs (Rs.)	8,125	9,900	12,439	5,855
3. Variable Cost (Rs.)	10,889	11,092	23,532	3,290
4. Total Costs (Rs)	19,014	20,992	35,971	9,145
5. Gross Income (Rs.)	27,800	32,580	65,000	13,889
6. Net Income (Rs.)	8,786	11,588	29,029	4,744
7. Investment Recovery period (Years)	3	2	2	4
8. Input : Output Ratio	1 : 1.46	1 : 1.55	1 : 1.81	1 : 1.31
9. Fixed cost Output Ratio	1 : 3.42	1 : 3.29	1 : 5.23	1 : 2.37
10. Variable cost Output Ratio	1 : 2.55	1 : 2.94	1 : 2.76	1 : 4.22

Table 13.6: Economics of 100 Layer Farm (Purchased at Point of Lay)

Small Farmer
Subsidy 25 percent
Interest 15 percent

	Rs.
I. Capital Investment	
Cost of 100 hybrid layer	
Purchased at point of lay (22 weeks) Rs. 60/bird	6,000.00
II. Building:	
Layer house 2½ sq. ft/bird250 sq. ft. @ Rs. 40/sq. ft.	10,000.00
III. Equipment – waterers	
Feeders etc. Rs. 10/bird	1,000.00
1,500.00	
Total Capital Investment	17,000.00
Total Capital Investment Term Loan for 6 years	15,000.00
@ 15% interest subsidy 25 percent	3,750.00
Effective Loan	11,250.00
Annual Repayment	1,875.00

Fixed Costs	Rs.
I. Interest @ 15%	
(a) on term loan	2,550.00
(b) working capital of Rs. 7,500 (for 6 months)	562.50
II. Insurance 5.3% of Purchase value of bird	18.00

III. Miscellaneous expenses		250.00
IV. Depreciation on		
(a) housing @ 10%		1,000.00
(b) Equipment @ 10%		100.00
Total		4,780.50

Variable Costs	Rs.
1. Feeds & Feeding	
100 layers-40 kg/bird @ Rs. 4/kg.	16,000.00
2. Cost of electricity charges	
Vitamins and medicines @ 10/bird	1,000.00
Total	17,000.00

Income	Rs.
I. By sale of eggs@ 260 eggs/bird26,000 eggs @ Re 1/egg	26,000.00
II. By sale of culled bird@ Rs. 25/bird	2,500.00
III. By sale of manure 100 layers—2 tonnes@ Rs. 350/tonne	700.00
IV. By sale of 50 gunny bags @ Rs. 20/bag	1,000.00
Total	30,200.00

Net Surplus
Net Surplus = Total income-(FC+VC)
= Rs. 30,200 – (4,780 + 17,000) = 8,420

Viability of the Enterprise=

$$\frac{\text{Initial Investment}}{\text{Net Surplus}} = \frac{17,000}{8,420} = 2.02$$

The enterprise can pay back within three years.

Annual Surplus and Income Statement

Year	*1*	*2*	*3*	*4*	*5*	*6*
Net Income						
Gross Income	30,200	30,200	30,200	30,200	30,200	30,200
Total Expenses	22,972	22,401	22,010	21,618	21,227	20,806
Net Surplus						
Income per year	7,228	7,799	8,190	8,582	8,973	9,394
Income per month	60.23	64.99	68.25	71.52	74.78	78.28

Table 13.7: Economics of 100 Broiler

Small Farmer
Subsidy 25 percent
Interest 15 percent

	Rs.
I. **Capital Investment**	
Bird: cost of 100 Broiler chicks @ Rs. 10 each	1,000.00
II. **Building:** Broiler house 1sq.ft/bird 100 sq.ft @ Rs. 40/sq.ft.	4,000.00
III. **Equipment – waterers**	
Feeders etc. Rs. 10/bird	1,000.00
Total Capital Investment	6,000.00
Loan @ 15% interest	6,000.00
Term Loan for 6 years Subsidy 25 percent	1,500.00
Effective Loan	4,500.00
Repayment in 5 instalments of Rs. 900 each at 8 weeks interval.	

Fixed Costs	*Rs.*
I. Interest @ 15% on term loan (8 weeks)	112.50
(b) working capital of Rs. 2,500.00 (for 1 months)	31.25
II. Insurance 5.3% of Purchase value of bird	53.00
III. Miscellaneous expenses	100.00
IV. Depreciation on	
(a) housing @ 10%	400.00
(b) Equipment @ 10%	100.00
Total	796.75

Variable Costs	*Rs.*
1. Feeds & Feeding	
4 kg/bird per 8 weeks, i.e. 400 kg. @ Rs. 4/kg.	16,00.002.
2. Cost of electricity charges, Vitamins	
and medicines @ 10/bird	1,000.00
Total	2,600.00

Income	*Rs.*
I. By sale of bird on an	
Average live weight of 1.5 kg @ Rs. 30/kg & 150 kg.	4,500.00
II. By sale of manure 2 kg/bird = 200 kg @ 30 paise/kg.	600.00
III. By sale of 8 gunny bags @ Rs. 20/bag	160.00
Total	5,260.00

Net Surplus
Net Surplus = Total income – (FC + VC)
= Rs. 5,260 – (796.75 + 2600.00) = 2,863.50

Viability of the Enterprise=
$$\text{Initial Investment} = \frac{6,000.00}{2,863.50} = 2.10$$
The enterprise can pay back within three period of eight weeks each.

Annual Surplus and Income Statement

Year	1	2	3	4	5
Net Income					
Gross Income	5,260	5,260	5,260	5,260	5,260
Total Expenses	4,296	4,224	4,151	4,076	4,007
Net Surplus	964	1,036	1,109	1,184	1,253
Per day	16.07	17.27	18.48	19.73	20.88
Per bird	9.64	10.36	11.09	11.84	12.53

Annual Costs

Item/period	1	2	3	4	5
1. Instalment	900	900	900	900	900
2. Interest on Loan (8 weeks)	112	90	67	45	23
3. Interest on working capital for one month	31	31	31	31	31
4. Insurance	53	53	53	53	53
5. Depreciation	500	450	400	350	300
6. Miscellaneous Expenses	100	100	100	100	100
7. Total	1,696	1,624	1,551	1,479	1,407
8. Variable Costs	2,600	2,600	2,600	2,600	2,600
Total Expenses	4,296				

14

Emerging Trends in Consumption of Livestock Products

Growing human population, rising per capita incomes, urbanization and for changing lifestyles are responsible rapid growth in demand for food of animal origin. Projections towards 2020 indicate a considerable increase in demand for food of animal origin (Bansil 2003, Kumar 1998, Bhalla et al. 1998, Delgado et al. 1999, Birthal and Parthasarathy Rao 2000).[1] The estimates however differ considerably particularly for the milk demand depending on the model used for estimation and magnitude of income elasticity and growth in population and per capita income. While the estimates by Kumar, and Delgado et al. are on the lower side, estimates by Bhalla et al. are on the higher side. Birthal and Parthasarathy Rao's estimates lie somewhere in between. They have estimated demand for milk at 191 million tonnes, for meat 11 million tonnes and for eggs 4.6 million tonnes. In other words, demand for milk will increase by a factor of 2.4, for meat by 2.3 and eggs by 2.7 over that in 2001. To meet the future demand, milk production has to increase at an annual rate of 4.3 percent,

[1]Birtha¹, P.S. and P. Parthasarathy Rao. 2002. Increasing Productivity of Livestock in Mixed Crop Livestock systems in South Asia. ICRISAT, Patancheru, and NCAP, New Delhi.

Bhalla, G.S., P. Hazell and J. Kerr. 1999. Prospects for India's Cereal Supply and Demand to 2020. Food, Agriculture and the Environment Discussion Paper 29. International Food Policy Research Institute, Washington, D.C.

Delgado, C., M. Rosegrant, H. Steinfeld, S. Ehui and C. Courbois. 1999. Livestock to 2020: The Next Food Revolution. Food, Agriculture and the Environment Discussion Paper 28. International Food Policy Research Institute, Washington, D.C., Food and Agriculture Organization, Rome, and International Livestock Research Institute, Addis Ababa.

Kumar, Praduman. 1998. Food Demand and Supply Projections for India. Agricultural Economics Policy Paper 98-01. Indian Agricultural Research Institute. New Delhi.

Bansil, P.C. 2003, Economic Problems of Indian Agriculture, 6th Edition, CBS Publishers and Distributors, New Delhi – 110002.

meat production 4.1 percent and egg production 4.8 percent (Birthal and Parathasarathy Rao, 2002). In the past, India has comfortably met the rising demand through domestic supplies with little dependence on imports. Milk production increased from about 32 million tonnes in 1980 to about 81 million tonnes in 2001 at an annual growth rate of 4.8 percent, meat production increased from 2.6 million tonnes to 4.9 million tonnes at an annual growth rate of 2.9 percent and egg production increased from 0.6 million tonnes to 1.9 million tonnes at an annual rate of 6 percent. The growth has however been driven largely by numbers. About half of the growth in milk production, and almost entire growth in meat production was due to increase in the number of animals milked/slaughtered.

If the current production trends were to continue, demand for animal food will be adequately met through domestic supplies. This is however ambiguous. India has huge livestock population in relation to feed and fodder availability. Feed and fodder availability in India has always remained short of requirement. Area under cultivated fodders has hardly ever exceeded 5 percent of the gross cropped area, and common grazing lands have been deteriorating quantitatively as well as qualitatively. With rising population of both human and animals, and declining per capita land availability competition for land is likely to intensify. The number driven growth may not sustain for long. Further, the scale of production is small and subsistence oriented. Livestock is largely concentrated among small landholders (<2 ha) that comprise about two third of the total rural households. For these households livestock is an important source of income and employment. The changes in future demand and supply as envisaged will have implications for organization of livestock production, efficiency and sustainability of livestock production, equity, poverty and food and nutritional security.

With this backdrop, this chapter examines long-term changes in consumption of livestock products by income classes, location of the households (rural and urban) and region. This has been divided into four parts. Part I takes a panoramic view of the consumption basket of rural households and changes in the consumption pattern from 43rd Round of NSSO. While Part II goes into a detailed discussion about the changes in the consumption pattern of various livestock products at the all India level among different economic classes. Part III concentrates primarily on milk and milk products and Par IV presents a scenario of modern dietary transition and its outcomes.

MEAT IN TRADITIONAL AGRICULTURAL SOCIETIES

Gradual adoption of sedentary farming, the process that started about 10,000 years ago and took thousands of years to complete, greatly boosted the maximum population density – by as much as four orders of magnitude – but in most instances this gain was paid for by a marked decline in the average quality of nutrition. Lowered intakes of meat almost always meant generally lower availability of complete protein as well as of several vitamins (A, B, D) and minerals (above all iron). These declines were reflected in diminished statures of sedentary populations. Quantifying these shifts is another matter. Archeological findings and written documents offer a wealth of information about the composition of diets in antiquity, but the anecdotal and fragmentary nature of this evidence precludes its conversion to any coherent summaries of secular trends. These records do not improve noticeably before the seventeenth century, and even afterward it is impossible to extrapolate detailed information for certain localities or socioeconomic groups to large-scale or national averages.

The only solid generalization in accordance with documentary and anthopometric evidence is the absence of any persistent trend in per capita meat consumption. A cautious quantification may be phrased as follows: average per capita meat intakes in traditional agricultural societies were rarely higher than 5-10 kg a year; in subsistence peasant societies of the Old World, larger than primate brains – at about 350 g the neonate brain is twice as large as that of a newborn chimpanzee , and by the age of five it becomes more than three times as massive as the brain of the closest primate species – we do not have more metabolically expensive tissues (i.e., internal organs and muscles) than would be expected for a primate of our size. This discrepancy led to argue that the only way to support larger brains without raising the overall metabolic rate was to reduce the size of another major metabolic organ. With relatively little room left to reduce the mass of liver, heart, and kidneys, the gastrointestinal tract is the only metabolically expensive tissue whose size can vary substantially depending on the dominant diet.

Obligatory herbivores subsisting on phytomass that combines low energy density with poor digestibility require relatively large gastrointestinal tracts to process large amounts of feed. Voluminous and elaborated fermenting chambers of folivorous ruminants are well known, but the extreme examples are koalas (Phascolarctos cinereus), marsupials whose adults weigh as little as 6-8 kg but eat up to 1.5 kg of leaves a day and digest them for as long as several days in their extraordinarily long (1.8–1.5 m) intestines. Even so, this poor nutrition allows them to be on the move only about 1 percent of the time. Consequently, a fructivorous primate of human size would have to eat 3-5 kg of sweet fruits and a folivorous one more than 10 kg of leaves a day, and even then this bulky plant diet would cover no more than about half of the essential protein requirements and would have little room for vigorous activity.

Obligatory carnivores subsisting largely on easily digestible protein can dispense with cumbersome metabolic arrangements and devote a great deal of energy to rapid pursuits (felids) or to persistent running (canids). Evolution had clearly shifted human capabilities in that direction. The human gastrointestinal tract is about 40 percent smaller than it would be in a similarly sized primate, and the most obvious explanation is that the reduction resulted from progressively larger inclusion of foodstuffs of higher energy density and easier digestibility. In those environments where nuts and seeds which also have relatively high protein content, were readily available, pre-agricultural foragers could obtain adequate diets by remaining overwhelmingly vegetarian. But where the energy-dense seeds were absent (in tundras), scarce, or difficult to reach (in arid grasslands or in high canopies of boreal forests), animal foods supplied large shares of overall food needs.

Carcass weight (the method of meat supply reporting preferred by the Food and Agriculture Organisation) amounts to as much as 90 per cent of live weight in poultry. It averages 74 per cent of body mass in American pigs but only 62 percent in beef cattle and 59 percent in dairy steers. Carcass cutting yield (the share that ends up as meat) depends on fatness and muscling of the animal as well as on the amount of boneless cuts and on the quantity of fat remaining on retail portions. Retail weight (the method of meat supply reporting preferred by the US Department of Agriculture) any amount to as little as 29 percent of live weight for a very fat beef animal butchered into closely trimmed boneless steaks and roasts and into lean ground beef – or to as much as 62 percent for a heavily muscled market hog turned into bone-in chops and roasts and regular ground pork for sausages. By far the most accurate, but only rarely available, figure is the actual intake at table (retail weight minus cooking and table waste), which can be reliably determined only by expensive household consumption studies such as Japan's National Nutrition Survey.

Choice of the reporting method makes a substantial difference to average annual aggregates, as indicated in Table 14.1 whatever the actual totals may be, humans have always consumed much more than the highly proteinaceous muscles. Some cultures eat (or at least used to before most of their people became more choosy or more squeamish) every internal and external organ, from a bull's testes to his tripe and from a cock's comb to his feet. Internal organs (offal: heart, lungs, kidneys, liver) may or may not be included in reported carcass or retail totals of meat supply. But it is to be included in reported carcass or retail totals of meat supply.

Table 14.1: Differences Between Live Weight, Dressed Carcass, Retail Weight, and Actual Consumption Illustrated with the Example of us Beef

Category	Explanation	Weight (kg)	Percent of live weight
Live weight	Typical US steer	540	100
Carcass weight	Dressed cold carcass	330	61
Saleable retail weight	Bones and fat included	250	46
Edible weight	Boneless steaks and roasts closely trimmed and lean ground meat	205	38
Actually consumed	Edible weight minus cooking and table waste	185	34

Sources: Typical share and total weights from Wulf (1999) and USDA (222a).

HOUSEHOLD SPENDING ON NON-FOOD ITEMS

One may call it a demonstration effect caused by the opening up of the economy to the global market. The consumption pattern of Indian households has undergone perceptible changes during the post liberalisation years. The great Indian consumer market may yet remain a myth, but the share of nonfood items in the individual's consumption basket has increased steadily during the late nineties. Given our low per capita consumption base, food and beverages continue to account for the larger part of any households final consumption expenditure, but what is significant is that its share has come down sharply in the nineties. The distribution of consumption expenditure between food and nonfood items reflects the economic well-being of the population. In general, poor households are expected to spend substantially more on food items as against nonfood items. The share of expenditure on food items is expected to decline with development and economic prosperity.

This is exactly what has happened in the nineties. The share of expenditure on food in total private consumption expenditure has declined from 63.2% in 1993-94 to 59.5% in 1999-2000 in rural areas. The share of expenditure on nonfood items has increased correspondingly during the same period from 36.8% in 1993-94 to 40.6% in 1999-00.

The decline in the share of food items was even sharper in urban households — down by 6.6 percentage points from 54.6% in 1993-94 to 48% in 1999-00. This was largely because the consumption expenditure itself has grown at a healthy rate in the nineties. Per capita monthly consumption expenditure has grown by 10.3% annually compounded during the period — 11% in urban areas and 9.5% in the rural sector. This was substantially higher than the growth rate of either GDP or that of per capita income. Per capita income grew by an annual compound rate of 4.6% during 1993-94 to 1999-2000.

The change in consumption pattern, of course, has been a continuous process for the last two decades and the share of food in the total final consumption expenditure has been declining steadily. It accounted for 65.6% and 58.7% of the per capita consumption expenditure of the rural and urban households, respectively, in 1983 and came down to 63.2% and 54.6% in 1993-94. At the individual state level the degree of change was, however, quite at variance. The eastern states, for example, have failed to reach the national average even in 1999-00. The share of food items in aggregate consumption expenditure of rural households of three of the four eastern states, namely Assam, Orissa and West Bengal was estimated at more than 65% each compared to 59.4% at the national level. The share was 64.1% in Bihar. The performance of urban households in these states was not very different. The share of food items in aggregate consumption was higher than that of the national average in each of these states. At 57% the share of food items in Orissa was more than 9 percentage points higher than that of the national average. Among the major states, Gujarat, at the other end has witnessed the sharpest decline in the share of food items in total consumption expenditure during the period — down by 7.3 percentage points from 67.1% in 1993-94 to 59.8% in 1999-00. This is significant, for, rural Gujarat, in fact, witnessed an increase in the share of food items in the early nineties — up from 66.7% in 1983 to 67.1% in 1993-94 (Table 14.2).

Demand for Milk and Dairy Products

Milk, meat, eggs, hides and skins and wools are the most important livestock products in India. As the livestock population increased, output from most livestock also grew. The spectacular growth in livestock production was fostered by the rising demand for these products due to a rapidly increasing population and rising income. Reliable time series data on consumption of various livestock products are currently not available. Bulk of the production ranging from 90 to 95 percent of total output of various livestock products are consumed within the country. Data on consumption of milk, eggs, and meat per household and percentage of households consuming these items during different survey rounds of NSSO are summarized in Table 14.3.

Market demand for milk and milk products has expanded considerably during the last two decades. This has been due to increase in population, urbanization, increased income, availability of relatively cheap subsidized liquid milk through government run milk plants in various metropolitan cities and the awareness for better and nutritious diet. India has largest domestic market for milk and dairy products. These products are widely consumed in all regions, both in rural and urban areas as well as among most socioeconomic classes. Total apparent consumption of milk is estimated to have increased from 19 million tonnes in 1960/61 to around 64 million tonnes in 1997/98. The annual compound rate of growth during the past 38 years comes to 3.5 percent. According to data collected by National Sample Survey (NSSO), per capita consumption for 30 days of milk (liquid), which includes milk products such as curds and ghee (but not milk-based sweetmeats) prepared from milk, increased since 1987/88 by about 600-700 ml. in both rural and urban areas. Despite this increase per capita milk consumption remained under 4 litres (i.e. about 130 ml per day) in rural areas and under 5 litres (about 165 ml per day) in urban areas. Moreover, one-third of rural households and one-fifth of all urban households reported no consumption of milk during the recall 30 days period. These proportions have not changed greatly since 1987/88. However, there is a considerable regional variation in milk consumption in the country. Consumption level is much higher in northern and northwestern states (Punjab, Haryana, Himachal Pradesh, Jammu & Kashmir, Rajasthan) than in the rest of the country. As regards the share of the market in the total per capita consumption, at the all India level, in urban areas as much as 88 percent to purchased; whereas in rural areas only 26 percent is obtained from market.

Table 14.2: Share of Non-food Items in Rural India's Consumption Basket.

State	Per Capita Monthly Consumption Expenditure (Rs)									Compound annual growth rate (%)					
	1999-2000			1993-1994			1983			1999-2000			1993-94/1983		
	Rural	Urban	Comb.	Rural	Urban	Comb.	Rural	Urban	Comb.	Rural	Urban	Comb.	Rural	Urban	Comb.
Andhra Pradesh	453.61	773.52	550.53	288.70	408.60	322.28	115.58	59.55	126.27	7.8	11.2	9.3	9.6	21.2	9.8
Arunachal Pradesh	647.92	765.91	672.31	316.85	494.11	343.75	0.00	0.00	0.00	12.7	7.6	11.8	-	-	-
Assam	426.12	814.12	473.42	258.11	458.60	280.42	113.03	160.48	117.87	8.7	10.0	9.1	8.6	11.1	9.1
Bihar	384.72	601.89	417.18	218.30	353.00	236.78	93.76	139.50	99.53	9.9	9.3	9.9	8.8	9.7	9.0
Goa	868.77	1155.45	1014.78	487.24	519.33	501.40	169.12	222.99	187.20	10.1	14.2	12.5	11.2	8.8	10.3
Gujarat	551.33	891.68	678.27	303.30	454.20	356.87	119.25	164.06	133.59	10.5	11.9	11.3	9.8	10.7	10.3
Haryana	714.37	912.07	767.89	385.00	473.90	407.67	149.14	183.97	157.03	10.9	11.5	11.1	9.9	9.9	10.0
Himachal Pradesh	684.50	1242.93	737.82	350.63	746.92	386.23	150.05	257.09	158.51	11.8	8.9	11.4	8.8	11.2	9.3
Jammu & Kashmir	677.23	952.85	746.74	363.31	541.58	406.84	128.11	155.19	134.02	10.9	9.9	10.6	11.0	13.3	11.7
Karnataka	499.78	910.99	638.81	269.40	423.10	318.47	118.12	168.11	132.81	10.8	13.6	12.3	8.6	9.7	9.1
Kerala	765.70	932.61	816.76	390.40	493.80	419.08	145.24	178.31	152.13	11.9	11.2	11.8	10.4	10.7	10.7
Madhya Pradesh	401.50	693.56	478.92	252.00	408.10	289.83	101.78	148.39	111.61	8.1	9.2	8.7	9.5	10.6	10.0
Maharashtra	496.77	973.33	697.42	272.70	529.80	371.54	110.98	187.56	138.57	10.5	10.7	11.0	9.4	10.9	10.4
Manipur	537.79	707.77	596.36	299.57	319.55	305.59	131.45	138.20	133.25	10.2	14.2	11.8	8.6	8.7	8.6
Meghalaya	563.64	971.87	639.13	356.98	530.55	390.00	0.00	0.00	0.00	7.9	10.6	8.6	-	-	-
Mizoram	721.83	1056.64	935.53	389.55	549.51	472.59	119.81	192.31	142.73	10.8	11.5	12.0	12.5	11.1	12.7
Nagaland	941.30	1242.39	1005.99	441.45	510.02	454.48	0.00	196.46	0.00	13.4	16.0	14.2	-	10.0	-
Orissa	373.17	618.48	413.71	219.80	402.50	245.94	97.48	151.35	104.06	9.2	7.4	9.0	8.5	10.3	8.9
Punjab	742.43	898.82	792.07	433.00	510.70	456.59	170.30	184.38	174.26	9.4	9.9	9.6	9.8	10.7	10.1
Rajasthan	548.88	795.81	611.19	322.40	424.70	346.60	127.52	159.96	134.50	9.3	11.0	9.9	9.7	10.2	9.9
Sikkim	531.68	905.69	559.97	298.72	518.44	321.12	0.00	222.81	0.00	10.1	9.7	9.7	-	8.8	-
Tamil Nadu	513.97	971.61	681.37	293.60	438.30	344.31	112.19	164.15	129.43	9.8	14.2	12.0	10.1	10.3	10.3
Tripura	528.41	876.59	589.50	343.93	489.94	367.43	0.00	0.00	0.00	7.4	10.2	8.2	-	-	-

State															
Uttar Pradesh	466.68	690.68	516.99	273.80	389.00	297.62	104.25	137.84	110.45	9.3	10.0	9.6	10.1	10.9	10.4
West Bengal	454.49	866.60	571.66	278.80	474.20	333.36	104.60	169.94	122.03	8.5	10.6	9.4	10.3	10.8	10.6
Andaman & Nicobar	780.21	1114.27	873.28	495.90	907.19	608.07	156.75	240.79	0.00	7.8	3.5	6.2	12.2	14.2	-
Chandigarh	989.20	1435.36	1382.87	463.03	1028.00	975.18	199.41	289.55	0.00	13.5	5.7	6.0	12.9	13.5	-
Dadra & N Haveli	561.18	1207.34	636.82	234.28	441.86	253.40	93.33	0.00	0.00	15.7	18.2	16.6	9.6	-	-
Daman & Diu	901.48	979.43	976.04	452.48	474.98	463.33	169.12	222.99	187.20	12.2	12.8	13.2	10.3	7.8	9.5
New Delhi	917.21	1383.46	1316.30	605.22	794.95	777.01	208.81	230.43	228.64	7.2	9.7	9.2	11.2	13.2	13.0
Lakshadweep	876.19	1018.25	967.35	526.32	515.17	0.00	0.00	0.00	0.00	9.3	12.3	11.1	-	-	-
Pondicherry	597.63	784.3	731.90	347.96	419.84	396.53	96.02	160.34	132.00	9.4	11.0	10.8	13.7	10.1	11.6
All States	486.08	854.96	690.98	280.40	458.00	328.18	112.31	165.80	125.75	9.5	11.0	10.3	9.6	10.7	10.1

State	Composition of Consumption Expenditure (%) – Rural						Composition of consumption expenditure (%) - Urban					
	1999-2000		1993-1994		1983		1999-2000		1993-94		1983	
	Food	Non-food	Food	Non-food	Food	Non-food	Food	Non-food	Food	Non-food	Food	Non-food
Sikkim	56.78	43.22	65.65	34.35	0.00	0.00	47.53	52.47	55.18	44.82	55.17	44.83
Tamil Nadu	58.74	41.26	62.84	37.16	65.17	34.83	45.61	54.39	54.60	45.40	58.40	41.60
Tripura	65.20	34.80	64.85	35.15	0.00	0.00	56.18	43.82	56.96	43.04	0.00	0.00
Uttar Pradesh	57.42	42.58	41.47	38.53	63.54	36.46	50.49	49.51	55.99	44.01	59.13	40.87
West Bengal	65.90	34.10	66.82	33.18	73.94	26.06	52.28	47.72	55.93	44.07	60.90	39.10
Andaman & Nicobar	61.56	38.44	63.28	36.72	66.30	33.70	51.26	48.74	43.78	56.22	0.00	0.00
Chandigarh	47.82	52.18	56.08	43.92	59.89	40.11	38.82	61.18	35.79	64.21	0.00	0.00
Dadra & N Haveli	60.09	39.91	65.46	34.54	66.67	33.33	47.72	52.28	62.68	37.32	0.00	0.00
Daman & Diu	59.26	46.24	63.11	37.89	65.88	36.12	63.70	46.30	62.79	57.21	59.18	40.82
New Delhi	44.41	55.59	63.46	36.54	54.86	45.14	41.04	58.96	48.58	51.42	54.00	46.00
Lakshadweep	62.09	37.91	64.49	33.51	0.00	0.00	60.03	39.97	67.14	32.86	0.00	0.00

Table 14.2: Share of Non-food Items in Rural India's Consumption Basket (Contd.)

| State | Composition of Consumption Expenditure (%) – Rural | | | | | | Composition of consumption expenditure (%) – Urban | | | | | |
| | 1999-2000 | | 1993-1994 | | 1983 | | 1999-2000 | | 1993-94 | | 1983 | |
	Food	Non-food	Food	Non-food	Food	Non-food	Food	Non-food	Food	Non-food	Food	Non-food
Pondicherry	56.61	43.39	61.37	38.63	67.67	32.33	51.00	49.00	57.71	42.29	56.09	43.91
All States	59.18	40.59	63.18	36.82	65.36	54.44	48.06	51.94	54.65	45.35	58.69	41.31
Andhra Pradesh	60.50	39.50	59.58	40.42	60.24	39.76	47.44	52.56	53.84	46.16	54.57	45.43
Arunachal Pradesh	55.60	44.40	61.63	38.37	0.00	0.00	57.65	42.35	60.62	39.18	0.00	0.00
Assam	67.63	32.37	72.26	27.74	73.37	26.63	55.38	44.62	59.68	40.32	63.77	36.23
Bihar	66.54	33.46	71.00	29.00	73.63	26.37	57.24	42.76	62.92	37.08	66.14	33.86
Goa	54.20	45.80	56.62	43.38	63.88	36.12	51.33	48.67	59.09	40.91	59.18	40.82
Gujarat	59.82	40.18	67.10	32.90	66.73	33.27	49.58	50.42	58.41	41.59	61.75	38.25
Haryana	55.51	44.49	60.05	39.95	64.03	35.97	45.87	54.13	53.87	46.13	57.80	42.20
Himachal Pradesh	56.00	44.00	60.02	39.98	63.09	36.91	45.34	54.66	42.45	57.55	54.00	46.00
Jammu & Kashmir	62.60	37.40	61.78	38.22	69.46	30.54	55.51	44.49	56.41	43.59	64.00	36.00
Karnataka	59.08	40.92	61.95	38.05	63.31	36.69	46.32	53.68	55.71	44.29	57.88	42.12
Kerala	53.70	46.30	60.45	39.55	61.64	38.36	49.04	50.96	53.93	46.07	58.96	41.04
Madhya Pradesh	58.09	41.91	61.19	38.81	65.95	34.05	47.60	52.40	52.85	47.15	58.99	41.01
Maharashtra	54.71	45.29	59.48	40.52	61.32	38.68	45.31	54.69	53.02	46.98	57.53	42.47
Manipur	63.12	36.88	67.48	32.52	71.38	28.62	56.40	43.60	63.82	36.18	71.56	28.44
Meghalaya	60.44	39.56	60.83	39.17	0.00	0.00	47.02	52.98	56.38	43.62	0.00	0.00
Mizoram	59.36	40.66	61.24	38.76	66.10	33.90	52.04	47.96	54.14	45.86	58.90	41.10
Nagaland	58.93	41.07	64.99	35.01	0.00	0.00	47.64	52.36	58.85	41.15	64.64	35.36
Orissa	64.11	35.89	68.06	31.94	73.72	26.28	56.95	43.05	57.79	42.21	65.13	34.87
Punjab	52.29	47.71	57.92	42.08	58.67	41.33	47.12	52.88	53.03	46.97	55.92	44.08
Rajasthan	59.50	40.50	62.28	37.72	60.52	39.48	50.85	49.15	56.65	43.35	57.58	42.42

Source: NSSO

Table 14.3: Monthly Consumption of Milk, Eggs & Meat Per Household and Percentage of Household Consuming these Items:: (ALL INDIA)

N.S.S. Rounds	Milk				Egg				Meat			
	Quantity of consumption per HH (litres)		% of HHS reporting consumption		Quantity of consumption per HH (No.)		% of HHS reporting consumption		Quantity of consumption per HH (No.)		% of HHS reporting consumption	
	Rural	Urban	Rural	Urban	Rural	Urban	Rural	Urban	Rural	Urban	Rural	Urban
43rd Rounds (July 87 to June, 98)	16.25	20.06	62	78	2.64	6.73	17	32	0.51	0.94	32	43
47th Round (July-Dec., 1991)	18.71	22.80	64	79	0.74	1.21	43	49	3.72	7.66	26	38
48th Round (1992)	18.54	23.20	62	79	0.73	0.07	42	49	3.65	8.03	25	39
49th Round (Jan-June, 1993)	17.50	21.47	61	78	0.69	1.00	41	48	3.26	6.11	24	33
50th Round (1993-94)	19.29	21.79	66	80	3.13	6.59	22	35	0.64	0.89	20	28

Note: Quantity figures have been derived by multiplying per capita consumption with average household size.
Source: Sarvekshana, various issues.

Although milk production has extended considerably, the share of quantities sold at the market has also risen markedly. Currently at the all India level around 60 percent of milk production in India is sold in the market. The rest is consumed at the producer (urban and rural) household level. These estimates are supported by the findings of the research study commissioned by the World Bank on Livestock. According to the survey carried out for the study in the three states viz. Rajasthan, Gujarat and Kerala, milk consumption within the producing households in these three states averaged 43 percent. However, there are significant variations across states. In Kerala, which has a much more developed milk economy, only about 14 percent of the milk production was consumed at home with a share of home consumption increasing from 13 percent for the bottom 40 percent households to 20 percent in the top 40 percent. A similar trend prevailed in the Gujarat, although the average consumption of milk at home was higher (approximately 50 percent). In Rajasthan, only about 20 percent of the milk production was sold and there was little difference in this respect between poor and rich households[1]. Following the increased output, per capita availability of milk had increased from 124 grams per day in 1950/51 to 211 grams in 1998/99.

In 1993/94, 36 million tons of milk were marketed, of which 13 million tonne (36 percent) were channeled through the organized sector (Operation Flood, Cooperatives government milk schemes, and large private processors) and 23 million tonne (64 percent) went through the unorganized sector (small private dealer, and processors). Operation Flood, cooperatives and government schemes account for 17 percent of milk marketing and private processor account for 19 percent. Milk in the organized sector is processed in 275 dairy plants and 83 milk product factories operated by cooperatives, private dairy processors and government milk schemes. Milk channeled through Operation Flood cooperatives is generally processed in rural dairy plants and transported into cities and towns. The unorganized sector includes private milk vendors and milk dealers. Milk dealers supply milk either to bigger milk dealers or to private dairy factories. Small dealers generally collect milk from a small number of villages that serve as part of a large procurement scheme operated by a bigger milk dealer or processor. The large processors set a fixed price according to fat content and nonfat solids, leaving it to the suppliers to set prices for farmers. The processors usually integrate forward marketing channels by establishing or leaving ice factories to chill the milk, enabling them to seek the best price for their milk from private dairy factories within or outside the state.

Meat Consumption

Total consumption of meat, which is almost wholly accounted for by four categories of meat, viz. goat meat, mutton, beef and chicken, increased from 1.13 million tonnes in 1975 to 2.26 millions tonne in 1995. The annual rate of growth was 3.6 percent during the last two decades. Among these categories, the most rapid growth, as discussed below, has been in consumption of poultry meat, which increased by almost 6 times. The rate of growth in goat meat and beef was around 3 percent per annum. There is a great deal of regional variation in the consumption of meat. At the all-India level, during 1987/88 to 1993/94 consumption of goat meat, mutton and chicken remained unchanged at about 80 grams per person per month in rural sector and about 140-150 grams in the urban areas. However, there has been a shift in urban consumption habits away from goat meat and towards chicken.

An Indian may prefer rogan josh and murg makhani over beef but they consume more beef per head than either mutton or chicken. According to trade estimates, the per capita consumption of beef (considered the poor man's meat) is estimated at 1.8 kg. On the other hand, the consumption of sheep/goat meat is only 700 gm per capita, while that of chicken is about 800 gm per capita[1]. Although cow slaughter is banned in all states except two, there are relatively fewer restrictions on the humble buffalo. As a result, Indian beef is mainly buffalo meat or carabeef.

Poultry Meat and Eggs

With the development of poultry industry production and consumption of poultry meat has increased considerably. Poultry is a choice meat in India. It being considered as white meat contains less fat and is said to be easily digestible than other meat. Economic growth and urbanization has resulted in restricting the availability of red meat. Also despite many fold increase in prices during the last two-decades, price of poultry meat is lower than of the red meat. Consequently it has captured part of the red meat market. An examination of the wholesale price index reveals that prices of poultry meat have registered the lowest increase.

Consumption of eggs increased both in rural and urban areas. In the rural areas per capita consumption rose by 23 percent during 1987/88 to 1993/94, while the proportion of households reporting egg consumption increased from 17 to 22 percent. Similarly, per capita consumption of egg in urban areas increased by 4 percent and the proportion of household reporting its consumption rose from 2 percent to 35 percent during this period in urban sector. Nevertheless, per capita consumption of eggs remained low per person per month in the urban areas, even though this figure is more than twice the consumption in the rural sector. Market share (i.e. cash purchases) for eggs during 1993/94 was 70 percent for rural areas and 97 percent for urban areas. Homegrown eggs accounted for 30 percent in rural areas and only 3 percent in urban areas[1]. NSSO Survey data on monthly consumption of milk, eggs and meat per household and percentage of households reporting consumption of these items, are summarized in Table 14.4.

---

[1]Ministry of Planning: Department of Statistics: Per Capita Consumption of selected Commodities: Sàrvekshana: Issue No. 2. Vol. XX. No. 2, October-December 1996: pp. 50.028-62 and S0.02 Statistical Tables S-1 to S-7.

Table 14.4: Consumption of Milk and Milk Products, Eggs and Poultry Products Per Person for 30 Days

Item	1987-88 (43rd Round)			1993-94 (50th Round)		
	Total kg	Cash Purchase (kg)	% cash of total	Total kg	Cash Purchase (kg)	% cash of total
RURAL INDIA						
Milk liquid (Litre)	3.20	0.88	27.5	3.94	1.00	25.4
Goat meat	0.05	0.05	100.0	0.05	0.05	100.0
Mutton	0.01	0.01	100.0	0.01	0.01	100.0
Beef	0.02	0.02	100.0	0.02	0.02	100.0
Buffalo meat	0.01	0.01	100.0	0.02	0.02	100.0
Total meat	0.09	0.09	100.0	0.10	0.10	100.0
Chicken	0.02	0.1	50.0	0.02	0.01	50.0
Eggs (no.)	0.52	0.34	65.4	0.64	0.45	70.3
URBAN INDIA						
Milk liquid (Litre)	4.26	3.73	87.5	4.89	4.32	88.3
Goat meat	0.11	0.11	100.0	0.09	0.09	100.0
Mutton	0.02	0.02	100.0	0.02	0.02	100.0
Beef	0.03	0.03	100.0	0.03	0.03	100.0
Buffalo meat	0.04	0.04	100.0	0.03	0.03	100.0
Total meat	0.20	0.20	100.0	0.17	0.17	100.0
Chicken	0.02	0.01	50.0	0.03	0.03	100.0
Eggs (no.)	1.43	1.38	96.5	1.48	1.44	97.3

Source: Sarvekshana, October-December 1996.

The market prospects for future growth for poultry meat and eggs seem to be bright. A part of the increase in demand will be economically driven, with expected increase in the household incomes. Moreover the expected product diversification and composition, such as cut up parts and processed products, will help increase demand. For instance the demand for skinned and boneless poultry which are very low in fat, high protein and low cost, will result in considerable use of poultry meat in a variety of institutional and value added consumer products, as has happened in U.S.A. Moreover, the size of the Indian population can guarantee a demand, which may dazzle the biggest poultry consuming country. Assuming that half of the current population of India is non-vegetarians, there are over 500 million potential egg and poultry meat consumers. Another characteristics of the Indian industry is that 80 percent of the demand for poultry products comes from rural areas. However, only 20 percent of the poultry products find its way to rural India. The problem here is of accessibility. Also the demand for poultry products in India is determined more or less by location i.e. whether it is rural, urban or seasonality. Nevertheless supply keeps on increasing every year. When demand slumps during summer months and religious festival periods, prices of poultry products decline sharply, especially of eggs. As a result of this, the suppliers are worst affected, particularly the smaller ones. This requires some kind of coordination between the producers, processors and the state and the central governments.

Domestic market demand for poultry products including poultry meat is increasing rapidly among households, institutions, and gained increasing popularity especially of poultry meat during social functions, conferences, seminars and workshops, and sports and athlete meets. Based on the expected growth in income and population in demand and these trends, a steady growth in demand of around 10 percent in poultry meat is envisaged. This would mean a production target of 6.5 million tonnes of poultry meat by the year 2030. This implies a per caput availability of around 4.5 kg, per annum, just half the National Institute of Nutrition (NIN) recommendation of 9 kg, and the nutritional requirement of II kg per caput.

Overall Consumption Levels

Despite the continuing increase in supply and in aggregate consumption, per capita consumption of livestock products in India is still considerably lower than that in developed countries. For example, per capita consumption of milk is about half the level in Australia and the United States, while per capita poultry meat consumption is 12 percent of the level in China. Consumption of beef and veal is extremely low as compared to that of other countries. However, this is primarily due to sociocultural factors. For religious reasons, a large section of the population does not consume them. Moreover, the impact of these sociocultural factors spill over to the consumption of buffalo meat.

Annual per capita consumption of eggs (30) and poultry meat (0.43 kg) is still significantly lower in India than that in other countries, and thus offers opportunities for growth. Moreover, over 75-80 percent of eggs and poultry meat are consumed in urban and semi-urban areas, which account for only about a quarter of the country's population. Egg consumption in urban area is about 90 eggs per capita, while rural consumption is about 13 eggs per capita. Factors contributing to the higher consumption in urban areas include higher purchasing power of consumers and the transport costs from peri-urban to rural areas, which contribute to higher rural prices. Consumers preference is also implied by the fact that egg consumption increased even though the ratio between the price of eggs and the price of other livestock products (milk and meat) declined.

Poultry meat is becoming a popular source of affordable protein for the (largely urban) Indian population. In addition, broiler meat consumption is increasing faster than other types of poultry (duck, quail) meat. In 1993, broiler production accounted for 56 percent of total poultry production. By the year 2000, it accounted for about 70 percent.

High Income Elasticity of Demand for Livestock Products

The demand for livestock products in India is highly elastic. Recent estimates of expenditure elasticity for milk and milk products range from

1.14 to 1.47 for rural households and 0.61 to 1.09 for urban households. The demand for meat, and eggs is more elastic in rural households (0.92 – 1.18) than urban households (0.54 – 0.88). Presently, animal products (dairy, meat, eggs and fish) are already an important component of consumer budgets. Dairy products account for a large share of rural (4-22 percent) and urban (7-21 percent) consumer spending, with the percentage share increasing significantly with expenditure budget levels. Meat, egg and fish account for five to six percent of rural and two to seven percent of urban consumer expenditures. Even poor consumers spend a large share of per capita budgets on livestock products (5-15 percent rural areas and 11-19 percent in urban areas). Sustained economic growth and attendant increases in income will therefore continue to boost livestock product demand in the future.

Two trends will shape future livestock demand:
- An increasing shift from vegetarianism of diets that include meat (poultry-mutton-goat).
- The high income and price elasticities of demand for livestock products. Experience from other countries indicates that consumption will increase with increasing per capita gross domestic product (GDP). Decreasing product prices due to increased supply and improved market efficiency would have the same effect.

DEMAND FOR LIVESTOCK PRODUCTS[1]

Data and Method

This part makes use of information from the four major rounds of National Sample Survey (NSS) covering the years 1983 (January-December), 1987-88 (July-June), 1993-94 (July-June) and 1999-2000 (July-June). These rounds are numbered as 38th, 43rd, 50th and 55th respectively. Both the rural and urban households have been classified into four major income classes namely, very poor, poor, non-poor and rich on the basis of poverty line adopted by the Planning Commission, Govt. of India. Households below 75 percent of the poverty line are classified as 'very poor' and those above 75 percent and up to poverty line are classified as 'poor'. Households falling between the poverty line and 150 percent above the poverty line are designated as 'non-poor', and those above 150 percent of the poverty line are defined as 'rich'.

As the consumption patterns vary from region to region, the analysis is also done at the regional level. The entire country is divided into five regions namely east (Assam, Bihar, Orissa and West Bengal), west (Gujarat, Rajasthan, Madhya Pradesh and Maharashtra), north (Haryana, Punjab, Uttar Pradesh), Hill (Jammu and Kashmir, and Himachal Pradesh) and south (Andhra Pradesh, Karnataka, Kerala and Tamil Nadu).

---

[1]Praduman Kumar, Indian Journal of Agricultural Marketing, Conference No. 2004

Trends in Consumption of Livestock Products

Level of consumption and changes therein are analyzed in terms of budget shares of livestock products and their per capita consumption by income class, location, and region.

Share in Total Consumption Expenditure

In 1999-2000, food of animal origin accounted for 12.79 percent of the total consumption expenditure (Table 14.5). This is slightly higher than that in 1983 (12.11 percent). The share of food of animal origin in total consumption expenditure however increased in the intermittent years. It increased to 13.41 percent in 1987-84 to further 13.79 in 1993-94. Milk is the most preferred food of animal origin, sharing about 70 percent of the total expenditure on livestock products. Meat stands next with a share of 17 percent, followed by fish, and eggs. This pattern of expenditure allocation across products has remained almost stable over the last seventeen years. This implies that whenever there is an increase or decrease in the budget allocation to food of animal origin, households allocate expenditure to different livestock products in a set proportion.

Analysis of budget shares across income classes shows a positive relationship between income and share of food of animal origin. In the very poor households, food of animal origin accounted for 7.91 percent of

Table 14.5: Share of Livestock Products in Household Consumption Expenditure (%)

Products	Year	Income class				
		Very poor	Poor	Non poor	Rich	All
Milk	1983	3.68	6.06	8.37	10.01	8.40
	1987-88	4.86	6.77	9.28	10.18	9.28
	1993-94	5.01	7.17	9.65	10.46	9.64
	1999-00	4.56	5.82	8.02	9.68	8.92
Meat	1983	1.46	1.84	2.14	2.17	2.05
	1987-88	1.73	1.91	2.20	2.33	2.22
	1993-94	1.69	2.07	2.18	2.25	2.19
	1999-00	1.79	1.89	2.08	2.13	2.09
Eggs	1983	0.15	0.22	0.29	0.43	0.33
	1987-88	0.20	0.26	0.32	0.43	0.37
	1993-94	0.22	0.30	0.35	0.40	0.37
	1999-00	0.32	0.38	0.42	0.42	0.41
Fish	1983	1.18	1.38	1.45	1.29	1.34
	1987-88	1.30	1.58	1.73	1.48	1.54
	1993-94	1.22	1.56	1.76	1.55	1.59
	1999-00	1.24	1.40	1.56	1.31	1.56
Livestock + fish	1983	6.47	9.50	12.25	13.90	12.11
	1987-88	8.08	10.52	13.52	14.42	13.41
	1993-94	8.15	11.09	13.95	14.46	13.79
	1999-00	7.91	9.48	12.05	13.54	12.79

Source: NSSO

their total consumption expenditure in 1999-2000, while it was 13.54 percent for the rich households. For all income classes, the share of food of animal origin increased till 1993-94, but fell during 1999-2000. These relationships hold true irrespective of food items under consideration. An interesting point that emerges from the temporal changes in shares is that the share of animal food in total expenditure in case of non-poor and the rich households in 1999-2000 was less than that in 1983. For very poor households, the change was positive and for poor households this remained stable.

Pattern of expenditure allocation to different livestock products varies considerably across income classes. The share of milk increases with increase in income, while share of meat and fish increases. Very poor households allocate about 60 of the total expenditure to milk, and the rest to meat, eggs and fish. On the other hand, the rich households spend about 72 percent on milk, and the rest on meat, egg and fish. A comparison over time indicates little if any change in this pattern of allocation.

Per Capita Consumption

Between 1983 and 1999-2000, there have been considerable changes in per capita consumption of different food items of animal origin (Table 14.6). Per capita annual milk consumption increased from 43.04 kg to 73.54 kg, meat consumption increased from 2.38 kg to 3.1 kg, fish consumption from 2.45 kg to 3.47 kg, and number of eggs consumed from 9.22 to 19.48. However, there was considerable variation in consumption of these items across income classes. There was a strong positive association between quantity of milk consumed and income level. In 1983, per capita consumption of milk by the rich was about 11 times more than that by the very poor, and 5 times more than by the poor. A similar pattern follows is observed for egg. The association is somewhat weak in case of meat and fish. Meat consumption by the rich was higher by 4 and 2.6 times over the very poor and the poor. The gap in consumption of almost all items has however reduced during 1999-2000.

Amongst various types of meat, goat and sheep meat are the most preferred, followed by beef (cattle and buffalo meat), poultry and pork. During 1990s, per capita consumption of goat and sheep meat however has declined, while consumption of beef, poultry and pork has increased. Maximum increase has taken place in consumption of poultry meat; it increased from 0.32 kg/capita/annum in 1983 to 0.71 kg/capita/annum in 1999-2000. Pork consumption also got doubled from 0.16 kg/capita/annum in 1983.

Besides income, consumers' tastes and preferences, and price of product and availability of substitutes are other important determinants of the consumption pattern. This is observed in case of meat. In India, beef and pork are much cheaper compared to mutton and poultry meat. Table 14.3 shows that per capita beef consumption is much higher compared to other meats among the very poor households. Among the poor households also

Table 14.6: Per Capita Consumption of Different Livestock Products (Kg/capita/annum)

Products	Year	Income class				
		Very poor	*Poor*	*Non poor*	*Rich*	*All*
Milk	1983	9.36	22.03	40.16	89.68	43.04
	1987-88	12.42	23.77	43.76	97.89	54.37
	1993-94	13.42	26.54	48.01	99.01	58.56
	1999-00	13.83	23.47	46.68	115.61	73.54
Goat meat and mutton	1983	0.31	0.63	1.06	2.12	1.09
	1987-88	0.34	0.57	0.89	1.89	1.10
	1993-94	0.32	0.56	0.79	1.55	0.97
	1999-00	0.45	0.40	0.83	1.30	0.96
Beef and buffalo meat	1983	0.48	0.55	0.58	0.83	0.62
	1987-88	0.59	0.56	0.60	0.95	0.71
	1993-94	0.51	0.63	0.63	0.81	0.69
	1999-00	0.69	0.63	0.78	1.00	0.85
Pork	1983	0.05	0.05	0.14	0.33	0.16
	1987-88	0.06	0.08	0.14	0.36	0.19
	1993-94	0.05	0.11	0.18	0.47	0.26
	1999-00	0.07	0.10	0.14	0.37	0.24
Chicken	1983	0.11	0.22	0.31	0.60	0.32
	1987-88	0.09	0.17	0.28	0.67	0.37
	1993-94	0.08	0.16	0.26	0.72	0.39
	1999-00	0.18	0.26	0.47	1.09	0.71
Total meat	1983	1.04	1.62	2.26	4.18	2.38
	1987-88	1.17	1.46	2.00	4.05	2.49
	1993-94	1.03	1.54	1.95	3.66	2.39
	1999-00	1.43	1.43	2.35	4.37	3.10
Eggs (Numbers)	1983	1.92	4.09	7.25	21.31	9.22
	1987-88	2.78	4.95	8.02	23.33	12.05
	1993-94	3.33	6.10	9.70	22.52	12.97
	1999-00	5.62	8.85	13.55	28.74	19.48
Fish	1983	1.35	1.98	2.43	3.73	2.45
	1987-88	1.32	2.01	2.55	4.02	2.78
	1993-94	1.14	1.84	2.64	4.34	2.93
	1999-00	1.32	2.16	3.11	4.44	3.47

Source: NSSO

beef consumption is higher compared to other meats. In 1999-2000, beef accounted for 48 percent and 45 percent of the total meat consumed by the very poor and poor households respectively. On the other hand, rich households consume more of goat and sheep meat, followed by beef and poultry meat. Their shares in total meat consumed in 1999-2000 stood at 30, 23 and 25 percent respectively. Further, there is a discernible trend in per capita consumption of different meats in different classes. Goat and sheep meat consumption showed an increasing trend in the very poor and rich categories, while it showed a decreasing trend in other categories. Trend in consumption of all other types of meat was increasing but with gyrations. This indicates that the poor households consume more of inferior meats, but as their income increases they substitute these with quality meats.

A comparison of changes in budget shares and quantity of different livestock products consumed brings out that with rising per capita incomes, consumption of different livestock products has increased over the last two decades, but overall share of livestock products in household consumption expenditure has not increased much. In recent years per capita consumption of cereals has declined. This coupled with a stable share of livestock products in total consumption expenditure indicates that households allocate more of their incremental incomes towards consumption of livestock products.

Rural–Urban Disparities

Rural-urban disparities in consumption of food of animal origin are analyzed in terms of the share of livestock products in total household consumption expenditure and quantity consumed. Table 14.7 presents the shares of livestock products in total consumption expenditure of rural and urban households. In 1999-2000 livestock products accounted for 12.92 percent of the total household consumption expenditure of rural households. This is slightly higher than that of urban households (12.65%). In rural areas, share of livestock products increased from 11.02 percent in 1983 to 13.08 percent in 1987-88 and to 13.85 percent in 1993-94. In urban areas, however it increased slightly during 1980s, but declined during 1990s.

Both the rural and urban consumers spent about 70 percent of the total allocations to livestock products on milk. Meat and fish are next in the order with a share of about 17 and 10 percent respectively. And this pattern has not changed much over time particularly in the urban areas. The share of milk in rural areas increased between 1983 and 1993-94, but fell in 1999-2000. A similar pattern is observed for all other products. On the

Table 14.7: Share of Livestock Products in Total Consumption Expenditure of Rural and Urban Consumers (%)

Products	1983	1987-88	1993-94	1999-2000
Rural				
Milk	7.59	9.02	9.69	8.96
Meat	1.86	2.14	2.14	2.08
Eggs	0.24	0.30	0.32	0.40
Fish	1.33	1.63	1.70	1.47
Total	11.02	13.08	13.85	12.92
Urban				
Milk	9.54	9.65	9.60	8.88
Meat	2.32	2.33	2.24	2.10
Eggs	0.47	0.47	0.42	0.42
Fish	1.35	1.42	1.46	1.25
Total	13.67	13.86	13.71	12.65

Source: NSSO

other hand, in urban areas the relative shares of different products did not change much.

Table 14.8 compares per capita consumption of different livestock products of rural and urban consumers and changes therein between 1983 and 1999-2000. Consumption rates of different products have been higher in urban areas. In 1983, mean per capita annual consumption of milk, meat and fish in rural areas was 36.96 kg and 1.96 kg and 2.39 kg respectively compared to 55.46 kg, 3.24 kg and 2.58 kg in urban areas. The consumption rates have kept on increasing. In 1999-2000, per capita milk consumption in rural areas increased to 63.33 kg, meat consumption to 2.44 kg and fish consumption to 3.38 kg. The corresponding figures for urban areas are 90.70, 4.22 and 3.63.

Table 14.8: Per Capita Consumption of Livestock Products in Rural and Urban Areas (Kg/Annum)

Products	1983	1987-88	1993-94	1999-2000
Rural				
Milk	36.96	49.42	54.73	63.33
Meat	1.96	2.14	2.05	2.44
Eggs	5.91	8.26	9.32	15.10
Fish	2.39	2.73	2.77	3.38
Urban				
Milk	55.46	64.59	65.24	90.70
Meat	3.24	3.22	2.99	4.22
Eggs	15.99	19.89	19.34	26.85
Fish	2.58	2.90	3.21	3.63

Source: NSSO

The comparison between rural and rural consumption rates over time brings out that consumption patterns of rural and urban populations are heading towards convergence. This was observed particularly in late 1980s and early 1990s, when the gap between rural and urban consumption rates was very small. This was because of faster growth in rural consumption rates than urban consumption rates. What this implies that though urbanization will continue to be an important source of growth in demand for food of animal origin, sustained growth in per capita rural income will fuel further growth in it.

Regional Disparities

At the regional level, there are considerable differences in the shares of livestock products in total consumption expenditure (Table 14.9). In 1983, the percent of consumption expenditure on livestock products was maximum (16.4) in the hill region, followed by northern (15.23%), western (12.50%), southern (11.05%) and eastern (9.65%) regions. Except in the hill region, the proportional budget allocation to livestock products increased till 1993-94, and declined thereafter. In the hill region, the

Table 14.9: Share of Livestock Products in Total Consumption Expenditure by Region (%)

Products	1983	1987-88	1993-94	1999-2000
Eastern				
Milk	4.68	5.83	6.07	5.42
Meat	1.85	2.11	2.11	2.06
Eggs	0.36	0.43	0.49	0.62
Fish	2.75	3.22	3.12	3.08
Total	9.65	11.59	11.79	11.18
Western				
Milk	10.21	11.41	11.94	10.06
Meat	1.45	1.50	1.41	1.29
Eggs	0.23	0.25	0.21	0.23
Fish	0.60	0.62	0.63	0.52
Total	12.50	13.78	14.18	13.10
Northern				
Milk	13.52	14.58	15.16	13.20
Meat	1.26	1.09	1.18	1.01
Eggs	0.22	0.18	0.18	0.22
Fish	0.24	0.15	0.16	0.17
Total	15.23	15.99	16.67	14.60
Southern				
Milk	5.37	6.08	6.35	6.10
Meat	2.59	2.56	2.80	2.62
Eggs	0.47	0.53	0.55	0.55
Fish	1.62	1.91	2.07	1.87
Total	11.05	11.08	11.78	11.14
Hills				
Milk	12.58	11.83	13.95	13.04
Meat	3.35	3.40	1.26	2.76
Eggs	0.33	0.35	0.21	0.34
Fish	0.14	0.16	0.02	0.06
Total	16.40	15.73	15.43	16.20

Source: NSSO

scenario was reverse; the share of livestock products declined till 1993-94, but improved in 1999-2000. Almost a similar pattern is observed for the individual products.

There are also considerable regional differences in expenditure shares of individual products. Milk is important in northern, western and hill regions with a share of 90, 80 and 77 percent respectively in total expenditure on food of animal origin in 1999-2000. In southern and eastern regions, its share was 55 and 48 percent respectively. In these states, meat and fish are important.

Table 14.10 presents regional differences in per capita consumption of animal products and changes therein between 1983 and 1999-2000. In 1983, per capita milk consumption was the highest (74 kg/annum) in the hill region and it increased to 129.13 kg/annum in 1999-2000. Northern region

Table 14.10: Per Capita Consumption of Livestock Products by Region (Kg/Annum)

Products	1983	1987-88	1993-94	1999-2000
Eastern				
Milk	20.64	26.05	29.30	32.82
Meat	1.95	2.02	1.82	1.98
Eggs	8.23	10.66	13.79	22.22
Fish	3.49	4.33	4.41	5.11
Western				
Milk	49.59	61.08	69.48	77.30
Meat	1.71	1.68	1.57	1.65
Eggs	6.46	8.52	7.73	11.08
Fish	1.00	1.14	1.21	1.23
Northern				
Milk	72.29	96.52	102.64	103.55
Meat	1.89	1.71	1.86	2.17
Eggs	6.27	6.38	6.07	10.53
Fish	0.50	0.30	0.29	0.47
Southern				
Milk	31.44	40.11	43.50	51.52
Meat	2.99	2.86	2.97	3.62
Eggs	15.02	20.28	23.38	32.54
Fish	4.99	5.39	5.50	6.14
Hills				
Milk	74.00	83.22	102.33	129.13
Meat	3.49	3.65	1.47	4.20
Eggs	10.95	13.88	7.92	19.93
Fish	0.30	0.34	0.05	0.21

Source: NSSO

has followed it closely. Compared to these regions, per capita consumption of milk has remained very low in the eastern and southern regions. Per capita meat consumption has also remained highest in the hill region throughout the period, followed by southern, northern, eastern and western regions. Meat consumption rate in eastern and western regions remained also unchanged during the last two decades; in northern, southern and hill regions it has increased substantially. Fish is an important food of animal origin in southern and eastern regions with an average per capita consumption of 6.14 kg and 5.11 kg a year respectively. Fish consumption rate kept on increasing throughout.

Two important inferences are drawn form analysis of regional pattern of demand for livestock products. First, there are considerable regional differences in the pattern of consumption of different livestock products, and the differences have persisted over time. This is because of regional differences in the availability of a product, and tastes and preferences. For example, easy availability of fish in the eastern and southern regions (coastal), compared to milk makes fish a preferred consumption item. Conversely, milk is the most preferred food of animal origin in northern, hill and western region, mainly because it is easily available. Second, households try balancing their animal protein requirement through substitution of one product with another depending on their availability and prices.

Vegetarianism and Level of Meat Consumption

India being a predominantly a Hindu country is considered to have a majority of its inhabitants as vegetarians. And this is offered as an explanation for low level of per capita meat consumption. Estimates of non-vegetarian population have been arrived at to test this hypothesis (Table 14.11).

Table 14.11: Non-Vegetarian Population in India (%)

	1983	1987-88	1993-94	1999-2000
Total	56.74	58.68	60.02	58.85
Location				
Rural	54.79	57.37	58.88	57.55
Urban	60.73	61.38	62.00	61.05
Income class				
Very poor	49.41	52.47	50.77	55.71
Poor	56.98	58.02	60.30	59.05
Non poor	60.23	59.64	61.26	59.71
Rich	58.42	60.78	61.91	58.70
Region				
Eastern	72.98	78.65	78.60	80.07
Western	39.22	39.19	41.35	38.30
Northern	31.01	29.56	33.84	31.79
Southern	74.81	74.06	76.48	76.10
Hills	50.83	59.66	32.61	52.22

Source: NSSO

In 1999-2000, about 59 percent of the population in the country were that of non-vegetarians. This figure does not include egg eating population. The population of non-vegetarians has been rising though at a slow rate. It increased from 57 percent in 1983, to 60 percent in 1993-94. A disaggregated analysis by type of locality (rural or urban) indicates a slightly higher proportion of non-vegetarians in urban population, compared to in rural population. In 1999-2000, non-vegetarians comprised 57.55 percent of the rural population and 61.05 percent of the urban population.

The proportion of non-vegetarians does not differ much across income groups. In 1999-2000, it ranged between 55.71 percent in the very poor category to 59.71 percent in the non-poor category.

Across regions, the highest proportion (80.07%) of non-vegetarians in 1999-2000 was in the eastern region, and followed by southern region (76.10%). The proportion of non-vegetarians in other regions has remained below the national average. In northern and western regions,. non-vegetarians comprised only 31.79 percent and 38.30 percent of the total population. The population of non-vegetarians has been increasing in eastern and southern regions, and in other regions it has almost remained stagnant.

The per capita consumption of meat and fish get inflated if calculated for the non-vegetarian population (Table 14.12). While per capita milk consumption gets reduced slightly. This holds true across income classes, locations and regions. The proportion of non-vegetarian is less in the northern and western regions. Per capita consumption with non-vegetarian population as denominator shows substantial improvement in consumption of meat and fish in these regions.

Table 14.12: Per Capita Consumption of Livestock Products by Non-Vegetarian Population (Kg/Annum), 1999-2000

	Milk	Meat	Egg	Fish
Total	61.08	5.27	30.42	5.90
Location				
Rural	49.27	4.24	24.04	5.87
Urban	79.77	6.91	40.52	5.94
Region				
Eastern	32.07	2.48	26.81	6.38
Western	56.32	4.31	25.41	3.20
Northern	83.00	6.82	25.43	1.48
Southern	48.75	4.76	40.11	8.07
Hill	126.95	8.04	33.50	0.40
Income class				
Very poor	11.68	2.56	8.75	2.38
Poor	20.30	2.42	13.26	3.66
Non-poor	36.39	3.93	20.60	5.20
Rich	97.28	7.44	45.40	7.56

Source: NSSO

The changes between 1983 and 1999-2000 suggest a slow and steady increase in population of non-vegetarians in the country. Low level of consumption of meat and fish are primarily due to lack of their availability and affordability on a regular basis. These are consumed on some special occasions such as festivals and feasts.

Implications of Growing Non-Vegetarianism

Over the last two decades, per capita consumption of various livestock products in India has increased considerably. Per capita consumption of milk and egg almost doubled. Growth in per capita consumption of meat and fish was relatively slow. The relative shares of different food items in total consumption expenditure on livestock products have however not undergone any significant changes. Consumption rates and consumption pattern vary widely across income classes. There is a wide gap in the consumption rates of different food items between the rich and poor. The gap is higher for milk, compared to meat and fish. This however is narrowing down with the passage of time. There are also considerable differences in consumption rates of rural and urban consumers; per capita consumption is higher in urban areas. The pattern of allocation of expenditure to different livestock products does not differ much. Further, the disparities in consumption rates of the rural and urban population are weakening. On the other hand, substantial disparities exist in consumption pattern across regions. Milk is the most preferred livestock product in almost all the regions, but with substantial differences. It shares over 80 percent of the expenditure on livestock products in northern, western and hill regions. In the eastern and southern regions, meat and fish are as important as milk. In all the regions, per capita consumption of different livestock has increased, but the pattern of consumption has not changed much over time.

The level and pattern of consumption of different livestock products are influenced by income, price of the product and its substitutes, availability of the products and tastes and preferences. There exists a strong positive relationship between income and per capita consumption of livestock products. Poor households consume more of inferior types of meat. Differences in regional consumption patterns are mainly due to availability of the product. In India about 60 percent of the population is of non-vegetarians, but the per capita consumption of meat has remained much below than in the developed countries. Vegetarianism, as is often claimed, does not seem to be responsible for low level of meat consumption. It is the availability and affordability that determine the level of meat consumption.

Demand plays an important role in the growth of livestock sector. In the past, growth in livestock sector was mainly demand driven, and is likely to remain so. Emerging trends in level and pattern of consumption of livestock products have some important implications for the growth of livestock sector. First, the evidences indicate that if the current production trends continue, future demand for food of animal origin will be adequately met through domestic supplies. The production of food however is likely to come under heavy pressure. Increase in production might come from increase in number of animals and their productivity. The first option does not seem to be practical considering chronic scarcity of feed and fodder, and declining per capita land availability, besides its adverse effects on environment. Given the feed and fodder resources, second option implies a need for optimization of livestock population commensurate with the feed resources, and generation and dissemination of yield-enhancing technologies. At present, productivity of different species of livestock is low compared to the world average. For example average milk yield of Indian bovines is about 50 percent of the world average, and mutton yield is about 70 percent and pork yield is about 50 percent. This indicates that there is a considerable scope to raise the production through yield improvement measures.

Secondly, the emerging trends in meat consumption imply that the structure of meat production will gradually shift towards monogastrics (poultry and pig) with the rising per capita incomes.

Thirdly, there are significant interpersonal disparities in consumption of livestock products. The consumption levels of the poor are much below the consumption levels of the rich, though gap is narrowing down. Similarly, the gap in consumption levels of urban and rural population is also heading towards a convergence. With sustained growth in rural incomes and reduction in poverty, demand for livestock products is expected to increase faster, as there is little if any difference in the proportion of non-vegetarian populations across income classes and between rural and urban areas. This implies a need for faster growth in production of livestock products.

Lastly, demand driven growth in livestock production will help reduce poverty, as livestock wealth is largely concentrated among the small landholders. Evidences suggest that livestock makes substantial contributions to the income and employment of the small landholders.

MILK AND MILK PRODUCTS[1]

Organised milk marketing has been expanded to over 800 urban markets. The underlying assumption of the programme was an increasing urban demand for liquid milk and milk products, owing to increasing urbanisation and rising disposable incomes, offering an opportunity for the rural milk producers to expand their production and earn cash incomes. However, the producing households are themselves consumers as well though their existing incomes levels may warrant sell rather than self-consumption of milk. However, as incomes rise, the demand for liquid milk in the rural milksheds would also rise, the extent of which, among others, would depend on how income elastic is their demand for liquid milk. The present note is an exercise to estimate such elasticity for such State's urban and rural population, to provide inputs to future milk marketing strategies in India.

Methodology

Household surveys generally provide the data necessary to analyse the relationship between consumption of different commodities (in terms of quantities or expenditure) and disposal income (or total expenditure). The functional relationship between household expenditure (or as a proxy to income) in a family budget and consumption expenditure of different items is analyzed through appropriate forms of Engel's Law of Demand (as income increases the expenditure on different items in the budget has changing proportions, and the proportions devoted to urgent needs, such as food decrease, while those devoted to luxuries or semi-luxuries increase).

[1]T.N. Datta and B.K. Ganguly: An analysis of Consumption Expenditure Pattern in Indian States with special reference to milk and milk products, Indian Dairyman, September 2002

Commodities with income elasticity greater than unity are termed as luxury goods, those with less than unity but greater than zero as necessities and those with negative elasticity are called inferior goods. In terms of sensitivity, luxuries are most responsive to changes in income; inferiors encounter negative response while the necessities respond less than proportionately to any unit change in income under normal conditions.

Among the nine forms of Engel's curve, FAO has fitted three forms (double-log, semi-log and log-inverse) for milk products for estimating demand elasticity. Linear form does not yield a good measure in extreme cases of income (lowest and highest). Gandhi and Mani (6) used the log-quadratic form of Engel curve to estimate demand elasticity, while Sinha and Giri (7) adopted double-log method to estimate elasticity coefficient. Coondoo and Majumdar (8), like Swamy and Binswanger (9) studied household consumption through analysis of Engel's curve and estimation of adhoc equation system, regardless of price effects or cross price relationship which are essential in applied policy analysis. Radhakrishna and Murty (10) focussed on the demand system while Roy (11) used broadly aggregated commodity groups such as clothing, food and other nonfood items. Babu's (12) exercise relate to demand for food and nutrition for disaggregated commodity groups such as rice and wheat on the basis of Almost Ideal Demand System (AIDS) to State level data and provided demand elasticity even for different population groups. Jain et al (13) also used AIDS to estimate food demand system for rural and urban areas using pooled time series and cross-sectional data. Saxena (14) computed net demand elasticity for milk considering changes in milk prices, food grains prices and own income elasticity for all-India demand projection.

The present paper estimates demand elasticity for liquid milk (LM), milk products (MP) and milk and milk products (MMP), through double-log, semilog and linear forms of Engel's curve, for 32 States/UTs, for rural and urban areas.

Data Source

The National Sample Survey data on consumer expenditure, 43rd Round (1987-88) provided, for the first time, disaggregated data on quantity consumed and expenditure incurred per person across 12 expenditure classes. Earlier, it was not possible to accurately estimate Engel's curve and income elasticity of demand since NSS provided aggregated data.

Allocation of Household Budget

On average, per capita expenditure (PCE) in the urban areas is one and half times higher (more so in case of "other food and non food") than that of the rural PCE (Table 14.13). Nearly two-thirds of the rural PCE is spent on food (56% in urban). Of the food items, cereals constitute the single largest item of expenditure both in rural and urban areas followed by LM (7.6 to 7.9%). Household budget allocated to milk products is relatively insignificant— less than 2%. Edible oils constitute about 5% of the PCE, in both the areas.

Table 14.13: *Per Capita Monthly Expenditure (PCE)*

Items	Rural (Rs)	%	Urban (Rs)	%
Total Cereals	41.3	26.1	36.9	14.7
Milk	12.1	7.6	19.7	7.9
Milk Products	1.5	1.0	4.1	1.6
Animal Food	5.1	3.2	8.8	3.5
Edible Oils	8.8	5.5	13.2	5.2
Other Food	32.0	20.2	57.0	22.8
Total Food	100.8	63.7	139.7	55.9
Total Non-food	57.2	36.3	110.2	44.1
Total Expenditure	158.1	100.0	249.9	100.0

Source: NSSO

Given the expenditure pattern in Table 1, the natural question is what are the differences in the PCE across income levels? Using PCE as a proxy to income (1, 6), Table 14.14 presents interesting expenditure behaviour.

Table 14.14: *Variations in PCE Across Income Groups*

(Rs/ month)	Cereal	Milk	MP	MMP	Animal food	Edible oils	Food	Non-food	%	All (Rs)
URBAN										
<90	34.3	4.8	0.3	5.1	3.5	6.0	72.5	27.5	100	74.9
90-110	30.8	5.8	0.5	6.3	3.3	6.2	71.3	28.7	100	100.8
110-135	27.7	6.7	0.7	7.4	3.9	6.2	69.7	30.3	100	122.4
135-160	22.8	7.5	1.0	8.5	3.9	6.3	67.5	32.5	100	147.2
160-185	21.4	8.1	1.1	9.2	3.8	6.3	64.8	35.2	100	172.5
185-215	18.5	8.9	1.4	10.3	3.8	6.3	63.4	36.6	100	199.7
215-255	16.4	9.1	1.6	10.7	3.9	6.2	62.0	48.0	100	234.1
255-310	14.2	9.4	2.0	11.4	3.9	6.0	59.5	40.5	100	279.9
310-385	11.9	9.2	2.0	11.2	3.6	5.5	55.6	44.4	100	343.9
385-520	9.4	8.4	2.1	10.5	3.8	4.8	51.5	48.5	100	439.3
520-700	7.2	7.9	2.4	10.3	3.1	4.2	47.2	52.8	100	593.6
>700	4.2	5.0	1.9	6.9	2.4	2.7	32.1	67.9	100	194.3
RURAL										
Rural < 65	43.8	1.9	0.2	2.1	1.9	4.8	73.5	26.5	100	53.7
65-80	42.6	2.7	0.3	3.0	2.5	5.2	74.3	25.7	100	73.2
80-95	39.7	4.2	0.3	4.5	2.7	5.4	73.8	26.2	100	87.8
95-110	37.4	4.7	0.4	5.1	3.0	5.5	72.5	27.5	100	102.6
110-125	34.6	6.0	0.5	6.5	3.2	5.5	71.7	28.3	100	117.5
125-140	31.7	7.2	0.7	7.9	3.3	5.4	70.3	29.7	100	132.6
140-160	29.4	7.7	0.8	8.5	3.5	5.4	68.7	31.3	100	149.3
160-180	26.6	8.6	1.0	9.6	3.5	5.2	67.1	32.9	100	169.8
180-215	23.5	9.8	1.2	11.0	3.5	5.0	64.5	35.5	100	196.4
215-280	19.7	10.4	1.4	11.8	3.5	4.8	60.8	39.2	100	242.8
280-385	15.9	10.3	1.4	11.7	3.3	4.3	55.2	44.8	100	322.0
>385	9.9	7.2	1.6	8.8	2.9	4.0	41.7	58.3	100	628.5

Source: NSSO

Expectedly, food items take the bulk share of PCE and tend to decline as incomes rise and as non-foods take prominence, especially in the urban. Cereals constitute the single major expenditure item, declines as income rises (rather steeply in the urban). Among lower income groups, the rural people spend greater part of their PCE on cereals than their urban counterparts (suggesting greater coverage of PDS in urban areas). Edible oils constitute the second major group (4-6% of PCE), higher in urban areas compared to rural. It is observed that the shares, albeit marginally, tend to fall after initial rise. About 2-4% of PCE is on animal foods, it tends to rise (more rapidly in the rural from a lower base) only to decline after certain levels. Significantly, the milk group (LM, MP and MMP) occupies prominence in the food basket and rises steadily with income in both areas, tends to become more prominent than edible oils and animal foods. Especially in the rural areas, it takes off from a lower level and tends to attain the urban levels in terms of share in PCE though absolute urban PCE on MMP is nearly two times than rural PCE (even at lower incomes).

Per Capita Monthly Expenditure (PCE)

Overall PCE is estimated at around Rs 188 (Table 14.15) — urban PCE being 1.6 times to rural. Though the regional PCEs vary between Rs 175-207, wide subregional fluctuations are observed. In the east, except for West Bengal, major states like Bihar, Orissa and Assam have less than regional PCE. Delhi's high PCE (Rs 474) pulls the region's average to Rs. 207, offsetting the lower PCE of populous UP (Rs 168). In the south, Kerala has PCE (Rs 227) higher than Karnataka (Rs 180) or Tamil Nadu (Rs 200). In the west, MP's PCE (Rs 169) is well behind Maharashtra (Rs 216) or Gujarat (Rs 195).

PCE on Liquid Milk (LM), Milk Products (MP) and Milk and Milk Products (MMP) — Per Capita Consumption (PCC) of Liquid Milk (gm/Day)

An average Indian about Rs 17 a month or about 9% of his PCE on MMP (about 8% on LM and rest 1% on MP) — urban PCE on MMP is 1.8 times to that in the rural. The ration of urban/rural LM price is around 1.2:1. Regional disparities in PCE on MMP are very clear — it swings from Rs 29 in north (15% of PCE) to Rs 9 in the east (5% of PCE) ...(Table 14.16).

Generally PCC in urban and rural areas are positively correlated (r=0.87, significant at 1%). Overall PCC of LM is 120 grams a day (bought at Rs 4.1 a litre) — quantity in the urban (144 grams) is higher than in the rural area (108 grams). Except in the north, this disparity in LM consumption is observed in all the regions. Northern PCC of LM (214 grams) is the sharp contrast to that of east (54 grams) and south (88 grams). Relatively, people in the east, be urban or rural, spend more on MP than elsewhere (26% and 19% of MMP, respectively). In major states of West Bangal, Bihar, Assam and Orissa, PCC of LM varies between 35-60 grams and urban PCC is

Table 14.15: Per Capita Expenditure (PCE) on Liquid Milk (LM), Milk Products (MP) and Milk and Milk Products (MMP) — Rs/Month

State	Urban				Rural				All India			
		% to PCE				% to PCE				% to PCE		
	PCE	LM	MP	MMP	PCE	LM	MP	MMP	PCE	LM	MP	MMP
All India	**250**	**8**	**2**	**10**	**158**	**8**	**1**	**9**	**188**	**8**	**1**	**9**
A & N Island	420	1	4	6	272	3	3	6	304	4	5	9
Arunachal	240	6	3	9	204	2	2	4	209	3	2	5
Assam	70	15	8	23	154	4	1	4	136	4	1	5
Bihar	186	7	1	8	137	5	1	6	147	4	1	5
Manipur	200	1	1	2	191	1	1	1	195	1	1	2
Meghalaya	331	4	1	6	174	2	0	3	211	4	1	4
Mizoram	324	4	2	6	246	3	2	4	270	5	3	7
Nagaland	367	4	2	7								
Orissa	225	5	1	6	128	2	0	2	149	2	0	3
Sikkim	278	7	2	10	170	12	1	13	208	11	2	12
Tripura	271	4	2	5	194	4	1	5	205	4	1	5
WB	249	5	1	6	150	4	0	4	186	4	1	5
East	**225**	**5**	**2**	**7**	**158**	**4**	**1**	**4**	**175**	**4**	**1**	**5**
Delhi	485	8	3	11	372	21	8	29	474	22	9	31
Haryana	252	16	3	19	215	22	3	25	226	24	4	27
HP	346	9	3	12	210	12	1	14	231	14	2	16
J & K	271	10	3	13	204	8	1	10	223	11	2	13
Punjab	270	14	2	16	244	17	1	18	254	21	2	23
Rajasthan	238	11	4	15	178	15	3	18	196	14	3	17
UP	218	10	2	12	149	10	1	11	168	9	1	10
North	**264**	**11**	**2**	**13**	**182**	**13**	**1**	**14**	**207**	**13**	**2**	**15**
AP	230	6	1	7	160	5	0	5	185	5	1	6
Karnataka	228	7	1	8	149	6	1	7	180	6	1	7
Kerala	266	5	1	6	211	4	0	5	227	6	1	6
Lksh'dwp	229	2	3	4	263	1	2	2	248	2	3	4
Pondi	214	5	1	6	156	3	1	4	180	4	1	5
TN	249	5	1	6	154	3	0	4	200	5	1	6
South	**240**	**6**	**1**	**7**	**168**	**4**	**0**	**5**	**196**	**5**	**1**	**6**
Dadra NH					114	3	1	3	114	2	0	2
Goa D & D	329	6	1	8	184	3	1	4	241	6	1	8
Gujarat	241	11	3	14	161	12	2	14	195	12	2	14
MP	236	8	2	11	142	7	2	8	169	7	2	8
Mhrstra	279	8	1	9	161	6	0	6	216	8	1	9
West	**260**	**9**	**2**	**10**	**152**	**7**	**1**	**8**	**194**	**8**	**1**	**10**

Source: NSSO

1.8 times, if not higher, to rural PCC. Urban/rural PCC disparities are more in Orissa than in the other three major states. Leaving aside smaller states, southern PCC of LM varies between 80-107 gram; urban/rural ration is around 1.6:1. Though its 5.9% of PCE on MMP is marginally higher than the east, bulk of it is on LM. North has an average PCC of LM at 214 gram

Table 14.16: Liquid Milk Per Capita — Monthly Qty (Ltr), Value (Rs) and Per Capita Consumption (Grams/Day)

State	Urban			Rural		
	Qty	Price	PCC	Qty	Price	PCC
All India	4.3	4.56	144	3.2	3.75	108
A & N Island	1.1	5.17	35	1.7	5.03	58
Arunachal	2.5	5.60	83	1.1	4.03	36
Assam	2.0	5.05	67	1.3	4.29	44
Bihar	2.5	5.21	84	1.6	4.37	52
Manipur	0.3	4.15	9	0.3	3.69	12
Meghalaya	3.7	4.06	123	1.1	3.59	38
Mizoram	3.3	4.16	109	1.6	4.12	55
Nagaland	2.9	5.19	96			
Orissa	2.4	4.35	80	0.7	3.58	23
Sikkim	4.6	4.36	155	5.1	3.98	170
Tripura	2.0	5.17	65	1.7	4.51	57
WB	2.7	4.65	90	1.3	4.11	43
East	**2.4**	**4.75**	**80**	**1.3**	**4.22**	**45**
Delhi	8.2	4.52	274	6.1	4.82	537
Haryana	8.2	4.80	272	1.5	4.07	383
HP	7.9	4.09	264	7.1	3.65	237
J & K	6.3	4.32	211	4.9	3.52	163
Punjab	8.9	4.13	297	2.9	3.26	430
Rajasthan	6.1	4.38	204	6.9	3.87	231
UP	4.8	4.58	160	4.3	3.50	144
North	**6.4**	**4.41**	**213**	**6.4**	**3.59**	**215**
AP	3.4	3.86	112	2.3	3.16	77
Karnataka	3.9	3.96	129	2.8	3.33	92
Kerala	3.1	4.62	102	2.2	4.19	72
Lksh'dwp	0.9	5.09	29	0.4	4.17	14
Pondi	3.2	3.69	105	1.6	3.27	52
TN	3.3	4.12	110	1.6	3.48	52
South	**3.4**	**4.06**	**112**	**2.2**	**3.47**	**72**
Dadra NH				0.6	4.88	20
Goa D & D	4.1	5.05	137	1.0	5.27	33
Gujarat	5.5	4.76	183	4.5	4.37	152
MP	4.2	4.77	139	2.3	3.99	78
Mhrstra	4.3	5.30	142	2.2	4.06	75
West	**4.5**	**5.02**	**150**	**2.6**	**4.14**	**88**

Source: NSSO

a day — while it is below 200 grams in J & K and UP, it exceeds 300 gram in Delhi, Haryana and Punjab. Overall, limited urban/rural disparities are observed in PCC and PCE pattern in the north. Nearly 15% of the region's PCE on MMP is on MP, second to the east. In the west, average PCC of LM is 112 gram — it is higher at 165 gram in Gujarat but both Maharashtra and MP, the two other big states, have lower than regional average, however marginally. Gujarat devotes higher PCE on MMP, has lowest urban/rural disparity in PCE and LM price.

Urban-Rural Variation in PCC

Though urban PCC is higher compared to rural PCC, it is of interest to analyse the possible factors, which influence a proportionately higher urban consumption. The factors considered are PCE, PCELM and Price — all in terms of ratio of urban and rural. Urban-rural variation in PCC with respect to ration of urban-rural PCE, PCELM and Price is captured in the multiple regression analysis.

$$PCC = 1.83 + 0.91 \; PCELM - 1.64 \; Price - 0.011 \; PCE$$
$$(7.1)^* \qquad\qquad (42.2)^*(-8.4)^* \quad (-0.23) \quad R^2 = 0.98$$
$$N = 28$$

* significant at 1% parentheses figs indicate t valves;

It significant that both PCELM and Price influence PCC significantly — the former positively and the latter inversely. In terms of sensitivity, 1% increase in urban-rural ration of PCELM lead to 0.91% increase in PCC while 1% increase in urban-rural ration of PRICE leads to 1.64% decreases in PCC. In other words, under a more favourable relative price regime, the urban consumption of PCC would increase, given a constant PCELM.

Elasticity of Demand for Liquid Milk (LM)

Elasticity of demand has been estimated (Table 14.17) on Linear, Semilog and Double log methods; separately for rural/urban and State/UTs at their respective mean values of income (expenditure). Jain et al (13) has estimated such elasticity, pooling cross-sectional data across the States. However, Double-log estimates are considered better (though it assumes a constant elasticity) than Linear estimates as it assumes endless and proportionate growth in consumption with income, contrarily to the behaviour of a rational consumer. Following sections, therefore, centre on the Double-log estimates.

The rural elasticity of demand for LM for the country is higher (1.60) than urban elasticity (1.05). FAO (1) also observed higher rural elasticity (1.78) compared to the urban (1.25). This signifies that the rural LM demand is more sensitive to change in income compared to the urban. Barring notable states like Kerala, Karnataka, Maharashtra and Tamil Nadu, higher rural elasticity is observed compared to urban. Significantly, rural income-elasticity in the north is greater than unity while except for Haryana, the remaining states have inelastic urban LM demand (which could perhaps be explained by its high PCE, PCE on LM and PCC). On the contrary, eastern states (except ones like Sikkim) have elastic urban as well as rural demand. Thus, this region overwhelmingly portrays a very stimulating demand scenario for LM, so also the western regional states.

Table 14.17: Coefficients of Elasticity of Demand for Liquid Milk (LM)

State/UT	RURAL						URBAN					
	Linear		S-LOG		D-Log		Linear		S-Log		D-Log	
	ELAS	R²	ELAS	R²	ELAS	R²	ELAS	R²	ELAS	R²	ELAS	R²
A & N Island	1.07	0.92	1.70	0.95	1.45	0.88	1.63	0.94	2.31	0.80	2.03	0.81
Arunachal	2.12	0.63	1.94	0.46	2.64	0.43	0.69	0.49	0.94	0.72	0.94	0.57
Assam	0.95	0.83	1.14	0.93	1.39	0.90	0.51	0.72	0.93	0.92	1.00	0.79
Bihar	1.00	0.81	1.30	0.94	2.04	0.82	0.77	0.89	0.98	0.97	1.30	0.82
Manipur	1.12	0.86	1.84	0.85	1.32	0.69	0.12	0.01	0.11	0.01	0.33	0.06
Meghalaya	0.87	0.80	1.04	0.85	1.16	0.82	0.81	0.77	1.14	0.95	1.67	0.65
Mizoram	1.46	0.87	1.98	0.91	2.69	0.64	0.80	0.80	0.94	0.54	0.60	0.53
Nagaland							1.24	0.87	2.85	0.77	1.47	0.88
Orissa	1.36	0.96	1.56	0.89	1.77	0.96	1.16	0.95	1.28	0.90	1.57	0.91
Sikkim	0.64	0.54	0.90	0.78	0.81	0.52	0.41	0.30	0.55	0.50	0.77	0.33
Tripura	1.41	0.95	1.72	0.93	2.41	0.67	1.58	0.89	1.61	0.80	1.95	0.90
WB	1.10	0.91	1.40	0.94	1.76	0.89	0.88	0.90	1.09	0.97	1.40	0.88
Delhi	1.10	0.97	2.52	0.91	1.40	0.93	0.43	0.73	0.68	0.97	0.75	0.83
Haryana	0.90	0.87	1.11	0.95	1.30	0.90	1.06	0.94	1.14	0.80	1.13	0.94
HP	0.86	0.87	0.99	0.94	1.05	0.92	0.84	0.97	1.04	0.91	0.79	0.95
J & K	0.46	0.59	0.79	0.90	1.09	0.64	0.61	0.81	0.75	0.98	0.92	0.83
Punjab	0.90	0.91	1.12	0.94	1.10	0.96	0.69	0.90	0.78	0.98	0.89	0.93
Rajasthan	0.94	0.91	1.15	0.95	1.43	0.92	0.62	0.92	0.85	0.96	0.85	0.93
UP	0.94	0.68	1.12	0.67	1.30	0.62	0.73	0.86	1.14	0.97	0.99	0.93
AP	1.03	0.89	1.27	0.95	1.57	0.90	0.78	0.89	1.03	0.95	1.06	0.95
Karnataka	0.66	0.83	0.90	0.97	0.96	0.92	0.62	0.81	0.89	0.97	0.97	0.90
Kerala	0.52	0.19	0.84	0.36	0.81	0.33	1.05	0.82	1.18	0.80	1.16	0.64
Lksh'dwp	0.86	0.49	1.46	0.64	0.78	0.59	1.15	0.59	1.55	0.43	1.20	0.39
TN	1.29	0.97	1.56	0.91	1.77	0.94	0.66	0.28	0.76	0.32	1.23	0.63
Pondi	0.40	0.32	0.71	0.60	1.01	0.57	0.94	0.98	1.15	0.84	1.06	0.88
Dadra NH	2.06	0.85	2.14	0.63	2.37	0.84	0.00	0.00	0.00	0.00	0.00	0.00
Goa D & D	1.66	0.93	2.21	0.82	1.73	0.88	1.12	0.93	1.47	0.89	1.33	0.82
Gujarat	1.08	0.96	1.20	0.94	1.49	0.90	0.66	0.84	0.84	0.97	0.91	0.93
MP	0.97	0.88	1.20	0.95	1.45	0.90	0.67	0.76	0.86	0.90	1.02	0.85
Mhrstra	0.63	0.81	1.00	0.98	1.05	0.88	0.85	0.90	1.02	0.94	1.13	0.95
All India	**1.06**	**0.91**	**1.33**	**0.97**	**1.60**	**0.91**	**0.71**	**0.87**	**0.92**	**0.98**	**1.05**	**0.92**

Source: NSSO

Elasticity of Demand for Milk Products (MP)

It should be noted that the NSSO data on MP only includes Ghee and, as such, could be an underestimate, as households consume both traditional/ modern products like Dahi, Peda, Butter, sweetmeats and Milk Powder. Generally, rural elasticity of MP is much higher than urban elasticity, almost twice at the aggregate (2.02 vs 1.04 at all-India level). Regionally, the East has highest elasticity, both in rural and urban, followed by the West. Large variations between rural/urban elasticity are observed in all the major milk producing states of the North and the West (Tables 14.18 and 14.19).

Table 14.18: Coefficient of Elasticity of Demand: Milk Products (MP)

| State/UT | RURAL | | | | | | URBAN | | | | | |
| | Linear | | S-LOG | | D-Log | | Linear | | S-Log | | D-Log | |
All India	ELAS	R^2	ELAS	R^2	ELAS	R^2	ELAS	R^2	ELAS	R^2	ELAS	R^2
A & N Island	1.04	0.80	1.72	0.88	1.49	0.67	1.630	0.93	2.32	0.80	2.03	0.82
Arunachal	-0.55	0.01	0.23	0.04	2.16	0.96	0.69	0.49	0.93	0.70	0.95	0.57
Assam	2.15	0.95	2.11	0.72	2.16	0.96	0.51	0.72	0.92	0.92	1.00	0.79
Bihar	1.42	0.79	1.72	0.81	2.21	0.89	0.77	0.89	0.98	0.98	1.30	0.82
Manipur	0.97	0.50	1.55	0.45	0.37	0.56	0.12	0.01	-0.11	0.06	0.33	0.06
Meghalaya	1.61	0.98	0.00	0.00	0.00	0.00	0.88	0.75	1.23	0.92	1.76	0.67
Mizoram	0.05	0.00	0.17	0.00	0.00	0.00	0.80	0.79	0.94	0.54	0.60	0.53
Nagaland	0.00	0.00	0.00	0.00	0.00	0.00	1.24	0.87	2.85	0.77	1.47	0.88
Orissa	1.53	0.96	1.72	0.86	2.31	0.88	1.20	0.95	1.33	0.91	1.49	0.86
Sikkim	1.28	0.60	1.60	0.70	1.53	0.73	0.55	0.32	0.70	0.50	0.63	0.22
Tripura	1.87	0.98	2.12	0.83	1.74	0.87	0.57	0.89	1.60	0.80	1.95	0.90
WB	2.42	0.91	2.48	0.61	2.04	0.97	0.88	0.90	1.08	0.97	1.40	0.88
Delhi	1.32	0.90	3.78	0.97	1.64	0.95	0.48	0.66	0.78	0.94	0.56	0.85
Haryana	1.62	0.97	1.76	0.82	2.01	0.76	1.06	0.93	1.13	0.80	1.13	0.94
HP	1.09	0.85	1.22	0.86	1.50	0.70	0.83	0.97	1.04	0.90	0.79	0.95
J & K	0.90	0.94	1.18	0.86	1.67	0.52	0.61	0.81	0.75	0.98	0.92	0.83
Punjab	1.40	0.94	1.64	0.87	1.78	0.71	0.69	0.90	0.78	0.98	0.89	0.93
Rajasthan	1.68	0.97	1.74	0.74	1.80	0.96	0.62	0.92	0.85	0.96	0.85	0.93
UP	1.29	0.20	1.78	0.25	2.44	0.82	0.73	0.86	0.88	0.97	0.99	0.93
AP	1.21	0.97	1.31	0.80	1.18	0.94	0.78	0.89	1.03	0.94	1.06	0.95
Karnataka	1.16	0.92	1.39	0.83	1.40	0.81	0.62	0.80	0.88	0.97	0.97	0.90
Kerala	0.61	0.19	0.95	0.32	0.12	0.00	1.08	0.82	1.23	0.82	1.25	0.62
Lksh'dwp	-0.15	0.02	0.02	Negl	2.40	0.41	1.15	0.59	1.54	0.43	1.20	0.39
TN	1.04	0.74	1.41	0.89	1.40	0.81	0.66	0.27	0.75	0.32	1.23	0.63
Pondi	0.82	0.55	1.26	0.75	1.44	0.72	0.93	0.98	1.15	0.84	1.06	0.88
Dadra NH	2.06	0.96	2.10	0.58	2.67	0.74	0.00	0.00	0.00	0.00	0.00	0.00
Goa D & D	1.39	0.75	2.00	0.77	1.41	0.62	1.12	0.84	1.47	0.89	1.33	0.82
Gujarat	2.05	0.96	2.01	0.73	2.44	0.97	0.66	0.84	0.83	0.97	0.91	0.94
MP	1.63	0.97	1.78	0.84	2.19	0.88	0.70	0.75	0.91	0.90	0.92	0.82
Mhrstra	1.22	0.92	1.75	0.90	1.91	0.82	0.84	0.90	1.02	0.94	1.13	0.95
All India	**1.58**	**0.99**	**1.79**	**0.85**	**2.02**	**0.96**	**0.71**	**0.87**	**0.92**	**0.98**	**1.04**	**0.92**

Source: NSSO

The State/UTs have been classified by their degree of elasticity (Table 14.20). In terms of population, it is observed that over 66% of the country's rural population have high/very high income elasticity of demand for LM (mainly in the north and West, higher in the South), 52% have very high elasticity for MP (in the North and the West) while another 25% have very high elasticity for both LM and MP (mainly Eastern States of Bihar and WB).

Table 14.19: Coefficient of Elasticity of Demand: Milk and Milk Products (MMP)

State/UT	RURAL						URBAN					
	Linear		S-LOG		D-Log		Linear		S-Log		D-Log	
All India	ELAS	R^2	ELAS	R^2	ELAS	R^2	ELAS	R^2	ELAS	R^2	ELAS	R^2
A & N Island	1.06	0.88	1.70	0.94	1.59	0.83	0.900	0.79	1.34	0.88	1.17	0.81
Arunachal	1.61	0.74	1.57	0.60	1.83	0.60	1.12	0.89	1.23	0.84	1.35	0.81
Assam	1.21	0.96	1.35	0.93	1.53	0.95	0.49	0.73	0.91	0.98	1.01	0.78
Bihar	1.07	0.82	1.37	0.92	2.11	0.83	0.78	0.88	1.00	0.98	1.32	0.83
Manipur	0.94	0.83	1.50	0.84	1.16	0.67	1.76	0.66	1.98	0.51	1.65	0.77
Meghalaya	0.98	0.86	1.16	0.89	1.27	0.85	0.79	0.75	1.13	0.95	1.42	0.74
Mizoram	1.41	0.85	1.93	0.92	2.82	0.62	0.80	0.86	0.96	0.79	0.61	0.70
Nagaland							1.13	0.89	0.31	0.70	1.06	0.82
Orissa	1.39	0.97	1.58	0.89	1.82	0.92	1.12	0.93	1.26	0.91	1.63	0.90
Sikkim	0.69	0.59	0.95	0.83	0.88	0.57	0.58	0.54	0.70	0.74	0.90	0.51
Tripura	1.49	0.97	1.79	0.92	2.48	0.67	1.24	0.83	1.24	0.72	1.31	0.72
WB	1.33	0.99	1.59	0.90	1.83	0.93	0.97	0.95	1.16	0.96	1.42	0.92
Delhi	1.15	0.96	2.83	0.92	1.67	0.94	0.64	0.87	0.93	0.98	0.97	0.89
Haryana	0.99	0.91	1.18	0.95	1.38	0.93	1.07	0.97	1.18	0.86	1.24	0.96
HP	0.88	0.87	1.02	0.94	1.09	0.92	0.94	0.99	1.23	0.93	0.95	0.97
J & K	0.52	0.70	0.84	0.96	1.14	0.66	0.79	0.93	0.91	0.98	1.04	0.91
Punjab	0.93	0.92	1.15	0.94	1.13	0.93	0.81	0.94	0.90	0.98	1.01	0.95
Rajasthan	1.06	0.96	1.24	0.96	1.49	0.93	0.77	0.95	1.03	0.93	1.03	0.94
UP	1.03	0.88	1.28	0.96	1.66	0.87	0.81	0.91	0.95	0.97	1.07	0.94
AP	1.04	0.91	1.27	0.95	1.52	0.92	0.82	0.91	1.06	0.94	1.08	0.96
Karnataka	0.71	0.86	0.95	0.97	0.99	0.93	0.65	0.82	0.92	0.97	1.01	0.90
Kerala	0.53	0.19	0.85	0.36	2.70	0.32	1.02	0.91	1.16	0.91	1.28	0.95
Lksh'dwp	0.51	0.42	0.91	0.67	1.30	0.43	0.72	0.57	0.95	0.46	0.92	0.88
TN	1.27	0.97	1.53	0.92	1.76	0.93	0.71	0.30	0.80	0.34	1.30	0.64
Pondi	0.46	0.39	0.80	0.69	1.10	0.63	0.92	0.96	1.15	0.86	1.07	0.91
Dadra NH	2.03	0.83	2.12	0.63	2.44	0.83						
Goa D & D	1.59	0.95	2.16	0.87	1.77	0.84	0.98	0.91	1.31	0.92	1.25	0.81
Gujarat	1.22	0.99	1.27	0.92	1.59	0.93	0.73	0.85	0.92	0.97	1.02	0.93
MP	1.12	0.93	1.33	0.94	1.58	0.92	0.75	0.78	0.96	0.95	1.16	0.86
Mhrstra	0.68	0.83	1.06	0.98	1.10	0.88	0.92	0.92	1.09	0.93	1.22	0.96
All India	**1.13**	**0.93**	**1.39**	**0.94**	**1.65**	**0.92**	**0.81**	**0.91**	**1.02**	**0.97**	**1.15**	**0.93**

Source: NSSO

Table 14.20: Classification of State/UTs by Elasticity

	RURAL			URBAN		
Low	High	Very High	Low	High	Very High

Liquid Milk

Sikkim	Assam				
Karnataka	Manipur				
Lkshdwp	Meghalaya				
	Delhi				
	Haryana				
	J & K				
	Punjab				
	Rajasthan				
	UP				
	Gujarat				
	MP				
	M'hrstra				

Milk Products

Low	High	Very High	Low	High	Very High
Manipur	AP	A & N Island	MP	Orissa	M'hrstra
Meghalaya	Karnataka	Assam			
Mizoram	TN	Sikkim			
Nagaland	Goa, D & D	Delhi			
Kerala		Haryana			
Dadra, NH		J & K			
		Punjab			
		Rajasthan			
		UP			
		Lksh'dwp			
		Gujarat			
		MP			
		M'hrstra			

Liquid Milk and Milk Products, Both

Low	High	Very High	Low	High	Very High
Kerala	A & N Island	Arunachal	Arunachal	Assam	Meghalaya
	HP		Manipur	Bihar	Tripura
	Pondi		Mizoram	Nagaland	
			Sikkim	WB	
			Delhi	Haryana	
		Bihar	HP	AP	
		Orissa	J & K	Kerala	
		Tripura	Punjab	Lksh'dwp	
		WB	Rajasthan	Pondi	
			UP	TN	
			Karnataka	Dadra, NH	
			Gujarat	Goa, D & D	

As for the country's urban population, 21% have high elasticity for LM (mainly in the Western States of MP and Maharashtra, 38% have high elasticity for both LM and MP (the South and the Eastern States in the main) while 38% have low elasticity for both LM and MP (includes the Northern states of Punjab, Delhi, HP, J&K, Rajasthan and UP, Gujarat and Karnataka).

Table 14.21 provides a historical review of demand elasticity of milk and milk products (MMP) as a composite sector. On the whole, the results appear consistent, however, marginal slowing down of demand elasticity is observed in the present estimate than that of the estimate of FAO.

Table 14.21: Elasticities of Milk and Milk Products—Historical Review

Source	Year	Method	Reference	Rural	Urban
FAO	1972	Double log	All India	1.78	1.25
Gandhi	1995	Log quadratic	All India	1.70	1.06
Jain	1992	Almost Ideal Demand System	All India	1.41	0.61
Sinha & Giri	1989	Double log	Punjab	1.26	1.10
		Double log	Gujarat	1.86	1.38
NDDB	1997	Double log	All India	1.65	1.15

Concluding Observation

Leading rural milksheds of the country, in terms of organised milk procurement for urban supplies, lie in the state of Punjab, Haryana, Rajasthan, UP, Gujarat, Maharashtra, AP, TN while most of the eastern States (minor exceptions in Bihar and WB) are net consumers or importers. It is observed that most of the leading milk producing States has high rural demand elasticity for milk and milk products. Unless urban prices rise faster and if rural incomes constitute to rise, organised milk procurement for urban supplies may enter a stage wherein adequate marketable surplus of rural milk may not be available for procurement and supply to the urban markets. It is important therefore to initiate production enhancement programmes in the leading rural milksheds to offset any supply constraint in rural procurement in the future.

MODERN DIETARY TRANSITION AND ITS OUTCOMES

Major dietary change got underway in Europe only during the mid-nineteenth century, and its scope ranged from eliminating any threat of famine of the founding of highly frequented restaurants and the emergence of grande cuisine. Increased consumption of meat was among the most important markers of this dietary transition, which was driven by combined forces of improved agricultural productivity, rapid industrialization, and widespread urbanisation. The other universal components of that transition have been lower consumption of staple cereals and legumes, rising intakes of dairy and aquatic products and of sugar and fruits, and a wider choice in every food category (Popkin 1993; Poleman and Thomas 1995; Caballero and Popkin 2002).

The onset of these changes varied by more than a century, starting first in Western Europe during the latter half of the nineteenth century, noticeably affecting Mediterranean Europe only after 1900 and East Asia only after 1950. The pace of the worldwide dietary change accelerated after World War II as the increasingly mechanized agriculture began receiving higher energy subsidies (directly for field machinery, indirectly for agricultural chemicals and crop breeding) and converted from traditional, low yielding varieties to new high-yielding cultivars.

Higher yields made it possible to use a larger share of grain harvests in animal feeding. In 1900 just over 10 percent of the world's grain harvest was fed to animals, most of it going to energize the field work of draft horses, mules, cattle and water buffaloes rather than to produce meat. By 1950 the global share of cereals used for feeding reached 20 percent, and it surpassed 40 percent during the late 1990s (USDA 2001a). National shares of grain fed to animals now range from just over 60 percent in the United States to less than 5 percent in India. The continuing rise in the global demand for meat means that an even larger share of cereals will be fed to animals. Refrigerated shipments of meat began during the 1870s, and the world meat trade has grown steadily to account for nearly 10 percent of all red meat and poultry production (FAO 2002). Expectedly, the pace of the dietary transition has been highly country-specific as it progressed slowly in parts of Europe but moved rapidly in post-World War II Japan to reach a new equilibrium in less than two generations, and it was even more rapid in China after 1980 (Popkin et al. 1993).

Historical data allows a fairly reliable reconstruction of this progress for the past two centuries in France and Britain (Dupin, Hercberg, and Lagrange 1984; Perren 1985). French meat consumption remained unchanged during the first half of the nineteenth century, and then it took over 80 years to double the average annual rate to more than 50 kg (carcass weight) per capita; the second doubling took only 25 years between 1950 and 1975 (as seen in Figure I). British per capita consumption rates (also as carcass weight) rose faster during the nineteenth century, roughly tripling to a fairly high level of almost 60 kg by the year 1900. This was followed by stagnation until the late 1940s, and the subsequent growth lifted the average above 70 kg/year by 1970 but not above 80 kg/year by the century's end (Figure I).

Average US meat consumption (as edible weight) was far ahead of the European means throughout the nineteenth century, and only after 1950 did Europe's richest countries match the level reached by the United States 100 years earlier. A well-documented US record begins in 1909, with about 51 kg of boneless trimmed (edible) weight per capita (excluding edible offals and game) (USDA 2002a). Reversal of the subsequent stagnation and decline (to 40 kg by 1935) began during World War II and the average rate surpassed 70 kg (a typical adult body weight) by 1967 and reached about 82 kg by the end of the 1990s (see Figure 2). Japan's average rate surpassed 3 kg (carcass weight, including nearly a kg of whale meat) only in 1955, but thereafter the country's rapid economic growth propelled it to 12 kg by 1965, 25 kg by 1975, and to about 45 kg by 2000 (FAO 2002). Official Chinese statistics of meat production (in carcass weight) including an unprecedented rise from 11.2 kg/capita in 1975 to 25 kg by 1990 and to nearly 50 kg by the end of the 1990s (NBS 2000). If true, this would have been the fastest increase of meat eating in history. But the official statistical yearbook (NBS 2000) puts actual per capita purchases of meat during the late 1990s at about 25 kg/capita for urban households (unchanged in a decade) and the meat consumption of rural families at less than 17 kg, up from about 13 kg in 1990, a clear indication that output data for the 1990s became increasingly exaggerated. Unfortunately, FAO balance sheets (FAO 2002) calculate China's average per capita meat supply on the basis of clearly exaggerated production claims, putting it at nearly 49 kg/capita in 1999 (including, as all FAO statistics do, consumption in Taiwan). In addition, unimproved varieties of traditional Chinese pigs produce carcasses that contain more fat than meat.

Higher per capita rates of meat intake have been accompanied by changing patterns of consumption. Some of them have traditionally been highly country-specific, a variable shares of beef, pork, mutton, goat, poultry, and other meats reflected environmental conditions, agricultural and pastoral practices, cultural attitudes, and dietary taboos. One kind of meat was often dominant: Argentinian beef and Chinese pork are perhaps the two best examples. Gradual homogenization of meat consumption and the rising share of poultry in the total supply are two clear markers of dietary modernisation. Consumption of meats other than beef, pork, and poultry has been declining throughout the Western world. Mutton, goat, horse, and other meats supplied 15 percent of French consumption in 1960, but less than 10 percent now; the British have halved their mutton eating since 1960. Horsemeat is now a rarity in the West outside France, Benelux, Germany, Italy, and Spain.

Beef eating was declining nearly everywhere long before the scares about bovine spongiform encephalopathy (BSE), which may cause a variant Creutzfeld-Jakob disease (vCJD) in humans, led to abrupt drops in demand. In the United States, a country unaffected by BSE, beef's share of total meat consumption declined from a high of about 50 percent in 1910 to about 35 percent in 2000 (USDA 2002a;). In Britain, the country hardest hit by vCJD, beef consumption is down a third in absolute terms and 40 percent in relative terms (to just about a fifth of the total demand) when compared to 40 years ago. The decline of beef eating has been less steep in France, from about 37 percent of meat intake in 1960 to 26 percent in 2000 (FAO 2002). .

Pork may be retaining or even slightly increasing its absolute per capita consumption rate, but its relative share is down in many countries. In the United States, where the absolute per capita intake of pork remained remarkably constant throughout the twentieth century, its share fell from a high of 50 percent in the early 1930s to 27 percent by the late 1990s (Figure 3), and recently it has slipped even in China as mass-produced broilers have accounted for a fifth of all meat consumption. Poultry's share rose from 10 percent in 1900 to 37 percent by 2000 in the United States (Figure 3); in France it more than doubled to 25 percent since 1960; and the absolute demand more than quadrupled in Britain, where poultry now accounts for 36 percent of the meat total, the highest share among affluent countries.

Finally, some revealing global perspectives. With global annual output of nearly 500 million tonnes (Mt), cow milk is the most important animal food, far ahead of 80 Mt of pig meat (FAO 2002). But because fresh milk (about 87 percent water) has only 3.5 percent protein while moderately fat pig carcass has about 10 percent protein, cow milk now contains only about twice as much protein as the world's rising pork output; and total meat production, including poultry, now exceeds 200 Mt a year and it supplies more protein than do all milks. Poultry now produces more meat (nearly 60 Mt/year) than cattle (beef and veal), and demand for broilers continues to rise on every continent. Consumption of hen eggs is now at more than 40 Mt a year, and recent rapid growth of aquaculture (with combined freshwater and marine output now close to 30 Mt a year, equal to nearly a quarter of ocean catch) has put cultured fish, crustaceans, and mollusks ahead of mutton.

The global average of annual per capita meat supply (determined by the aggregation of national food balance sheets) was about 38 kg (carcass weight) in the year 2000, but in this dichotomous world very few countries actually consume this amount of meat. The mean for affluent countries is now close to 80 kg/year while FAO's mean for modernising countries is only about 27 kg/year, and the actual figure should be lower because of the inclusion of the exaggerated official Chinese claim of nearly 50 kg/year (FAO 2002). By the last century's end, the population of affluent countries represented only one-fifth of the global total, but these countries produced and consumed two-fifths of all red meat and three-fifths of all poultry.

The current list of top carnivorous countries (using FAO's average per capita supply in terms of carcass weight and including all offal) is headed not only, as might be expected, by the United States and Australia but also by Ireland, Spain, and Cyprus, all with annual availability between 115 and 125 kg (carcass weight). New Zealand, Denmark, France, Canada, and Argentina are not far behind. Meat supplies in these countries are an order of magnitude higher than in such poor populous countries as Indonesia, Pakistan, and Ethiopia. The lowest ranks are, at round 5 kg/year or less, occupied by Bangladesh, India, and a number of countries in sub-Saharan Africa. In contrast, Brazil's average annual per capita meat supply is, at about 80 kg, nearly twice the Russian mean.

In macronutrient terms, meat now supplies 10 percent of all food energy and more than 25 percent of all protein in rich countries, while the corresponding shares are, respectively, merely 6 percent and 13 percent for the poor world. But the relative importance is reversed for lipids associated with meat: in poor countries meat fat provides about 25 of all lipids, while the growing demand for lean meat has reduced that share to about 20 percent in the affluent world. Extending significantly higher meat intakes to the world's roughly one billion people with moderate incomes and then also to some 4 billion with low incomes would require a massive expansion of animal husbandry and hence a substantial increase of feed harvests. Better management of pastures, as well as their regrettable but inevitable expansion due to continuing deforestation in parts of Latin America, Africa, and Asia, will meet some of this additional need—but most of the additional feed will have to come from arable land.

As already noted, increasing levels of meat production necessitated a steady rise in the share of cereal and leguminous grains devoted to feeding Conversion of this plant energy and protein into meat is accompanied by large metabolic losses. As a result, grain harvests in highly carnivorous countries, or in countries producing feeds for export, must be multiples of those needed for direct human consumption, and the food demand of a modern urbanite has to be a multiple of the area claimed by an overwhelmingly (or entirely) vegetarian subsistence peasant. In order to understand the basic agricultural and environmental implications of this shift, we must recognise major metabolic differences among principal domesticated meat animals.

REFERENCES

1. FAO (1972). "Income Elasticities of Demand for Agricultural Products", (mimeo, No. CCP72/WP.1), ROME.
2. World Bank (1995). "India Livestock Sector Review", (mimeo).
3. Kurup, et al (1995). "India Livestock Sector Perspectives", Swiss Development Cooperation, New Delhi (mimeo).
4. Mishra & Sharma (1989). "Livestock Development in India – An appraisal Institute of Economic Growth, Studies in Economic Development planning, pp-142.
5. International Food Policy Research Institute (IFTRI, 1995), Washington, "Global Food Supply Demand and Trade to 2020", (mimeo).
6. Gandhi, Vasant P. and Mani, Gyanendra (1995). "Are Livestock Products Rising in Implementation? A study of the Growth and behaviour of their consumption in India", Indian Journal of Agricultural Economics Vol Jul-Sep 1995, No. 3 Bombay.
7. Sinha P. and Giri, A. K. (1989). "Consumption of Livestock Products – Analysis and comparison of data of NSS 32nd and 38th Rounds". Livestock Economy of India, Edited by Indian Society of Agricultural Economics, Bombay, PP 153-182.
8. Coondoo, D. and Majumdar, A. (1987). "A System of Demand Equations based on Price Independent Generalised Linearity", International Economic Review, 28: 213-228.
9. Swamy, G. and Binswanger, H. P. (1983). "Flexible Consumer Demand System and Linear Estimation: Food in India", American Jour. Agril Econ, 55: 675-84.
10. Radhakrishna, R. and Murthy, K.N. (1980). "An Application of Indirect Addlog System to Consumer Behaviour in India", India Econ. Jour, 27 (4): 28-52.

11. Ray, R. (1982). "The Testing and Estimation of Complete Demand Systems on Household Budget Surveys – An Application of AIDs", European Economic Review, 17: 349-369.

12. Babu, N.B. Suresh Chandra (1989). "An Analysis of Demand for food and nutrition in India", Unpublished Ph. D Thesis, Iowa State University, Ames. Iowa (USA).

13. Jain, D.K. et al (1992). "Food Demand Analysis in India, An Application of Almost Ideal Demand System", NDRI, Karnal (mimeo).

14. Saxena, R. (1996). "Demand for Milk and Milk Products in India", working paper, IRMA, Anand.

15

Demand and Supply Projections of Livestock Products for 2030

GROWTH OF THE SECTOR

The livestock sector has been among the few growth sectors in rural India and domestic demand for animal based food products is expected to grow rapidly with increasing incomes. Animal protein requirement is expected to grow faster than protein from other sources and to meet these requirements, the protein availability has to be doubled from the present 10 grams. For this to be achieved, the annual growth rates for milk, egg and meat production (averaging 4.3%, 4.7% and 4.1% respectively) have to be increased substantially. The increase in productivity shall be achieved using sustainable production systems while maintaining environment, and addressing concerns of animal bio-diversity, quality and safety of animal foods, human and animal health and animal welfare. The livestock population with growth rate of 1.14% per year would go up from 470 million (excluding poultry) in 1992 to 635 million in 2020. Shortage of feeds and fodder, shrinkage of grazing lands and environmental concerns specially of methane emission from ruminants call for stabilizing livestock numbers at present or even lower level and improving productivity per animal to meet present and future animal food needs using newer technologies.

With increasing incomes and high demand elasticity, there is a noticeable change in the consumer basket of an average Indian. A study of the NSSO data over the last 35 years shows interesting results- per capita consumption of cereals both in the rural and urban India is declining (Graph 15.1) and the constitution of the food basket is undergoing a drastic change in favour of non-cereal components – livestock products and horticulture (Graph 15.2). Nevertheless, per capita consumption of milk in rural areas is lower than in urban areas, despite the fact that the bulk of it is produced in these areas. Among states only in Haryana and Punjab per capita milk consumption in rural areas is higher. Per capita consumption of other livestock products also is lower in rural areas (Tables 15.1 and 15.2). Moreover, 75-80 percent of the eggs and poultry meat are consumed in

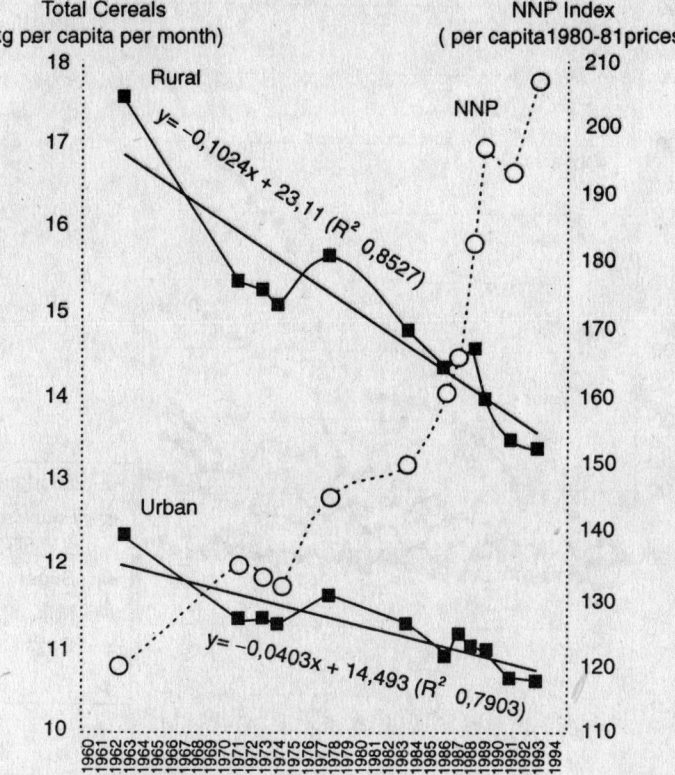

Graph. 15.1: *Consumption pattern of cereals*
Source: NSSO Survey of Consumer Expenditure various rounds

urban and semi-urban areas, which account for only about a quarter of the country's population. Per capita egg consumption in urban areas is about 90, while in rural areas consumption is about 13 eggs. Factors contributing to the higher consumption in urban areas include higher purchasing power of consumers and the transport costs of eggs and poultry meat from semi-urban to rural areas, which contribute to higher rural prices of these products. Consumer preference is also implied by the fact that egg consumption increased even though the ratio of the price of eggs relative to other livestock products (milk and meat) declined.

Poultry meat is becoming a popular source of affordable protein for the (largely urban) Indian population. In addition, broiler meat consumption is increasing faster than other types of poultry (duck, quail) meat. Presently, animal products, (dairy, meat, eggs and fish) are already an important component of consumer budget. Dairy products account for a large share of rural (4-22 percent) and urban (7-21 percent) consumer spending. With increasing disposable income, percentage share of dairy products will increase significantly. Meat, eggs and fish account for five to six percent of rural and two to seven percent of urban consumer expenditure. Even

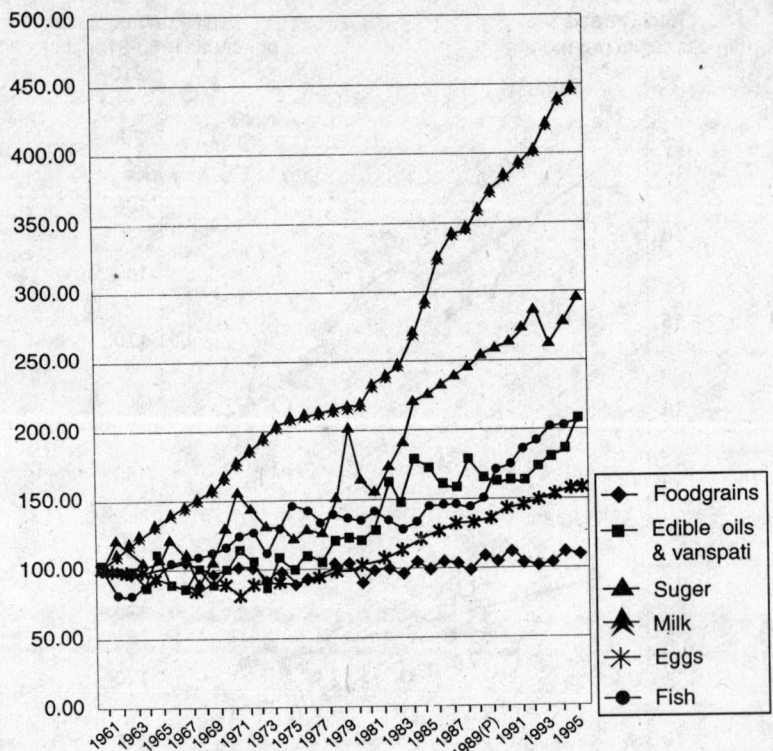

Graph 15.2: Per capita availability of various food items

poor consumers spend a large share of per capita budgets on livestock products (5-15 percent in rural areas and 11-19 percent in urban areas). Sustained economic growth and attendant increases in income will, therefore, continue to boost livestock demand in the future.

Demand Elasticities

Demand projections for various commodities are normally based on income elasticities. These elasticities are generally not valid, particularly for a long-term study like the one in hand. Beginning with the First Plan, elasticity for cereals, for example, has regularly come down from 1.0 in the fifties to 0.65 in the seventies and declined further to 0.3 in the eighties.

It is thus clear that any long-term projections based on this 'scientific tool' may not hold good. In fact the National Commission on Agriculture (1976) projected the demand for foodgrains for 2000 at 240 million tonnes based on an income elasticity of 0.65. However it could not be considered valid even by 1987-88 when the elasticity had already come down to 0.3. Similarly any long term projections based on such elasticities will not be valid 30 years hence. It is true for livestock products as well.

Table 15.1: Per Capita Consumption of Various Livestock Products –Rural: 1993-94
(Kg. for 30 days)

State	Milk	Goat Meat	Mutton	Beef	Buffalo Meat	Chicken	Eggs (No)
Andhra Pradesh	2.62	0.06	0.07	0.03	0.01	0.05	1.44
Arunachal Pradesh	0.43	0.01	0.01	0.15	0.01	0.12	1.02
Assam	1.21	0.03	0.00	0.04	-	0.08	1.12
Bihar	2.39	0.05	0.00	0.01	0.00	0.01	0.14
Goa	2.59	0.02	0.02	0.15	-	0.05	3.69
Gujarat	5.07	0.03	0.00	0.00	0.01	0.01	0.17
Haryana	13.82	0.02	-	0.00	0.04	0.00	0.08
Himachal Pradesh	7.52	0.09	0.00	-	-	0.00	0.22
Jammu & Kashmir	7.26	0.04	0.01	-	-	0.04	0.63
Karnataka	2.88	0.03	0.06	0.02	0.00	0.02	0.89
Kerala	2.61	0.01	0.01	0.12	0.07	0.03	2.00
Madhya Pradesh	2.76	0.04	0.00	0.00	0.00	0.02	0.15
Maharashtra	2.50	0.09	0.01	0.01	0.00	0.01	0.61
Manipur	0.12	0.00	0.00	0.13	0.06	0.06	0.84
Meghalaya	1.32	0.01	0.00	0.37	0.00	0.05	1.04
Mizoram	0.69	0.00	0.01	0.15	0.00	0.15	0.91
Nagaland	0.25	0.01	-	0.42	0.01	0.13	1.74
Orissa	0.77	0.03	0.00	0.01	0.00	0.02	0.29
Punjab	14.33	0.05	0.00	-	-	0.01	0.47
Rajasthan	10.41	0.05	-	-	0.00	0.00	0.07
Sikkim	4.77	0.07	0.01	0,21	0.00	0.04	1.73
Tamil Nadu	2.12	0.09	0.02	0.04	0.00	0.02	1.06
Tripura	1.43	0.02	0.00	0.00	-	0.06	1.48
Uttar Pradesh	5.44	0.05	0.00	0.00	0.06	0.00	0.21
West Bengal	1.54	0.04	0.00	0.06	0.00	0.03	1.69
A & N Islands	1.63	0.03	0.02	0.01	-	0.20	3.35
Chandigarh	8.64	0.06	-	-	-	0.20	0.31
Dadra & Nagar Haveli	1.08	0.04	-	-	-	0.03	0.35
Daman & Diu	3.35	0.20	-	-	-	0.04	0.90
Delhi	8.69	0.24	-	-	-	0.02	1.85
Lakshadweep	0.29	0.00	0.02	0.29	-	0.01	2.20
Pondicherry	2.99	0.11	0.01	0.06	-	0.02	1.09
All India	3.94	0.05	0.01	0.02	0.02	0.02	0.64

Source: NSSO, 50th Round, 1993-94.

There are four more theoretical problems with these elasticities. Firstly while the elasticities are calculated from consumption expenditure, for projecting the demand, income is being used as a proxy for expenditure. This is not in keeping with the facts. Graph 15.3 shows that total expenditure moves within the narrow band of Rs. 3000 to Rs. 6000 per capita per annum, irrespective of income. The gap between income and expenditure goes on widening once income crosses the Rs. 7500 mark at 1993-94 prices. As mentioned above, expenditure on cereals starts declining even earlier.

Table 15.2: Per Capita Consumption of various Livestock Products–Urban: 1993-1994
(Kg. for 30 days)

State	Milk (Litre)	Goat Meat	Mutton	Beef	Buffalo Meat	Chicken	Eggs (No)
Andhra Pradesh	3.92	0.05	0.11	0.02	0.00	0.05	2.13
Arunachal Pradesh	2.43	0.21	0.02	0.14	—	0.16	2.52
Assam	1.66	0.11	0.01	0.01	—	0.11	2.49
Bihar	3.49	0.11	0.00	0.02	0.01	0.02	0.90
Goa	3.25	0.03	0.07	0.16	0.01	0.04	3.35
Gujarat	6.21	0.06	0.01	0.01	—	0.01	0.43
Haryana	9.10	0.05	—	—	0.00	0.00	0.49
Himachal Pradesh	8.95	0.12	0.00	—	—	0.01	0.96
Jammu & Kashmir	9.11	0.16	0.01	0.00	—	0.05	1.73
Karnataka	4.42	0.06	0.10	0.04	0.00	0.03	1.59
Karala	3.27	0.01	0.01	0.11	0.06	0.05	2.49
Madhya Pradesh	4.08	0.09	0.00	0.00	0.02	0.02	0.81
Maharashtra	4.72	0.12	0.02	0.06	0.01	0.03	1.50
Manipur	0.17	—	0.00	0.05	0.00	0.02	0.81
Meghalaya	3.46	0.10	0.01	0.29	—	0.10	2.01
Mizoram	1.90	0.00	0.00	0.31	0.00	0.09	1.76
Nagaland	0.81	0.05	0.02	0.23	0.01	0.11	2.80
Orissa	2.20	0.13	0.02	0.02	—	0.02	1.32
Punjab	9.70	0.06	0.00	-	—	0.01	0.73
Rajasthan	7.53	0.10	—	-	0.00	0.00	0.37
Sikkim	5.41	0.07	0.02	0.29	0.01	0.08	2.10
Tamil Nadu	3.80	0.10	0.04	0.03	0.00	0.03	2.54
Tripura	2.29	0.08	0.01	—	—	0.07	2.31
Uttar Pradesh	5.63	0.07	0.00	0.00	0.19	0.00	0.64
West Bengal	2.73	0.08	0.01	0.06	—	0.06	2.61
A & N Islands	1.93	0.10	0.03	0.02	—	0.24	4.62
Chandigarh	9.84	0.11	-	-	-	0.06	1.83
Dadra & Nagar Haveli	3.57	0.14	0.00	-	-	0.06	0.54
Daman & Diu	5.75	0.18	-	0.00	0.04	0.04	0.64
Delhi	8.64	0.17	0.00	0.25	0.00	0.04	2.22
Lakshadweep	0.39	0.03	0.02	0.02	-	0.03	2.36
Pondicherry	4.10	0.11	0.01	-	-	0.03	1.90
All India	4.89	0.09	0.02	0.03	0.03	0.03	1.48

Source: NSSO, 50th Round, 1993-94.

Secondly, while elasticities have been calculated at constant prices, all income projections are at current prices of the target year.

Thirdly, there is a limit to the total calories, which an average human being can consume under given climatic conditions. There is no built in formula in the elasticities referred to above where elasticity coefficient becomes zero and takes negative value once the satiation point is reached. As an answer to this problem, demand studies centered around complete demand system taking into account mutual interdependence of a large

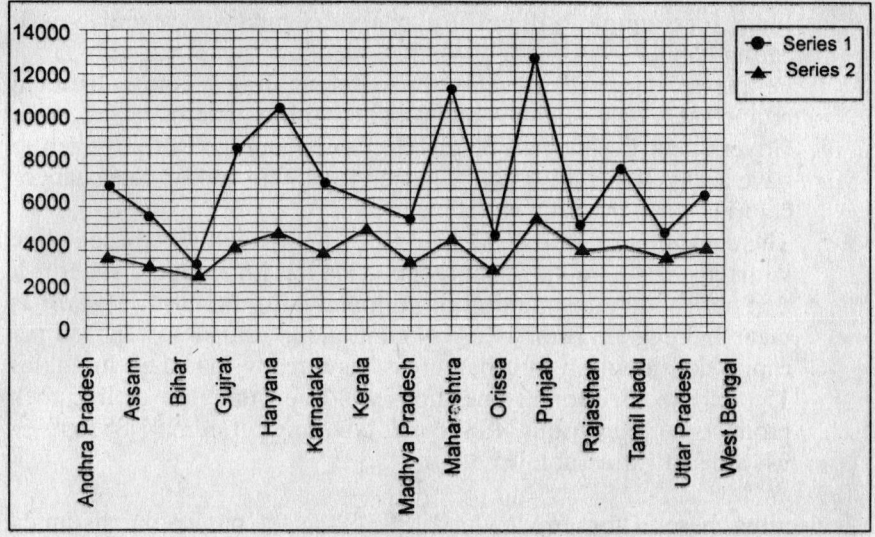

Fig. 19.3: Per capita income expenditure relationship

number of commodities in the budget decisions of the consumer were undertaken by some experts. The important models, which received considerable attention, are the linear expenditure system (Stone, 1954)[1] and 'almost ideal demand system (AIDS)' (Deaton and Muellbaur[2] 1980). These models were generally used for estimating demand equation for group of commodities and not for commodities at a disaggregate level. But they also do not allow increasing or decreasing income elasticities.

Fourthly, elasticities are being calculated from the same given source (NSSO data) by different methods. The results are widely different. While according to Bhalla demand elasticity for foodgrains is 0.3, the one by Praduman Kumar[3] who uses the Food Characteristic Demand System (FCDS) model, the corresponding figure is negative. This scientific tool may not therefore yield valid results for the long-term projections.

Demand Projections

For purpose of the present study, the normative approach has been used, with the following assumptions:

1. By and large absolute poverty will be eradicated by 2030.
2. Tastes and habits of the people at large will not undergo any drastic change other than the normal patterns as for the rural/urban areas.

[1]Stone, J.R.N. 1954: Linear Expenditure System and Demand Analysis: An Appreciation to the Pattern of British Demand: Economic Journal: 64: 511-527.

[2]Deaton, A., and J. Muellbaur: 1980. An Almost Ideal Demand System: American Economic Review: 70(3): pp. 312-26

[3]Praduman Kumar: Food Demand and Supply Projections for India: Indian Agricultural Research Institute. New Delhi.

India, for example, will not be at par with China with regard to meat eating habits.

3. People at large will have better understanding of the nutritional requirements for a healthy and productive life pattern.

4. Government Policy will be directed to encourage every citizen to have access to nutritive and balanced food with appropriate share of calories/ proteins from animal sources.

5. The consumption of livestock products are likely to increase in line with the present trends. In this connection it is important to underline, that per capita consumption of milk and dairy products, as well as meat and eggs in rural area will continue to remain lower than per capita consumption in urban areas (as already indicated in Tables 15.1 and 15.2). Monthly per household consumption of livestock products during various NSS rounds covering period 1987/88 to 1993/94, are shown in Table 15.3.

Keeping these factors in view and 1993-94 as the base, a reconstituted food basket has been drawn for 2020 and 2030 (Table 15.4). A projected population of 1311 million in 2020 and 1451 million for 2030, of which, 50% will be urban during 2030, it is projected that by 2030 an average Indian will have 2873 calories available daily against 2312 calories during 1993-94. This, of course, is the gross availability on the basis of total production of various commodities. Actual consumption after taking account of kitchen wastage, etc. at various levels will work out to be more than sufficient to meet the required nutritional norms. Similarly, of a total of 90.5 grams of proteins per day, the share of animal sources will be 40 grams (including 4.5 grams from fish) as against the present level of 15 grams.

In keeping with the recent experience of consumer behaviour, religious as well as climatic considerations, the consumption of meat as a group will continue to have a lower preference from among the various livestock products. Again from among the various components of meat, beef and pig will have much lower demand because of religious taboo of Hindus and Muslims, the two major population groups. Due to reasons of sociocultural background, majority of the Indian population, mainly inhabiting the North West and Southern regions, do not take meat, specially of cow and its progeny, buffalo and pig. However, the people living in the State of Kerala, West Bengal and North-Eastern are, by and large, non-vegetarian in food habit and the consumption of meat and fish is very common. Though, buffalo does not attract the religious sensitivity of majority of the people, its meat consumption is still region and community specific.

Drinking of milk on the other hand will continue to remain more popular and daily per capita availability is projected at nearly 350 grams. This includes direct as well as indirect (processed) component. Similarly the consumption of eggs is projected to increase from the present level of 31 eggs per day to over 100 during the coming 30 years. True, every one will

Table 15.3: Quantity of Monthly Consumption of Milk, Eggs & Meat per Household and Percentage of Household Consuming these Items. (All India)

N.S.S. Rounds	Milk				Egg				Meat			
	Quantity of consumption per HH (litres)		% of HHS reporting consumption		Quantity of Consumption per HH (No.)		% of HHS reporting consumption		Quantity of Consumption per HH (kg.)		% of HHS reporting consumption	
	Rural	Urban	Rural	Urban	Rural	Urban	Rural	Urban	Rural	Urban	Rural	Urban
43rd Round (July. 87 to June, 1988)	16.25	20.06	62	78	2.64	6.73	17	32	0.51	0.94	32	43
47th Round (July-Dec., 1991)	18.71	22.80	64	79	0.74	1.21	43	49	3.72	7.66	26	38
48th Round (1992)	18.54	23.20	62	79	0.73	0.07	42	49	3.65	8.03	25	39
49th Round (Jan- June, 1993)	17.50	21.47	61	78	0.69	1.00	41	48	3.26	6.11	24	33
50th Round (1993-94)	19.29	21.79	66	80	3.13	6.59	22	35	0.64	0.89	20	28

Note:
(i) Quantity figures have been derived by multiplying per capita consumption with average household size
(ii) Both Quantity and percentage of household figures for meat for 43rd round exclude chicken and other birds.
(iii) Quantity figures for meat for 50th round excluded birds other than chicken.
(iv) Percentage of households figures for-meat for 50th round includes only goat meat.

Source: National Sample Survey Organization, Deptt. of Statistics.

Table 15.4: Reconstituted Consumer Basket – 2020 and 2030

Item	1993 Production (population-884 million)	TE-ending 1993 Per capita availability				Total Demand Million tonnes		Per Capita Availability in 2030			
		Annual kg.	Gm.	Calories kg.	Proteins	2020 (nos)	2030 Gm.	Annual kg.	Gm.	Calories (nos)	Proteins gm.
Cereals*	123.30	139.48	382.1	1336	32.9	173.09	191.58	132.03	361.7	1266.0	31.2
Pulses	13.00	14.70	40.3	142	8.5	20.48	22.66	15.62	42.8	150.9	9.0
Milk	53.90	60.97	167.0	175	6.1	167.15	185.00	127.50	349.3	366.5	12.7
Oils	6.20	7.01	19.2	173	-	15.32	16.96	11.69	32.0	288.0	-
Egg	1.10	1.24	3.4	6	4.6	6.15	6.80	4.69	12.8	23.1	17.8
Meat	3.50	3.95	10.8	12	2.2	12.53	13.87	9.56	26.2	29.5	5.4
Fish	3.09	3.50	9.6	10	1.7	12.30	13.61	9.38	25.7	25.8	4.5
Fruits	24.12	27.28	74.7	56	0.8	69.64	77.08	53.12	145.5	108.9	1.5
Vegetables	43.02	48.66	133.3	82	3.5	153.64	170.04	117.19	321.1	198.1	8.4
Sugar**	20.36	23.03	63.1	250	-	41.79	46.26	31.88	87.3	346.2	-
Total			903.5	2242	60.3				1404.4	2803.0	90.5
Miscellaneous				70						70.0	
Grand Total				2312						2873.0	

* This is the actual consumption level for humans.

* * Includes jaggery

Population for 2020 is 1311 million and for 2030, it is 1451 million.

not eat eggs; it may still be lower than the accepted number of one egg a day for at least those who have no objection to eat eggs. Tables 15.5, 15.6 and 15.7 provide the resultant demand projections for milk, meat and eggs for the years 2020 and 2030.

Table 15.5: Demand Projections for Milk (million tonnes)

	1993	2000	2002	2007	2010	2020	2030
Cow	25.4	35.5	38.5	42.0	56.5	74.0	77.0
Buffalo	32.5	40.0	44.0	60.0	70.0	85.0	100.0
Goat	2.7	2.5	2.5	3.0	3.5	4.0	5.0
Processed	0.1	0.3	0.4	0.6	1.0	1.5	2.0
Total	60.7	78.0	85	105	130	163.0	182.0

Table 15.6: Demand Projections for Meat (million tonnes)

	1995	2000	2002	2007	2010	2020	2030
Human Population Million numbers	900	1000	1045	1120	1165	1311	1451
Beef	1.2	1.3	1.3	1.4	1.5	1.6	1.7
Buffalo	1.29	1.3	1.3	1.5	1.7	2.2	2.4
Sheep and Goat	0.65	0.68	0.7	1.0	1.3	1.5	1.8
Pig	0.42	0.43	0.4	0.6	0.8	1.0	1.2
Poultry meat	0.44	0.9	1.0	2.0	3.0	5.8	6.5
Total	4.0	4.61	4.7	6.5	8.3	12.2	13.6

Table 15.7: Projection of Egg Production

	1992	2000	2002	2007	2010	2020	2030
Egg Production (Billion)	22	35	42	55	60	90	120
Birds Producing Eggs							
Layers (Million)	200	200	220	250	280	360	435
Improved	65.1	127	148	175	200	275	360
Desi	134.9	73	72	75	75	75	75
Ducks and Duckial	22.0	22.1	21.0	20.0	20.0	20.0	20.0
Improved	1.7	1.75	1.8	2.0	2.2	2.4	2.6
Desi	20.3	20.35	19.2	18.0	17.8	17.6	17.4

* Includes Poultry meat

Supply Projections

The livestock sector in India is facing new challenges as well as opportunities. Projections dealt with above, indicate that a faster growth in demand for livestock products during the next three decades. Prospects for exports of some livestock products, as detailed in Chapter 12 on Foreign Trade, seem to be achievable. Indian livestock sector have been growing at an impressive rate of about 5 percent a year in the past few decades. The growth has been possible due to increasing numbers, technological change and better management of livestock wealth. However, it is apprehended that the recent trends in livestock sector growth may not sustain for long owing to the number of operating constraints. Though India has enormous and diverse livestock species adapted to varied agroclimatic conditions and farm typologies, the productivity of its livestock remain low compared to international standards. For instance, cattle milk yield is about half of the world average of around 2,100 kg/animal/annum. Productivity of species other than dairy and poultry has been stagnant at an extremely low level. The main reasons for low productivity are lack of appropriate technologies fitting to the different agro-ecologies and farm typologies, scarcity of feed and fodder resources in relation to livestock population and inappropriate disease management. Nevertheless, there is a considerable scope to raise productivity of livestock in different management systems of the land and livestock resources.

The livestock sector's future performance will also be significantly influenced by its international competitiveness. With trade liberalization, the sector needs to improve efficiency and lower costs. The underlying current trends in livestock production system present tremendous challenges—but they also offer opportunities. While some intensification is occurring in livestock production, especially among dairy and poultry producers, the sector is still dominated by low-input production systems operating at a low level of intensification than the crop sector. Intensification of production is further constrained by sociocultural factors, which prohibit the slaughtering of cows. The faster growth in consumption of livestock products however, would require greater intensification in the livestock sector.

Output increase in dairy sector will have to come from improvement in the quality of the animals and not, as in the past, from increases in animal population. Emphasis would, therefore, need to be placed on the use of improved buffalo and higher producing crossbred cows, while maintaining enough local genes to be able to function under prevailing smallholder conditions. Giving the existing price incentives for higher-fat milk, the buffalo population is expected to grow strongly. However, to keep the animal population within limits the old buffalo stock and additional male stock will need to be culled out. More intensive production and use of genetically superior animals will increase the use of stall-feeding and farm-produced fodder and improved crop residues. This ultimately should lead to a closer integration of cattle and buffaloes in the farming system. The use of bullock for farm operations can be expected to decrease further, as the quality of small-farm machinery continues to improve and price decline. More and more farmers, especially the younger ones, may switch on to tractors for cultivation.

In the small ruminant sector, increased meat production initially will have to come in the short term from increase in herd numbers, as no infrastructure exists to genetically improve meat production. Long-term opportunities exist in genetic improvement of local breeds. The development of intensive feedlots for sheep fattening will also offer an important means of increasing total meat production. Provided that its competitiveness improves, the poultry sector will be able to maintain its spectacular growth, especially for broilers. Growth will come from the expansion of intensive production systems, mainly operated by the private sector. The most critical factors governing these trends will be availability of high quality and low-priced feed, since this will determine the feasibility of stall-feeding, the opportunities of intensive feedlots, and the efficiency and international competitiveness of the poultry industry. These factors are further analyzed in Chapter 16.

Based on the factors discussed above supply projections for selected livestock products to the years 2010, 2020 and 2030, have been worked out. The production of milk will need to be increased by almost three times by the year 2030, and meat output by around four times, Among various meats, sheep and goat meat will need to record higher annual growth by 3.6 percent per annum. Poultry meat is projected to continue to increase at an impressive rate of over 8 percent per annum, while egg output is projected to increase by 5 percent (Table 15.8). A detailed meat balance is presented in Table 15.9.

Table 15.8: Supply Projections for Selected Livestock Products

(Million tonnes)

Commodity	Average TE 1997/98	Projected supply			Annual growth 2030 over base period (percent/year)
		2010	*2020*	*2030*	
Milk	68.7	135	180	200	3.1
Meat Total	4.33	9.0	13.7	16.7	4.0
of which Beef	1.37	1.6	1.9	2.3	1.5
Buffalo meat	1.38	1.9	2.5	3.4	2.7
Sheep and goat meat	0.65	1.5	1.8	2.3	3.6
Pig meat	0.44	0.80	1.00	1.20	3.0
Poultry	0.49	3.2	6.5	4.5	8.3
Eggs (Billion Nos.)	28	90	120	156	5.1

Projections computed by the Authors.

Table 15.9: Supply Projection for Meat: 2010, 2020 and 2030

Item	Unit	Cattle	Buffalo	Sheep	Goat	Pig	Layers	Broilers
I .	**Nos.**							
1992	Million	204.5	84.2	50.8	115.3	12.79	200	307
2010	"	190	80	60	135	20	250	1800
2020	"	170	70	65	149	22	400	3700
2030	"	160	65	70	160	24	430	4000
II. Slaughtering Ratio								
1992	Percentage	6	10	31	39	99	100	100
2010	"	7	20	32	40	100	100	100
2020	"	8	25	35	45	100	100	100
2030	"	• 9	28	40	50	100	100	100
III. Yield								
1992	kg./animal	100	100	15	10	35	2	1
2010	"	115	120	20	15	40	2.2	1.2
2020	"	135	150	25	18	45	2.5	1.5
2030	"	150	180	30	25	50	2.8	1.6
IV. Meat Output								
1992	Million tons	1.23	0.84	0.16	0.45	0.44	0.40	0.31
2010	"	1.60	1.90	0.84	1.0	0.8	0.5	2.70
2020	"	1.90	2.5	0.65	1.2	1.0	0.8	4.2
2030	"	2.3	2.9	0.86	1.4	1.2	1.0	6.0

16

Consumption and Supply of Feed and Fodder

Due to pressure on the land for growing foodgrains, oilseeds and pulses, adequate attention has not been given to the production of fodder crops and pasture grasses/legumes. As a result there is an acute shortage of nutritious green/dry fodder in India. Thus, ensuring an adequate supply of reasonable quality feed and fodder is one of the major challenges facing the Indian livestock sector. In fact, quantitative and qualitative insufficiency of feeds and fodder in the country is one of the main impediments in the way of improvement of livestock production. The chronic shortage of feeds and fodder has in general lowered the productive capacity and fertility of the Indian livestock and has brought about their degeneration. While there is some debate on the exact size of the current deficit, there is a general agreement that the volume and quality of future feed supply will be of vital importance in sustaining the growth of the livestock sector. This chapter reviews the current status of the feed and fodder supply and identifies constraints that hamper its development. Structural problems and public sector policies influencing the performance of the sector are examined. The challenge of improving the genetic base in India, which could also increase the efficiency of feed use, is also discussed.

STATUS OF THE AVAILABILITY OF FEED

A number of studies have so far been carried out to assess the availability of livestock feeds in India. These estimates, however, vary quite widely as these are based on different assumptions. Nevertheless, all these studies indicate unequivocally that feeds available in India are quite inadequate for the existing livestock population even at their present low level of feed consumption. In fact, one of the main factors responsible for the overall deficiency of feedstuffs is the enormous population of livestock in the country. At present, land has to provide sustenance for over 1020 million human beings and has, in addition, to maintain huge number of animals of low productivity. Because of low productive capacity of livestock large numbers of them have to be maintained, which in turn creates greater shortage of feeds and fodder, resulting in further degeneration of the stock. It is therefore urgently necessary to enhance the availability of feed resources for increased production of milk, meat, eggs, wool, etc. as well as to properly maintain the efficiency of draught animals. The Famine Enquiry Commission (1945) had rightly stressed that "feeding was of crucial importance, for no lasting improvement could be brought about by breeding alone, since improved breeds deteriorate rapidly if not fed adequately". In point of fact, better breeding is no substitute for better feeding.

Feed Consumption in India

Green and dry fodder account for most feed consumption in India (Figure 16.1). Dry feeds, composed mainly of agricultural residues, cultivated green fodder and green fodder from grazing in forests and pastures together account for over 90 percent of livestock feed consumption. Grains and feed concentrates are only important in the intensive production system.

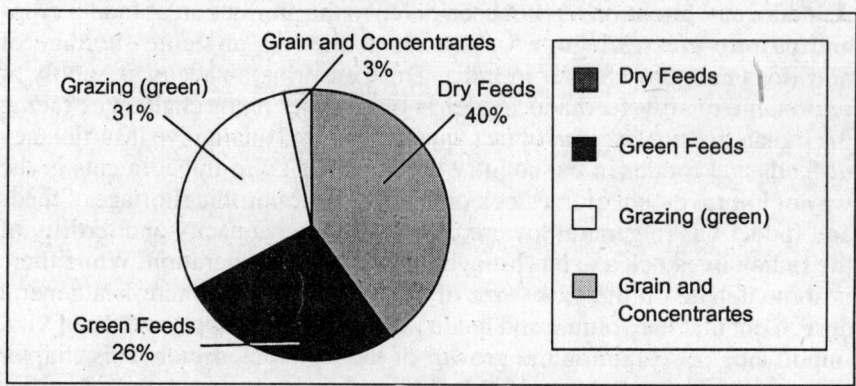

Fig. 16.1: Composition of Feed Consumption in India

Agricultural Residues

Agricultural residues consumed by livestock consist of two-thirds straw from wheat, rice, barley, maize, sorghum and millet and one-third hay from pulses and oilseeds. It is customary to collect residues immediately after harvest and pile them into heaps, either near the threshing yard or in backyards, for stall or supplemental feeding during the lean season. In some states (for example Punjab and Rajasthan) the complementarity between intensive cropping systems and livestock production is exploited through the migration of animals (mostly goats and sheep) to the wheat and rice growing areas after harvest to feed on the agricultural residues. Over the past decades, the quality and quantity of wheat and rice straw, the main ingredient in residues, have deteriorated because of the shift towards the production of "green revolution" varieties, which produce less and poorer quality straw. A number of technologies for on-farm treatment can improve the feeding quality of these straws.

Grazing and Cultivated Green Fodder

Grazing is the most important source of fodder for cattle and other ruminants. Most grazing takes place in forest areas, nonarable lands, permanent pastures and earmarked grazing area, and land under miscellaneous tree crops and groves. The total area covered by these land categories shrank by about 30 percent (23 million hectares) between 1950-51 and 1988-89. The area under green fodder totals about 8.3 million ha, or 5 percent of the total cultivated area, and is increasing in significance with the diversification of Indian agriculture. For example, fodder cultivation for dairy production is being increasingly introduced in the irrigated Punjab area. Most grasslands are severely degraded and overgrazed as a result of continuous grazing or harvesting of the grasses. Consequently, the soils are shallow, low in nutrients, and severely compacted. Moreover, the levels of palatable and nutritious grasses have fallen. In addition noxious weeds and bushes have invaded extensive areas.

Fodder from Forests

Tree leaves and grass undergrowth from forests constitute an important source of fodder, particularly in hilly and arid areas. Leaf fodder available from forest areas depends on several factors, including the proportion of fodder trees to the total growing stock, the density of the forests, the practice and intensity of harvesting of leaf fodder, and the distance of the forest areas from the village. In some parts of the country more animals feed on shrubs and trees in forest areas than on open grass and pasture land. Forests cover about 700, 000 square kilometers or about 21 percent of India's land area. About 90 percent of all forests are publicly owned and managed. The Ministry of Environment and Forests in 1993 estimated that about 90 million cattle and buffaloes graze in forest areas.

Forests areas are not equally distributed throughout the country, more than half of forest land is located in five states: Madhya Pradesh, Arunachal Pradesh, Andhra Pradesh, Orissa and Maharashtra. The area covered by forests in these states ranges from 15 to 30 percent, with the exception of Arunachal Pradesh with 82 percent. In contrast, in the mainly semiarid and arid states such as Gujarat and Rajasthan, only 4 percent of the area is covered by forest. Most forests are not large contiguous blocks, but rather small patches interspersed by habitations.

The pressure from grazing has contributed to degradation in many forest areas. Heavy grazing in the forest damages trees, compacts soil and inhibits regeneration. Livestock pressure on forests has built over time as the population has grown and traditional grazing lands have been turned over to crop cultivation. Both sedentary village livestock (mainly cattle and small ruminants) and migratory animals raised by nomadic livestock producers use forest lands.

Forests those are situated near habitations and villages have the heaviest incidence of grazing. Grazing and other activities, such as repeated annual ground fires and the removal of dry fuel wood and non-timber forest produce, have reduced vegetative cover, exposing the forest floor to erosion and thus further reducing its carrying capacity for grazing. The magnitude of livestock pressure is illustrated by a survey of 174 protected areas. The survey found that 67 percent of national parks and 83 percent of sanctuaries reported grazing incidence, despite laws prohibiting grazing in these areas. It was estimated in 19 84 that more than half (about 36 million hectares) of forest areas were degraded. A key challenge therefore is to find a more sustainable strategy for using these forest areas.

The cost of feed is the largest item of expenditure in the rearing of animals, and it becomes proportionately greater when labour and land are relatively cheap and where elaborate plant or buildings are unnecessary or to the minimum. Thus, it becomes all the more important to have some knowledge of the basic principles of feeding essential to maintain and increase productivity.

A mere classification of these food constituents, (shown in Figure 16.2 and Table 16.1) gives no indication of their relative importance either quantitatively or qualitatively but they must be considered in their relation to the function of the body and the manner in which one fits in with the other in the process of transformation. Each, therefore, will be discussed briefly and separately.

Roughages

Roughages are the feed stuffs which are bulky in nature and contain more than 18 per cent crude fibre, a material which makes their direct use by any

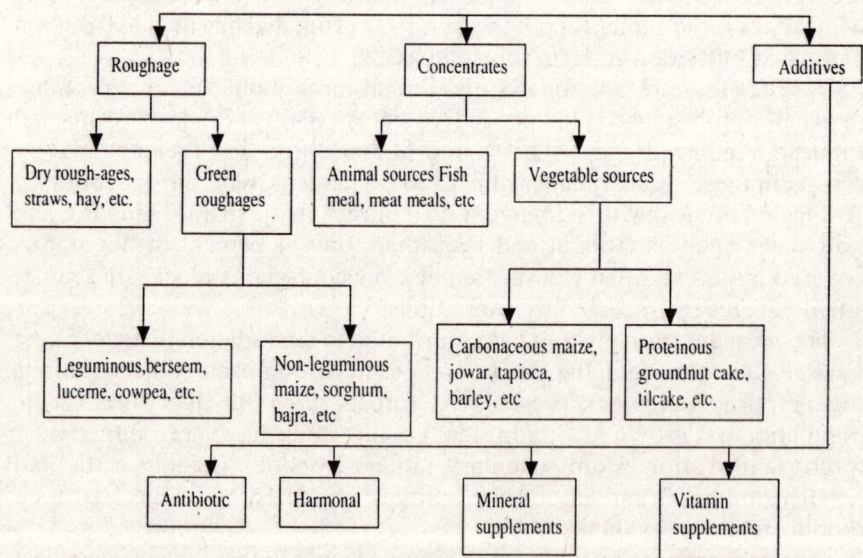

Fig. 16.2: Classification of feeding stuffs

Table 16.1: Classification of Feeding Stuffs

	Item			Example
R O U G H G A E S	1. Dry feeds	Hay	Leguminous	Berseem hay, lucerne hay,
			Non-leguminous	Napier hay
		Straw	Grain straw	Wheat or barley straw or paddy straw
			Pulses straw, Grasses	Arhar, urad, moong straw and Doob grass
		Uncultivated	Tree leaves, Bushes	Peepal, gular pakar leaves, Jharberi
	2. Green feeds	Cultivated	Leguminous	Lucerne, berseem, cowpea Maize, jowar.
			Non-leguminous	Oats, hybrid napier
	3. Silage			Maize and jowar silage
	4. Roots			Carrot, potato, sweet potato
	5. Kernels			Mango, jamun kernels
		Crushed grains		Barley, oat, maize, gram
CONCENTRATES		Grain byproducts		Wheat, bran, chuni, etc.
		Oil seeds		Cotton seeds
		Oil cakes		Linseed, groundnut cake, til cake
ANIMAL BYPRODUCTS				Bone meal
				Blood meal
				Meat meal
				Fish meal
INDUSTRIAL BYPRODUCTS				Sugar industry byproducts and Guar gum industry by-products Lemon grass oil industry byproducts Starch industry by-products Dairy industry byproducts Antibiotic industry byproducts
ANTIBIOTICS				Terramycin, penicillin, streptomycin, etc. Aurofac, TM5, boon-o-milk,
MINERAL SUPPLEMENTS				Milkmin, starmin, etc.

Source: Livestock and Poultry Enterprises for Rural Development.

other than herbivorous animals, impossible. The roughages are straws, kadhies, green fodders, bays, silage, etc. Roughages may be dry or green. Succulent roughages have more than 70 per cent water.

The feed and fodders fed to cattle can broadly be grouped under concentrates and roughages, depending upon the amount of crude fibre, digestible protein content and TDN value. Any feed high (over about 60 per cent) in crude fibre and low in TDN (under 20 per cent), on air dry basis is usually grouped under roughages. Any feed low (under about 20 per cent) in crude fibre and high (over about 60 per cent) in TDN on air dry basis is grouped under concentrates.

Thus, a variety of roughages and concentrates are available for feeding cattle. The roughages can be succulent or dry roughages depending on the moisture content. Succulent roughages are further classified into green fodder and silage. Greens include leguminous and non-leguminous fodder. Leguminous fodder consists of leaves and stems of a group of plants belonging to the group Leguminosae. They have a higher protein content and can form a major source of protein to farm animals. The important legumes are berseem, lucerne, cowpea, kudzu vine, soyabeans, crotalaria group.

Legumes may be either annual or perennial. Non-leguminous roughages contain lower percentage of protein. So, when fed to animals, the ration requires additional protein supplements. Cereal fodder crops, perennial cultivated grasses, indigenous grasses and introduced grasses are important roughages. The cereal crops are maize, sorghum, bajra, oats, teosinte; cultivated perennial fodder grasses are guinea grass, napier grass, hybrid napier, para grass, rhodes grass, sudan grass. Indigenous grasses include anjan grass, dhub grass, giant star grass, marval grass, sewan grass, masel grass. Grasses like signal grass, orchard grass, pangalo grass, etc., have been introduced from Africa, USA, Australia. Silage and hay are also commonly fed as roughages. They can be either from cultivated fodder grasses or legumes or mixture of these.

Dry roughages are commonly fed. Usually hay and straws are included in this category. Dry roughages can include both leguminous and non-leguminous crops and residues. Paddy straw, wheat straw or bhoosa, oats straw, barley straw, ragi straw are the commonly fed straws. As a rule, they are devoid of digestible crude protein and are usually taken for their TDN value. They may contain excess of salts of oxalates of sodium and potassium (paddy straw) and interferes with the Ca and P metabolism and adequate balancing is essential in the ration for these minerals when ration is mainly dependent on straws. Stovers of maize, bajra, sorghum are also fed and they are better than straws.

Pulse straw is comparatively better. They are urad, moong, moth, cowpea, massur, arhar, etc. Groundnut straw is superior to that of non-leguminous hays and is comparable to that of leguminous hay of cowpea. It can be safely fed along with wheat bran and wheat straw to meet the entire nutritional requirements of milch cows producing up to 4 to 5 kg milk daily.

Straws and Stovers

Intensity of rainfall, temperature, humidity, soil structure, surface elevation and gradient, flora and fauna all make a difference. The cropping pattern plays an equally important role, especially through the quality and quantity of feed nutrients associated with it. If rainfall is adopted as a crude index of topography the density of India's livestock population varies directly with it. As one moves from the relatively drier regions of the northwest and Deccan plateau towards eastern and southeastern India, the sub-Himalayan ranges and the western coast, the density of population increases from about 55 to 147 per 100 acres of area under cultivation. Animal productivity measured in work capacity or milk yield, is largely found to very inversely with density and, therefore, rainfall. The Deccan plateau, a region of medium rainfall and low productivity, is an exception because of such topographical factors as rocky soil and undulating surface. The average milk yield per day per cow in milk varies from about 2.3 kg in Punjab to 0.50 in Orissa, a state falling in heavy rainfall zone. In the case of buffaloes, the corresponding yield figures are about 4 kg for Punjab, and 1.5 kg in Orissa. It is interesting to note that animal and human population densities move together as the high rainfall areas are generally rice growing capable of sustaining higher human density. At the same time neither rice straw nor rice husk is rated high for animal nutrition leading to the inevitable consequences that in these areas poor animal productivity tends to be counteracted by larger stock size.

Straws and stovers are the staple livestock feed for Southeast Asia, and interest in their use as livestock feed in many other parts of the world is increasing as the prices of better quality feeds go up. They are essentially energy feeds containing very little protein or minerals. The digestibility of their energy is only 40-50 per cent. Further, they have excess salts of exalates, especially of calcium and of potassium. These interfere with the mineral metabolism, especially that of calcium and phosphorus. Voluntary intake of the roughage is also low, so that the maximum possible energy intake of livestock on straws diets is only about 150 Kcal/kg BW[1] .75, which is only enough to meet the maintenance requirements of animals. Any treatment of straws, that could increase their energy yield by even 10-20 per cent would add tremendously to the world's livestock feed resources, especially with small and marginal farmers, the by-product of agricultural activity is primarily straws and stovers of cereal crops.

Digestibility of forages is limited by the cell wall composition and non-cell components being completely available. The greater the crude fibre in the roughages, the lesser the digestibility of nutrients. This is mainly due to the increase in lignin content or some other factors which increase with increase in age of the plant. Lignin interferes with hydrolysis of polysaccharides, partly due to physical encrustation of the polyaccharide and partly due to lignin (polysaccharide links unattacked by the enzymes).

---

[1]BW = Body Weight

Ensilage produces an almost anaerobic fermentation of part of the herbage carbohydrates, producing fatty acids that lower pH enough to cleave acid-labile lignin-carbohydrate bonds. Strong lignin carbohydrate or lignin protein complexes are unchanged in the faeces. Silica also seems to be structural in plants and is contained in cell wall and may behave just like lignin. The influence of silica and lignin is additive on the digestibility of fodders.

The Alkali Treatment of Straws

The alkali treatment of straws that can increase digestibility markedly, has been known for nearly a century. The chemical composition of straws varies with variety, location and cultural practices employed in growing the cereal crop from which they are obtained. Paddy straw leaves contain more silica than the stems (15.5 per cent silica in leaves and 8.1 per cent in stem). The lignin content of leaves is 5.6 per cent and of stem 7.8 per cent. Thus, the silica is more important in inhibiting the digestibility of paddy straw than lignin. Alkali treatment of roughages dissolves lignin, silica and hemicellulose. Cellulose is not dissolved. Cellulose swells when treated with alkali. The straw can be soaked or sprayed with sodium hydroxide. About 3 to 6 g/100 g roughage is considered desirable.

Factory Treatment of Straw

Workers in Denmark have taken a lead in this field. They have designed a continuous flow, horizontal mixture with high speed rotating blades into which a fine spray is injected. Uniform wetting can be achieved with as little as about 10-15 litres solution per 100 kg straw, giving a finished product (after mixing molasses and other dry ingredients) with about 85 per cent dry matter. The treated straw is mixed with molasses, minerals and other ingredients and immediately pelleted. It is claimed that the pressure and heat to which the material is subjected in passing through the die holes of the pelleter enhance the effectiveness of the alkali. We may have to adopt this technology to improve feeding value of straws and stovers. This also reduces bulk and facilities transportation also.

Valuable Feed from Straw

Until recently, the feeding of straw to cattle was considered backward in livestock farming. In the past decade, however, the consumption of straw as fodder has more than doubled in the USSR. Is it evidence of the backwardness in cattle farming or have some new ways to use straw as fodder been found?

Three years ago, the All-Union Biotechnical Institute proposed a biological method to process straw. If nature has not given animal ferments which are needed for feeding with straw, microbiology could give ferments to them. Researchers have proved this. Digestion begins, as it were, before straw gets into the stomach. The ferments are added shortly before the feeding. They transform the composition of the crude fibre, increasing the amount of protein by 2-4 times. Experiments have proved that the composition of the straw treated with ferments is close to that of meadow hay which is a 'delicacy' for cattle. It is essential that the ferments be absolutely harmless. Since neither high temperature, nor high pressure are needed, the technological process is rather simple. No special equipment is needed and the cost of the fodder is low.

Some farms in the Moscow and Voroshilovgrad regions and in the Krasnodar territory now prepare straw for feeding milk cows and for fattening cattle using the method proposed by the Biotechnical Institute. All the operations involved in the preparation of the feed are mechanised and they are carried out with the help of feed mixers produced by the industry in series. To ensure that fresh feed containing water up to 70 per cent retains its nutritive properties, it should be consumed within a day of its preparation. The institute has also worked out a reliable way to preserve fermented straw for a year. Farmers have noticed that cows like feed granules made of fermented straw and prefer them to ordinary silage. The dairy milk yield of a cow had also increased by 2 kg on an average and the fat percentage of the milk had also increased. The cost on producing a ton of feed was reduced by nearly 10 per cent.

Silage of Paddy Straw and Berseem

The paddy straw and berseem can be preserved as a silage. The paddy straw should be cropped to 2.5 to 4 cm by a chaff cutter and mixed before ensiling in the ratio of paddy straw:berseem 1:5 or 1:4. The material should be thoroughly pressed in the silo pi. After a period of 105 to 110 days, a silage of good quality will be available for feeding cattle.

The anhydrous oxalic acid in the paddy straw before ensiling was 2.11 per cent, whereas after ensiling it came down to 1.52 per cent. Thus, ensilage of paddy straw resulted in decrease of 27.66 per cent in oxalic acid content. In the feeding trials, it was observed that the crude fibre digestibility increased by 12.42 per cent and all animals showed positive nitrogen and mineral balances. The silage contained 2 per cent DCP and 16 per cent TDN on fresh basis. By feeding this silage, it is possible to meet the DCP, TDN and mineral requirements of animals having 250-300 kg body weight. The quality of silage can still be improved by the addition of additives and bacterial inoculation.

Balanced Concentrate Mixtures

These are less bulky and therefore contain less crude fibre (below 18 per cent). Concentrates may belong to any of the following three categories.

1. Concentrates which are rich in energy and are low in digestible crude protein, e.g. cereal grains, tubers, etc., carbonaceous concentrates.
2. Which are very rich in digestible crude protein like oil cakes proteinous concentrates.
3. Protein and energy are in medium range like brans, chunies, etc.

Because of poor quality of roughages, it has become necessary to feed a certain amount of concentrate mixture to maintain production. The concentrate mixture is prepared in order to balance for the DCP and TDN. Besides these, they are further balanced for their Ca, P and NaCl; so that deficiencies due to these can be minimised. This is generally done by the addition of one to two per cent of finely ground limestone or steamed bone meal or good quality mineral mixture and one per cent is also added. This is done, because, concentrate mixtures are usually poor in calcium. Similarly, both concentrates and roughages are very poor sources of common salt. A properly balanced concentrate mixture will be rich in phosphorus, especially when bran is added. One kg may contain as much as 4 to 5 gm of phosphorus and 1.5 to 2.0 gm of calcium. When seasum cake (til cake) is used as one of the ingredients, the concentrate mixture becomes rich in calcium when introduced at the rate of 20 per cent of the concentrate mixture, one kg of the mixture should provide very nearly 6 g of Ca, since one kg of mixture corresponds to 2.5 kg of milk, addition of seasum cake in the manner shown above satisfies the requirements.

Depending upon the ration, i.e., growth, maintenance, pregnancy, milk production and dry period, the DCP and TDN in the concentrate mixture varies. For milk production, the concentrate mixture should have at least 16 per cent DCP and 72 per cent TDN and 1 kg is sufficient to meet the DCP and TDN requirements for 2.5 kg of milk produced. Some of the commonly used concentrate mixtures are given below.

Composition of Concentrate Mixtures
(76 per cent TDN and 16 per cent DCP)

Ingredients			
1. Maize	30%	2. Maize	25%
Rice bran	30%	Oats	25%
Groundnut		GNC	25%
Cake (GNC)	20%	Wheat	20%
Wheat bran	20%	Gram husk	5%

Technologies for More Efficient Use of Fodder Resources

New technologies have been developed in India to improve the utilization of crop residues. Fodder production and cut-and-carry systems offer an alternative to communal grazing. The quality of crop residues (i.e. straw) may be improved by urea treatment to improve its nutritive value. Similarly, urea-molasses blocks have been improved through research conducted by ICAR, Agricultural Universities and the NDDB. Increased milk yields of 20 percent as a result of using urea-molasses blocks have been reported. The application of bypass protein technology in combination with straw[1]

---

[1]Bypass protein technology refers to the use of special protein sources (e.g. brewer's grain, corn gluten meal, cotton seed cake, soybean meal) and processes (e.g. heating) to reduce the digestive losses in the rumen and improve the efficiency of protein utilization.

has been found to quadruple the efficiency of supply of amino acids from feed to milk production. Bypass protein technology, under experimental conditions, has reportedly allowed the reduction of concentrate requirement by 40 percent, the increase in the conversion of protein in dry matter by over 30 percent and the reduction of dry matter requirement by 24 percent.[2] Important constraints to the utilization and dissemination of these technologies remain. These include the applicability of these technologies to high yielding crossbred cows only, their commercial production and utilization potential, and weaknesses in the existing technology transfer system, which could introduce such technologies to farmers. However, genetic improvement of millet and sorghum crop residues has not been explored much hitherto. It is possible that genetic variation in the quality of sorghum and millet stover could be exploited to develop improved crop germplasm with stover of higher nutritive value. Small increases in roughage digestibility have been reported to result in considerable increase in milk and meat yields.[3]

Sorghum and millet breeders, however, joined hands with animal nutritionists for developing a collaborative research project in this area. The initial and basic work was planned at ICRISAT, and was applied at four places in the country. The JAVA feed-animal performance simulation model on the expected increases in milk yield and draught power of livestock from increased digestibility of crop residues of sorghum and millets, showed an average increase of 3.2 percent in buffalo milk yield and 3.4 percent in cow milk yield in one domain (southern part). In the second domain (northern part), the increase in milk yield was much higher (6.3 percent in case of buffaloes and 10.7 percent in case of cows). The feed model also indicated a 8.4 percent increase in the draught hours of bullocks. The ex-ante assessment of the returns to this research project indicated that it was economically viable and justified. The internal rate of return of the project was found to be 18.71 percent.[4] This internal rate of return is reasonably high. There is an urgent need to adopt such technologies to improve the digestibility of crop residues from sorghum and millets.

Current policy of the Government of India for increasing the production of fodder crops and pasture grasses/legumes consists of the dissemination of high yielding foundation/certified seeds of these crops[5]. For this purpose, several regional stations and a Central Fodder Seed Production Farm have been established to undertake their production and propagation. Regional stations have been established at Mamidipally, Hyderabad (Andhra

[2]Chatterjee, A.K., and Acharya, R.M. Heading for 21st Century: in Dairy India: 1992.

[3]International Livestock Research Institute: Implementation of Rumen Ecology into Tropical Feed Utilization Programme: 1995, Nairobi, Kenya

[4]Rao, K.P.C., Krisjanson, P.M., and Zerbini, E. Genetic Enhancement of Sorghum and Millet Residues fed to Ruminants: An Ex-ante Assessment., in Birthal, Pratap S., et al: Livestock In Different Farming Systems in India: 2002

[5]Department of Animal Husbandry & Dairying: Annual Report 2001-2002, pp. 24-25

Pradesh), Gandhi Nagar (Gujarat), Hisar (Haryana), Suratgarh (Rajasthan), Sahema (Jammu and Kashmir), Alamadhi (Tamil Nadu) and Kalyani (West Bengal). These stations are catering to requirements of the farmers of different agroclimatic regions. The Central Fodder Seed Production Farm is located at Hesserghatta. In addition, a scheme for fodder mini-kit demonstration aims to educate the farmers on new high yielding fodder varieties and improved agronomic practices through field demonstrations. This is also being implemented in the regional stations and the Central Fodder Seed Production Farm. Fodder seed supply is also an important constraint. To increase the availability of improved fodder seeds, the provision of incentives to registered seed growers in different states to take up the production of seeds needs to be more vigorously pursued.

Concentrate Feed

Concentrate feed in India is supplied by the organized and unorganized sectors. The original feed compounding industry (plants with capacity greater than 100 ton/day) in the cooperative and private sector currently produces nearly 3 million tonnes of feed annually. The bulk of the feeds are produced in the Western and Southern regions of the country. Another two million tonnes of feed is produced by the unorganized sector (10-30 tons/day plant capacity). Concentrate feeds largely utilize domestically produced feed ingredients.

ENZYME SUPPLEMENTATION IN POULTRY RATIONS—AN OVERVIEW

Enzymes have emerged as a latest biotechnological tool and have a potential to revolutionise the animal feed industry. Possibility of making available hitherto in digestible cell wall materials and neutralization of various anti-nutritional factors into poultry rations is likely to open up new vistas in poultry feed formulation by way of incorporating many cheaply available feed ingredients into poultry rations thereby economizing the poultry production on one hand and reducing competition between man and poultry for same staple feed on the other.

Number of enzymes are available and are being used in wide variety of combinations along with a variety of feed stuffs. Enzymes are specialized proteins, enhancing specific chemical reactions in biological systems without being changed themselves. Almost all the reactions in the biological systems are facilitated by enzymes, many of them acting in concerted manner to bring about biochemical changes that are necessary for metabolism. The specific three dimensional structure of enzymes ensure that they act at a specific reaction conditions (temperature, pH and humidity), substrate concentration as well as in presence of activators and inhibitors.

The recent advances in biotechnology has facilitated the commercial production of enzymes thereby making them available cheaply in large quantity. Large scale expansion of poultry industry (both layers and broilers) has increased the pressure on the conventional feed ingredients. Presently India ranks 4th in egg production and 19th in broiler production. In spite of spectacular increase in production per capita availability of eggs and poultry meat is much below the ICMR recommendation. To make poultry meat and eggs available to general masses the industry has to grow manifold in the coming years. One of the impediments in this is the availability of feed which accounts for 70% of the cost of production.

With the production of conventional feed ingredients remaining static, the search for novel methods to improve the nutrient availability of feedstuffs along with search for the alternate non-conventional feed stuffs is imperative. Use of non-conventional feed ingredients not only economises the production by way of decreasing the feed cost but it also reduces the competition between poultry and man in terms of sparing staple feed ingredients like maize for human consumption.

Poultry being monogastric lacks fibre degrading enzymes that could degrade the complex molecules like cellulose, hemicellulose, pectin etc. The use of exogenous enzymes facilitates degradation of these polymers thereby making available the nutrients which would otherwise be excreted for want of degradation. Besides, use of non-conventional feed ingredients has a limitation for the presence of certain anti-nutritional factors (Table 16.2), which have adverse effect on the performance of birds.

Various types of enzymes find use in poultry diets that are relatively specific for certain substrates and their chemical bonds. However most of the enzymes prepared for use in animal feeds have relatively a broad spectrum of activity. These enzymes are sufficiently impure to possess certain activities in addition to their own and act in synergy. These additional activities or apparently unrelated aspects of enzyme activity may cause unexpected beneficial effects e.g. the supplementation of diets with carbohydrates improve the deposition of vitamins and fatty acids in chicken tissues.

Table 16.2: Problem Compounds Present in Some Commonly used Poultry Feed Ingredients

Ingredient	Problem Compound
Maize	Lectins, phytate, resistant starch
Wheat	Arabinoxylans, wheat germ agglutinins, phytate, resistant starch
Barley	B-glucans, resistant starch
Rice	Phytate, arabinoxylans
Sorghum	Tannins, resistant starch
Rye	Arabinoxylans, polyphenols
Soyabean Meal	Oligosaccharides, NSPs trypsin inhibitors lectins.
Peas	Resistant starch, proteins and saponins
Beans	Tannins, trypsin inhibitors, lectins, oligosaccharides NSPs
Lupins	Oligosaccharides, NSPs proteins
Rapeseed meal	Oligosaccharides, NSPs, tannins, glucosinolates
Sunflower meal	Oligosaccharides, NSPs

The improvement of feed utilization due to enzyme activities occurs in two ways:-

1. The young birds in early life lacks enzymes needed for maximum utilization of feed nutrients, hence exogenous enzymes supplement the host enzyme systems.
2. Nature of diet is such that enzyme supplementation facilitates better nutrient utilization.

Due to economic pressure, spiraling feed cost, the interest in feed enzymes has grown in recent years and has resulted in development of specific multienzyme mixtures and custom designed for particular feed in order to improve the productive value of feeds and to allow the use of more novel feed stuffs with profitability. Significant improvement in body weight and feed conversion ratio was recorded in broilers fed on low energy and high fibre diets supplemented with multienzyme mixture. In many cases it has been observed that there is significant improvement in performance of broilers when the diets containing maize, groundnut cake, soyabean meal, and rice polish were supplemented with a commercial enzyme containing protease, amylase, cellulase, lipase and pectinase.

The common enzymes used as feed additives along with their activity are listed in Table 16.3. The beneficial effect of enzyme supplementation of poultry diets was demonstrated for the diets based on barley. Following success in the barley based diets there is an increasing interest in application of enzymes to the diets based on other cereals. Since a compound feed is often a blend of various ingredients of plant and animal origin, the mixture of enzymes rather than a single enzyme proves to be more beneficial. Most of the enzyme products used in poultry either singly or as a cocktail can be categorized into two groups:-

a. Enzymes hydrolyzing Non starch Polysaccharides
b. Phytases
c. NSPs hydrolyzing enzymes:

The NSPs present in the cell walls of cereals like rye, barley and wheat are mainly glucan and pentosans (arabinoxylans), which are poorly digested by the chickens and possess antinutritive properties resulting in depressed performance, especially the soluble B-glucans increase digesta viscosity, has a negative impact on the digestibility of nutrients. It influences the passage time and can cause sticky and wet droppings. In addition cell wall substances such as cellulase can cause a so called cage effect. Digestible nutrients are attached to the inert substances and are therefore not accessible for the digestive enzymes. Further, there is a strong negative correlation between the content of NSP and the apparent metabolisable energy (AME) of the cereals. Therefore the feeds like rye and barley which have higher level of NSP respond better to enzyme supplementation as compared to diets like maize and sorghum which contains lower NSP levels. The removal of antinutritive effect of NSPs by adding enzyme followed depolymerization

Table 16.3: Major Feed Enzymes and their Action

Enzyme	Substrate	Function
Cellulase	Cellulose	Break down of cellulose in high fibre diets and release of energy.
Hemicellulase	Hemicellulose	Breakdown of hemicellulose (arabans, xylans and galactans) and release of energy.
Phytase	Phytate	Release of bound phosphorus in plant material thereby increasing the phosphorus availability
Protease	Protein	Weakens protein starch matrices and improves digestion.
Glucanase	Glucans	Decrease glucans and decrease the viscosity and improve the digestion, useful in the diets based on barley, oats, jowar, sorghum, milo, wheat etc.
Amylase	Starch	Improves starch digestion
Tannase	Tannins	Break down of tannins in the diets like sorghum
Pectinase	Pectin	Breakdown of pectins for better utilization

effect of NSPs by enzyme action. The enzyme supplementation of diets with lower NSP levels produced effects in same direction but differences fail to be of any statistical significance.

Due to varying nature of feed stuffs used, and variation in the enzyme properties, different workers have reported different results. The results are as diverse as ones reporting no effect of enzymes on one end, to significant improvement in body weight FCR, livability etc. The variation could be explained by the wide variation in feed stuffs, genotype of birds used, enzymes used, nature of mixing, feed manipulation and many other micro-macro environmental condition. The Table 16.4 summarizes the observations of various workers on the use of fibre degrading enzymes in the poultry ration.

Phytase

The main part of plant phosphorus is present at phytic acid and phytases (myoinositol – hexaphosphate) which is poorly available for poultry. The supplementation of phytase in the feed improves the utilization of phosphorus from the phytates and improves the utilization of other minerals which are bound to phytate complex. As a consequence of the improved utilization of phytates like phosphorus excretion is reduced and the use of inorganic phosphorus in the diet could be reduced significantly. Phytate can increase the phosphorus availability in the grains and oilseed meal by 25-50% and reduce the phosphorus excretion by 15-40% in grain based poultry feed. The positive effect of phytase supplementations in broiler diets in terms of nitrogen retention, energy retention, higher Ca availability reduced P excretion, more tibial ash, high serum Ca and inorganic P, more availability of Mn and Zn etc. has been demonstrated. One of the greatest benefits of phytase supplementation seems to be the maintenance of liability at a lower dietary

Table 16.4: Effect of Enzyme(s) Supplementation of Different Poultry Rations

Sl. No.	Type of poultry	Enzyme(s) used	Ration	Effect
(1)	(2)	(3)	(4)	(5)
1.	Broiler	Cellulase	Guar meal based diets	Increased LWG. Better FCR
2.	Broiler	Glucanase	Barley based diets	-do-
3.	Broiler	Cellulase (extract from Iprex lacteus	Barley based diets	-do-
4.	Broiler	Amylase (extract from Bacillus subtulis)	Barley based diets	-do-
5.	Broiler	Pectinase	Rye based diets	-do-
6.	Poultry	Cellulase	Wheat, Lucerene, rapeseed based diets	No effect
7.	Poultry	Cellulase	Maize, Soyabean diets	Improved LWG and marginal improvement in FCR
8.	Broiler	Hemicellulase	Guar meal based diets	Improved FCR
9.	Chicks, ducks, and geese	Hemicellulase and Pectinase	Maize, Soyabean and wheat based diets	No effect on LWG
10.	Layers	Kezyme (amylase, glucanase, cellulase, protease, lipase)	—	Increased EP and egg size
11.	Broiler	B-glucanase	Hulled and hull-less barley, oats and wheat based diets	Increased LWG and Improved FCR
12.	Broiler	Cellulase (extract *T. viridae*)	High roughage diets	+ve effect in BW, mortality not affected
13.	Broiler	Arabinoxylans	Barley and rye based diet	Increased LWG, FI and improved FCR
14.	Broiler	Provico (B-glucanase)	Barley based diets	Improved performance. No effect in faecal consistency
15.	Broiler	GP500 (B-glucanase, arabinoxylans)	High protein diets	Decreased wet dropping
		Novozym343 (B-glucanase, arabinoxylans)	Low protein diets	Improved performance
16.	Broiler	Ekanoza (B-glucanase, cellulase, hemi-cellulase) extract from <u>T. reesei</u>	Wheat and Barley based diets	Increased BW, better FCR no effect on survivability
17.	Broiler	Novozym 343	—	Better performance but the effect was apparent after 3-weeks of age.

18.	Broiler	Novozym 343	Whole barley diets	Increased LWG and improved FCR
19.	Broiler	B-glucans, Pentosans	Wheat, barley, rye and oats based diets	Increased AMEn and LWG, Better FCR
20.	Broiler	Roxazyme (Cellulase, glucanase, xylanase, pectinase, amylase from T viridae	Pelleted feed	Better FCR
21.	Layer	Biofeed	Wheat and Rye based diets	Increased viscosity in Jejunum and ileum, effect on fat digestibility.
22.	Layer	Cellulase, glucanase, xylanase	Barley	Increased energy utilization
23.	Poultry	Multienzyme mixture	Cereal based diets	Better performance and decreased viscosity of excreta
24.	Broiler	Multienzyme mixture (Cellulase, xylanase, B-glucanase, amylase and pectinase)	—	Positive effect on growth, FCR and carcass quality
25.	Layer	Enzyme mixture	Sorghum and soya based diets	Increased nutrient utilization
26.	Broiler	Xylanase	Wheat based rations	Improved AMEn, nutrient digestibility and FCR. Digesta viscosity decreased.
27.	Broiler	Enzyme mixture	Barley based diets	Growth increased with increased enzyme concentration
28.	Broiler	Galactosidase	Dehulled peas	FC increased LWG and FCR not affected
29.	Broiler	Pectinase	Dehulled peas	FC increased LWG and FCR not affected
30.	Chicks and ducks	Enzymes targeting NSPs	Rice bran based diets	No effect
31.	Broiler	Enzyme mixture	Wheat and Maize based diet	Improved LWG and FCR
32.	Broiler	Enzyme mixture	Wheat based diet	Effect observed when wheat content is more than 80 g/kg
33.	Broiler	B-glucanase	Barley and Wheat based diets	Improved LWG, and FCR, Increased water intake
34.	Broiler	Xylanase and Protease	Barley and Wheat based diets	No effect on LWG, Poor FCR
35.	Broiler	Enzyme mixture	—	Increased dressing%. Decreased P and ALP

Table 16.4: *Effect of Enzyme(s) Supplementation of Different Poultry Rations* (Contd.)

Sl. No.	Type of poultry	Enzyme(s) used	Ration	Effect
(1)	(2)	(3)	(4)	(5)
				activity
36.	Broiler	Allzyme Vegpro (Amylase, Protease, Xylanase)	Com and Soya based diets	Improved illeal digestibility of nutrients
37.	Quails	Grindazym	Wheat and Barley based diets	Improved performance and carcass yield
38.	Broiler	—	Whole barley based diets	Improved carcass traits
39.	Broiler	Xylanase and Pectinase	Sunflower Extract rich diets	Decreased viscosity Decreased litter moisture Marginal increase in BW
40.	Broiler	Xylanase and Cellulase	Sunflower Extract rich diets	Decreased viscosity Decreased litter moisture Marginal increase in BW
41.	Broiler	Maxigest (-amylase, galactosidase, pectinase, acid protease, diets cellulase, lipase, hemic-ellulase, phytase and invertase.	Maize, sunflower and fishmeal based diets	Increased performance and economy
42.	Broiler	—	Soya bean replaced with canola meal	Increased dressing %, breast, thigh, drumstick yield
43.	Layer	Enzyme mixture	Wheat and Barley based diets	Increased performance
44.	Broiler	Multi enzyme mixture	Apple pomace based diets	Masks depression caused by apple pomace supplementation
45.	Layer	Cellulase	High fibre layer ration	Cost of production decreased
46.	Layer	Cellulase	High fibre layer ration	Increased nutrient utilization
47.	Broiler	Avizyme	Maize replaced with different levels of Ajar seed meal	Masks depression caused by Ajar seed meal
48.	Broiler	Multi enzyme mixture	Standard broiler ration	Improved BW, LWG, FC and FCR and profit per bird

LWG - Live weight gain BW - Body weight FCR - Feed conversion ratio
FC - Feed Consumption AMEn - Apparent metabolisable energy

level of non-phytate phosphorus. Phytase supplementation is also known to increase the body weight and FCR of the broilers. Phytase is more efficient with a lower, than high non-phytate-phosphorus diet in broiler.

Factors affecting the efficacy of enzymes:

Substrate Binding

The enzymatic efficacy may be regulated by allosteric alternation of substrate binding affinity. Substrate binding induces a tertiary conformational shift in the catalytic subunits of an enzyme, which increases the subunits substrate binding affinity and thus increases the enzyme's catalytic efficiency.

pH

Enzymes being proteins, have properties that are quite pH sensitive. Most proteins in fact are active only within a narrow pH range, typically 5-9. In the same way efficacy of enzymes is maximum in the same pH range because in this range enzyme has lower K_m and higher V_{max} values. pH of reaction mixture changes efficacy by affecting through combination of factors viz.

(a) Binding of substrate to enzyme
(b) Catalytic activity of the enzyme
(c) Ionisation of the substrate
(d) Variation of protein structure

Temperature

The velocity of any reaction catalysed by an enzyme, increases with an increase in the temperature and it doubles approximately for every 10°C rise in temperature thus indicating that rise in temperature increases the efficiency of an enzyme by decreasing its Km (substrate concentration at half maximum velocity) and increasing Vmax (Maximum velocity) But at very high temperatures, loss of enzyme efficiency is due to thermal conformational change of this enzyme. Most enzymes are inactivated at temperature above 50-60°C.

Ionic Strength

Ionic concentration in the reaction mixture affects the active site of an enzyme thus modulating the enzyme's efficacy positively or negatively depending upon the type of ion and other modulating factors.

Methods of Enzyme Supplementation

The enzymes are added in form of
(i) powders
(ii) granules
(iii) liquids

Possible Effect of Enzyme Supplementation on Cereal Based Diets

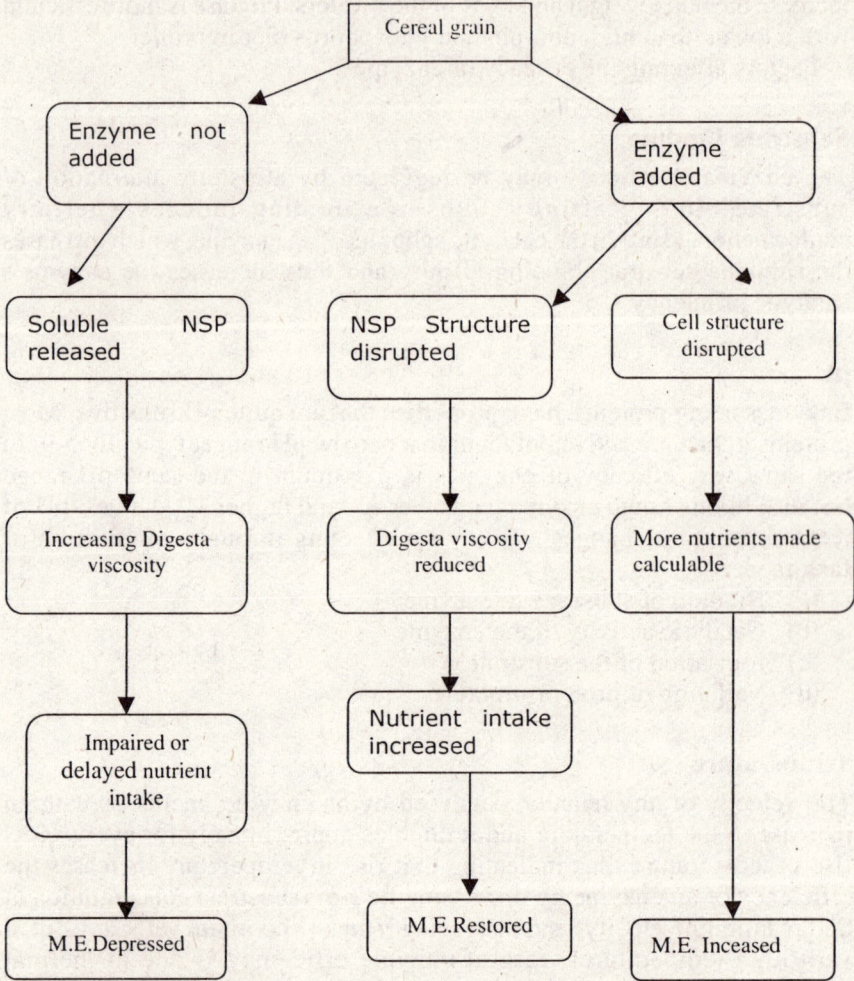

Fig. 16.3: Possible effect of enzyme supplementation

Powder and granules are mixed with diets before pelleting. This allows uniform mixing. However, many enzymes tend to be thermolabile at processing. High temperatures is likely to reduce their activity. This limitation can be overcome by coating liquid enzymes on surfaces of pellets or crump after processing.

Qualities of feed Enzymes

1. Should be potent
2. Should be available in adequate concentration
3. Should have a long storage life

4. Should be cheaply and easily available
5. Should be available in the form which can allow easy mixing with derived ingredients
6. Should not get inactivated by feed processing
7. Should be active in wide range of pH and temperature
8. Should be purchased from a reputed company and activity; composition etc. should be mentioned on the packing.

Animal Feeding Requirements

Feeding grain crops to animals always entails a loss of potential food output: food grains cultivated in place of feed crops would yield more digestible energy, as well as more protein, although meat protein is superior to that harvested in cereals or legumes. Energy and protein losses caused by inherent inefficiencies of animal growth and metabolism vary widely among domesticated species. The most common choice for calculating that inefficiency – in the United States as units of feed, expressed in terms of corn equivalents containing gross energy of 3,670 kcal/kg, needed per unit of live weight gain – misleads in several ways. Edible parts of meat supply range from less than 30 per cent to more than 60 per cent of live weight.

No commercial meat is produced with higher feeding efficiency and at a faster rate than that of chicken. In the United States the average time needed to produce a broiler was cut from 72 days in 1960 to 48 days in 1995, while the bird's average slaughter weight rose from 1.8 to 2.2 kg and the feed/gain rate fell by about 15 per cent. When chickens are fed a well-balanced diet (a mixture of corn and soybeans containing about 21 per cent protein), cumulative feed/gain ratios are as low as 1.5 – 1.8 for lighter birds slaughtered after 4-6 weeks, and between 1.8 and 2.0 for birds in the most common range of 2.0-2.5 kg. The USDA's long-term records on poultry production, available from the mid-1930s when broilers were produced no more efficiently than pigs, show the only instance of a steady improvement of average feeding efficiency among the country's meat animals.

Pigs make good meat animals because their basal metabolism is up to 40 per cent lower than expected for their body mass, while for cattle it is up to 15 per cent higher than expected. As a result, pigs at the midpoint of their growth will convert almost two-thirds of their metabolized energy into weight gain, while the share for a 300-kg steer is only around 45 percent. Moreover, pigs have a short gestation time (114 days) and a high reproduction rate (litter ranging from 8 to 18) and they grow rapidly, reaching slaughter weights (90 to 100 kg) just 100-160 days after weaning. The feed/gain rate for North American pigs from weaning to slaughter ranges between 2.5 and 3.5.

The addition of feeding costs of the breeding stock and adjustments for environmental stresses, disease, and premature mortality can significantly raise overall feed/gain rates. The long-term records of pig feeding kept by the US Department of Agriculture since 1910 show a nationwide feed/live weight gain ration of 6.7 in 1910, and after an initial decline it has fluctuated between 5.0 and 6.5 ever since. The main reason why continuous improvements in feeding have not resulted in better gain rates has been the quest for less fatty pigs. Leaner animals are inherently more costly to produce than lardy ones: the efficiency of metabolizable energy conversion to protein in pigs peaks at about 45 per cent, while conversion of feed to fat can be as much as 75 per cent efficient.

Calculations of overall feed/gain efficiency ratios for beef are complicated by a variety of arrangements under which meat production takes place. The two extremes are entirely grass-fed beef that requires no feed concentrates, and calves raised after weaning in a feedlot on a diet of grain combined with feed additives, growth promoters, and disease preventers (a minimal share of roughages must be included for normal ruminant digestion). The actual time that North American beef animals spend in feedlots on high-grain diets varies greatly. Calves born in early spring may remain with cows on pasture until November and then (weighing 200-300 kg/head) they are either moved to a feedlot or maintained on forage for another year and only then (as yearlings weighing 300-400 kg) put on a diet of concentrates. Feedlot animals gain between 1.0 and 1.3 kg a day – growing much faster than grazing animals, whose daily gains average no more than 0.5 kg – and they spend commonly up to 200 days in feedlots before reaching the market weight of around 500 kg.

While cattle are unmatched converters of roughages that can be digested only by ruminants they are relatively poor performers in turning grain feed into meat. Thus a leading expert on and proponents of cattle husbandry concluded that feeding grain to ruminants is biological and economic nonsense: it is a misuse of arable resources, a misuse of a ruminant animals objective potential, it is polluting, it is dependent on whims of economic policy and it is driven by commercial gain, not human need.

As already noted, cattle's basal metabolism is higher than expected, and their large body mass and long gestation and lactation mean that the feed requirements of breeding females in cattle herds claim at least 50 per cent more energy than required for pigs. For growing and finishing steer and heifers (calves and yearlings), North American and European feed/live weight gain ratios range between 6 and 9. Adjusting these rates for the costs of reproduction and growth and maintenance of sire and dam animals raises the feed/gain ratio of herds to over 10 and the USDA's feed/gain data for all of the country's cattle and calves show a pattern fluctuating between 9 and 14 kg of corn equivalents per kg of live weight gain. But because nearly all beef animals in North America spend only a part of their lives on a grain diet (they enter feedlots only after they reach 45-60 per cent of their final weight), this total should be adjusted downward for a more meaningful comparison with nonruminant animals whose diet does not include forages.

Using the typical USDA rates for entire animal populations and expressing the feeding efficiencies in units of concentrate feed per unit of edible weight only accentuates the differences among major kinds of meat produced from cereal and leguminous grains (Table 16.5). Broilers are by far the most efficient producers, pigs require roughly twice as much feed per unit of edible meat, and feedlot- fed beef needs five times as much grain per kg of meat as chickens. Chickens are also the best converters of plant-to-animal protein (about 20 per cent efficiency), beef cattle again the worst.

Table 16.5: Feed Conversion Efficiencies of Major Animal Foods

	Milk	Carp	Eggs	Chicken	Pork	Beef
Feed conversion (kg of feed/kg of live weight)	0.7	1.5	3.8	2.5	5.0	10.0
Feed conversion (kg of feed/kg of edible weight)	0.7	2.3	4.2	4.5	9.4	25.0
Protein content (% of edible weight)	3.5	18	13	20	14	15
Protein conversion efficiency (%)	40	30	30	20	10	4

Typical efficiencies of protein production via animal feeding are thus very wasteful: at least 80 per cent and as much as 96 per cent of all protein in cereal and leguminous grains fed to animals are not converted to edible protein. Metabolic imperatives dictate that any meat production exploiting mammalian or avian species must be a less efficient way of securing high-quality and easily digestible animal protein than is provided in milk and eggs. Consequently, if the delivery of superior protein was the only objective of animal husbandry, then all high-quality feed should be reserved for dairy cows and laying hens; and the only meat-producing animals that would not compete for arable land with humans would be ruminants, animals that are uniquely adept at converting feed that no other domesticated species can use, raised on grasslands that are not potentially suitable for conversion to crop fields. But people choose to eat specific foodstuffs, not generic nutrients, and their preference for meat causes many environmental disruption.

LIVESTOCK FEED INDUSTRY

The production of compound livestock feed in the country has made substantial progress with the increasing demand for cattle as well as poultry feed. The total production was hardly 39,400 tonnes in 1964, which touched 1.08 lakh tonnes in 1966, 2.09 lakh tonnes in 1971 and 4.02 lakh tonnes, it virtually jumped to 8.06 lakh tonnes in 1977. The uptrend in production could not be sustained and the production dropped to 6.54 lakh tonnes in 1978 before staging a partial recovery to 7.88 lakh tonnes in 1979.

It was after this that the past two decades have almost seen an upward trend in production from nine lakh tonnes in 1980 to 13.70 lakh tonnes in 1985, 21.61 lakh tonnes in 1990 and 28.10 lakh tonnes during 1995-96 (Table 16.6).

Table 16.6: Trend of Compound Feed Production in India

Year	Cattle and other feeds	Poultry feeds	Total
1970	125.4	84.3	209.7
1975	275.3	143.9	419.2
1980	549.9	350.8	900.1
1981	590.9	359.3	950.2
1982	618.9	325.3	944.2
1983	663.9	348.9	1012.8
1984	746.4	406.8	1153.2
1985	867.3	502.8	1370.1
1986	924.8	567.4	1492.2
1987	1208.9	630.3	1839.2
1988	1116.1	709.2	1825.3
1989	1151.3	772.5	1922.8
1990	1324.5	833.7	2161.2
91-92	1479.2	942.8	2422.0
92-93	1454.2	805.6	2259.8
93-94	1370.8	876.5	2473.3
94-95	1442.8	1063.6	2506.4
95-96	1542.8	1267.8	2810.6

Source: World Bank; India Livestock Sector Review. 1996

Of this, the production of cattle and other feeds have grown from 25,000 tonnes in 1964 to 1.25 lakh tonnes in 1970, 2.75 lakh tonnes in 1975, 5.49 lakh tonnes in 1980, 8.67 lakh tonnes in 1985 and 13.24 lakh tonnes in 1990. In 1995-96, the production was estimated to have reached 15.43 lakh tonnes.

In the case of poultry feeds, however, the production recorded a gradual increase until a decade ago and in fact there was a major growth during the period 1993-94 to 1995-96. Production of poultry feeds increased from 14,400 tonnes in 1964 to 84,300 tonnes in 1970, 1.43 lakh tonnes in 1975, 3.50 lakh tonnes in 1980, 5.02 lakh tonnes in 1985 and 8.33 lakh tonnes in 1990. The production touched 9.42 lakh tonnes in 1991-92 before declining to 8.05 lakh tonnes in 1992-93. Thereafter, it recovered to 8.76 lakh tonnes in 1993-94 and was up at 10.63 lakh tonnes in 1994-95 and further to a new high of 12.68 lakh tonnes in 1995-96. The growth in this industry could have been still better but for the constraints created by various authorities. Major among these were classification of animal feed supplements and additives for excise purpose, licensing requirement for the import of animal feed supplements, quality standards for feeds and its coverage under the Essential Commodities Act. Prior to the presentation of the 1996-97 Union Budget, dicalcium phosphate (DCP) was exempted from the excise for its use as an ingredient in the manufacture of animal feed supplements. However, 1996-97 Finance Bill sought to rescind many exemption notification and in the process the notification No. 7/94 CE exempting DCP from excise for feed was also rescinded.

Animal feed is a crucial and indispensable agri-input and accordingly is exempted from excise duty. DCP is an essential ingredient of a balanced animal feed. It is unfair to make the manufacturer pay the so-called potential revenue even if the department has doubts about classification. Proper steps like chemical analysis of the products, trade parlance and use, along with the opinions of experts can decide whether the classification of animal feed supplements under chapter 23.02 needs a change. The merits of the product should be tested before initiating any action leading to perforce payment of duty by the manufacturers of feed supplements.

Animal feed is also one of the commodity covered under the Essential Commodities Act of 1955. The total requirement of animal feeds in the country is estimated around 37 million tonnes comprising 30 million tonnes of cattle feed, six million tonnes of poultry feed and one million tonnes of other animals and aquatic feeds. In this, animal feed produced by the members of the Compound Livestock Feed Manufacturers' Association of India (CLFMA) represents a very small proportion of 1.5 million tonnes in the case of cattle feed accounting for around five per cent and 1.25 million tonnes in the case of poultry feed representing 21 percent of the total.

There are, however, a large number of manufacturers outside CLFMA membership who grind various raw materials and mix them with an intention to sell without branding, and they are currently out of the scope of any order to control the quality of animal feeds. In the absence of analytical laboratories or any means of analyzing various quality parameters, the feed supplied by them is totally substandard and of low quality, yet, they are not required to take any registration or licence and follow quality standards. Another section of manufacturers, who manufacture animal feeds without branding, barter these feeds with farmers. They also are not covered under any feed quality regulations. One more category of feed manufacturers who are not covered under any quality control standards are those who mix feeds as per the instructions of the purchasers.

These three types of animal feed manufacturers together account for the alarmingly large proportion of animal feeds production in the country. If they are not brought under the purview of the proposed legislation by the state governments who regulate and control the manufacture and sale of poultry and livestock feed, it would not only amount to discrimination but would also be self-defeating. The very purpose of bringing in legislation for controlling the quality of animal feed would be totally lost if it covers only a small percentage of registered feed manufacturers like CLFMA members and leave out a very large proportion of manufacturers.

This is a competitive industry and the private industry and trade can survive only if it meets the required standards and supplies feeds under various conditions of farming. Further, the genetic potentiality of livestock and poultry has been improving every year. The nutritional requirements and the parameters also have undergone tremendous changes over the past few years. For instance, a hen-housed egg production by the layer bird which was less than 250 around five years ago, has presently reached 310, and so have the nutritional needs of these high producing layers.

A major genetic improvement has happened to broilers the world over. The potential of broilers to attain a weight of 1.5 kg in five weeks is a very common occurrence. The nutrient requirements of these birds also have undergone a sea change. Similarly, the mere emphasis on minimum crude protein has also undergone a metamorphic change. Presently, research scientists have been expressing the birds' requirements in terms of digestible and available amino acids, which also have been dynamically changing. Under the circumstances, fixing up rigid standards without providing scope for such improvements may stifle research, innovation and advancements.

The Feed Deficit

Inadequate nutrition is the major constraint for raising animal productivity in India like many other developing countries. National feed balance calculations, such as those estimated by the Wasteland Development Board and the Ministry of Agriculture consistently project feed deficiencies of about 20-30 percent of requirements, equivalent to 250 million tonnes dry feed per year (Table 16.7).

More conservative estimates worked out by the World Bank, showed a total dry matter (DM) availability of about 480 million tonnes and a requirement of about 735 million tonnes in 19 95 (Table 16.8). Natural grazing is the most difficult to estimate and slight changes in the assumptions regarding natural grazing yields have considerable impact on the size of

Table 16.7: Estimated Feed and Nutrients Balance in India in 1991

Estimated Nutrient Availability and Requirements in 1991

Nutrient	Availability	Requirement million tonnes	Deficiency	Percent deficiency
Dry Matter	530.25	766.19	235.94	31
Digestible Crude Protein	15.10	35.82	20.72	58
Total Digestible Nutrients	283.16	412.80	129.65	31

Estimated Feed and Fodder Availability and Requirement in India 1991

Feed Components	Availability (million tonnes)	Requirement (million tonnes)	Deficiency	Percent deficiency
Straw/stovers	398.88	583.62	134.74	31
Green fodder	573.50	744.73	171.23	23
Concentrate	41.98	79.40	37.42	47

Source: Singh, P., and Majubar, A.B. Current Status of Feed and Forage in Management of Livestock: in Agricultural Situation in India: August 1992: pp. 375-382.

Table 16.8: Requirement and Availability of Feed in 1995

(Million tons dry matter)

Item	Type	Roughage	Concentrate Feed
Supply	Grazing	213	33.1
	Crops and crop residue	271	
Total		**484**	**33.1**
Requirements	Cattle and buffaloes	606	24.3
	Small ruminants	122	1.9
	Poultry	0	4.5
	Pigs	0.7	4.4
Total		**735**	**35.7**
Balance		**- 251**	**- 2.6**
Deficit as % of requirements		**41.4**	**7.2**

Source: World Bank: India Livestock Sector Review: Enhancing Growth and Development: May 23, 1996. Annex Table 3.2c, pp. 104-105.

deficit. For example, an increase of forest grazing yields of only one tonne DM per hectare per year would decrease the deficit by one third. For concentrate feeds, supply estimates can be more precise. Most estimates show an annual production of about 33 million tonnes. In the case of concentrates, the debate focuses on the requirements, and especially those of the traditional sector. Most national calculations show a feed deficit of about 50 – 60 million tonnes (15.0 percent of the requirements), mainly the result of the assumptions of 0.5–1.0 kg per animal consumption per day by the traditional sector. If, as is likely, farmers do not find this economically justified, the estimated deficit would be only 3 million tonnes.

Regional deficits are more important than the national deficit, especially for roughage, which is not economical to transport over long distances. According to the latest estimate available for the year 1991 from the National Wasteland Development Board, 43 out of the total 55 micro-regions exhibited deficits; only 12 micro-regions exhibited surplus. In the surplus regions, improved livestock are mostly stall-fed. In the hills and dry western regions of Rajasthan and Gujarat, the surplus is attributable to the large quantity of pasture grasses produced from the vast range and pasture lands. In most deficit states, the deficiency is due to the large livestock population, little or no area under fodder, and very low biomass from degraded/marginal lands (0.5-1 ton dry matter/hectare).

The deficit is likely to increase in the future. National feed balances predict a further widening gap in concentrate supply of about 60 million tonnes by the year 2016.[1] The rate of growth of the poultry industry will be an important factor influencing the feed demand pressure. A continuation

---

[1] Alpha Agritech Consultants Ltd.,, Feed and Fodder Production: Consultant's report prepared for the World Bank: 1994.

of the growth of the commercial broiler industry registered during the recent years (15 percent per year) would increase requirements of that sector by about 3.5 million tonnes per year. A doubling of the number of improved dairy cows over the same period would increase demand by another 10 million tonnes.

Tackling the Problem of Feed Deficit

Several factors contribute to the feed deficit. The continued growth of the livestock population has been fostered by increasing demand, sociocultural factors which inhibit the killing of cows, low output prices which slows down the uptake of more productive stock and increase in incentive to maintain larger herds compensate for low productivity, and a shift to small ruminants in the more degraded areas. Large livestock population combined with changes in government land policy, have contributed to the reduction in size of the common grazing areas and the breakdown of the traditional institutions managing these areas.

As a result of population growth, the pressure on the traditional grazing area (pastures and forests) has increased. Most natural grazing area (community pastures and grazing lands, community forests, and wasteland) is common property resources (CPR). Two important factors have contributed to the decline and subsequent degrading of the common property grazing areas: (i) the change in land policy of the GOI, initiated in the early 1950s and (ii) population growth.

A major factor contributing to the degradation of common property grazing areas has been their conversion into open access areas. This has been to a large extent due to changes in government land policy beginning in the 1950s. Because the government was unable to acquire adequate land for redistribution through land ceiling laws or voluntary donation, it decided to distribute some of the common lands instead. Privatization was carried out either through the formal distribution of common lands to the landless and other groups or through the legalization or illegal grabbing of such lands by more powerful groups. Both actions increased the pressure on the remaining common areas. The traditional management systems for CPRs (including usage regulation, enforcement of user obligations, and investments in conservation and development) were also seriously weakened in many areas when the traditional institutions were replaced by the administrative structures such as village panchayat system or elected village councils.

The increased use of concentrate feeds could reduce demand for fodder, but it is discouraged by government dairy policies and other market interventions. Demand for concentrate cattle feed remain limited in India. This is despite the fact the price of feed relative to milk prices is more favourable in India compared to other major milk producing countries. For cattle, a major factor contributing to the low demand is the predominance of low productivity animals, which makes the use of concentrate feeds less profitable. The adoption of improved and higher yielding animals, which would demand higher quality feeds, however, is slowed by low milk prices and poor availability of veterinary services in many areas. Inefficiency in the dairy-processing sector further contributes to low milk prices.

A number of regulations also inhibit the efficient distribution of feed ingredients. Movement controls on coarse grains and cereals under the Essential Commodities Act hinder arbitrage between surplus and deficit areas, while storage controls limit private interseasonal storage. Multiple central and state taxation increase marketing costs.

The weak domestic demand for concentrate feeds and heavy reliance on fodder has had a serious negative spillover effect on the environment. Overgrazing in many areas is causing serious degradation problems in many common grazing areas and forests. Another major constraint to the expansion of the feed concentrate sector is the small and highly volatile supply of quality feed ingredients. Feed manufacturing often face problems of adulteration of feed ingredients, such as when urea and sawdust are added to fishmeal. Poor post-harvest handling and storage of feed ingredients result in low quality inputs. Quality standards are available from the Bureau of Indian Standards, but no mechanism ensures that these standards are met by the industry for both ingredients and finished products.

It is also essential to address constraints in the poultry feed sector. Presently, the price of poultry feed relative to output is considerably higher in India in relation to other countries, such as US. For example, the value of one kg of broiler meat in the US is equivalent to 7.2 kg of broiler feed, compared with India's 4.9 kg of feed. Increasing domestic production of maize, a major ingredient in poultry feed, will likely contribute the reduction of poultry feed prices. An important factor contributing to the high cost of poultry concentrate feed is a 1977 regulation restricting poultry feed manufacture, with the exception of poultry feed in pellet form, to small scale enterprises. Only new units are subject to the regulation, however; medium-size and large units manufacturing poultry feed prior to the enactment of the regulation are exempt. The regulation does not apply to cattle feed manufacture, although the same processing facilities are often used to manufacture both feeds.

This restrictive policy inhibits the development of both the feed and poultry industry. Currently, the large capacity modern feed mills in both private and cooperative sectors have underutilized capacity. Moreover, firms cannot take advantage of economies of scale, thus increasing the cost of production. Since poultry feed preparation requires sophisticated technology and small enterprises do not have the capacity to make such investments, limiting poultry feed production to small-scale enterprises also hampers production of standardized high-quality feed products.

For addressing the feed sector's problems in India, the World Bank has recommended adoption of a four-pronged strategy that [1].

---

[1]World Bank: India Livestock Sector Review: Enhancing Growth and Development; May 23, 1996

- Improves incentives for adopting improved stock, both to increase productivity and feed efficiency and to remove the incentives to keep large herds of low-productivity animals;
- Improves the management of the environmentally fragile areas to restore and increase their productivity;
- Eliminates economic barriers to the increased availability of concentrate feed; and
- Increases integration of crop and livestock production systems, and promotes more efficient use of crop byproducts.

Action will have to be taken by the GOI and the States to address the Resource Degradation Problem. To restore the productivity of the degraded common grazing areas and common fodder supply sources, efforts should be made to establish or strengthen grassroot community and user groups who would be responsible for managing the common property areas. A comprehensive approach would involve:

- At the Central Government Level: Establishing national guidelines for allowing user groups to manage the common property grazing areas.
- At the State Level: Enacting legislative reforms to allow user groups to manage common property grazing areas. Adopting mechanisms (such as a microplanning approach and collaboration with nongovernmental organizations) to identify common property areas and, in cooperation with users and user groups, develop area management plans. Alternative management approaches could include cut-and-carry and stall feeding systems in the rural areas, and introduction of grazing fees, and rotational grazing; and
- Formulating supportive mechanisms (such as initial matching grants and loans) to compensate user groups for the temporary closure of degraded grazing areas until productivity is restored.

Liberalizing the Domestic Concentrate Feed sector

is important for increased use of concentrate feed. The domestic marketing of feeds and feed ingredients needs to be further liberalized to reduce their costs, increase their availability, and help ease the pressure on fodder sources. This would involve eliminating laws that impose storage and movement restrictions on feed ingredients and limit poultry feed (except feed in pellet form) and oilseed manufacturing to small-scale enterprises.

The Compound Livestock Feed Manufacturer's Association, with government cooperation, also should review the marketing and feed quality problems and examine ways to improve the distribution and feed quality standards and control.

17

A Comparative Study of Feed/ Roughage Production and Utilization in the Asian Region

Asian region comprises of 82 countries spread over varying agro economic zones, habitats and ecosystems ranging from dry hot to humid tropics and cold deserts. The literacy standards vary from very low to almost 100 percent. On the basis of economic development, there are developed countries like Japan, and Korea. Rest are at varying levels of development and growing economically very rapidly. Japan and Korea is a net importer of feed grains, Japan also imports roughages. While Thailand and India are net exporter of grains, others are marginally self sufficient or net importers. Based on agro ecosystems and farming practices, four countries are selected *for* an in-depth study, namely China, Thailand, Indonesia and India. They represent 70% of the bovine and poultry population of the region. Basic data on production of important commodities and productivity of livestock products in these countries are given in Tables 17.1 and 17.2.

With increasing demand for livestock products on the one hand and uninterrupted increasing human population, and shrinking land area on the other, future hopes of feeding the millions and safeguarding their food security will depend on intensification of agriculture and new breakthrough in food/feed biotechnology. In this context, it is essential to evolve (i) scientific systems to project the demand for foodgrains production and utilization, (ii) for livestock feed and fodder, over short/long periods. This would help in evolving appropriate development policies and a technology agenda for their production/availability. While reasonably strong data base is available about production and human consumption of foodgrains in a major part of the developing world, there is hardly any study available which can help to provide any empirical basis for the present consumption pattern of livestock feed (feedgrains, concentrates and roughages) or project the demand for the same in the major parts of the region.

Table 17.1: Agricultural and Livestock Production in Selected Countries

(Thousand tonnes)

Crop	India		China		Indonesia		Thailand	
	2000	2002	2000	2002	2000	2002	2000	2002
Rice	85,020	75,720	126,542	117,560	34,598	34,386	17,229	17,073
Wheat	76,369	71,814	99,636	90,290	-	-	1	1
Coarse Cereals	31,097	26,355	117,886	133,367	9,677	9,527	4,687	4,435
Total	**192,486**	**173,889**	**344,064**	**341,217**	**44,275**	**43,913**	**21,917**	**21,509**
Total Milk	**81,030**	**84,020**	**12,402**	**17,141**	**798**	**823**	**520.6**	**580.8**
Cow	34,000	35,300	8,632	13,356	498	521	520	580
Buffalo	44,600	46,200	2,650	2.650	-	-	-	-
Sheep	-	-	890	892	100	102	-	-
Goat	2,430	2,520	230	243	200	200	0.6	0.8
Total Meat	**5,001**	**5,339**	**56,707**	**57,888**	**2,048**	**2,074**	**1,797**	**2,092**
Goat & Sheep	697	702	2,386	2,465	84	95	57	59
Beef	1,442	1,462	4,990	5,480	340	324	167	180
Buffalo	1,421	1,443	360	387	46	44	52	58
Pigmeat	469	472	39,946	40,188	760	790	430	475
Poultry Meat	972	1,260	9,025	9,377	818	821	1,091	1,320
Total Eggs	1,749	2,000	22,826	25,010	192	217	807	804
Hen	1,749	2,000	19,433	21,288	51	48	514	500
Others	-	-	3,393	3,722	141	169	293	304

Source: FAOSTAT DATA

CHANGES IN DIETARY PATTERNS

The four countries studied have diverse dietary habits. Indonesia has a significantly large percentage of Muslim population for whom eating pork is a taboo. In India, predominant Hindus regard cattle as sacred and the majority of Indians are vegetarian who obtain their major share of protein from pulses and dairy products. While eating of beef is prohibited for Hindus and pig for Muslims, the consumption of poultry (egg and chicken) is fast increasing in these countries. Chinese food is characterized by a relatively large consumption of pork *and* fried vegetables. For Asian countries, rice can be regarded as the common staple food. However, many depend on other starchy food, such as roots and tubers, in their daily diet. Moreover, in North China and some states of India, rice is not a staple food. Despite these diverse eating habits and customs, certain common changes have taken place in dietary patterns of all these four countries. Most important of these changes is shift from mainly cereals to larger consumption of livestock product.

Table 17.2: A comparative Study of Productivity Levels of Various Livestock Products

Items	China			India			Indonesia			Thailand		
	No.	Prod.	Yield	No.	Prod.	Yield	No.	Prod.	Yield	No.	Prod.	Yield
Cow milk												
2000	4,936	8,632	1,749	36,000	34,000	944	352	498	1,412	201	520	26
2002	5,143	13,356	2,597	37,600	35,300	941	358	521	1,454	230	580	25
MeatBeef & Veal												
2000	36,128	4,990	1,381	14,000	1,442	1,030	1,695	340	201	837	167	200
2002	39,874	5,480	1,374	14,200	1,462	1,030	1,708	324	190	900	180	200
Buffalo meat												
2000	3,605	360	1,002	10,300	1,421	1,380	224	46	205	205	52	253
2002	3,866	387	1,002	10,460	1,443	1,380	209	44	210	230	58	253
Goat meat												
2000	83,328	1,083	13	46,700	467,000	10	4,489	449	10	43	0.6	15
2002	85,160	1,107	13	47,000	470,000	10	5,099	570	10	53	0.8	15
Pig Meat												
2000	510,846	39,946	78	13,400	469	35	13,820	760	55	8,600	430	50
2002	515,230	40,188	78	13,486	472	35	14,364	790	55	9,500	475	50

No.: '000 heads. Prod.: '000 MT, Yield: kg per No.
Source: FAOSTAT DATA for 2000 and 2002.

Regarding the share of food in the total monthly per capita expenditure, the data available for the four countries are for different years (Table 17.3) but by and large the food expenditure shares in the four countries confirm Engel's Law that as income or expenditure increases, the food expenditure

Table 17.3: Food Expenditure Share (in US dollar)

Year	China, 1988		India, 1993-94		Indonesia,	Thailand,
	Rural	Urban	Rural	Urban	1993	1988
Monthly/capita expenditure (US $)	10.67	24.73	10.8	17.6	32.26	44.35
Food expenditure share (%)	53.41	51.36	63.2	54.7	36.2	39.80
Cereal	36.55	13.34	24.2	14.0	24.3	27.3
Meat	16.83	30.03	3.3	3.4	5.2	28.4
Dairy product	N.A	N.A	9.5	9.8	5.0	6.4
Vegetable	11.59	12.47	6.0	5.5	8.8	6.9
Fruit	N.A.	N.A.	1.7	2.7	4.7	19.0*

Source: NSSO, 50th Round for India; Office of Agricultural Economics for Thailand; Guoqiang 1997 for China; Gunawan 1997 for Indonesia.
Note: In India meat includes meat, eggs and fish. In Thailand monthly expenditure per capita and food expenditure share are those of production workers. The shares are percentages in the food expenditure.

share decreases. Among these four countries, the highest share of expenditure on food is in rural India (63.2%), while that of Indonesia is the lowest at 36.2%. Socioeconomic profiles of these countries reflect the changes in social structure which determines the feeding patterns.

There is a clear contrast in the long-run trend of direct consumption of certain livestock and dairy products. A decreasing trend of cereal consumption is observed in all the countries except for rural areas in China. This may be due to the overall early stage of rural socioeconomic development there where cereal consumption has not yet reached its satiation point. The most remarkable decrease in cereal consumption is in urban areas of China where per capita cereal consumption decreased from 145.4 kg/capita/year in 1978 to 97.8 kg/capita/year in 1993. As for Thailand and India there is a relatively large decline in cereal consumption which fell by more than 10% during the early or middle 1970s to the latter half of 1980s. Indonesia, however, is the only country among this group where per capita consumption of cereals has increased.

An analysis of the Thai dietary pattern shows that meat is becoming more important in the daily diet. Therefore, it is expected that demand for meat will increase. Using the RAPA data base (from a study undertaken in Thailand by FAO) for function types and parameters, the demand for meat, eggs, and milk in 2001 was estimated. The estimation was done under the assumption that the population grows at a rate of 1.04% annually and per capita income expenditure growth rate is 7.18 %. The projected quantities of these commodities were converted to demand for feed through the number of livestock

As income increases, the Thai population increases its consumption of meat, eggs and milk. Demand for pork, chicken meat, eggs and milk is estimated to have increased from 382.8, 736,686.8 and 1,226 thousand tonnes in 1996 to 433, 832, 769 and 1,713 thousand tonnes in 2001, respectively. The quantities of meat demand in 2001 were converted to live animals by 5.28, 700.25, 41.02, and 0.68 million heads of swine, chicken, hens and dairy cows, respectively. As a result, feed requirement for the whole livestock industry total 5.4 million tonnes in 2001.

Consumption of other foods, especially meat and milk is low compared to other Asian countries in Indonesia. Besides their relatively high price, this is probably due to the eating habits of most Indonesians who prefer vegetable protein to animal protein. Cereals are the largest source of calories and protein for most of the population, more so than in other countries with similar economic conditions. Surveys on food consumption trends from the 1970s to the 1990s in each of the countries show a shift away from cereal consumption towards meat and dairy products. People in these countries are likely to consume more meat and dairy products as their income improves.

The above discussion would highlight the fact that livestock feeding practices and norms will primarily be effected by changes in dietary pattern of human population and the production systems. While poultry meat is produced under the intensive system every where, systems for producing other types of meat-beef, buffalo, sheep, goat and pig etc.- vary from country to country. China produces nearly 57 million tonnes of meat, of which more than 84 percent is from piggery and poultry (major part in the semi organised extensive sector). Total meat production in India, on the other hand, is estimated at 5.4 million tonnes, of which hardly 10 percent of poultry meat is the contribution of organised sector. The position in Indonesia and Thailand is also similar to China where meat production, although in small quantities, is produced in the organised sector.

WORLD ESTIMATES FOR FEEDGRAINS

The FAO's estimates of world utilization of total cereals, wheat, coarsegrains and rice, for food, feed and other uses, for selected years, are shown in Table 17.4. According to these estimates, as much as 36.4 percent of world cereals production was used for animal feed increased by 88 million tonnes to 710 million tonnes in 2002-03, from 622 million tonnes in 1984-85. Comparative data for world cereal utilization for fees for the FAO and USDA are available only up to 1995-96. These two estimates differ. For instance according to the FAO source, the estimates of cereal utilization for feed for the year 1994-95 was 27 million tonnes higher than for 1995-96, despite lower world production of milk, meat and eggs in 1994-95. The respective figures were 647 million tonnes and 620 million tonnes in 1995-96. The story is however, different, as described below, as per the USDA sources.

According to the USDA data use of the wheat and coarse grains in 1995-96 totaled 641 million tonnes (Table 17.5), against 613 million tonnes estimated by the FAO. According to USDA no rice is fed to animals as feed. Unfortunately, the USDA data for the recent years are not available to the authors. However, in all probability, the difference in the two estimates would have continued.

Data from the two sources do not tally which is possible because the methodology in each case may be different. But what is important in the two sources is that while according to FAO the total quantity of coarse grains, wheat and rice fed to animals came down from 622 to 620 million tonnes during the 11 years period, corresponding figures for USDA are 608.7 and 641.9 million tonnes. A long time data series of USDA shows that the consumption of wheat for feed increased from 60.6 to 97.2 million tonnes (62.3%) and coarse cereals from 336.4 to 568.4 million tonnes (59.2%) during 1968-69 to 1995-96. There is a steady increase up to 1987-88 when estimated feed (wheat and coarse grain) peaked at 661.5 million tonnes. Eight years later (1995-96), the estimate is only 641.9 million tonnes-nearly 20 million tonnes less than the base 1987-88.

According to USDA, rice is not being fed to animals anywhere in the world, but FAO shows that this has increased from 7.0 to 9.0 million tonnes during the same period. Our studies show that small quantities of rice are being consumed by livestock in India. While in China during 1993 as much

Table 17.4: World Cereal Utilization (million tonnes)

Items	Cereals total				Wheat				Coarse grain				Rice			
	84-85	95-96	2001-02	2002-03	84-85	95-96	2001-02	2002-03	84-85	95-96	2001-02	2002-03	84-85	95-96	2001-02	2002-03
Food	768	912	963	967	332	400	424	427	163	190	178	175	273	332	361	365
Feed	622	620	714	710	99	93	105	109	516	518	595	589	7	9	13	12
Other uses*	203	250	263	264	63	72	71	70	112	146	156	159	28	32	36	35
Total	1,593	1,792	1,940	1,941	494	564	600	606	790	855	929	923	308	373	411	412
Feed as % of Total	39.0	34.6	36.8	36.6	20.0	16.5	18.0	18.0	65.3	60.6	54.4	63.8	2.27	2.4	3.2	2.9

*Other uses include seed, industrial uses and waste.
Source: Food Outlook, FAO various issues.

Table 17.5: Consumption of Foodgrains for Feed (Million MT)

	Total production	Feed consumption	Feed as % of total
Wheat, 1995-96	534.7	94.3	17.6
Coarse Grains, 1995-96	787.4	547.6	69.5
Total*	1322.1	641.9	48.6

Source: Grain, World Market & Trade, May 1996, USDA
*According to USDA, no rice is fed to animals as feed.

as 20.0 million tonnes of rice was consumed by the animals. A study by IFPRI shows that the estimated consumption of paddy for feed use was 32.0 million tonnes representing 8.0 per cent of production during 1980. Total consumption of cereals according to the IFPRI study during that year as feed was 681.0 million tonnes representing 43.5 per cent of total production.

A comparison of these three sources of data FAO, USDA and IFPRI depicts a rather confusing picture. IFPRI does not give any annual data series. But for 1980 its estimate was 681.4 million tonnes as against 559.6 million tonnes by USDA. Again for 1984, FAO estimate was 622 million tonnes against USDA 582.2 million tonnes. Besides such varied estimates, one striking feature is that while cereal feed consumption according to FAO and USDA has come down during the last 10-11 years, world production of eggs, meat and milk increased many fold during the same period. With this type of data before us from the three highly respected sources, one would wonder what sanctity can be attached to all these estimates. The only conclusion which one can derive from all this is that none of these organisations which, of course, depends on country information, has any empirical basis for estimating the demand for feedgrains either at the national or international levels. Every one of the players in the game is depending on guess work. IFPRI appreciates that the use of cereals for livestock feed is growing rapidly in developing countries and is reaching significant proportions and that this fact has profound implications for food security of low-income people, employment, and the size of markets available to exporters of cereals and has undertaken a few studies, but no one has tried to find the real ground situation which has its own peculiarities.

Taking the case of China, the largest consumer of feedgrains, we find that besides the national sources, estimates are available from FAO, USDA and IFPRI. None of these however make any sense in the context of livestock products produced by the country. We provide here a comparison of various estimates (Table 17.6).

COUNTRY PROFILE

Indonesia

In the case of Indonesia where per capita consumption of meat is just 0.5 kg. per annum and eggs only 0.3 Kg., FAO Food Balance sheet shows a

Table 17.6: Consumption of feedgrains in China (000 tonnes)

	Rice	Wheat	Maize	Other Cereals	Total
FAO (1992-94)	2,340	3,000	53,667	3,826	62,833
USDA (1993-94)	-	2,700	7,170[1]	-	74,400
National Sources (1993)2	2,000	-	80,000	12,410	124,100
IFPRI (1990-92)	11,000	4,000	56,000	6,000	77,000
(2020)	-	-	-	-	232,000
World Bank	46,300	21,600	-	138,200	206,100
(2020)					

1. Represents total coarse grains,
2. Separate for wheat is not available. This possibly includes all other cereals.

utilization of 739 thousand tonnes of rice and 3050 thousand tonnes of maize during 1992-94 for feed. USDA estimate of total feedgrains used during 1992-93 is 2930 and for 1993-94,3190 thousand tonnes. FAO Food Balance sheet shows a consumption level of 204.8 kg. per annum per capita during 1993-94 and the corresponding figure according to national sources is only 123.2 kg. There is no mention of wheat in the human consumption pattern, although imports have touched nearly 4 million tonnes in recent years- all for human consumption. Calculated on the FAO basis, human consumption of cereals works out to 38.1 million tonnes, leaving a few thousand tonnes for feed, and wastages. At the same time, the country is a net exporter of 0.5 million tonnes of rice and coarse cereals.

All these data have no relation with the National sources. Reliable data on utilization of each commodity for different purposes such as feed, food industries, and human consumption are not available in Indonesia. The time series Food Balance Sheet (FBS) data provide information on the average availability of each crop per capita per year and the use for feed and food industries as well as for human consumption. These data are published by Ministry of Agriculture (MOA) and Central Bureau of Statistics (CBS). Production, export and import on the supply side are regarded as accurate, but the data on feed and food industries which are usually estimated as percentages of total supply are generally very poor. In FBS data, the portion of commodity for seed is estimated as 5%, waste around 20%, and feed 2%. Hence, it is difficult to estimate the trend in demand for industry for a particular commodity using FBS data.

Indonesia produces about 40 million tonnes of cereals, of which around 32.0 million tonnes is rice. According to national sources, 2 per cent of cereals is used for feed. On the basis of total production, it will calculate to 0.8 million tonnes and if restricted to coarse cereals alone, it would mean 0.16 million tonnes. The FAO Food Balance Sheet as against this shows 3.8 million tonnes as feed consumption. Human consumption of maize in Indonesia is around 6 kg per capita per annum. For a total population of 190 million, this will calculate to only 1.14 million tonnes during 1994. Indonesia produced a total of 6.9 million tonnes of maize and imported another 0.5 million tonnes. If the total human, livestock and industrial consumption was hardly 1.3 million tonnes, what happened to the remaining quantity. In nutshell, we will not, therefore, be wrong to assume that, there is a major problem with the collection and interpretation of data about the consumption patterns, not only of feed, but also of human consumption.

Thailand

Thailand produced 3.4 million tonnes of maize during 1993, of which 3.2 million tonnes was used for industry and seed. Industry means primarily feedgrains. National sources give norms for calculating feed requirements which are in terms of concentrates. Total quantity of such concentrates required for 1996 has been calculated as 4.5 million tonnes and 5.4 million tonnes for 2001 (Table 17.7). As against this, FAO Food Balance sheet shows the quantity of foodgrains used for feed during 1992-94 as 4.1 million tonnes, of which 3.5 million tonnes is maize and the balance is rice, although according to national sources no rice is fed to livestock. National sources also calculate the demand for maize for the feed industry as 3.68 million tonnes during 1994. What is the basis of norms fixed as given above is not clear. Even otherwise, although different estimates vary between 3-4 million tonnes, the difference is quite significant in a country where total human consumption is only 12.0 million tonnes.

India

India, is perhaps the only country where feedgrains estimates are lumped together with seed and wastages. A fixed rate of 12.5 per cent has been adopted by the Govt. of India for a period of nearly 50 years for feed, seed and wastages without any empirical basis. This is neither scientific nor does it make any sense. A survey conducted by Techno Economic Research Institute, New Delhi during 1986-87 showed that the total consumption of feedgrains was 10.32 per cent for the northern region with a wide variation (8.22 to 12.01). Some of the scholars in India have estimated feed requirements for the year 2000. Praduman Kumar by counting total livestock production in LOU (Livestock Output Units) concluded that total feed available during TE 1992 was 14.5 million tonnes, of which share of foodgrains was only 2.7 million tonnes.

There are 3 international sources, FAO, World Bank and IFPRI whose estimates are available. FAO Food Balance Sheet gives 1730 thousand tonnes of foodgrains used as feed during 1992-94. As against this, World Bank shows that, during 1995, of the total supply of 33.7 million tonnes of concentrates, against a demand of 31.6 million tonnes, 22.0 million tonnes was from brans of foodgrains and the balance of 11.0 million tonnes from oil cakes. IFPRI estimates, on the other hand calculate the requirements of feedgrains as 52 million tonnes for the year 2000. We tried to approach this problem for the year 1993-94 according to the residual method and found that a total of 10.2 million tonnes of food grains were consumed by livestock in that year. (Table 17.8).

Table 17.7: Meat Demand, Livestock Numbers and Feed Requirement in Thailand

Year	Meat demand (000 tonnes)				Livestock numbers (million head)				Feed requirement (million tonnes)				
	Pork	Broiler	Egg	Milk	Swine	Broiler	Layer	Dairy cattle	Swine	Broiler	Layer	Dairy cattle	Total
1996	382.8	736.1	686.8	1226.0	4.668	619.613	36.629	0.490	1.284	2.231	0.134	0.916	4.565
1997	395.4	756.0	704.0	1322.0	4.822	636.364	37.547	0.529	1.326	2.291	0.137	0.989	4.743
1998	407.7	775.6	720.8	1419.0	4.972	652.862	38.443	0.568	1.367	2.350	0.140	1.062	4.910
1999	419.8	794.8	737.2	1516.7	5.120	669.024	39.317	0.607	1.408	2.408	0.144	1.135	5.095
2000	431.7	813.5	753.3	1614.9	5.265	684.764	40.176	0.646	1.448	2.465	0.147	1.208	5.268
2001	433.2	831.9	769.1	1713.1	5.283	700.252	41.019	0.685	1.453	2.521	0.150	1.281	5.405

Source: Office of Agricultural Economics; Thailand

Table 17.8: Consumption Pattern of Foodgrains in India During 1993-94

	Million tonnes
Human Consumption	
Rural (675 @ 168 kg. per anum.)	111.34
Urban (225 @ 132 – do -)	29.70
Total (900 @ 159 – do -)	141.04
Pulses (Total production)	13.30
Poultry	1.85
(1.54 @ 1.2 tonnes per million)	
Seed of foodgrains	5.00
Wastage (@ 1.5 % for total production + net imports	2.73
(181.9 million tonnes)	
Total	163.92
Total availability 179.48-9.6 (public sector stocks)	172.28
169.88 + 2.4 imports	
Balance for milk & other meat and Work animals	8.36
Work animals	2.5
Breeding Bullocks	0.8
Other meats	1.5
Total	4.8
Balance for milk	3.56
Total production of milk during 1993-94	60.60
Milk produced per kg. of foodgrains consumed: (kgs)	17.0

In the absence of any empirical evidence available to calculate the actual quantity of foodgrains consumed as feed, we have adopted a residual approach based on the following assumptions:

1. Total population as on March 1994 was to 914.1 million. This is based on the 1991 revised figure of 861.4 million and 2% annual growth.
2. With the base population of 896.17 million on March 1993, estimated population fed during 1993-94 is taken as 900 million, of which 225 million at 25 % is calculated as urban.
3. According to the 50th Round (1993-94) NSSO Survey, per capita consumption of cereals was around 168 kg per annum for rural and 132 kg. per annum for urban areas. Adding to this the total production of pulses (13.3 million tonnes), total human consumption comes to 154.34 million tonnes constituting 86 per cent of total production.
4. Based on our study, 1.2 million tonnes of foodgrains are required to produce one million tonnes of chicken/eggs.
5. Seed requirements have been calculated for 122.75 million hect. area under food grains.
6. Since a part of the wasted grain is consumed by livestock, a total of 1.5 per cent of total production and net imports is taken as the grain which is actually wasted. Over 66 percent of wasted grain was used for livestock feeding.

7. Total availability of grain in circulation during 1993-94 is taken as total production (179.48) minus changes in public sector stocks (9.6) plus net imports (2.4 million tonnes).

8. Balance left, 8.35 million tonnes, was fed to animals to produce 3.1 million tonnes meat, 60.6 million tonnes of milk produced during 1993-94, and rest used for work animals and for other livestock etc.

9. India has a special place for Draught Animal Power (DAP) and this aspect of the feed requirement has actually been ignored by practically every body (national/international researchers). This is peculiar to India and its neighbours where animals form a major part of the economy. DAP produces energy equivalent to 6 million tonnes of petroleum, has to have proper energy sources. Assuming that animals have to be fed concentrates say for 100 days in a year and an average of 30 kgs of foodgrains are given per animal per year, requirements of foodgrains for a total of 82.0 million work animals would calculate to 2.5 million tonnes.

10. There are over 12.0 million (including half a million cross bred) non castrated male cattle and about a million male buffaloes kept for breeding. This 13 million or odd breeding bovines, the recommended norm is 0.3 kg per day per animal. Requirement of this group of animals should then be around 0.8 million tonnes.

11. The feed requirements for meat other than chicken has been worked out as 1.5 million tonnes. All the meat from female cattle is a by product. Nearly half (about 7.0 million) buffalo males, around 1.5 million crossbred sheep out of a total of about 50.0 million, some of the 100 million goats, about 1.0 million crossbred pigs (out of a total of over 10.0 million) are getting some concentrates. In the absence of any information available, we assume 1.5 million tonnes of foodgrains for all the 3.1 million tonnes of meat produced other than poultry.

12. Out of a total of 8.5 million tonnes left with us for livestock feeding other than poultry, we are now left with 3.56 million tonnes for milk. This when calculated for 60.6 million tonnes of estimated milk production during 1993-94, gives us a conversion factor of 17.0 kg of milk for one kg of foodgrains (Table 17.8). This appears to be reasonable as compared with our Regional Survey estimate of 14.0 kg milk for one kg. foodgrains for North India where animals are wellfed. It must be appreciated that of the 25 million or so of cattle in milk less than 7% are cross bred. Most of the non descript animals who produce less than 2-2.5 kg of milk no concentrates are fed to them. Proportion of animals producing less than 22.5 kg. of milk is quite high. (Table 17.9 and 17.10).

On the basis of above examination of the published data, from national and international sources, on estimates for livestock feeding (grains and roughages) and projections for 2000 AD, there is neither any basis for

Table 17.9: Number of Milch Cows and Average Milk Yield During 1998-99—State-Wise

States/UTs.	Animals in milk (000 Nos.)		Milch animals (000 Nos.)		Average milk yield per animal in milk per day (kgs.)		Total production (000 tonnes)			
	N.D.	C.B.	N.D.	C.B.	N.D.	C.B.	N.D.	C.B.	Total	%
1	2	3	4	5	6	7	8	9	10	11
Andhra Pradesh	1305.0	165.0	2251.0	220.0	1.80	6.75	859	407	1266	4.2
Arunachal Pradesh	26.6	11.6	40.9	15.3	1.30	7.67	13	32	45	0.1
Assam*	1214.0	99.0	2251.0	160.0	1.05	3.81	466	138	604	2.0
Bihar	1856.0	126.0	6159.0	188.0	1.63	4.91	1105	226	1331	4.4
Goa	16.4	5.1	0.0	0.0	1.85	5.41	11	10	21	0.1
Gujarat	1263.0	98.0	2060.0	133.0	3.00	8.05	1383	287	1670	5.5
Haryana	306.0	134.0	451.0	193.0	4.22	6.70	471	328	799	2.6
Himachal Pradesh	308.7	105.5	562.0	137.0	1.74	3.39	197	129	326	1.1
Jammu & Kashmir*	—	—	—	—	—	—	—	—	0	0.0
Karnataka	1973.0	447.0	3076.0	541.0	2.11	6.25	1520	1020	2540	8.3
Kerala	293.0	856.0	400.0	1224.0	2.55	6.23	273	1947	2220	7.3
Madhya Pradesh	4395.0	103.0	7971.0	201.0	1.32	5.59	2115	210	2325	7.6
Maharashtra	1879.0	625.0	0.0	0.0	1.59	7.07	1087	1613	2700	8.9
Manipur	44.8	11.9	102.0	22.0	1.45	6.50	24	28	52	0.2
Meghalaya	86.5	10.4	182.9	13.4	0.75	8.81	24	33	57	0.2
Mizoram	23.9	4.6	32.1	5.9	1.05	6.39	9	11	20	0.1
Nagaland*	—	—	—	—	—	—	—	—	0	0.0
Orissa	1719.5	189.8	3812.0	316.4	0.51	3.93	317	272	589	1.9
Punjab	183.9	564.0	333.0	880.0	2.79	8.70	187	1792	1979	6.5
Rajasthan*	2215.0	32.0	4467.0	47.0	2.78	5.31	2248	62	2310	7.6

Table 17.9: Number of Milch Cows and Average Milk Yield During 1998-99 — State-Wise (Contd.)

States/UTs.	Animals in milk (000 Nos.)		Milch animals (000 Nos.)		Average milk yield per animal in milk per day (kgs.)		Total production (000 tonnes)			
	N.D.	C.B.	N.D.	C.B.	N.D.	C.B.	N.D.	C.B.	Total	%
1	2	3	4	5	6	7	8	9	10	11
Sikkim*	—	—	—	—	—	—	—	—	0	0.0
Tamil Nadu	1264.0	667.0	2166.0	880.0	2.48	5.90	1144	1435	2579	8.5
Tripura*	—	—	—	—	—	—	55	18	73	0.2
Uttar Pradesh	3555.8	421.5	6174.0	654.0	2.14	6.13	2776	943	3719	12.2
West Bengal	2835.8	366.6	4828.0	511.0	2.07	7.24	2147	969	3116	10.2
A & N Islands	15.0	1.0	27.0	3.0	2.29	4.52	13	2	15	0.0
Chandigarh	0.4	3.4	0.5	3.9	3.50	7.40	1	9	10	0.0
D & N Haveli*	—	—	—	—	—	—	—	—	0	0.0
Daman & Diu*	—	—	—	—	—	—	—	1	1	0.0
Delhi	—	28.0	—	33.0	—	5.61	11	57	68	0.2
Lakshadweep	0.5	0.3	0.5	0.3	3.00	5.00	1	1	2	0.0
Pondicherry	2.0	19.0	3.0	29.0	2.38	4.79	2	32	34	0.1
Total@	26782.8	5094.6	47358.9	6411.2	1.89	6.46	18459	12012	30371	100.0

*Details not available.

@Total of only those States/UTs. for which data are available.

Source: Basic Animal Husbandry Statistics, 2002.

Table 17.10: Details of Estimates of Milk Production from Buffaloes—1998-99 Statewise

States/UTs.	No. of animals in milk (000 Nos.)	No. of milch animals (000 Nos.)	Average yield per animals in milk per day (kgs.)	Estimates of milk production (000 tonnes)
1	2	3	4	5
Andhra Pradesh	3335	4462	2.939	3577
Arunachal Pradesh	—	—	—	—
Assam*	129	205	2.006	94
Bihar	1340	3193	3.354	1640
Goa	16.38	0	3.292	20
Gujarat	2194	3323	3.963	3174
Haryana	1716	2551	5.79	3627
Himachal Pradesh	319.62	474	3.069	359
Jammu & Kashmir*	—	—	—	—
Karnataka	1713	2265	2.66	1662
Kerala	36	50	5.71	75
Madhya Pradesh	2522	4675	2.995	2758
Maharashtra	1962	0	3.699	2650
Manipur*	11	23	3.25	13
Meghalaya	5.448	11.78	1.8	4
Mizoram*	—	—	—	—
Nagaland*	—	—	—	—
Orissa	209.06	402.16	1.845	141
Punjab	2320	3620	6.322	5355
Rajasthan	2610	4460	4.107	3913
Sikkim*	—	—	—	—
Tamil Nadu	1221	1937	3.8	1694
Tripura*	—	—	—	1
Uttar Pradesh	6369.6	9889	3.901	9069
West Bengal	150.7	216	5.716	314
A & N Islands	4	8	2.59	4
Chandigarh	14.04	16.98	6.5	33
D & N Haveli*	—	—	—	—
Daman & Diu*	—	—	—	1
Delhi	110	125	5.766	233
Lakshadweep*	—	—	—	—
Pondicherry	2	2	3.75	2.74
Total@	28310	41909	3.91	40413

*Details not available.

@Total of only those States/UTs for which data are available.

Source: Basic Animal Husbandry Statistics, 2002.

these estimates, nor any type of agreement between the calculated numbers by different agencies. The variation between them is so wide that no reconciliation is possible. Since the importance of livestock products is increasing in human consumption patterns, we recommend that a reasonable empirical basis is established to determine the requirements of feedgrains and projections for future.

To meet the demand for green fodder, a new hybrid is showing promising results. Interspecific hybridisation between bajra (*Pennisetum typhoides*) and napier grass (*Pennisetum purpureum*) was initiated at the Punjab Agricultural University with the objective of combining high quality and faster growth of bajra with the deep root system and multicient habit of napier grass. Though specific hybridisation, a promising bajra-napier hybrid, PBN 233, was developed and released by the State Variety Release Committee in 1999. This hybrid produces 1500 quintal green fodder per acre in seven cutting in a year. It yields higher than the earlier released hybrids, NB 21 and PBN 83. It regularly supply fodder throughout the year, except during its short dormancy (December 15 to end of January).

PBN 233, unlike NB 21 and PBN 83, is photosensitive and flowers only in winter. Due to this characteristic, it remains in the vegetative stage throughout the year, except in winter, when it is dormant. The continuity of its vegetative stage provides succulent, palatable and highly digestible fodder on cutting at the right stage. Further, there is relatively less decline in its quality in comparison to other bajra-napier hybrids on delay in cutting. Delays are mostly observed at the end of rainy season when the growth is fast. It is better to cut it at the right stage and its silage than to cut it as fodder at a late stage.

Up to 70 percent of the daily expenditure in dairy farming is on feeding the animals. This cost could considerably be reduced by growing multi-cut hybrid PBN 233, which regularly supplies fodder for 10 months in a year. The hybrid once planted supplies fodder continuously and regularly for a period of three years, thus the expenditure on ploughing and sowing is reduced by 20 times. The cost of production is almost half that of single-cut crops. The production per unit area and time is approximately double than conventional fodders. Being multi-cut, it can be harvested at the optimum stage, thus maximum nutrients without any loss can be harvested.

PBN 233 contains 20.1 percent dry matter when harvested at the right stage. On dry-matter basis it contains 10.9 percent crude protein, 10.2 percent ash and 29.2 percent crude fiber. It also contains 7.99 percent digestible crude protein and 68.7 percent total digestible nutrients, and has nutrients ration of 1:7.6. PBN 233 has become very popular in certain districts of Punjab. Due to higher production and regular supply of quality fodder for a long time, some farmers in these districts are raising it on an area of 10 acres at their farms and exclusively using this fodder. There is a big demand for root-slips or stem-cuttings of PBN 233 because this hybrid maintains its quality for a long time. It flowers in winter and enters the reproductive stage. On flowering, the fodder becomes lignified, unpalatable and less digestible. However, farmers of certain other districts know little about this hybrid. It is time for agricultural extension agencies to popularise it among the farmers of these districts.

This interspecific hybrid is sterile and does not produce seed. It is vegetatively propagated by root ships and by stem-cuttings. Its introduction, distribution and propagation is difficult in the initial stage but its spread is very easy after its introduction because every farmer will have its root-slips at his own farm for the subsequent year. Vegetative propagation also helps preserve its genetic purity. There is thus no need to replace its seed.

China

In China, feed is conventionally divided into three types: feed grains, oilcakes and bran. Feed grains include maize (which is the major grain), rice, tubers and roots. Tubers and roots in China refer to field crops including potato and sweet potato, but taro, cassava and other tubers and roots used as vegetables and grown in suburbs are excluded. Presently, there are no formal statistical data of feed in China. Feed data in China are generally calculated by two methods: one method is to take food, seed, the part for industry, stocking, the difference between import and export and the losses from the total grain production, and consider the remainder as feed grain. The other method uses the yearly livestock and fishery output to calculate feed by a certain feeding ratio. Both methods are based on estimated data or data from sampling surveys. The estimated food consumption in the first method tends to be a little higher because food is always oversupplied in both urban and rural areas and rural consumers usually use the remainder as feed. On the other hand, with the second method, it is not easy to determine the feeding ratio. Two feeding patterns for livestock and fisheries exist now in China, namely, household raising and large scale raising. Household raising accounts for the majority production and its feed type, nutrition and husbandry vary greatly. Consequently, it is very difficult to calculate a set of feeding ratios for household raising.

The first method of calculation is based on grain and it gives the available amount of feed, while the second is based on the production of livestock and fish and it gives the consumption of the feed. The gap between the two methods is considerable, but it is generally believed that the first is more realistic (Table 17.11). Because of the difficulty in accessing statistical data directly, the total level of feed grain availability is generally based on its share in the output of grain. In 1990, feed grains accounted for about 25% of grain production compared to about 15-20% before the reforms and opening up to the outside world, which amounts to 100 million tonnes more feed grain. In 1994, this proportion reached more than 30%.

According to the nutrition requirements of livestock and poultry, the protein content in the feed should be up to 14.5% while in China now, it is only about 10%. Although the output of oilcake has increased to a certain extent in recent years, it only constitutes 3.8% of the total feed production. The shortage of protein feed supplements causes an imbalance between

Table 17.11: Domestic Demand for Feed in China

(In million tonnes)

Item	Feeding ratio	1990-1992	2000 Trend projection	Demand systems
Domestic demand for livestock products				
Pork	3.50	24.56	36.13	35.64
Beef	3.20	1.53	2.09	1.98
Mutton	3.20	1.17	1.70	1.51
Poultry	2.10	3.91	7.23	6.86
Egg	3.00	9.12	24.90	13.79
Milk	1.84	5.21	14.37	6.43
Domestic demand for feed				
Feed demand for				
Pork	85.96	126.46	124.74	
Beef	5.36	7.32	6.93	
Mutton	4.10	5.95	5.29	
Poultry	13.69	25.31	24.01	
Egg	31.92	87.15	48.27	
Milk	18.24	50.30	22.51	
Total domestic demand for feed	159.25	302.47	231.74	
Annual growth rate (%)		7.39	4.26	

energy and protein feeding and thus influences the feeding ratio. Protein mainly comes from the high protein oilcakes; only 30% of oilcake output was used as feed in China in 1980. In 1993, the output of oilcake was 21 million tonnes, of which 15 million tonnes was used as feed, accounting for about 71 %.

Statistical analysis indicates that total bran production accounts for 21 % of food consumption of raw grains, of which 62% can be used as feed. In 1993, the output of bran feed in China was 36 million tonnes . From the limited statistical data, we cannot get details of the share of feed grains. Calculations based on related available data indicate the following: feed grains make up the largest share, about 70%, oilcakes 8% and bran 20%. Maize, rice and tubers and roots account for the major proportion of feed grain output. Some recent research demonstrated that about 58 million tonnes of maize output and the 13.32 million tonnes of rice were used for feed, but these estimates may be somewhat on the low side.

The output of industrial feeds rose at a rate of 10% each year, the demand still cannot be satisfied. It is important to note that the additives used in concentrates and premix feed have to be imported. Based on the demand for livestock products, the requirement for feed was estimated for the year 2000 (Table 17.11).

There is a big variation in the feed requirement by the year 2000 obtained by the trend projection and demand system methods. The trend line method projected the demand for feed at about 302.47 million tonnes in the year 2000 with an annual compound growth rate of 7.39%. On the other hand, the consumer demand system projected the feed demand at 231.74 million tonnes in the year 2000 with a growth of 4.26% per annum. Looking at the actual growth rate in availability of feed during 1980 to 1992 (6.1%), the projections derived from the demand system approach appear to be more realistic. Thus, China should plan for meeting the annual domestic demand for feed of about 231.74 million tonnes in the year 2000.

The projected annual growth in domestic demand for feed is 3.22% for maize, 5.65% for soybean meal, 0.88% for rice and 0.13% for grain equivalent for sweet potato and potato during the period 1991 to 2000. The demand as animal feed in the year 2000 will be about 73.98 million tonnes of maize, 3.08 million tonnes for soybean meal, 21.94 million tonnes for rice, 15.46 million tonnes of grain equivalent for sweet potato and potato. In the year of 2000, the demand as animal feed is estimated about 103.82 million tonnes of maize, 6.03 million tonnes for soybean meal, 25.95 million tonnes for rice, 19.47 million tonnes for grain equivalent of sweet potato and potato. Looking at the actual feed composition in availability of feed in the early 1990s and comparing the results of demand projections, the demand projections as animal feed for maize, soybean meal, rice, sweet potato and potato (Table 17.11) appear to be more realistic. Thus, these products together would meet about 67% of the projected total feed demand (231.74 million tonnes) for the year 2000. The other share of future feed demand has to be met from other sources.

ROUGHAGES

Roughages include grass and grazing, crop residues, industrial byproducts, (sugarcane, fruits, vegetables distilleries) cultivated fodders, weeds and fodders from trees. One would have very much liked to have complete information on each and every one of these sources of livestock feeds as available and being utilised by the animals. Since quantity and productivity levels of animals certainly depends on the quality of fodder, available for feeding and importantly absorptive capacity of the animal, it is necessary that these two parameters be ensured in the feed, as most livestock with small holders are raised on straws and supplemental grazing. The level of feeding thus be in direct relationship with the output. Some idea in this respect about the countries studied can be made from the unit productivity levels (Table 17.12, 17.13) which cannot be quantified. It, however, highlights the manifold systems of mixed crop/livestock farming in the different countries (Table 17.14).

Use of the crop residues as livestock feed is a common practice. There is in fact, an enormous potential for a better utilisation of crop residues as livestock feed. Here again, some standard conversion factors have been applied to come to these numbers, but very little information is available

Table 17.12: Land use Patterns in 1993 and Changes in Relative Proportions of Each Land use Type Since 1974/76

| Country/ region | Land use patterns in 1993* | | | | | | | | | Changes since 1974/76(%) | | |
| | Area | AL | PC | PP | F/W | Other | A+PC | PP | F/W | A+PC | PP | F/W |
	(1,000 ha)						(% of total area)					
China	932,640	92,708	3,267	400,000	130,496	306,169	10	43	14	-1	12	2
India	297,319	166,100	3,550	11,400	68,500	47,769	57	4	23	1	0	1
Indonesia	181,157	18,900	12,087	11,800	111,774	26,596	17	7	62	6	0	-6
Thailand	51,089	1,760	3,200	800	13,500	15,989	41	2	26	8	1	-10

* AL-arable land, PC-permanent crops, PP-permanent pastures, F/W-forest and woodland, A+PC-arable land and permanent crops.

Source: FAO, 1984, 1994

Table 17.13: Estimated Crop Residues Availability (000 tonnes fresh weight) in 1993*

Country	Wheat	Rice	Barley	Maize	Rye	Oats	Millet	Roots & tubers	Sorghum	Pulses (total)	Soyabean	Groundnut (in shell)	Sugar cane
China	138,314	233,968	4,550	309,138	1,400	910	15,844	22,448	28,990	23,828	61,292	33,984	33,984
India	73,791	152,168	1,958	28,959	0	0	34,576	47,212	4,449	52,580	18,488	30,504	56,963
Indonesia	0	62,635	0	19,380	0	0	0	0	3,971	2,016	6,836	4,272	8,250
Thailand	1	25,892	3	9,984	0	0	0	832	4,084	1,760	2,052	0	9,456

*Based on conversion factors in Kossila. The availability of crop residues in developing countries in relation to Livestock Population:

Source: FAO, Production yearbook: In Reed, J.D., Capper, B.S.: al Neate, P.J.H. (Eds): Plant Breeding and the Nutritive Value of Crop Residues. Proceedings of a Workshop, 7-10 December 1987, International Livestock Centre for Africa (ILCA) Addis Ababa, Ethiopia.

Table 17.14: Main Agricultural Systems in Different Countries

Main agricultural systems				
Country/ region	*Classification of zone (mm annual rainfall m attitude)*	*Main crops*	*Livestock[2]*	*Main livestock products*	*Predominant*
China	Pasturing area (northern China)	NA	C,S,G, camel	Meat, milk, wool, trans- port, fuel	Grazing
	Cropping- pasturing area	NA	C,S,G	Transport, draught Manure, fuel, meat, milk, wool	NA
	Cropping area (southern China)	Rice, wheat, maize soyabean, rapeseed groundnut, sugarcane sugarbeet, Linseed	C,S,G,B	Meat, milk, draught	NA
India	Arid (Rajasthan and surroun- dings)	Millet, pulses, cotton Oil- seed, wheat	D,G,C,B,S,	Milk, wool, hair, meat, draught	Grazing/ Feeding millet leave
	Sem-arid (south and central)	Rice, wheat, sugarcane pulses, oil- seed, sorg- hum, cotton	D, G,C,B,S, camel	Milk, wool, hair, meat, draught	Grazing, Stall feeding of straws, Feeding stover grasses
	Humid/sub humid Tracks	Rice, wheat, sugarcane pulses, oil- seed, sorg- hum, cotton	D,C,B,S,G	Milk, wool, hair, draught	Grazing, stall feeding of straws chopped green stover, grasses
	Subtropical/ temperature	Rice, wheat (forest)	S,G,D,C	wool, meat, milk	Mainly grazing, stall feeding of stover and straws
	(Humalayan foothills) Highlands	Rice, buck- wheat, small millets,	S, G	Wool, meat, milk	Grazing, partly stall feeding of

| | | | | |

Table 17.14: **Main Agricultural Systems in Different Countries** *(Contd.)*

Country/ region	Classification of zone (mm annual rainfall m attitude)	Main crops	Livestock[2]	Main livestock products	Predominent
	(alpine/ subalpine tracts)	vegetable (forest)			chopped fodders
	Coastal region	Rice, coconut, cassava, small millet		Wool, meat, milk	Grazing, partly stall feeding with chopped straws and other fodders
Indonesia	Lowland (<100m)	Rice, maize, cassava vegetable, sugarcane, oilpam, coconut, rubber	B, C, S Calves	Draught, meat residues	Grazing and cut-and carry tree- livestock system
	Upland (> 500 m)	Maize, rice, potato, sweet potato	C, G	Draught, meat	Cut-and- carry, limited grazing of crop residues crop- live- stock system
Pasture	(100-5-m)	Rainfed rice, Maize	C, B, G	Tramping meat	Mainly grazing natural crop residues Crop-live- stock system
Thailand	Subhumid lowlands	Rice, maize	B,C, D,C	Meat milk	Grazing and cut-and carry, Rice, straw concen trate, crop residues
	Humid lowlands	Fruit tree plants	B,G,C, S, G	Meat	Grazing and cut-and carry, tree, fodder

B= Buffalo: C= Cow: D= Duck: G= Goat: S= Sheep

Main agricultural systems

about the qualitative aspect. The relative importance of crop residues has inter and intra country as well as regional variations depending upon agro-ecological conditions and various other allied aspects. Some idea about the relative importance of crop residues in the total diet composition of livestock can be formed from the scattered information available (Table 17.15). Crop residues are generally of low nutritive value. One way of improving the quality of the diet is to supplement them with other feed resources which are richer in energy and protein and/or superior in digestibility or intake.

An attempt has been made to tabulate this information for the four countries (Table 17.13) Cereal straws have, no doubt, been the main focus of attention as the main source of livestock feeding. But unfortunately hardly any progress has been made by the farmers to adopt available technologies like urea ammonia treated straw enriched with molasses. Some of the key factor associated with this are:

Too much emphasis on the characterization and pretreatment of cereal straws. (i) inadequate project design, lacking in a systems approach, ensuring effective priority setting in accordance with farmer's needs, farmers participation in technology design, on farm evaluation with farmers, and appropriate mechanisms for technology no clear demonstration of the economic benefits of this technology to farmers. Without such benefits, farmers acceptance and adoption are likely to remain insignificant.

An attempt has been made here to provide information about the potential available in the 4 countries from grazing as well as stall feeding. A study of Land Use Patterns (Table 17.12) in different countries can give a comparative picture of the available grazing facilities. China is the only country in the region which has the maximum (43%) area under permanent pastures, while Indonesia is on the top with regard to forests and woodlands. How much of these areas are available for livestock grazing and what is their capacity of feeding is, however, be made by an understanding of the major agricultural systems. (Table 17.14).

These countries will perforce have to give up animal production and become net importers of animal foods (milk, meat, eggs). There is, however, a silver lining which could change the future of animal production in this region. This calls for total reexamination of available technology options in respect of major raw material ingredients available for livestock feeding (i) Crop residues and industrial byproducts; (ii) Oilcake, oil meals from cultivated oil seed crops, oil meals from forest produce and (iii) By-product of petroleum industry.

These are ingredients which have been used for feeding of livestock. The present research on animal nutrition and physiology has reached a stage that traditional feeding system will not deliver the higher productivity levels as these two basic raw materials have a low digestibility of (hardly 2-3%) and are short on available/usable energy and protein. It has however, a major reserve of energy in the untapped plant cell wall in terms of lignocellulose complex and will yield enough energy to feed all the one billion livestock if released.

Table 17.15: Feeding System in the Selected Countries

Products	India	China	Thailand	Indonesia
Milk	Mainly dry and green fodder and waste foodgrains. Concentrate only to hybrid milch cattle primarily in the organised dairy sector	Total production hardly 12-13% that of India and major part in the organised sector. A by-product of beef.	Practically no milk production A by-product of beef	Practically no milk production. A by-product of beef
Beef	Mainly dry and green fodder and waste food grains besides grazing. A by-product of dairy.	Major part in the organised sector depending on adequate concentrate feeding.	Stall feeding with concentrate	Stall feeding with concentrate
Pork	Scavanging waste food grains. Concentrates only to crossbred pigs numbering about 1 million which are stall fed	Pork meat production is 97 times that of India and productivity three times. This calls for appropriate stall feeding with concentrate.	Stall feeding	Pork production double than that of Thailand and 25% higher than that of India. Mostly stall fed.
Poultry product	Concentrate to the organised poultry farms. Rest on kitchen waste and scavanging around.	Chicken production based on concentrates only. But total production 20 times of India. Major part of egg production in the extensive sector from improved local breeds with concentrate feeding.	Organised sector with concentrate	Organised sector with concentrate

This will however, require large investments in research on feed biotechnology, of manipulating and constructing microbes through genetic engineering which can digest the lignin ring and release the sugars for animal feeding. The current nutrition and biotechnology research has to focus research goals on only this area.

The source of protein in oil meals and cakes etc. produced from oil seed crops and forest produce, unfortunately is bound by various chemical moieties like tannin and other antigrowth factors and this protein is not readily available to animals, a method has to be found that these chemicals are removed from these oil meals so that the abundant protein in these meals is available to livestock.

If we are able to address these two problems within the next 25 years we should be able to solve the problem of livestock feed to meet the targets of 2020 to feed the human population.

COW SLAUGHTER

Today 16 out of every 100 cows in the world are in India, not to speak of 57 out of every 100 buffaloes. But while the population is impressive, fodder availability is not. Cattle is already facing an acute shortage of fodder, with availability falling to just 50% in the last couple of years. So, despite government's pious intentions, the ban on slaughter could eventually mean serious hurt to the 9.8 million small farmers whose livelihood depends on them.

The Planning Commission believes fodder availability is "grossly inadequate" even for maintaining the existing cattle population. If more numbers are added due to a ban on slaughter, it would further aggravate the problem. A complete ban on the slaughter of all cattle would tend to increase their number further and to jeopardize the well being of the limited number of good cattle, which the country possesses, the Planning Commission has pointed out in its midterm review of agriculture in the Tenth Plan.

Consequently, it has advised caution. "In defining the scope of bans on the slaughter of cattle, states should take a realistic view of the fodder resources available and the extent to which they can get the cooperation of voluntary organizations to bear the main responsibility for maintaining unserviceable and unproductive cattle with a measure of assistance from the government and general support from the people. The above recommendations made in the Second Plan are valid even today, the Commission has said. As the livestock sector contributes more than 23% to India's farm GDP, this is a warning the government can scarcely choose to ignore.

The problem of fodder scarcity could, in fact, become the biggest stumbling block in the development of this sector. The area under permanent pasture and grazing land has been estimated at 11.06 million hectares. However, actual availability appears to be much less. It is estimated that during 2000, the availability of fodder remained in short supply by about

COW ROWS
- 1994, 1996: Bill by K.R. Rana
- 1999: Bill by Aditya Nath
- 2000: Bills by U.V. Krishnamaraju
- S.S. Ahluwalia, Prahlad Patel
- 2001: National Commission on cattle appointed
- 2003: MP CM seeks ban. BJP promises bill in Budget Session

In 2000-02 India exported 2,43,355,58 metric tonnes of beef. Cow urine is sold for Rs 5 per litre in Bhopal and Indore.

The National Commission on Cattle Says

The ban to be included in the Fundamental Rights Central law banning cow slaughter. Violation of this law should be a non-bailable offence. Government should set up Rashtriya Goseva Ayog. Completely ban export of beef and veal: Central Cattle Protection – Rapid Task Force should be set up. Penal laws like POTA should be amended to tackle cow smugglers/mafia.

47%. Dry fodder was scarce by 22%. Worldwide, grain is the one of the biggest sources of cattle feed. However, in India less that 3% of the grain produced is used as cattle feed. Crop residues are the other biggest source of food. The three major sources of fodder supply are: crop residues (paddy straw, wheat bhusa), cultivated fodder and fodder from forests, permanent pastures and grazing land.

On the other hand, the main recommendation of the Lodha Committee report, submitted in June, 2002, to the government is to make a constitutional amendment and include ban on cow slaughter in the fundamental rights so that it is obligatory. At present it is part of the directive principles. The stated rationale is to protect cows essentially for economic reasons, as their population is depleting. "Cows should be protected by setting up more gaushalas and panjara poles across the country, apart from banning slaughter.

COW FACTS
- India has nearly 69 million cows, one-sixth of the world's cow population
- From 1997 to 2001, cattle population has fallen by 10 million
- Nearly 15 million cows have been slaughtered during the same period.

Cow slaughter is banned in most states in India except West Bengal, Kerala and the North East. Around 2,000 cattle are butchered every day in West Bengal to meet the requirement of cheap protein. Kerala has never had a law banning cow slaughter. In fact, according to the Vegetarian Congress, it has 95 per cent of the 30 million people meat-eaters. It imports several hundred heads of cattle everyday from Karnataka, Tamil Nadu and Andhra Pradesh. No political party here has ever had demanded a ban. The Shiv Sena, which has only a notional presence in Kerala had organized agitations against cruelty to cattle at various entry points and enroute to the Sabarimala Pilgrimmage. The Vishwa Hindu Parishad has launched a campaign and petitioned the Kolkata High Court to stop cow slaughter in West Bengal. The Forward Bloc, a Left Front Partner, says that cattle slaughter has never created a problem in West Bengal and the party is against any move to amend the Constitution to stop the practice.

Conclusions

1. A comprehensive study of the production and consumption patterns of the four major countries of the Asian Region shows that while the production estimates of foodgrains (cereals in particular) by different national as well as international sources are more or less in agreement with each other, estimates of quantities used as feedgrains for livestock are nothing more than guestimates in all these countries.

2. Picture is not very clear even with regard to human consumption. National source estimates in this respect are based primarily on consumer surveys, but international data (particularly FAO Food Balance Sheets) provide diagrammatically opposite trends. In the case of India, while NSSO data shows a consistent decline in per capita consumption of foodgrains, FAO Feed Balance Sheet gives an increasing trend.

3. At the World level, there is no consistency in the estimates given by the different agencies on the one hand and on the other, even for the same agency, there is no relationship between foodgrains consumed and livestock products produced from year to year.

4. At the national level, there is a confusion between concentrates and feedgrains. It has to be clearly understood that other than roughages, animal nutritionists have laid down specified quantities of DCP (Digested Crude Proteins) and TDN (Total Digestible Nutrients) in formulating concentrates. But these are also of indicative nature. The farmer rarely goes by these recommendations. He is invariably guided by his instinct, traditions and above all availability and economics of the various feed components. It is, therefore, extremely necessary that we should have the composition of various feeds and concentrates that are fed and utilized by the farmers to have a clearer picture.

Our comments for different countries are as follows:

(a) Feed data in China are generally calculated in two ways: one way is to take food, seed, the part for industry, stocking, the difference between import and export and the losses from the total grain production, and consider the remainder as feed grain; the other way uses the yearly livestock and fishery output to calculate feed by feeding ratio technique. Both ways are based on estimated data/ data from sampling systems. The estimated food consumption in the first method tends to be a little higher because food is always oversupplied and rural consumers usually use the remainder as feed. With the second method, it is not easy to determine the feeding ratio. Two feeding patterns for livestock and fisheries exist, namely, household raising and large scale raising. Household raising accounts for the majority of output and its feed, nutrition and husbandry vary greatly. Consequently it is very difficult to calculate a set of feeding ratios for household raising. This is the theoretical approach. But the real position is different. Estimates of feedgrains used for livestock in China during 1992-94 vary from 62.8 to 112.4 million tonnes.

(b) In India, official estimates assume 12.5 percent of gross production as feed, seed and wastages as well as industrial uses. It has no empirical basis, most importantly, none of the component has any relation with the production of foodgrains and it is quite incorrect to use a constant denominator over a period of 50 years, while all relationships have changed. All future projections made by various researchers make their own assumptions – the result is confusion worse confounded.

(c) In Thailand, some conversion rates are given for feed (concentrates). According to these norms, total concentrate required was 5.4 million tonnes in 2001. This estimate for 1994 for maize was 4.68 million tonnes. FAO Food Balance Sheet (FBS) for 1992-94 shows a feedgrain consumption of 364 thousand tonnes of rice and 3498 thousand tonnes of maize. National source balance sheet for paddy does not allocate anything for industrial uses. Soya meal, national sources shows 1.16 million tonnes and FAO (FBS) nil.

(d) Reliable data on utilization of each commodity for different purposes such as feed, food industries, and human consumption are not available in Indonesia. The time series Food Balance Sheet (FBS) data provides information on the average availability of each crop per capita per year and the use for feed and food industries as well as for human consumption. These data are published by Ministry of Agriculture (MOA) and Central Bureau of Statistics (CBS). Production, export and import on the supply side are regarded as accurate, but the data on feed and food industries are generally very poor. Data on seed, feed and food industries are usually estimated as percentages of total supply. In FBS data, the portion of commodity for feed is estimated as 5%, waste around 20%, and feed 2%. Hence, it is difficult to estimate the trend in demand for industry for a particular commodity using FBS data.

BIBLIOGRAPHY

1. Anonymous. 1994. Statistical Abstract of United States Situation, United States Department of Commerce, Washington D.C.
2. Anonymous. 1995. Livestock and Poultry; World Markets and Trade, U.S.D.A. Beltsevilla Máryland, USA.
3. Anonymous. 1996. Cereal, Feed Use in the Third World: Past Trends and Projection to 2000, Research Report 57. IFPRI Washington. D.C.
4. Anonymous. 1997. Livestock Products in the Third World: Report 49. Past Trends and Projections to 1990 and 2000, IFPRI, Washington. D.C.
5. Bansil, P.C. 1959. Future Feed, Seed and Wastage Rates, Indian Journal of Agricultural Economics, Vol 21(2): 2733.
6. Bansil, P.C. 1987. Feed, Seed and Wastage Rates in India, A Regional Study, Techno Economic Research Institute, New Delhi, Memograph notes pp 29.
7. Bansil, P.C. 1997. India's Demand for Foodgrains in 2000 AD – Simple Incremental Demand Model. Indian Farming, 46 (2): 2332.
8. Bansil, P.C. 1997. Feed grains for livestock. Indian Farming 47 (7): 3843.
9. Bhalla, G.S. 1994. Economics Liberlisation and Indian Agriculture. Institute for Studies in Industrial Development, New Delhi.
10. Bhat, P.N. 1994. Livestock Policy in India, Draft Paper Department of Animal Husbandry and Dairying, Ministry of Agriculture, Krishi Bhawan, New Delhi.
11. Bhat, P.N. 1995. Bovines in India Working paper No. 28, Department of Animal Husbandry and Dairying, Ministry of Agriculture, Krishi Bhawan, New Delhi.
12. Bhat, P.N. and P.C. Bansil. 1996. Poultry Development in India, Perspectives. and Approaches, Indian Journal of Animal Production, 28 (S): 1240.
13. Bhat, P.N. 1997. Science and Technology in Agricultural Development – A key to the Future 2nd Indian Agriculture Science Congress, NAAS, New Delhi 3140.
14. Cheng, Guoqian. 1997. Market Prospects for Upland Crops in China, Working Papers series, The CGPRT Centre, Jakarta, Indonesia.
15. Devendra, C. 1992. Non-conventional Feed Resources in Asia and the Pacific: Strategies for Expanding Utilisation at the Small Farm Level. Fourth revised edition. Regional Office for Asia and the pacific (RAPA), Food and Agriculture Organisation of the United Nations (FAO), Bangkok, Thailand.
16. FAO. 1994. FAO Production Yearbook, vol. 48. Food and Agriculture Organisation of the United Nations, Rome, Italy.
17. Government of India. 1976. Report of the National Commission on Agriculture part III: Demand and Supply, Ministry of Agriculture and Irrigation, New Delhi.
18. IFPRI. 1984. Assessment of Food Demand-Supply Prospects and related Strategies for Developing Member Countries of the Asian Development Bank. International Food Policy Research Institute, Washington, D.C., Mimeo.
19. Kossila, V. 1988. The availability of crop residues in developing countries in relation to livestock populations. In Reed, J.D., B.S. Capper and P.J.H. Neate 9eds), Plant Breeding and the Nutritive Value of Crop Residues. Proceedings of a Workshop, 710 December 1987, International Livestock Centre for Africa (ILCA), Addis Ababa, Ethiopia, pp. 2939.

20. Kumar, P., W.R. Mark and E.B. Howarth. 1996. Demand for Foodgrains and other Food in India. Indian Agriculture Research Institute, New Delhi and International Food Policy Research Institute, Washington, D.C., Mimeo.

21. Kumar, P. 1997. Market prospects for uplands crops in Thailand, Working Paper Series, The CGPRT Centre.

22. Machal, J. H. H. 1997. A synthesis of country reports presented at the workshop on Crop residues in sustainable Mixed Crop/Livestock Farming Systems (Ed) Renard C. ICRISAT. Hyderabad, India.

23. Mamed, G. 1997. Market Prospects for Upland Crops in Indonesia, Working Paper 25, The CGPRT Centre, Jakarta, Indonesia.

24. Mishra, S.N. and R.K. Sharma. 1990. Livestock Development in India – An Appraisal, Vikas Publishers, New Delhi.

25. Patel, R.K. (1994) Draught Animal Power, Journal of Rural Energy, 2 (24) : 2933.

26. Radhakrishna, R. and C. Ravi. 1991. Food Demand Projections for India, Centre for Economic and Social Studies. Hyderabad.

27. Radhakrishna, R. and C. Ravi. 1992. Effects of Growth, Relative Price and Preferences on Food and Nutritions, Indian Economic Review, Vol. 27: pp. 303.

28. Radhakrishna, R. and C. Ravi. 1994. Food Demand in India: Emergence trends and perspectives, Paper presented at the International Conference on economic Liberalisation in South Asia, Australia South Regional Centre, Australia National University, 30 November December, 1994.

29. Ranjhan, S.K. 1994. Feed and Fodder Requirement, Consultancy Report, Dept. of Animal Husbandry and Dairying, Ministry of Agriculture, New Delhi.

30. TAC. 1992. Review of CGIAR Priorities and Strategies, Part 1. Technical Advisory Committee of the Consultative Group on International Agriculture Research (CGIAR), Rome, Italy.

31. Van Soest, P.J. 1988. Effect of environment and quality of fiber on the nutritive value of crop residues. In: Reed, J.D., Capper, B.S. and Neate, P.J.H. (Eds), Plant Breeding and the Nutritive Value of Crop Residues. Proceedings of a workshop, 7-10 December 1987, International Livestock Centre for Africa (ILCA), Addis Ababa, Ethiopia, pp. 7196.

32. Verma, J. M. 1994. Food Exports and Food Requirement, Economic and Political Weekly, 2 (35): 2261.

18

Livestock and Livestock Product Marketing

MARKETING CHANNELS FOR LIVE ANIMALS

India has more than 2,000 markets where livestock and livestock products are traded. All livestock markets are under the jurisdiction of state governments and union territories, although direct operation and supervision generally fall to local bodies, such as village panchayat and municipal corporations. There are a few privately owned markets.

The market for live animals is not very developed. There are no separate markets for different species of animals. Farmers usually bring their animals to the weekly or fortnightly village markets on foot or occasionally on trucks, where they are assembled in the market yard. Cattle and buffaloes, milching and draught, are assembled in the same yard, with most exchanges facilitated by brokers. Because of the lack of contacts in the terminal markets and/or access to transportation, local traders primarily perform the assembling function for wholesalers. The animals brought to the village markets are sold by haggling over prices. Secondly, agents, middlemen or wholesale dealers visit rural areas and advance cash to the farmers. The animals are collected later for sale. Vertical linkages between processors/ butchers and livestock producers are quite rare. Farm-wholesale marketing margins amount to about 20-30 percent of the consumer price. Market facilities are generally inadequate or if available are poorly maintained. In most markets, for instance, weighbridges are not available. Figure 18.1 shows marketing channels for livestock in India.

Grading standards are currently only applied to livestock product for exports, to meet international requirements. In practice, buyers perform animal grading with the assistance of brokers and commission agents. Prices are based on such factors as breed, age, body structure and appearance, milk yield, lactation number, estimated meat yield etc. Prices are arrived at through negotiations, directly or indirectly through brokers and commission agents or, in a few cases, through auction.

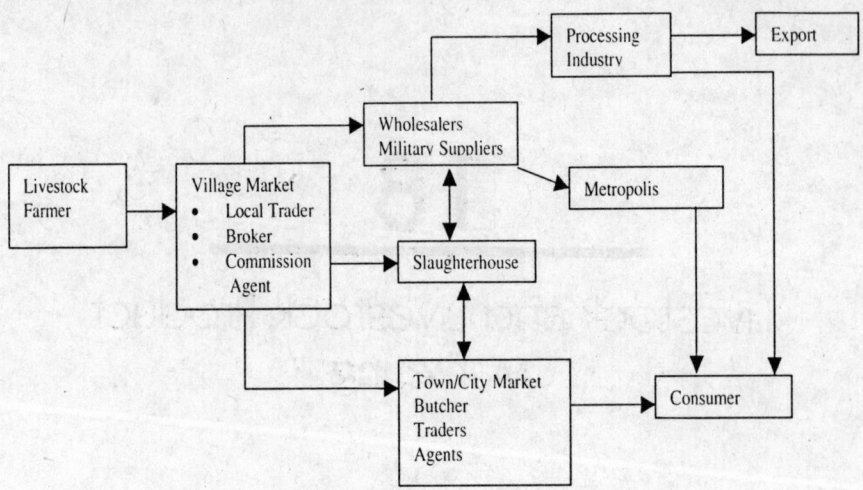

Fig. 18.1: Marketing Channels for Livestock in India

Marketing of Fodder

The market for green and dry fodder is not yet well developed. In areas with surplus dry fodder from agricultural residues, the fodder is primarily marketed in nearby deficit areas. Sometimes, they are baled and sent to distant locations by rail. The sale of dry fodder in the weekly markets is quite common. Green fodder is also cut and transported over short distances for marketing, particularly to nearby urban areas. Large-scale organized markets for fodder are few; they only operate in Mumbai, Ahmedabad, Delhi and Kolkata.

Marketing of Dairy Products

About 60 percent of milk production in India is sold in the market. The rest is consumed at the producer (urban and rural) household level. In 1993/94, 36 million tonnes of milk were marketed, of which 13 million tonnes (36 percent) was channeled through the organized sector (Operation Flood, cooperatives, government milk schemes, and large private processors) and 23 million tonnes (64 percent) went through the unorganized sector (small private dealers and processors). Operation Flood, cooperatives and government schemes account for 17 percent of milk marketing: private processors account for 19 percent. Milk in the organized sector is processed in 275 dairy plants and 83 milk product factories operated by cooperatives, private dairy processors, and government milk schemes. Milk channeled through Operation Flood cooperatives is generally processed in rural dairy plants and transported into cities and towns.

The unorganized sector includes private milk vendors and milk dealers. Milk dealers supply milk either to bigger milk dealers or to private dairy factories. Small dealers generally collect milk from a small number of villages that serve as part of a larger procurement scheme operated by a bigger milk dealer or processor. The large processors set a fixed price according to fat content and on-fat solids, leaving it to the suppliers to set prices for farmers. These processors usually integrate forward by establishing or leasing ice factories to chill the milk, enabling them to seek the best price for their milk from private diary factories within or outside the state. Total milk production in the fiscal year 1997 was estimated at 70.8 million tonnes. About 45 percent of milk production is consumed as fluid milk. About 35 percent is processed into butter or ghee, 7 percent is processed into paneer (cottage cheese) and other cheeses, 4 percent is converted into milk powder, and the rest is used for other dairy products such as curd (yogurt) and sweet meats. In recent years, ice cream production has been increasing, although domestic and foreign investments in the ice cream industry have been constrained by the restriction of ice cream production to small-scale industries. Annual production of milk powder and infant food is estimated at 160,000 tonnes, malted milk food at 45,000 tonnes, cheese at 3,000 tonnes, and condensed milk at 8,500 tonnes. Annual butter and butter oil production totals about 1.2 million tonnes, most of which is produced by small businesses and households.[1]

The role and impact of Operation Flood in milk collection and marketing has already been dealt with in Chapter 5. The primary objective of Operation Flood (Of) launched in 1970, was the creation of farmer owned and farmer controlled organization based on the Anand pattern of cooperative development. Of has been successful in spreading the dairy cooperatives and providing an important demonstration effect on the potential for dairy development in India. As on 31 March 1998, 9.9 million member farmers (estimated to be 36 percent of the total dairy farmers) were supplying about 11 million litres of milk per day to 77,531 milk cooperative societies, who in turn delivered the milk to 170 milk unions for processing and marketing.[2] The success of the dairy cooperative movement has encouraged private sector participation in the dairy industry. The noncooperative private dairy processing sector currently handles about 80 percent of marketed milk. The cooperative movement has also served as a check and balance for private dairy marketing activities. Despite commendable achievement, the cooperatives suffer from a number of deficiencies. For instance, in the 1990s, a large number of cooperatives were performing too poorly. A 1994 World Bank Review of ll7 cooperatives receiving assistance under the World Bank National Dairy Project II found that 52 percent incurred losses. Their combined losses for the two years 1993/94 were Rs. 1.1 billion ($ 37 million), which had to be covered by budgetary transfer from the central and state resources. The continued subsidization of the diary cooperatives is not sustainable.

---

[1] USDA: India Agricultural Situation: 1994: AGR No. IN4084
[2] Basic Animal Husbandry Statistics, 1999, p. 114.

Although the Milk and Milk Products Order (MMPO) was amended in 1993, several key regulations were retained, which inhibit incentives for increased competition and efficiency in the dairy industry. The continued protection of the dairy processing industry, especially the cooperative sector, has fostered inefficiencies in the processing and marketing of milk products. Although producer milk prices in India are significantly lower than in the United States and Western Europe, dairy product prices (butter and whole and skimmed milk powder) were substantially higher (20 to 50 percent) than international market prices. Only during the mid-90s, the rupee devaluation and a sharp rise in world dairy prices - as a consequence of a production shortfall in major dairy producing countries, narrowed the gap between Indian dairy product prices and world market prices. Fluid milk marketing margins are high in India - for example it is about 67 percent higher than in the United Kingdom.

Moreover, state intervention and consequent diversion from the original farmer-controlled cooperative concept, contributed to the poor performance of many cooperative unions. For example, social pricing policies implemented in some states resulted in negligible or zero processing margins. Other than state intervention, weak management and poor market orientation resulted in the poor economic performance of some cooperatives. Lack of flexibility in adapting to changing market conditions, poor quality control, over staffing, under-utilization of capacity due to limited milk market, processing inefficiency and weak marketing and commercial orientation further contributed to the poor financial performance of these cooperatives and resulted in their continued dependence on state financial transfers/ subsidies. Increased efficiency of the dairy industry is critical in many respects. It is essential to create a level playing field for all market participants. For this a World Bank Team had recommended adoption of a package of reforms revolving around the four key areas:

   (i) Elimination of all state interventions in Cooperatives:

  (ii) Lifting of MMPO:

 (iii) Establishing mechanism to monitor milk market to ensure fair competition: and

 (iv) Strengthening of Public Monitoring and Enforcement of Hygiene Standards.[1]

Growing Milk Market

Milk market is expected to grow to Rs. 100,000 crore in the next five years—and in areas as varied as butter, ice-creams and dahi, the Gujarat Cooperative Milk Marketing Federation (GCMMF) is already feeling the heat.

---

[1]World Bank: India: Livestock Sector Review: Enhancing Growth and Development: May 23, 1996.

Consider the cheese market. Till a few years ago, Amul had 55-60 per cent share of the 9,000-tonne annual cheese sales. Britannia, which entered the market in July 1997, now accounts for more than 20 per cent of the market, thanks to its aggressive marketing techniques. A threatened Amul has countered by launching new variants such as Emmenthal, Gauda and Mozzarella, and plans to introduce cheese sauces and dips.

Even its traditional stronghold of milk is under MNC threat, with Britannia's Milkman—a "tribute" to the man often referred to as India's Milkman, Kurien—and Nestle's UHT Milk and Slim Milk venturing into the market. Amul, in response, has entered the Nagpur and Pune markets— earlier, its polypacks were available only in Gujarat and Mumbai—and its long-life tetrapack milk is said to be doing very well in milk-deficit areas like Kolkata, the Northeastern states, Andamans, etc. Health concerns may have led to a sluggish 6-7 per cent growth in the butter market, but that hasn't deterred Britannia from taking on the Amul bull by its horns. Amul still commands nearly 75-80 per cent of the national market as the only all-India brand, while local products like Parag (Uttar Pradesh), Verka (Punjab), Vijaya (Andhra), Vita (Haryana), etc., account for between 3-6 per cent.

TRADE LIBERALIZATION AND INDIAN DAIRY INDUSTRY

In the 1990s, Government of India introduced major trade policy reforms, which had important implications for the dairy sector. First, the dairy industry, which was reserved mainly for the cooperative sector, was delicensed in 1991 and the private sector companies including multinationals were allowed to set up milk processing and product manufacturing plants. Second, India signed the Uruguay Round Agreement (URA) of the General Agreement on Tariffs and Trade (GATT), now vested in the World Trade Organization (WTO), which makes it mandatory for its members to open their agricultural sector to the world markets. Moreover, the import and export of dairy products, which was restricted through quantitative measures (canalization, licensing, quotas, etc.) and other non-tariff barriers, was brought under the Open General Licence (OGL) and import tariffs for most dairy products were significantly reduced in the second half of the 1990s. For example, in March 1995, import of milk powders and butter oil was decanalized and delicensed. In 1999, whole milk, yogurt, grated or powdered cheese of all kinds, blue-veined cheese, buttermilk, whey, curdled milk and acidified milk and cream were shifted to OGL. All these developments expose the Indian dairy sector to an open economy environment, which have a significant bearing on the Indian dairy sector.

MEAT MARKETING AND PROCESSING

Under the prevailing conditions, the marketing of meat involves many agencies, intermediaries and middlemen. It is difficult to assess their exact number in an entire operational chain. The middleman, in most cases earns the major part of the total price charged to the consumer. The entire marketing of livestock as well as carcasses is on a unit basis graded subjectively. The total marketing cost between producers and consumers amount to 40 to 50 percent of the cost of animal. The profit made by intermediaries is around 50 to 55 percent, the maximum profit being made by the retailer.[1]

Municipal bodies manage most slaughterhouses. In 1996, there were 3,650 slaughterhouses. The four states with the largest number are Karnataka (860), Kerala (715), Tripura (397), Maharashtra (387). In addition, there are almost over 10,000 unorganized slaughterhouses. State governments operate most slaughterhouses, with the exception of a few private facilities catering to the export market. The slaughter of cattle is prohibited in all but a few states (Kerala, West Bengal and several northeastern states). Buffaloes are not subject to the same religious sensitivities and are slaughtered at a variety of weights (average about 300 kg live weight) and ages. However, only few slaughterhouses offer facility for slaughter of buffalo. All slaughterhouses, except few private ones, operate as service abattoirs; there the butchers slaughter animals for a nominal fee and the municipal meat inspectors certify the carcasses suitable for human consumption. In addition to municipal abattoir at Deonar in Mumbai, modern state owned meat complex have been set up in Goa, Durgapur (West Bengal), Hyderabad, Bangalore, Chennai and near Ambala in Haryana. There are plans to set up modern abattoirs in Kolkata, Delhi, Srinagar and some other cities. When completed these projects will supply wholesale meat to the consumer and support a meat export trade. Management, marketing and slaughtering are traditional and require scientific improvement. A number of privately owned and operated abattoirs have also been set up.

Despite an innate ability for better conversion of coarse roughage, nutritional superiority and good quality of meat, it is paradoxical that buffalo is yet to be developed for commercial meat production on lines of beef cattle production. As indicated by Dr. Bhat and Dr. Lakshmanan, the gap between the present situation of salvaging meat as an end product and the goal of producing it as a principal commodity, as has been the case with milk, is too wide. The authors contend that the situation was fast changing in recent years.[2]

POULTRY MARKETING

Broilers are sold live, fresh dressed, dressed chilled, or frozen. The first two categories account for bulk of total sales. The marketing channels for broilers are illustrated in Figure 18.2. Broilers farms are generally located

---

[1] Bhasin, N.R.: Marketing of Buffalo Meat, in Indian Journal of Animal Production vol.30, No.1-4, January-December 1996, p.85.

[2] Dr. P.N.Bhat and V. Lakshmanan: The Buffalo Meat Industry in India: An Overview: published in Buffalo Production and Health: by ICAR, 1988. pp.186.

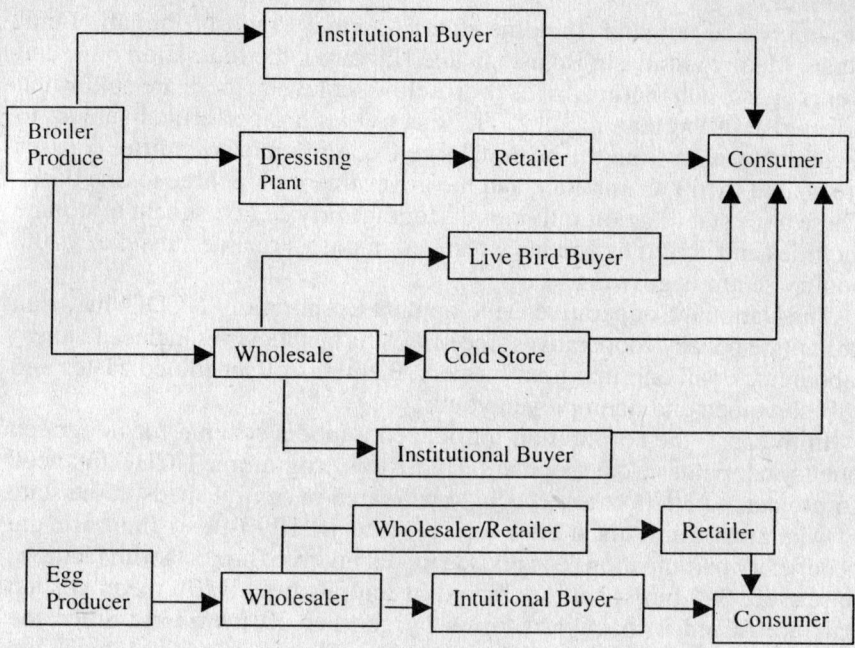

Fig. 18.2: Marketing channels for broilers and eggs in India

within an 100 km radius of big cities. In certain markets auctions are held daily. In others, framers sell the birds to traders or processors. Egg marketing on the other hand, is primarily handled by traders and commission agents.

The poultry-processing sector in India is still underdeveloped. In 1998, only about 6 percent of domestic poultry production was processed in modern plants; the balance was processed in small retail meat shops or households under unhygienic conditions. Processing of broilers in rural markets is uncommon due to storage and distribution problems. A number of private export oriented egg processing projects are in pipeline. One egg powder processing plant has been operational in Mumbai since the seventies.

Further development of poultry industry should focus on more hygienic slaughtering plants and cold storage facilities supported by mechanical dressing plants and cold storage facilities. Increased private sector investments in these technologies will be greatly influenced by both macro and sectoral policies to the extent that they affect the profitability of the ventures.

Persistent mistrust of private trader behaviour and the strong commitment by the central and state Governments to control prices have led to a variety of interventions in the poultry market. Several government parastatals are involved in poultry marketing.

The National Agricultural Cooperative Marketing Federation stabilizes egg prices. Prices fluctuate considerably in some states due to the seasonality of supply and demand. In some states (Andhra Pradesh, Punjab, Tamil Nadu. Madhya Pradesh, Rajasthan and Haryana), the federation buys and stores eggs when market prices drop below set levels; these are sold when prices rise in the lean months. These activities are performed subject to recommendation from the National Egg Coordination Committee. Losses are shared by the Committee and the government on a three to one basis. These price stabilization activities discourage private investment in storage facilities and activities and have resulted in unsustainable subsidies as the poultry sector is growing.

The National Cooperative Development Corporation (NCDC) has been promoting poultry cooperatives since 1979. Its beneficiaries include landless labourers, small and marginal farmers, members of scheduled castes and tribes, women and unemployed youth.

In the past, the corporation introduced a model scheme for integrated poultry cooperative development. Under this programme NCDC financed 25 projects of 30, 000 birds each, to be reared in central sheds in the state of Maharashtra. This model was revised in 1990-91 to increase the beneficiary participation. The revised model involved projects with facilities to rear 60, 000 birds; half are reared in central sheds by 30 members and half are raised in backyard farms by another 30 members. Since the programme is targeted at the vulnerable segments of society, loans are provided at concessional differential rates of interest, lower rates for cooperatives in underdeveloped states and slightly higher rates for cooperatives in other states. These rates are generally below the current market rate of interest. Additional poultry projects were undertaken in the Eighth and Ninth Five Year Plans.

State Level Poultry Corporations

Poultry Corporations have also been established in several states. These corporations were designed to help farmers by supplying good quality feed at reasonable prices, assisting in the marketing of eggs, and so on. Because they were established as autonomous bodies, the corporations were viewed as being better able to perform these functions than government departments. The Corporations, however, have performed poorly and are incurring heavy losses. The Punjab Poultry Development Corporation, for example, witnessed feed production decline from 18, 600 tonnes in 1976/77 to 8, 600 tonnes in 1992/93. Its remaining production was designated primarily for government poultry, diary and piggery farms. The corporation's egg sales fell from 72.6 million pieces in 1982/83 to 13.9 million in 1992/93, while dressing plant and egg-tray manufacturing plants were closed.

Economic Performance of Poultry Cooperatives

The performance of the poultry cooperatives varies considerably. Several cooperatives operate successfully in Maharashtra. Their success can be attributed to good management, effective leadership, and a strong cooperative spirit among the members. These cooperatives have expanded the operations of the "central unit" to 50, 000 to 60, 000 commercial pullets, which are distributed among members, whose average flock size is about 1,000 birds. The central unit for the production infrastructure arranges loans and subsidies from the government. The society centrally procures and sells inputs (feed, equipment), provides technical advice, and markets the eggs and culled hens. The poultry-raising activities in the "daughter units" are mainly handled by women; the average profit from egg production is about Rs. 2 per bird per month. In view of the commercial success of these farmer cooperatives, continued public sector subsidies are no longer economically justified. However, cooperatives in other states have not been successful mainly because of management problems.

The Failure of a Poultry Cooperative

The Sutlej Poultry Cooperative Society in Ludhiana (Punjab) was organized in the late 1970s and began with 100 farmer units. Poor production (overcrowding of cages, poor disease control, poor feed) and financial management (no provision for working capital needs) resulted in the closure of about 80 farmer units within five years. Despite efforts by the society (additional credit) to bail out poorly performing farmers, by 1990 there were only 16 operating units, of which ten had expanded layer operations and six were converted into medium-sized (6,000-10, 000) broiler units.[1]

MARKETING OF WOOL

The marketing channels for wool, shown in Figure 18.3, are quite similar to those for meat, although the government and the Wool Marketing

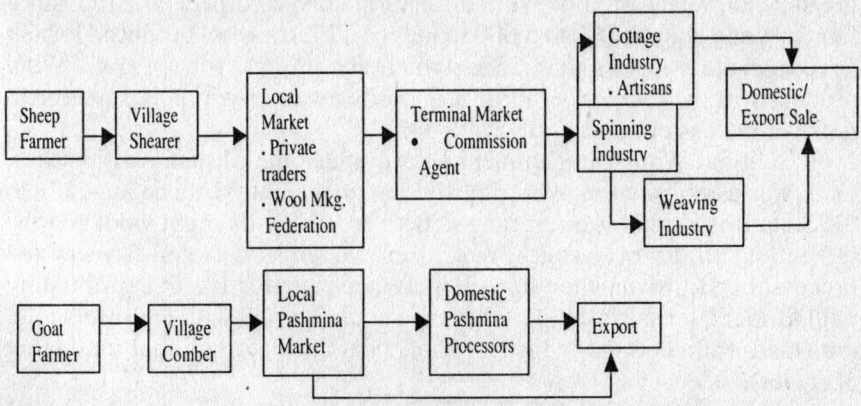

Figure 18.3: Marketing Channels for Wool and Goat Hair

---

[1]Alpha Agritech Consultant Ltd., "Poultry Development", Consultant's report prepared for the World Bank: 1994.

Federation intervene more extensively in the wool market. The government buys 10-15 percent of marketed wool. There are 61 wool markets situated in 13 states in India, with 40 percent of the wool trade occurring in Rajasthan. The farmer's share of the price of unprocessed wool is about 80 percent. The remainder is accounted by the cost of shearing (8-10 percent), transport (about 3 percent), local taxes (about 3 percent), commission charges (about 3 percent), and miscellaneous costs (about 2 percent). It is estimated that on an average, the profit margin of the yarn merchant is 5-20 percent (Table 18.1).

Table 18.1: Percentage Breakdown of Yarn Processing Margins

Cost Category	% Share
Yarn Sale Price	100
Cost of clean wool	65-80
Spinning cost	7-8
Wastage	8-10
Transport and Packing	1-1.4
Profit Margin	5-20

Source: Alpha Agritech Consultant: Small Ruminant Development Report: 1994

Wool quality: Grading facilities are available only in a few states, such as Rajasthan, Uttar Pradesh, Gujarat and Punjab, but the grading systems followed are not uniform across states. The lack of grading facilities in other areas further hampers the standardized pricing of raw material. Wool is graded on the average diameter of wool fibers and percentage of hairy fibers.

The quality of wool and hair produced in India (most with a diameter greater than 30 u) are more suited for furnishings, carpets, and industrial fabrics. Only about 3,000 to 5,000 tonnes (8-12%) of wool produced locally have diameters of less than 25 u, which are suitable for apparels. Wool produced in the temperate north and northwestern regions is superior to those of the eastern and southern regions.

A National Wool Development Board under the Ministry of Textiles, GOI, was established in 1989. It provides financial assistance annually to the State Boards and Corporations. There are currently eight wool boards/federations in different states, which serve as links between farmers and processors. However, they have largely been ineffective in coordinating with farmers, farmer's cooperatives and societies and with end-users (e.g. the small-scale cottage industry, wool mills and international marketing agencies).

Wool Processing Industry: The wool processing industry is small compared to the cotton, art silk and man-made fiber industries. The vertically integrated (combing, spinning, weaving, and machine carpet production) sector complements the decentralized (hosiery, power looms, hand-knotted carpets, handloom, and khadi) sector in meeting domestic and export market demand. During 1997/98, domestic wool production was estimated at 45,590 tonnes, while wool processing demand was estimated at 82,000 tonnes. The deficit had to be met through imports. These amounted to 45,000 tonnes of wool, 25,000 tonnes of rags, and waste, and 1000 tonnes of wool and hair tops, valued at over Rs. 3.5 billion.

MARKETING OF HIDES

Hides and skins are traditionally collected from villages, towns and cities and transported to major terminal markets. In recent years, tanneries are also obtaining skins at the district level markets. The major terminal markets for hides and skins are Chennai, Kolkata, Kanpur, Delhi, Mumbai and Hyderabad. However, because most of India's animal slaughter takes place in small villages and peri-urban units, the quality of the hides and skins retrieved following slaughter is very poor.

MARKET PRICE BEHAVIOR

Internal Prices

Wholesale price of fluid milk, beef, and mutton prices exhibited an increasing nominal trend from 1980-98 (Table 18.2). Their behaviour varied considerably, in real terms. Real milk prices registered smaller increase compared to other livestock products. This may be attributed to the doubling of supply and direct and indirect fixing of prices by the government and cooperatives. Real beef prices have risen since the late 1980s. Mutton prices, which remained almost stable in the 1980s, have risen most followed by butter.

There have been no significant long-term relative price changes between dairy, beef products and mutton to encourage cross-commodity shifts in consumption and resources. The ratio of milk prices to beef and mutton prices has remained essentially unchanged although the price of mutton relative to beef has improved. The declining costs of broiler meat relative to beef, mutton and milk during 1980-98 have also favoured increased poultry meat consumption.

Poultry Price Seasonality

Egg prices exhibit distinct seasonality. As illustrated by wholesale prices in the Chennai, Delhi, Mumbai markets, egg prices generally reach their lowest point in April and remain low throughout summer, after which they rise, peaking in November-December. Several factors, including seasonal changes in consumption and feed supply contribute to the seasonality of egg prices. In addition, egg consumption typically drops during festival and summer months, contributing to lower egg prices. To insulate producers from such seasonality, the states, with central government support, finance price stabilization activities.

Egg and broiler prices have declined in real terms as the industry has become more established. The real price of eggs declined by 5 percent

Table 18.2: Index of Wholesale Prices of All Commodities, Food Articles and Livestock Products (Base 1981-82 = 100)

Sl. No	Commodity	1984-85	1985-86	1986-87	1987-88	1988-89	1989-90	1990-91	1991-92	1992-93	1993-94	1994-95	1995-96	1996-97	1997-98	1998-99	1999-2000
1.	All Commodities	120.1	125.4	132.7	143.5	154.2	165.7	182.7	207.8	228.7	247.8	274.7	295.8	314.6	329.8	352.4	363.1
2.	Food Articles	131.8	134.1	147.8	161.1	177.1	179.3	200.6	241.1	271.0	284.4	312.7	335.7	375.1	388.0	440.9	457.7
3.	Milk	132.6	140.4	147.4	162.3	184.4	201.1	209.2	236.4	264.8	279.9	307.7	313.8	319.0	348.6	376.7	403.2
4.	Tinned Milk Powder	132.2	155.5	153.9	153.0	184.8	201.5	203.6	230.1	305.2	304.2	312.1	322.2	350.5	365.9	412.6	442.7
5.	Skimmed Milk Powder	120.4	126.3	128.1	151.3	187.7	198.8	178.6	220.9	289.9	258.5	253.6	344.1	358.6	372.0	352.3	385.6
6.	Baby Food (All Kinds)	125.2	132.8	132.0	135.8	159.0	170.6	179.5	198.5	211.4	210.5	221.3	262.0	319.4	380.2	410.4	423.1
7.	Butter	122.8	125.3	135.5	161.8	182.8	203.3	216.7	245.6	262.6	160.1	319.0	371.7	381.2	400.6	435.9	452.1
8.	Ghee	130.1	114.3	134.8	157.7	167.3	176.3	188.7	227.2	239.1	235.8	310.4	325.2	326.5	342.7	382.5	400.4
9.	Cattle Feed	111.0	113.5	119.1	128.1	134.3	140.8	155.0	172.8	195.8	206.9	222.0	247.5	273.5	289.2	303.7	335.5
10.	Poultry Feed	114.1	125.7	152.2	153.9	165.1	175.1	201.1	234.0	257.3	257.8	286.0	327.8	363.3	373.1	366.7	403.5
11.	Fodder	105.5	151.3	169.2	194.0	207.7	165.0	224.4	269.4	245.4	252.8	291.1	326.3	374.2	417.3	437.3	428.1
12.	Eggs	123.0	125.0	131.3	143.5	157.4	147.7	160.0	197.6	219.1	239.0	265.6	272.2	295.0	323.1	308.8	325.1
13.	Poultry Chicken	131.7	139.9	138.4	145.4	158.7	161.5	158.5	192.3	228.2	254.2	276.2	256.8	310.5	300.9	318.0	299.2
14.	Mutton	126.2	142.3	167.8	176.6	189.4	203.8	219.0	244.5	275.1	304.3	377.7	436.3	511.4	545.5	577.7	581.9

Table 18.2: Index of Wholesale Prices of All Commodities, Food Articles and Livestock Products (Base 1981-82 = 100) (Contd.)

Sl. No	Commodity	Year															
		1984-85	1985-86	1986-87	1987-88	1988-89	1989-90	1990-91	1991-92	1992-93	1993-94	1994-95	1995-96	1996-97	1997-98	1998-99	1999-2000
15.	Pork	131.8	144.2	149.3	154.2	177.1	215.0	243.0	273.3	267.4	270.5	279.6	362.5	414.9	425.7	424.0	430.9
16.	Fish	125.8	146.0	151.1	156.9	165.5	172.0	202.0	224.5	286.0	341.9	483.2	513.7	434.5	524.5	589.3	595.1
17.	Hides Raw	118.9	150.7	153.9	130.1	147.1	186.2	230.7	261.4	269.3	318.8	370.8	453.1	526.0	485.3	418.2	370.7
18.	Skin Raw	128.2	169.9	212.7	259.5	320.7	339.8	370.0	336.9	306.6	373.8	455.5	608.7	669.1	637.2	626.4	632.4
19.	Raw Wool	88.7	91.0	144.1	161.8	153.7	166.2	155.1	166.5	161.4	219.0	318.8	343.3	361.7	263.1	228.1	230.7
20	Sheep and Goat Skin	101.2	102.4	102.0	106.6	140.4	148.9	185.0	166.6	127.5	133.3	143.7	153.3	150.4	147.8	147.8	125.6

Source: Basic Animal Husbandry Statistics 2003, Department of Animal Husbandry & Dairying.

between 1985 and 1993, while the real price of broilers declined by 8 percent. The rapid production growth during the late 80s and early 90s (14%) per year explain the greater decline in broiler prices. In contrast, the price of day-old layer chicks increased 23 percent and day-old broiler chicks increased 10 percent during the same period. Trade protections afforded by high tariffs contribute to the high domestic prices of day-old chicks. Poultry and egg prices in the rural areas tend to be higher than in urban areas. This could be attributed to transportation costs, since production is undertaken in peri-urban areas, and differences in consumer preferences for different breeds of poultry. In particular, the price of the traditional free-range *desi* breeds is generally higher than the hybrid broilers.

19

Role of Women and Children in Livestock Farming

Currently no data or material is available to assess the impact of the development of livestock on income distribution among those engaged in this activity. The only information available relates to the number of different livestock species and value of different livestock products. However, it will be useful to collect such data which would help to evaluate the achievement of different programmes and if need be, to take appropriate measures to achieve the objective of equity in growth and deal with the gender issues such as those relating to women and children engaged in the livestock sector in the countryside.

Although the policies and the development of intensive livestock farming in India seem so far to have little adverse impact on the traditional animal husbandry farming, the importance of growth with equity is, however, well recognized by the official agencies in India. Official support for the social dimensions of development is thus very strong. Those working in the livestock sector are concerned with poverty reduction by raising income earning within the sector and by increasing employment in input and downstream processing and marketing. They are aware that there may be cost in achieving such objectives within the sector with tariffs and subsidies, which raise the cost of living to other poor consumers. There are also trade-offs (in the use of professional staff and funds) between direct intervention in livestock cycles and indirect intervention through infrastructural investment.

In India rural household depends on livestock farming as one of the important sources of income, total or supplementary, and nutrition. More than 630 million people (74 percent of the population) live in rural areas, and 237 million (38 percent) of them are poor. In 1986/87, 73 percent of the rural household owned livestock. Small and marginal farmers account for three-quarters of those households owning livestock. These small and marginal farmers accounted for 56 percent of the bovine (cattle and buffalo) and 62 percent of sheep population. Ownership of livestock is more evenly distributed amongst landless labourers, small and marginal farmers vis-à-vis agriculture per se. The livestock sector employs 8 percent of the total labour force, including small and marginal farmers, women and landless workers. The livestock sector is central to the livelihood of the rural poor in the country. Small-scale backyard livestock production enables the family including women and children to earn income from animals grazed on common property pastures or fed on household wastes. In fact, livestock products enable farmers to diversify income, helping them to reduce income variability especially in semi arid regions. In many cases, livestock farming provides the only source of income in the rural areas. Income from livestock farming accounts for 15-40 percent of the total farm household income in the country.

ROLE OF WOMEN AND CHILDREN

In India about 80 per cent of the female population live in rural areas and 86 per cent of the rural women work in agriculture and allied activities (Borah, 1998). Female involvement in farming activities is a common feature in Indian rural setting. Women perform a variety of roles, of which many are of greater economic significance (Bhople and Palki, 1998).

Role of women in agricultural sector, especially as keepers of livestock, greatly improves world food security by enhancing health and livelihood of individual families (Sinn et al, 1999). Women provide much of the unpaid family labour to agriculture (Thakar and Patel, 1998) including animal husbandry. Having been highly employed in livestock rearing activities (Birader, 1986 and Bhogal et al, 1988), rural women were found to devote 90 per cent of their time on cattle care, making it more or less a female domain (Veena et al, 1986).

The contribution of rural women, though not less than that of men in terms of time and effort, and invisible because they are largely unpaid and home based. Their contributions are continued to be given lesser importance while formulating livestock/rural development programmes. Though the association between women and livestock production needs productive exploitation, especially while aiming at rural development through livestock development, lack of empirical evidence on the magnitude of the female participation and the extent and nature of their association in livestock farming operations, however, limit our efforts in exploiting this linkage.

Livestock raising is an intensive labour activity. Rural women and children play a very significant role in livestock management and participate actively in areas such as feeding, breeding, maintaining and providing health care to the animals. Women constitute about 71 percent of the labour force in livestock whereas in crop farming they constitute only 33 percent of the work force. On an average, a typical household has to spend about six to seven hours per adult person per day in livestock raising in India, which is only second in time spent on domestic activities. Almost this entire requirement is met by family labour. Incidence of hired labour for livestock raising is rather limited. In the three states surveyed under the World Bank study, women spent relatively more time than men on livestock raising.

Time spent by women and men on livestock raising per day in Kerala for instance, was 4 hours by women against only 1.8 by men. In Gujarat women devoted 3.7 hours per day against 2.5 hours by men folk while in Rajasthan the differential was the lowest 4.5 hours per day by women compared to 2.5 by men.[1] In some districts of Haryana like Mahendragarh, time spent by rural women for dairying activities goes even up to 6-7 hours per day. Women dairy farmers play a vital role in the economy of their home in particular and country as a whole.

Caring animals is considered as an extension of domestic activities in Indian social system, and most of the animal husbandry activities like bringing fodder from field, chaffing the fodder, preparing feed for animals, offering water to animals, protection of animals from ticks and lice, cleaning of animals and sheds, preparation of dung cakes, milking, ghee-making and marketing of produce are performed and decided upon by women (Puri, 1974). They play a significant and crucial role in agricultural and allied activities including livestock production (Jain and Verma, 1992).

There is limited and understatement of statistical data on women working on household farms (Wijaya, 1993). Hence, a systematic valuation of time spent by females for household activities including animal care attention for policy intervention (Guleria and Agnihotri, 1985).

The Department of Animal Husbandry and Dairying and the National Dairy Development Board (NDDB) have finalised a proposal to train young boys and girls from at least 50 backward districts in the tribal belts of eastern Uttar Pradesh, Bihar, Madhya Pradesh, Orissa, West Bengal and the north eastern states in different disciplines of animal husbandry. The training programme will continue for three weeks in general and would be imparted in Patna and Siliguri.

The programme will include training in animal healthcare, artificial insemination, fodder management, livestock upgradation, dairy development, piggery and poultry. The selection of candidates would be done by the concerned district magistrates. The Technology Mission for Dairy Development would be involved in the process. Apart from the 50 earmarked districts, eight districts of Bihar like Samastipur, Madhubani, Darbhanga, East and West Champaran, Khagaria, Nalanda and Saharan has been selected for such training.

Although children in rural India make significant contribution to the livestock sector, only limited quantitative information based primarily on some surveys is available. According to a field survey carried out on labour employment in diary enterprises among different categories of progressive farmers in Haryana (North India), on an overall basis, children contributed 22 percent to the total employment per household estimated at 302 mandays per annum. Their share varied from 22.4 percent in the case of medium

---

[1]Vinod Ahuja et al: Agricultural Services for the Poor: Case of livestock Health and Breeding Services in India, p 40.

farmers to 23.6 percent for small farmers and 23.7 percent for large farmers. Women's contribution to the total employment per household a 38 percent was only slightly lower than for men about 40 percent. For different categories of farming holding, women participation in the tota employment per household ranged from 31 percent in the case of large farms to 35.5 percent for the small farms (Table 19.1).

Table 19.1: Total Labour Employment in Dairy Enterprises Among Progressive Farmer.
(Mandays/household/year

S. No.	Particulars	Small	Medium	Large	Overall
1.	Male	83.06	112.82	200.56	120.49 (39.84)
2.	Female	72.05	112.11	135.63	115.31 (38.13)
3.	Child	47.81	64.90	104.21	66.64 (22.03)
4.	Total Labour Employment per: i) Household	202.94	289.83	4 40.40	302.44 (100.00)
	ii) Dairy animal	98.60	83.80	70.32	86.22

Note: Percentage to total employment per household indicated in parenthesis.
Source: V.P. Sharma and Raj Vir Singh (1994) NDRI, Karnal.

Poultry Development and Women

Women in villages can better manage poultry pens and cattle shed. The also get children enthusiastically involved in these activities. According t the National Sample Survey (NSS) data of the Government of India (38tl Round, Report No. 341)[1], as high as 84 per cent of all active rural womei are employed usefully in agriculture. A study by UNICEF sponsorec Applied Nutritional Programme (ANP) revealed that rural women:

- Are better apt to handle delicate chicks;
- Have traditionally managed poultry; and,
- Successfully get eggs accepted among the vulnerable groups.

A key factor in the failure of rural poultry units is the inability of government extension agencies to mobilize women's potential. A propei training programme, focused on the needs of rural women, can help them take up new ideas and innovative practices in poultry raising.

Two motivating factors for rural women to take to poultry raising are that it gives them pin money for supplementing the family income and provides nourishing food for better health of their family.

Livestock production is an integral part of crop farming and contributes substantially to poverty alleviation and creates employment opportunities. Thus the concept of development of dairy, piggery and other sub-sector in

---

[2]According to the survey carried out for study on Agricultural Services for the Poor, the total number of cows and buffaloes (.i.e. milch stock) per household were only 1.34 in Kerala, 2.75 in Gujarat and 3.88 Rajasthan. Op. cit. p. 38.

India is quite different compared to the developed countries. The expansion of livestock sector in India during the last five decades or so has been based mainly on the raising/rearing of bovine and other species on the traditional system. Under this system a very small number of livestock herd per household[2] are raised mainly on low cost agro-byproducts as nutritional inputs, using traditional technologies for production through underemployed family labour – mostly female workforce. This practice is more or less the same with regard to poultry in the rural areas. The growth in the livestock sector has helped to raise both employment and income of the most of the livestock raising households. The sector has a great potential for bringing about socioeconomic transformation in the lives of the rural masses and improving their standards of living. For instance annual gross net income per additional cow is estimated at Rs. 1071 and Rs. 1400 per buffalo.[1] Unfortunately data are not available concerning the benefits derived by various classes of livestock owners due to increased production of livestock product in India. However, the expansion of livestock sector seems to have generated generally equitable income and employment in the countryside. Moreover, there seems to have been no adverse impact on income and employment for women and children in the rural areas, as there has been practically no development of intensive livestock sector. Even in the poultry, where organized sector has played an important role and now large commercial poultry enterprises have come up, it had however, no adverse impact on women and children in rural areas, where still backyard poultry rearing continues to exist and grow. In fact, the introduction of commercial poultry helped the small poultry keeping farmers in rural area to upgrade local stocks with introduction of exotic hybrid cockerels, supply of parents stocks and follow up scientific breeding in eggs and broiler strains.

Census 2001

It is heartening to note from the latest census report that rural women work force have doubled during the last three decades. In 1971, the participation of rural females was just over 15 per cent of the rural employment, in India. This, according to the report, has doubled to 31 per cent by the year 2001.

The key facts are that out of total Indian population, 48.1 per cent are women. The female illiteracy is 62 per cent. In rural India, agriculture and allied industry employ as much as 89.5 per cent of the total female labourers. Women have extensive workloads with dual responsibility for farm and household production. Women's work is getting harder and more time-consuming due to ecological degradation and changing agricultural technologies and practices.

---

[1] Rough estimates derived on the basis of milk per cow and buffalo and cost of production in Maharashtra and Uttar Pradesh. Cf. Indian Journal of Animal Production: Special Supplement On Buffalo. Vol. 30, no. 1-4, January-December 1996.

Women have an active role and extensive involvement in livestock production, forest resource use and fishery processing. Women contribute considerably to household income through farm and nonfarm activities as well as through work as landless agricultural labourers. The report further identifies that there have been high degrees of interstate and intrastate variations in gender roles in agriculture, environment and rural production. According to the report, while the overall female participation has gone up, there has been evidence of under employment. Besides, the increase has been higher in the category of the marginal work force as compared to the main work force. The marginal category refers to those workers who work for less than half of the year. The ratio of the main and marginal work force has dropped from 35.8 per cent in 1991 to 31 per cent in 2001. In fact, the marginal workers amongst female have increased from 30 per cent in 1991 to 46 per cent in 2001.

In India Women comprise about 32% of the labour force. Although better than Pakistan's, this proportion is much lower than that in China and Bangladesh. US and Thailand occupy the top spot, with 46% of total labour force comprising women.

Although, dairying is a sub-sector of agriculture, but it provides round the year rural employment in comparison to the other sectors. Therefore, the marginal work force is comparatively lower in the dairy sector. The women play a predominant role in livestock sector, particularly in rearing of milch animals, general health care, milking and distribution. The dairy cooperative movement, in India, has enhanced women participation, both in terms of their becoming the member of the cooperatives as well as milk-pourers. The NDDB has been doing pioneering work in empowering rural women through organising cooperatives as well as by providing them various inputs, which also include training and management, etc.

According to the Annual Report (2000-2001) of NDDB, it has contemplated to enhance women membership from the present level of around 20 to 50 per cent by the year 2010. Amongst the dairy milk suppliers, in the cooperative system, according to an estimate, approximately 70 lakh women have been maintaining their livelihood by supplying milk into the system, round the year. Although the dairy sector is one of the major sources of rural employment and in particular the women work force, requisite policy support has hardly been provided to the sector. Somehow, under the different plans of the government of India, the allocations provided to this sector have been insignificant as compared to its growth potentials! Instead of generating more employment, industrial recession is piling up unemployment in India. Over and above, if we continue to ignore the potentials of the rural sector, it would lead to a greater socioeconomic disparity. Therefore, the need of the hour is a refocus in our policies, commensurating with the situational needs.

IRDP

Integrated Rural Development Programme of the Government initiated over 25 years back puts special emphasis on giving increased income to women through livestock projects. Concurrent Evaluation Study of the Fifth Round for Haryana, for example, says in the agriculture sector, maximum beneficiaries were in animal husbandry scheme, particularly of dairy units/ milch cattle' where percentage of beneficiaries ranged between 18 in Mahendergarh district and 45 in Rohtak district. The State average was a high as 31.69 per cent. There were also quite an appreciable number of beneficiaries under 'sheep units' scheme. In fact, as high as 24 percent beneficiaries were under the scheme in Sirsa district followed by 23% in Hissar district, 14% in Jind district and 12% in Bhiwani district. In rest of the districts the beneficiaries under the scheme varied between 1 per cent in Faridabad district and 8 per cent in Rewari district. However, in Karnal district there was none under the scheme. There were a few other schemes under animal husbandry where also a small percentage of beneficiaries existed. The percentage distribution of beneficiaries under these schemes in the districts varied between 2 and 6 save in Bhiwani, Hissar, Kaithal, Mahendergarh, Panipat and Sirsa districts where there was none.

RIGHTS TO LIVESTOCK—EMPOWERING WOMEN

More than 70 per cent of rural people own livestock. It provides a higher share of household income among poorer and landless families, especially for women, than among wealthier ones. Demand for livestock products is expected to double in developing countries in the next twenty years, making it the fastest growing agricultural sector. To maintain and expand the benefits this growing sector can bring to resource-poor women, new policies and practices must protect women's ownership and use rights, favour small-scale operations, and provide strong training programmes in group development and the production, processing, and marketing of animals and products.

Women's livestock projects in developing countries are increasing. When rural women have access to cash or microcredit, they usually choose to invest in livestock, which provide food, cash, draft power, and fertilizer, and gain value through reproduction. With increasing male outmigration and the feminization of rural poverty, women have a greater need and desire for livestock to improve their food security and income levels.

Livestock may be distributed to alleviate malnutrition, because foods of animal origin, including milk, eggs, and meat, contain high-quality protein and needed calories, vitamins, and minerals. Livestock have important cultural meanings, and their exchange through gifts builds social capital. It is increasingly recognized that animals under women's control are more likely to improve family nutrition and education than similar assets held by men. Heifer Project International (HPI), an international nongovernmental organization with nearly sixty years of experience with grassroots-based livestock development, has found that with careful planning women's livestock projects can lead to both economic success and empowerment.

Animal Ownership

Women benefit most when they have decision-making authority about the animals they manage, even without legal ownership rights. Women's rights vary by culture, class, and type of animal. Asserting claims to smaller species such as goats, sheep, poultry, and pigs, rather than cattle, camels, or buffalo, is usually easier for women. Micro-livestock (guinea pigs, silkworms, snails, honeybees, and rabbits) are especially important. It is easier to operate a productive enterprise with smaller animals, since the initial costs are lower: Profits may be low, but so are the risks, and men are less likely to interfere. When possible, women prefer to own larger animals such as dairy cattle, because they are more profitable and bring greater personal status.

Women often have access to livestock through family ties. A man may own a donkey but permit his wife to use it to carry water or vegetables, increasing her productivity by saving time and labour. A man with a dairy cow may sell the morning milk but permit the women to use the evening milk for household consumption.

However, livestock projects that distribute animals to families do not necessarily benefit the women in the household. Women usually provide most of the labour for stall-fed dairy cattle and other animals kept near the home, but may not realize benefits commensurate with their contribution, limiting their incentive to increase production. Traditional usufruct rights and ownership are in transition due to privatization and commercialization, so project planning must intentionally include labour and benefit analysis for all family members.

With privatization women often lose traditional rights to both household animals and land, since ownership and decision-making become concentrated in a single, usually male, individual. This is a real risk when women's traditional activities such as dairying or poultry production are commercialized, and there is no replacement of their income. Policies encouraging privatization should consider gendered impacts, so that poor women are not further disadvantaged.

Joint ownership is a strategy to protect a woman's right to household livestock after a husband's death. Heifer Project requires the wife as well as the husband to sign its livestock contract, to prevent "property grabbing" by the man's relatives when he dies. Local authorities are asked to enforce the contract. Projects with polygamous families decide on the most equitable contracts to protect women's future livelihoods.

Some livestock schemes allocate animals only to women, assuming they make decisions independently and will improve their bargaining position by bringing wealth into the household. The projects are most successful when men are included in discussions of workload and benefits, so that the project does not increase women's workload but her husband takes the income. As with any form of microcredit, appropriation or domestic violence may occur when men's interests are not addressed. In Kenya, some women's groups maintain legal ownership of animals and may remove them from homes where a husband treats his wife badly.

Constraints faced by Women

All the constraints to women's access to public programmes and commercial transactions with the 'outside' have been operative in the livestock sector. The common pattern is for women to handle most of the production aspects and for the men to control the cash income and assume ownership/membership of organizations if any. There are a number of problems associated with this traditional 'inside/outside' division of labour. Some affect the overall efficiency of production; others affect the welfare returns to the family and to the women producer herself. Women, for example, do not usually gain access to training in modern livestock management and techniques, which is available to men through the institutional structure. Instead, they must learn second hand through the men or continue with traditional practices, both of which lower their efficiency and reduce returns to investments in training

For women from poor households the greatest disadvantage is, however, that they have no control over income, which is collected by the male household member. In cases where the women used to deal with traditional traders who came to household compound, they lost what small degree of economic autonomy they had when marketing arrangements were formalized through the institutional structures. The fact that milk payments to cooperative members in many villages are, for efficiency reasons, now made less frequently and, hence, payments in larger sums, have apparently increased the likelihood that at least some of the money is diverted by the men before essential household expenses are met. In short, for nonmember women producers, Operation Flood has often meant more dairy work but no increase, and sometimes even a decrease, in their access to dairy income.

The critical bottlenecks to progress in subsistence and near subsistence farming often do not lie in the sector itself, but on the absence of roads, access to water and other simple infrastructural facilities. The poorest areas of any country, almost by definition, are those not accessible by year round transport. These are also the areas without schools and health services, let alone animal health services. Providing basic infrastructure will enable the farmers to bring in inputs, reach consumers and make their own production decisions and markets will develop. A reliable water supply and rural electrification will also reduce drudgery and increase productivity, particularly for rural women.

Working with Groups

Women's empowerment is strengthened through group action and support. Group discussion help communities explore women's decision making power, especially over large and valuable animals, so that men do not feel threatened. Facilitation by a respected leader or professional helps clarify the benefits of livestock to all family members.

Heifer project requires a written contract with all project recipients to "repay the loan" through "passing on the gift". This involves giving the first female offspring (or cash equivalent) from a cow, goat, or other animal to another needy family in the same group. The payback is essential for active participation in group training and other activities. Projects that hand out animals without requiring repayment usually fail. Projects have better success where animals are managed by individual families rather than by groups, unless there is a strong tradition of group herding.

Commercialization

Managing their own small-scale livestock enterprises provides rural women with more benefits than paid employment as unskilled workers on large-scale commercial operations typically managed by men. Also, serious environmental and animal welfare problems associated with large-scale confinement operations can usually be avoided on small-scale farms.

Women are the majority among the increasing number of peri-urban livestock producers providing milk and meat to informal urban markets. Many governments try to regulate their activities due to legitimate public health concerns. Including women when planning sanitation or marketing improvements is critical so that they do not lose their livelihood to industrial-scale producers.

Women's livestock activities have the potential for great financial success, but they need strong financial training to avoid losing control to men when expanding their enterprises. Cooperatives have also helped many small-scale male farmers market their products, but may disadvantage women. If meetings are held when women are busy with other tasks, they cannot effectively participate in decision making. Sometimes women form their own cooperatives. Other solutions include electing women to the coop managing committee, or changing the rules regarding membership, payment, and meeting times. In Uganda and India, women opened group bank accounts that only they could access to receive their dairy payments.

Commercialization of livestock production can affect family nutrition and women's status if all of the milk, rabbits, or chickens are sold rather than used for home consumption. This risks increasing women's financial dependence on men by having to ask for money to purchase food they once produced.

Some livestock programmes include human nutritional education and should address both men and women. Men can determine food distribution patterns, while women often only control food preparation. Out of respect, a woman in Tanzania or Bangladesh would not limit the high-quality food of animal origin she offers to her husband in order to improve her own or her children's diets. Often, husbands, when well fed themselves, are not aware that other household members receive less. In times of nutritional stress, women typically reduce their own food intake the most. Thus, although nutritional education is traditionally a women's programme, targeting men can benefit the entire household.

Training

Animal distribution or credit schemes without technical training have limited success. Technical training helps women ensure that their rights to livestock lead to increased food, income, and decision me making power. Training programmes that are held in the local language and provide child-care and meals increase the chances of meaningful participation by women. One day of village-based, hands-on, and participatory training is best for illiterate women with restricted mobility. Follow-up, refresher courses and farm visits are also important. Single-sex groups often help women improve their confidence with unfamiliar tasks, such as working with large animals. without interference from men.

Training in animal health and management, and access to veterinary care can control animal diseases that reduce productivity, especially with exotic or crossbred animals. In developing countries, most veterinarians and livestock extension specialists are men and target their expertise to other men. One solution is to recruit and train more women as professionals, another is to train and reward all professional staff for providing outreach to women. Existing women extension agents – now mostly home economists – can be trained in animal husbandry, which is important to all rural women.

In remote areas, community animal health workers may provide the best type of animal health care. When women are selected and trained, they perform as well as men and increase other women's use of animal health services. Unfortunately, the number so far are small. Successful recruitment strategies target older women with fewer domestic responsibilities or husband and wife teams, when contact with the opposite sex is severely restricted. Having women work in pairs is also helpful.

Finally, most women owning livestock report that the animals provide food security, income, and status in the community. They are more portable than land and crops and are a "living savings bank" that may be used throughout the year. Women with limited resources who receive animals through group distribution schemes also note that the group itself provides numerous benefits, such as increased confidence and leadership skills. In general, women prefer to work with all-women groups until they feel confident enough to speak in the presence of men. Membership in mixed groups offers access to additional valuable assets. By joining community-level committees, women begin to influence more of the decisions that affect their lives.

Livestock projects can be the entry point for other types of group-based interventions on health and sanitation, education, and land rights. Training in animal reproduction increases groups' ability to discuss human reproduction and health. Group savings can increase women's potential to invest in other enterprises. The social contact builds trust and mutual support for crisis times. In HPI's experience, the attraction of livestock and their tangible benefits create the economic opportunity, while the social impacts provide the most significant and long-lasting results.

TAMIL NADU STUDY[1]

This study was planned to fill gap, arising out of the dearth of documented evidence on female participation in livestock farming.

The specific objectives of the study were:

- To study the functions carried out by farm women in livestock farming;
- To study the time spent by farm women in different activities of livestock care.

Methodology

Villupuram District of Tamil Nadu was purposively selected for the study, for this district has the highest cattle population and ranks third across the districts of the State in total livestock population (Livestock Census, 1994) and 92.56 per cent of total women population of this districts reside in rural areas (Director of Census Operation, Tamil Nadu, 1991). Multistage random sampling technique was used to select the respondents. The chosen districts comprised 22 blocks of which, two blocks, viz., Kallakurichi and Thiyagadurgam were randomly selected. In the next stage, two villages from each selected block were chosen randomly. In total, 120 farmers were chosen again randomly from the selected four villages, 30 from each village, and it was ensured that the sample represented all the land holding class categories. The study was taken up during the months of April and May, 2000 and the data collected from the sample units related to the year 1999-2000. Relevant data were collected from the chosen respondents through personal interview using a pretested interview schedule. Cross checks were made to minimise the errors due to recall bias and also to ensure reliability of the information provided by the respondents.

Findings

The functions carried out by females in livestock keeping are listed out in Table 19.2. The major functions included feeding, watering, housing, breeding, health care, milking, hygiene and marketing, with regard to livestock farming were found to be performed by farm women. Average

---

[1]R. John Christy, Role of Farm Women in Livestock Keeping, Indian Dairyman, 2002.

Table 19.2: Animal Related Tasks Carried out by Farm Women

Tasks		Sub-Tasks
Feeding	(a)	Feeding concentrates
	(b)	Feeding roughages
	(c)	Feeding greens
	(d)	Bringing animals for feeding
	(e)	Taking animals for grazing
	(f)	Storing feeds
	(g)	Bringing greens from the field
	(h)	Managing and feeding vessels cleaning
Watering	(a)	Fetching water
	(b)	Bringing animals for watering
	(c)	Vessels cleaning
Housing	(a)	Housing the animals
	(b)	Penning and Depenning the animals
Breeding	(a)	Identifying animals in heat
	(b)	Sending/taking animals for service
	(c)	Caring pregnant animals
Animal Health Care	(a)	Identifying sick animals
	(b)	Sending/taking animals to hospital
	(c)	Sending/taking animals for vaccination
	(d)	Sending/taking animals for Mass Contact Programmes (MCP)
	(e)	Maintaining sick animals
Milking	(a)	Bringing animals for milking
	(b)	Udder cleaning
	(c)	Hand and udder disinfection
	(d)	Cleaning milking vessels
	(e)	Milking
	(f)	Keeping milk safe
Hygiene	(a)	Cleaning animals
	(b)	Cleaning animal house
	(c)	Disinfecting animal house
Marketing	(a)	Selling milk and products
	(b)	Transporting milk and products
	(c)	Storing milk and products
	(d)	Processing milk and product making
	(e)	Collection of money for milk and products sold

time spent on these tasks by farm women labour in livestock keeping is illustrated in table 19.3. On an average, females spent about 294.34 minutes and 87.17 minutes daily for large and small ruminates keeping respectively. Of the time spent for large ruminates, they spent about 46 per cent of the time for feeding, 21 per cent for milking and 12 per cent for marketing the milk and milk products, while for small ruminantes, they spent about 74 per cent in feeding tasks and around 7 per cent each for watering, housing and hygienic maintenance:

From Tables 19.2 and 19.3, it could be concluded that most of the tasks related to livestock keeping were performed only by the farm women. These findings were in line with the findings of Puri (1974b), Singh and Bhati (1985), Sisodia (1985), Susheela et al. (1991), Jain and Verma (1992), Nisha (1996) and Saikia (1999). Imputed economic value of the time spent on animal based tasks by farm women was calculated to be Rs. 24.53 and Rs. 7.26 per day per household in large and small ruminants keeping respectively. This measure underlines the economic importance of the functions carried out by farm women in the rural economy and in livestock farming.

Table 19.3: Average Time Spent on Animal Based Tasks by Farm Women

Tasks	Average time spent per day per household (in minutes)	
	Large ruminant keeping	*Small ruminant keeping*
Feeding	134.54 (45.71)	64.51 (74.00)
Watering	24.91 (8.46)	6.82 (7.82)
Housing	9.14 (3.16)	6.73 (7.72)
Breeding	7.02 (2.38)	0.80 (0.91)
Animal Health Care	9.25 (3.14)	1.42 (1.63)
Milking	60.73 (20.63)	—
Hygiene	13.15 (4.47)	6.89 (7.90)
Marketing	35.60 (12.47)	—
Total	**294.34 (100)**	**87.17 (100)**
Imputed economic value of the time spent (in Rs.) per day per household*	**24.53**	**7.26**

Note: Figures in the parenthesis indicate percentages to their respective totals.* Imputed economic value was calculated at the rate of Rs. 40/- per 8 hours of work.

The relationships between operational land holdings and the time spent by females in livestock based tasks are presented in Table 19.4. Female farmers in landless, marginal, small and large categories spent about 304.08, 269.12, 300.04 and 300.15 minutes per household per day respectively in tending large ruminants. These figures for small ruminantes keeping were 44.14, 91.33, 92.33 and 120.31 minutes respectively. The females spent more or less equal time for large ruminants keeping, except those in marginal farmer households who spent relatively lesser time. It might be due to the fact that they possessed lesser number of animals than that of other categories of farmers. The results are in line with the findings of Susheela et al. (1999) and Borah (1998) who observed that landholding did not influence the time spent by farmwomen on animal husbandry.

In small ruminants keeping, the time spent by female increased with the increase in land holding. This could be attributed to the fact that women with larger land holding could afford to spend their time in lighter tasks

Table 19.4: Relationships between Land Holding and Average Time Spent by Farm Women (Minutes per day per household)

Activities	Landless		Marginal (0-2.5 acres)		Small (2.6-5.0 acres)		Large (5.1 and above)		Overall	
	Ruminants		Ruminants		Ruminants		Ruminants		Ruminants	
	Large	Small	Large	Small	Large	Small	Large	Small	Large	Small
Feeding	141.58 (46.56)	34.29 (46.62)	125.46 (77.68)	58.33 (63.87)	135.21 (45.06)	71.67 (77.62)	135.92 (45.28)	93.75 (77.92)	134.54 (45.71)	64.51 (74)
Watering	24.96 (8.21)	5.29 (11.98)	21.73 (8.07)	5.83 (6.38)	26.72 (8.90)	8.33 (9.02)	26.23 (8.74)	7.81 (6.49)	24.91 (8.46)	6.82 (7.82)
Housing	8.81 (2.90)	2.57 (5.82)	8.08 (3.00)	4.83 (5.29)	10.10 (3.37)	7.50 (8.12)	9.58 (3.19)	12 (9.97)	9.14 (3.10)	6.73 (7.72)
Breeding	6.85 (2.25)	0.29 (0.66)	6.27 (2.33)	0 (0)	7.38 (2.46)	1.17 (1.16)	7.58 (2.52)	1.75 (1.45)	7.02 (2.38)	0.80 (0.91)
Animal Healthcare	9.46 (3.09)	1.57 (3.56)	8.15 (3.03)	1.67 (1.23)	9.17 (3.06)	1.17 (1.16)	10.23 (3.4¡)	1.25 (1.04)	9.25 (3.14)	1.42 (1.63)
Milking	65.15 (21.42)	0 (0)	58.73 (21.82)	0 (0)	58.90 (19.63)	0 (0)	60.12 (20.03)	0 (0)	60.73 (20.63)	0 (0)
Hygiene	13.12 (4.45)	0.14 (0.32)	10.19 (3.79)	21.17 (23.18)	14.21 (4.74)	2.50 (2.70)	15.08 (5.02)	3.75 (3.11)	13.15 (4.47)	6.89 (7.90)
Marketing	38.15 (12.53)	0 (0)	30.50 (11.33)	0 (0)	38.34 (12.78)	0 (0)	35.42 (11.80)	0 (0)	35.60 (12.09)	0 (0)
Total	304.08 (100)	44.14 (100)	269.12 (100)	91.33 (100)	300.34 (100)	92.33 (100)	300.15 (100)	120.31 (100)	294.34 (100)	87.17 (100)
Imputed Economic Value (in Rs.)	25.34	3.68	22.43	7.61	25.00	7.69	25.01	10.02	24.53	7.26

Figures in the parentheses indicate percentages to total.

like taking small ruminants for grazing which alone took more than 75 per cent of the time spent by females in small ruminants keeping. The imputed economic value of the time spent on large ruminants care by farm women were found to be Rs. 25.34, Rs. 22.43, Rs. 25.00 and Rs. 25.01 per households respectively and the same for small ruminants care were found to be Rs. 3.68, Rs. 7.61, Rs. 7.69 and Rs. 10.02 respectively.

The results of the study revealed that many of the tasks related to livestock keeping were performed by the farm women. On an average farm women spent about 294.34 and 87.17 minutes per day per household on large and small ruminantes keeping respectively. Imputes economic value of the time spent on animal based tasks by farm women was calculated to be Rs. 24.53 and Rs. 7.26 per day per household in large and small ruminates keeping respectively. Landholding did not influence the time spent by farm women for large ruminant's care in the study area but had a positive influence on the time spent by farm women on small ruminant's care.

Policy Suggestions

The results emanating from the study produce well-documented evidence that farm women have a close association with livestock farming in the State. These results tend to suggest a more active role for this segment of the rural society so as to achieve rural development through combining women and livestock development. In the light of these results the following policy suggestions are made to fully and productivity exploit the women-livestock linkage.

- Channels of information, credit, inputs and access to markets have to be aimed at women as they played a very important role in livestock keeping and decisions related to livestock productions.

- Extension assistance regarding livestock rearing have to be directed towards women to enhance their productive use of labour. The gender compositions of extension offices make it difficult for women farmers to obtain extension advice. Hence appropriate female frontline extension staff have to be employed to interact with the female farmers.

- Bringing the services available to rear the animals physically closer to women.

- Suitable training programmes for the skill development of rural farmwomen on animal keeping may be organised so that their earning potential may be increased and improve the efficiency of the farmwomen. Their participation in such programmes is likely to bring forward the real and practical problems that need immediate attention of the policy makers.

- Promoting intensive livestock rearing in rural areas may encourage female to participate more in livestock keeping as this practice did not require farm women to take animals for grazing far away from home.

Encouraging the formation of rural women livestock farmer's co-operative society may increase female participation in livestock rearing.

RAJASTHAN EXPERIENCE[1]

Rajasthan State is divided into nine agroclimatic zones on the basis of soil type, cropping pattern, access to irrigation etc. For the purpose of present study zone known as 'Humid South Eastern Plain' covering the districts of Kota, Bundi, Jhalawar and part of Swaimadhopur was choosen. From the selected zone, Bundi district was purposively selected as the district shares remarkable State's area of paddy, soyabean, mustard, wheat and sugarcane which are labour intensive crops. The source of irrigation plays a crucial role in the extent and magnitude of female participation in agriculture. The selected district was, therefore, divided into two parts on the basis of sources of irrigation. i.e. (i) solely well irrigated areas (ii) canals as well as well irrigated areas. Well irrigation augments labour use and in well irrigated areas most of the holdings fall under the category of marginal and small where female participation is expected to be high. The present study is confined to well irrigated situation in Bundi district only. Among the villages having adequate access to well irrigation, three village were randomly selected for the present study. In all 45 cultivators representing different farm size classes were selected from the three selected villages to collect the primary data for the crop year 1997-98.

Results and Discussions

Characteristics of Selected house holdings

The average size of holding was 2.8 hectares of which about 71 per cent was irrigated and the remaining 29 per cent was unirrigated (Table 19.5). In the sample farms, the average number of animals kept were 5.78 of which milking and non-milking animals were 25.95 and 74.05 per cent, respectively. Average number of workers per farm were 3.83 of which 54 per cent were males and the remaining were females.

Table 19.5: Average Holding, Animals and Labour Force on Sample Farms

Particulars			Total
Land (ha)	2.06 (irrigated)	0.83 (unirrigated)	2.89
	(71.28)	(28.72)	(100)
Animals (Nos.)	1.50 (Milking)	4.28 (Non-milking)	5.76
	(25.950)	(74.05)	(100)
Workers (Nos.)	2.05 (Male)	1.78 (Female)	3.83
	(53.52)	(46.48)	(100)

Figures in Parentheses are percentages of totals.

---

[1]Study by D.C. Paul; Role of Farm Women in Humid South Eastern Plain of Rajasthan, Bihar Journal of Agricultural Marketing, March 2001.

Female Labour Utilization in Crop Husbandry

It is evident from Table 19.6 that out of the total 292.46 days work per farm in all the crops, female labour worked for 171.44 days, i.e., 58.62 per cent. Among the various operations performed on the fields, there was no participation of female labour in ploughing and in the transportation of fertilizers. Removal of bushes, FYM application, seed treatment and sowing, irrigation, fertilizer, application of insecticides and pesticides, transportation of harvested crop of threshing floor and transportation of main and by-product were the operations in which female participation varied from 33.61 to 51.68 per cent. Female labour participation was very high in interculture, threshing and in harvesting/picking operations. It was 85.19, 80.95 and 75.97 per cent in these operations, respectively.

Table 19.6: *Extent of Female Labour Utilization in Crop Husbandry*

(Days/farm/year)

Day = hours

Particulars	Male	Female	Total
Removal of Bushes	1.55	1.41	2.96
	(52.37)	(47.63)	(100)
FYM application	8.12	7.51	15.63
	(51.95)	(48.05)	(100)
Ploughing	17.44	—	17.44
	(100.00)		(100)
Seed Treatment and sowing	5.01	2.72	7.73
	(64.91)	(35.19)	(100)
Irrigation	34.50	20.01	54.51
	(63.29)	(36.71)	(100)
Fertilizer transport action	1.70	—	1.70
	(100.00)		(100)
Fertilizer application	2.51	2.46	4.97
	(50.50)	(49.50)	(100)
Interculture operation	6.80	39.11	45.91
	(14.81)	(85.19)	(100)
Application of insecticides / pesticides	1.62	0.82	2.44
	(66.39)	(33.61)	(100)
Harvesting/picking	18.26	57.74	76.00
	(24.03)	(75.97)	(100)
Transportation to threshing floor	7.20	7.70	14.90
	(48.32)	(51.68)	(100)
Threshing	5.60	23.79	29.39
	(19.05)	(80.95)	(100)
Transportation of main & by-product	10.71	8.17	18.88
	(56.73)	(43.27)	(100)
Total	121.02	171.44	292.46
	(41.38)	(58.62)	(100)

Figures in parentheses are percentages of totals.

Female Labour Utilization in Animal Husbandry

In rearing the animals 214.42 days of labour per farm annually was required of which 55.54 per cent (119.08 days) was the share of female labour (Table 19.7). Item-wise, in animal grazing, health care and in breeding operations the share of female labour was less than male labour while in the milking operation female served for 46.75 days which is 82.38 per cent of the total requirement of labour.

Table 19.7: Female Labour Utilization in Animal Husbandry

(Days/farm/year)

Day = hours

Particulars	Male	Female	Total
Animal grazing	78.72	69.58	148.30
	(53.08)	(46.92)	(100)
Health Care	4.12	1.00	5.12
	(80.47)	(19.53)	(100)
Breeding	2.50	1.75	4.25
	(58.82)	(41.18)	(100)
Milking	10.00	46.75	56.75
	(17.62)	(82.38)	(100)
Total	95.34	119.08	214.42
	(44.46)	(55.54)	(100)

Figures in parentheses are percentages of row totals.

Female Labour Utilization in the Collection of Inputs

In the collection of inputs for crops and livestock 226.76 days per farm per year were required in which the male and female participation was almost equal, i.e., 49.14 and 50.86 per cent respectively (Table 19.8). In crop husbandry female served only for 28.31 days which is 34.63 per cent of the total labour required for the collection of inputs for crops. The share of female in storing and taking care of the stored material was high (i.e., 66.11%) while their share in the collection of seeds, insecticides/pesticides, FYM and fertilizers was less than 40 per cent of the total labour required for respective item. The utilization of female labour was 87.01 days which is 60.01 per cent of the total labour required in the collection of inputs for animal husbandry. In harvesting of green fodder and collection of fodder and concentrates the females served more to male while in chaffing the fodder there was no use of female labour.

Female Labour Utilization in Marketing of Farm Produce

It is evident from Table 19.9 that the total labour required for marketing of crop and livestock product annually per farm was 52.64 days of which the female labour served for 29.46 days (i.e. 55.97%). The requirement for labour in marketing of crop produce was less (8.02 days) compared to

Table 19.8: Female Labour Utilization in the Collection of Inputs for Crop and Animal Husbandry

(Days/farm/year)
Day = 8 hours

Particulars	Male	Female	Total
I Crop Husbandry			
Seed	13.56	1.46	15.02
	(90.28)	(9.72)	(100)
Culture	0.46	—	0.46
	(100.00)		(100)
Insecticides/Pesticides	3.00	1.92	4.92
	(60.98)	(39.02)	(100)
FYM	19.04	9.08	28.12
	(67.71)	(32.29)	(100)
Fertilizers	10.12	1.67	11.79
	(85.84)	(14.16)	(100)
Other (Storing, taking care etc.)	7.27	14.18	21.45
	(33.89)	(66.11)	(100)
Sub Total I	53.45	28.31	81.76
	(65.37)	(34.63)	(100)
II Animal Husbandry			
Harvesting of green fodder	36.53	69.44	105.97
	(34.47)	(65.53)	(100)
Collection of fodder and Concentrates	11.88	17.57	29.45
	(40.34)	(59.66)	(100)
Chaffing	9.58	—	9.58
	(100.00)		(100)
Subs Total II	57.99	87.01	145.00
	(39.99)	(60.01)	(100)
Total (I + II)	111.44	115.32	226.76
	(49.14)	(50.86)	(100)

Figures in parenthesis are percentages of row total

marketing of livestock product (44.62 days). In marketing of crop and livestock product female used for 2.46 days and 27 days, respectively. It is 30.67 and 60.51 per cent of the total labour required in marketing of crop and livestock product, respectively. Among the items in marketing the produce the female participation is equal to male in the preparation of crop produce for sale and it was 75.76 per cent in the preparation of dairy product for sale.

Female, Labour Utilization in off Farm Activities

On an average 86.38 days work was available on the nonfarm of which farm female labour was utilized for 5.14 days (Table 19.10). It means that about 6 per cent nonfarm work was performed by female and the rest was performed by male workers. Activities wise in crop production and in animal

Table 19.9: Female Labour Utilization in the Marketing of Crop and Livestock Product

(Days/farm/year)

Day = 8 hours

Particulars	Male	Female	Total
I Crop Produce			
Preparation of produce for sale	1.96	1.96	3.92
	(50.00)	(50.00)	(100)
Packing	1.10	0.33	1.43
	(76.92)	(23.08)	(100)
Loading	1.46	0.11	1.57
	(92.99)	(7.01)	(100)
Miscellaneous	1.04	0.06	1.10
	(94.55)	(5.45)	(100)
Sub Total I	5.56	2.46	8.02
	(69.33)	(30.67)	(100)
II Livestock Product			
Preparation of dairy	8.00	25.00	33.00
Product for sale	(24.24)	(75.76)	(100)
Marketing of milk and	9.62	2.00	11.62
Other products	(82.79)	(17.21)	(100)
Subs-Total II	17.62	27.00	44.62
	(39.49)	(60.51)	(100)
Total (I + II)	23.16	29.46	52.64
	(44.03)	(55.97)	(100)

Figures in parentheses are percentages of totals.

Table 19.10: Female Labour Utilization in the Off-farm Work

(Days/farm/year)

Day = 8 hours

Particulars	Male	Female	Total
Crop Production	4.36	15.39	19.75
	(22.08)	(77.92)	(100)
Animal Husbandry	0.26	1.67	1.93
	(13.47)	(86.53)	(100)
Nonfarm Work	81.24	5.14	86.38
	(94.05)	(5.95)	(100)

Figures in parentheses are percentages of totals.

husbandry the share of female was (77.92 and 86.53% respectively), more than nonfarm work (5.95%).

Female Labour Utilization in all Activities on and Off Farm

It is evident from Table 19.11 that the workers (male and female both) per farm got a total of 894.34 days employment in a year on the farm and off farm activities. In this female labours got 457.50 days work, which is 51.16 per cent of the total employment.

Table 19.11: Female Labour Utilization on the Farm and Off the Farm

(Days/farm/year)

Day = 8 hours

Particulars	Male	Female	Total
On the farm	350.98	435.30	786.28
	(44.64)	(53.36)	(100)
Off the farm	85.86	22.20	108.06
	(79.46)	(20.54)	(100)
Total	436.84	457.50	894.34
	(48.84)	(51.16)	(100)

Figures in parentheses are percentages of row totals

The employment on the farm was 786.28 days while it was 108.06 days per year off the farm. The use of female labour was more on the farm (53.36% of the total employment on the farm) compared to off the farm (20.54% of total employment off the farm). The employment per worker is presented in Table 19.12.

Table 19.12: Per Workers Female Labour Employment

(Days/farm/year)

Day = 8 hours

Particulars	Male	Female	Total
On the Farm	171.21	244.55	205.30
Off the Farm	41.88	12.47	28.21
Total	213.09	257.02	233.51

On overall basis a farm worker got 233.51 days employment in a year. Per worker employment of female was higher (257.02 days) while off the farm employment was 41.88 days per male and 12 days per female worker in a year. Male and female on the farm got 171.21 days work and 244.55 days. Thus, it can be concluded that female got more per worker employment in a year on the farm and less on off farm compared to male.

CONCLUSION

In all the operations for crops, animal husbandry, management of inputs for crops and livestock, marketing of farm produce and in off farm work, the female participation was evident. Their participation was high in interculture, threshing, harvesting/picking, milking the animals and in the collection of inputs for animal husbandry. Female participation was more compared to male in marketing of livestock product while a reverse picture is seen in the marketing of crop produce. Per worker employment of female was higher (257.02 days) compared to male worker (213.09 days) in a year. On the farm and off the farm per female worker got employment of 224.55 days and 12.47 days respectively in a year.

BIBLIOGRAPHY

Bhogal, T.S., J.S Sharma and V.P.S. Arora (1988). Augmenting Income and Employment of Small and Marginal Farmers and Landless Labourers through Dairying in Western Uttar Pradesh. Indian Journal of Dairy Sciences, 4 (1): 101.

Bhople, R.R. and A. Palki (1998). Socio-Economic Dimensions of Farm Women labour, Rural India., Sep-Oct. 1998: 192-196.

Birader, R.D. (1986). Changing through Dairy Development – A Case Study. Dairy Guide., 8(3): 2-24.

Borah, R. (1998). Perceived Drudgery and Factors Influencing Time Spent in Agricultural Operations by Farm Women in Assam. Rural India., Nov. 1998: 214-221.

Guleria, A.S. and B. Agnihotri (1985). Contribution of Female Workers in the Farm Sector. Indian Journal of Agricultural Economics., 40: 271.

Jain, V. and S. K. Verma (1992). Nature and Extent of Involvement of men and Women in Animal Husbandry Operations. Indian Dairyman., 44(7): 332-337.

Marothia, D.K. and S.K. Sharma (1985) 'Female Participation in Rice Farming System of Chhatisgarh Region, 'Indian Journal of Agricultural Economics'. Vol. 40, July-September pp 235-239.

Nisha, P.R. (1996). Role of Farm Women in Dairy Cooperatives. Unpublished M.V.Sc. Thesis. Department of Extension, TANUVAS.

Puri, S. (1974a). Role of Women in Animal Husbandry. Indian Dairy Man., 22(23):9.

Puri, S. (1974 b). Rural Families and Decision Making Pattern. Indian Journal of Extension Education., VII (March-June): 66.

Saikia, A. (1999). Role of Farm Women in Agriculture and their Involvement in Decision Making — A Study in Journal District of Assam. Indian Journal of Agriculture Economics., 54(3): 301-302.

Singh, D.V. and J.P. Bhati (1985). Women in Hill Agriculture: A Case Study of Himachal Pradesh. Indian Journal of Agricultural Economics., 40: 269.

Sinn, R., J. Ketzs and T. Chen (1999). The Role of Women in the Sheep and Goat Sector. Small Ruminants Research., 34: 259-269.

Sisodia, J.S. (1985). Role of Farm Women in Agriculture: A Study of Chambal Command Area of Madhya Pradesh. Indian Journal of Agricultural Economics., 40: 223-230.

Susheela, H., L. Phadnis, H.S. Surendra and V. Acharya, (1991). Women in Agriculture Under Different Landholdings. Indian Journal of Social Research., (32): 272-276.

Thakar, R.F. and K.F. Patel (1998). Knowledge of Farm Women about Improved Agricultural and Animal Husbandry Practices. Rural India., March (1998): 73-75.

Veena, S.,I. Grover and S. Munjal (1986). Participation of Rural Women of Haryana in Home, Farm and Dairy Sector. A Report on ORP, NDRI, Karnal.

Wijaya, H.R. (1993). Developing Agriculture with a Women's Perspective: A Challenge. Invited Paper, 37th Annual Conference, Australian Agricultural Economic Society, University of Sydney, Feb. 9-11.

20
Livestock Processing Industry

Though the contribution of animal husbandry and dairying sector to total gross domestic product (GDP) of the country is around 6 per cent and the value of output of livestock and fisheries sector is nearly one-third of the total value of output of agricultural and allied sectors, livestock processing industry has still not made a significant stride. It is universally accepted that processing of livestock products adds value, enhance shelf-life and have large employment generation potential per unit of investment. The manufacturing processes of livestock products are concerned with addition of value which comes from the changing of form. For example, livestock and poultry converted into meat and meat products, eggs and egg powder, milk into infant milk food, malted milk food, condensed milk, milk powder, cheese, ghee, etc. A dynamic livestock processing sector plays a vital role in diversification and commercialization of livestock products, enhancing income of farmers and creating surplus for export of livestock foods.

Livestock products are all highly perishable and require immediate processing/preservation, to move them from production areas to demand centers. Processing and market linkage are therefore, prerequisites for value addition. The core livestock production sector in India are the small holder group and markets for livestock products are by and large, unorganized, traditional and fragmented, except for the organized milk, meat and byproducts sectors.

In the livestock industry, dairy is the largest sector. However, so far the government policy in the dairy sector has been to give preference to the establishment of milk processing plants linking rural milk producers to urban consumers through a network of cooperatives. No policy measures have been undertaken so far to give a fillip to the unorganized sector involved in the production of Indian dairy products like ghee, paneer, chhena, khoa, etc. which have tremendous potential in the export market in Asian and African countries. Similarly, though the Indian poultry industry has come a long way from a backyard activity to an organized, scientific and vibrant industry mainly as a result of initiatives taken by private sector for commercial pure-line breeding, the poultry processing sector has not come of age.

The livestock processing industry in India needs a priority attention, particularly in the era of economic liberalization where the private, public and cooperative sectors are to play their rightful role in the development of processing sector. External markets are an extremely important source of demand and these need to be tapped much more aggressively. In order to encourage export of processed products, licensing control for processing must be repealed and all restrictions on their exports removed. As the ownership of livestock is more evenly distributed with landless labourers and marginal farmers, the progress in the processing sector will enhance their net income and consequently ensure more balanced development of the rural economy. The Government is now taking lot of interest to invest in the processing industry (Table 20.1).

MEAT PROCESSING[1]

Meat processing in India is generally confined to slaughter and dressing of carcases for fresh meat output for direct consumption and this is often carried out in the open air under highly unhygienic conditions. There are over 3643 slaughter houses throughout the country, owned by the local self governments, most of them dirty and dilapidated, just for rendering fresh meat. Value addition in meat is rare and is limited to small quantities of meat meant for export, poultry products and to a much lesser extent, pork products.

Positive Characters of Indian Meat

The Indian meat and meat products are in great demand and their popularity is increasing as the livestock in India is reared naturally on green pastures and are not fed any growth promoting hormones, antibiotics and chemicals and the meat is therefore, wholesome and safe for human consumption. It is fresh/frozen produced and stored/transported under refrigerated conditions. It is free from radiation and is considered to be 93% lean and is, therefore virtually free from fat. Indian buffalo meat is exported frozen in boneless and deglanded form and is free from foot and mouth disease (FMD). The meat is available at very competitive prices.

The Indian Buffalo and Lamb meat has established itself in the markets of South East Asia, Middle East and African countries and several other countries in the other world without any complaint of quality. Moreover

---

[1]Thanks are due to Dr. M.A Haleem, Hind Agro Industries Ltd., for his original draft contribution for this section of the chapter.

Table 20.1: Details of Investment in the Processed Food Sector

(Since liberalization in July, 1991)

(Rs. in crores)

Sl. No	Sector	Industrial entrepreneur memoranda (till Dec. 2002)		Industrial approval oriented units/ industrial licence (till Nov. 2002)		Total		Foreign investment out of total investment (till Nov. 2002)
		No.	Invest.	No.	Invest.	No.	Invest.	
1.	Grain Milling and Grain Based Products	422	6008	107	1259	529	7267	1207
2.	Fruit and Vegetable	1745	3438	422	5180	2167	8618	1090
3.	Meat and Poultry Products	96	456	59	1394	155	1850	267
4.	Fish Processing and Aquaculture	116	463	192	2228	308	2691	549
5.	Fermentation Industry	672	9301	211	2073	883	11374	1094
6.	Consumer Industry Including Soft Drinks/ Waters/ Confectionery, etc.	869	7523	79	5836	948	13359	4432
7.	Milk and Milk Products	1119	13823	27	1182	1146	15005	1054
8.	Other including food additives, flavours, etc.	-	-	75	945	75	945	906
9.	Edible oil/oil seeds	1675	13416	-	-	1675	13416	..
	Total	6714	54428	1172	20097	7886	74525	10599

Source: Annual Report 2002-2003, Govt. of India, Ministry of Food Processing Industries.

Indian meat has never been a cause for outbreak of any livestock disease in the meat importing countries. Shelf life of meat during storage at different temperatures is indicated in shelf life of meat during storage at different temperatures is indicated in Table 20.2.

Table 20.2: Shelf Life of Meat During Storage at Different Temperatures

Product	Storage temperature	Shelf life
Meat product –cuts	4 ± 1C	5 days
	– 12 C	8 months
	– 18 C	8 months
Minced meat	4 ± 1C	3 days
	– 12 C	6 months
	– 18 C	10 months
Cooked products	2 – 4 C	15 days
	– 12 C	6 months
	– 18 C	10 months

Product Mix: Meat is mainly exported in deboned, deglanded and frozen from having a pH below 6. The various commercial buffalo meat cuts are—

Hind Quarter: Knuckle, Tender, Strip Loin. Top Side, Silver Side Rump and Eye Round.

Fore Quarter: Blade, Chuck Tender, Cube Roll and Muscles.

Mutton: Mutton is normally exported as chilled carcass, occasionally, there is a demand for assorted mutton cubes in 1 kg packs (18-20 pieces) in frozen form. There is a good demand for chilled mutton carcass weighing 8 kg.

Quality Control Aspects of Meat and Meat Products

The quality and safety of meat and meat products are important both for domestic consumption and for export markets. The developing countries also have the opportunity to have a say in the lucrative international meat trade by meeting the stringent requirements of meat importing countries. Unless stringent quality control and inspection are adopted, it will result in quality rejection and loss of produce. India has comprehensive legislation as well as an administrative setup to ensure the food safety and quality of the meat production for domestic consumption and export. The quality control and inspection include healthy and disease free animals as well as disease free meat and meat products, particularly within the tolerance limits laid down by the importing countries. The meat and meat products should also be graded as per mandatory standards of importing countries. Surveillance of product laboratory analysis is one of the essential requirements.

Each export establishment is to be approved by concerned regulatory authority of state/central government and should also be accredited by the importing nation's agencies. This includes abattoir, processing units, storage– chillers and freezers as well as factory buildings and surrounding environment for quality and safety of food products. Antemortem and postmortem examination procedures of animal are to be adopted by qualified and experienced veterinary doctors, microbiologist and food technologist.

The potential of meat and poultry industry can be gauged from the phenomenal growth of livestock over the past three decades. The consumption of meat is on the rise in the domestic market. Revenues from the export of meat, poultry and byproducts have substantially increased in recent years. Further, globalization of Indian economy has created new opportunities and potential for the export of meat and poultry products. Government of India has recognized meat and poultry as one of the important sectors of food industry.

The annual production of meat and poultry products in India is estimated to be almost 6 million tonnes per annum. Whereas about 1% of meat produced is converted into value added products and most meat is purchased by consumers in the country in the fresh/frozen form. India has huge potential of export of meat and meat products. The value of buffalo meat and by-product available is estimated to be about Rs. 1375.04 crores annually and sheep meat export was valued at Rs. 78.16 crores during the financial year 2000-01.

Consumer outlook is changing towards quality meat and meat products. The challenges before the Indian meat and poultry industry are disease control in livestock, improvement in the hygiene status of meat, effective recovery and utilization of the byproducts and value addition to the meat. To achieve these targets knowledgeable human resources are essential. Management of Quality Control assumes great significance during production, processing, preservation and distribution of meat and meat products. Therefore it is essential to introduce modern production practices in the meat processing industry of the country.

Livestock is an important segment in the Indian agriculture from the point of its contribution to the gross national product as well as the employment generation potential in rural areas. A survey of rural India by the National Sample Survey Organisation (NSSO) of the Government of India has revealed that the livestock development activities are preferred by rural folks as a source of supplementing their income besides regular farm activities.

Improved production methods, modern processing, packing and preservation techniques, adoption of HACCP (Hazard Analysis Critical Control Point) ISO 9000, SQF, FMS, ISO, 14000 and GMP (Good Manufacturing Practices), Chilling, Freezing, IQF (Individual Quick Freezing) and Food Irradiation, are some of the modern processing techniques. Emulsion Technology, Hurdle Technology and MAP (Modified Atmospheric Packaging) are some of the techniques essential in improving food quality, safety and value addition to the meat products.

Indian Food Processors adopt the standards prescribed by the Food and Agricultural Department of the Bureau of Indian Standards and Meat Food Products Order 1973 of the Government of India and by the Meat Food Production Advisory Committee. The first schedule is application of license under the Meat Food Products Order, 1973. The second schedule relates to sanitary and other requirements to be compiled with by a licensee. The third schedule deals with hygienic and other requirements to be compiled with by a licensee who also slaughter animals in his factory. The fourth schedule pertains to requirements to be compiled with regard to packaging, marking and labeling of meat food products.

The Agricultural and Processed Food Products Export Development Authority (APEDA) under the Ministry of Commerce, Government of India, monitors and provides guidelines to promote export of meat. It has constituted a technical committee which includes a member each from Ministry of Agriculture, Ministry of Food. Processing Industries, Export Promotion Council of Ministry of Commerce, Government of India, representative from Animal Husbandry and Veterinary Department of the State Governments and a member from APEDA. The Technical Committee annually inspects the meat processing plants and slaughtering and meat processing facilities at meat plants. After a thorough inspection, the plant is certified fit for export of safe and quality meat and meat products and a certificate of plant registration is issued to the exporting company running the plant. The issuance of this certification for export of meat and meat products is critical to successful international marketing. Products carrying no certification or with wrong certification will invariably be detained at the port of entry and will most likely the shipment will be rejected.

Research and Development in the area of food science and technology is likely to contribute to the creation of sound technological base for various essential development parameters. Among them are the current technology acquisition, improved productivity and food quality, product diversification and cost minimization in processing, energy conservation, by-product utilization and better marketing for both domestic and export markets. Therefore it is necessary to look into different aspects such as the development of modern facilities in food processing industries, Introduction of latest production techniques, effective production planning and easy availability of financial resources and effective marketing of safe and quality meat and meat products. This will require a combined effort of entrepreneurs, food processors, scientists and food technologist and officials from national and international agencies.

Meat Plant Standards

These include general sanitary requirements, civil construction, basic product chilling room, processing hall, cold storage, laboratory having facility of microbiological examination, qualified veterinary doctors, shipment and product record. These standards have been published in the gazette of the Government of India notification dated January 30, 1993 and also form the standard of Meat Plant issued by APEDA, Ministry of Commerce, Government of India.

Meat Plant Inspection Manual Includes Evaluation of

General hygiene & sanitation in the meat plant, personal hygiene of workers, condition of processing and packaging equipments, temperature in chiller, temperature in cold storage and status of implementation of HACCP. The Bureau of Indian Standards (BIS) has published the Indian Standards for Meat and Meat Products-Beef and Buffalo meat-fresh, chilled and frozen – Technical Requirements (First Revision) BIS 1995.

Processing

The main problem faced by the industry is availability of good infrastructure, roads, power and water for processing. Unless these problems are attended suitably the industrial growth will be hampered. There is no dearth of technology available in India, Banks and financial institutions however, do not substantially finance the development of new units. In general there are labour problems in meat industry which require careful handling in view of strong labour unions.

Meat Processing Plants – Location, Plant Capacity & Export Growth

The leading modern abattoir-cum-meat processing plants exporting halal buffalo meat from India are as follows :

1. Hind Agro Industries Limited , Aligarh, Uttar Pradesh
2. Indagro Food Limited, Unnao, Uttar Pradesh
3. Frigorifico Allana Limited, Aurangabad, Maharashtra
4. Al-Kabeer Exports Limited, Hyderabad, Andhra Pradesh
5. Arabian Exports Limited, Koregaon, Pune, Maharashtra
6. MKR Frozen Foods Limited, Nanded, Maharashtra,
7. Al-Nafees Frozen Foods Limited, Goa
8. Amroon Foods Pvt. Limited , Barabanki, Uttar Pradesh
9. Frigerio Conserva Allana Limited, Mourigram, West Bengal

The annual production capacity of few big plants is between 50000-75000 metric tonnes. The meat export growth from India in coming years is expected to be around 10-25% annually if congenial conditions prevail.

Halal Meat Concept

The animals under halal method are slaughtered according to Islamic Law under the supervision and presence of representative of Islamic organizations like Mahakama E-Sharia and Jamiat—Ulema-I-Hind. According to the Islamic law for halal meat, water is to be offered to the animals before slaughtering. The animal should not be slaughtered in front of the other animals. Thorough bleeding is essential in halal slaughter as the well bled animal carcass/meat has better shelf life. Almost 93% of

Indian meat exports consist of deboned and deglanded frozen buffalo meat (and the balance sheep/goat meat). This is a risk free product having pH below 6.0, which is achieved by compulsory chilling of the carcasses after slaughter for a minimum 24 hours at temperatures between 2-4 degree C. Organisation International Des Epizooties (OIE), Paris has confirmed that international trade in deboned and deglanded frozen meat, prepared in accordance with the guidelines formulated under the Zoo Sanitary Code (International Animal Health Code) ensure that there is no risk of transmission of FMD virus.

Abattoir Process

The healthy and disease free animals meant for slaughter undergo antemortem check up and are rested for 24 hours and provided with sufficient drinking water before slaughtering. After slaughter, deboned, deglanded carcass having a pH 6 undergo postmortem inspection and stamped by the veterinary doctors of the state government veterinary department.

Conditions of Chilling, Deboning, Freezing and Storage

After the slaughter the carcass is kept in chilling room before being transferred for deboning. The deep bone temperature is + 7°C when deboning takes place and the pH level of the carcass is lower than 6.0. After deboning and packaging, the meat is frozen in plate freezer/blast freezer at – 40°C. The packed frozen meat is kept at 18°C in a cold storage until the time of shipping.

Packaging and Freezing

The different parts of the carcass are trimmed during deboning. The deboned meat is poly-packed cut wise and is sent for freezing. The buffalo carcass is separated into two halves namely hindquarter and forequarter. Hindquarter contains knuckle, tenderloin, striploin, topside, silverside, rump and eye round while forequarter contains blade, chuck tender, cuberole and meat. The packed meat is put in the carbon and is also tagged in inner and outer cartons showing the type of cuts and name and place of production and date of production. Mutton carcass is usually exported in chilled condition. However, mutton cuts are normally frozen in packs, each containing 20 pieces in one kg pack.

The marketing and distribution of meat industry are well developed and sophisticated in view of WTO regulations and well packed quality products imported to India. Coordinated efforts of meat exporters are necessary to maintain the quality, production, packaging and competitive price of products in international markets.

Veterinary Service

Compulsory antemortem inspection of livestock, postmortem examination of carcasses and microbiological testing of the frozen meat is undertaken by the competent Government. Veterinary authorities ensuring the use of only healthy livestock for meat processing. Government of India provides comprehensive veterinary health services for livestock. Veterinary health care is provided through facilities like polyclinics, hospitals, dispensaries and first–aid centers. Control of infectious and contagious diseases of livestock is undertaken by systematic vaccination programmes. Epidemiological studies are conducted for monitoring and disease diagnosis. Latest knowhow on production of vaccines and immunologicals is applied for this purpose. There are movement restrictions of livestock in disease outbreak areas and movement regulations of livestock meant for trade. Indian livestock is free from the dreaded Bovine Spongiform Encephalopathy (BSE), commonly known as Mad Cow Disease. Unlike FMD, which does not affect the human beings, meat obtained from BSE infected cattle can cause form of CJD in humans, which is an incurable and fatal disease.

Quality Control Aspects of Meat and Meat Products

India has comprehensive legislation as well as a good administrative system to ensure the food safety and quality of the meat production for domestic consumption and export.

Meat Food Products Order 1973 Including Amendments up to 1994

The order is implemented by Directorate of Marketing and Inspection. It controls production, quality and distribution of raw and processed products.

Meat Food Products Advisory Committee

The committee comprises agricultural advisors to the Government of India. The function of the committee is to aid and advice on matters pertaining to meat food products.

Export Quality Control and Inspection Act (1963)

This act was promulgated to promote export trade by ensuring exports of international quality products. The Export Inspection Council has been established to ensure compulsory quality control and inspection of various commodities.

APEDA

Agricultural and Processed Food Products Export Development Authority (APEDA), Ministry of Commerce, Government of India, encourages export of agro and processed food products including meat and meat products. APEDA is engaged in determining the area of operation and its action plan in developing technical and analytical quality assurance capabilities. It also conducts specific training programmes for quality management systems such as HACCP, TOM and ISO 9002 series and so on.

Prevention of Food Adulteration Act (PFA Act, 1954)

This is the basic food act which empowers the Central Government to make rules and amend the existing ones. Central Committee for Food Standards (CCFS) is the main standardization and advisory body to make the food control system effective in terms of science based approach to develop standards for food and other implementation aspects of the food regulation. Central Committee for Food Standards (CCFS) has been constituted at the center to advise the Central and State Governments on matters related to administration of the act.

Bureau of Indian Standards Specifications (BIS)

BIS (Certification marks) Act 1952 provides third party assurance/guarantee for the consumers. Under this system BIS issues license to a food manufacturing unit which complies with the specifications laid down in the relevant Indian standards.

Codex Alimentarius

Codex Alimentarius has now established the benchmark for ensuring food safety and consumer protection. FAO's manual of food quality control and food for export has become standard reference in the improvement of quality of food for national and international trade. Continuous surveillance of product by way of sampling and laboratory analysis is essential to ensure that contaminant levels comply with those prescribed by importing countries.

Regulations

Both exporting and importing countries have their own regulations in place. In India BIS specifications are followed and in international markets Codex Alimentarius specifications are adhered to.

Phyto-Sanitary Regulations of Importing Countries

All phyto-sanitary regulations prescribed by Codex are universally practiced.

Hind Agro Industries Limited – A Case Study

Hind Agro Industries Limited (HAIL) has a 100% export oriented modern integrated abattoir cum meat processing plant situated at Aligarh, Uttar Pradesh. The plant is equipped with latest machinery and in-house R & D facilities to produce high quality branded meat products under brands like Eatcco, Sibaco, Al-Najah, Shahia and AI-Hind. HAIL is a government recognized trading house. It is India's leading processor and exporter of halal deglanded and deboned fresh and frozen buffalo and sheep meat and meat products. HACCP, ISO 9002 and SGS have been implemented at the plant to ensure the highest degree of hygiene and sanitary requirements of international standards. HAIL is firmly committed to supply superior quality meat and meat products to achieve highest level of customer satisfaction.

HAIL is the only company in the country to have a backward integration Animal Rearing project under the Hind Livestock Development Foundation. It encouraged the local farmers to rear buffaloes especially for meat processing by the company. The animals are bred and reared under guidelines set by the company itself. In turn, the company provides assistance to farmers by providing feed stock and veterinary services from experts belonging to Hind Agro Industries Limited.

Some of the Constraints and Action areas for Meat Industry

1. **Development of Modern Infrastructure :** India has to further strengthen and modernize its existing infrastructure in the area of establishment of new storage facilities and cold chains for meat and meat products, providing inspection facilities for food hygiene, slaughter and meat processing facilities for both domestic and export production of quality meat.

2. **Strengthening Quality Monitoring Setup :** There is an urgent need to induct modern monitoring facilities to carry out the testing and monitoring of meat product sample for pesticide residues, metals, veterinary drug residues and mycotoxins etc., At present Food Quality Control activities are undertaken by various agencies. These should be brought under one authority for effective monitoring.

3. **Need for Reference Laboratories :** There is a need to setup reference laboratory that should monitor the performance standards of the testing laboratories.

4. **Training and Education of Inspection Personnel :** Adequate training and educational facilities along with training gadgets are to be made available for the training of food scientists and technologists including food inspectors.

5. **Entry of Imported Food Products in Indian Markets :** It is estimated that imported foodstuff cover almost 6% of the Indian food market. There are no proper arrangements to monitor quality checks on imported food items in the country. In fact, it has been reported that some imported food products do not adhere to the Indian Food laws and package commodities regulation order. Our customs and regulatory mechanism need to be strengthened to check the inflow of the imported foodstuff as the import restrictions are being lifted gradually.

6. **Eradication of Foot and Mouth Disease (FMD) :** There is a need for eradication of Foot and Mouth disease in some areas of the country and this requires sustained efforts similar to eradication of

Rinderpest (RP) by Central and State governments in order to boost production of milk and meat and also to increase the productive capacity of animals and bring down their mortality rates.

7. **Rearing of Male Buffalo Calves :** Eighty percent of male buffalo calves need to be salvaged by educating the farmers about the modern animal rearing methods along the scientific lines to fatten them. These animals can fetch substantial remunerative prices after attaining body weight of 150 kg and sold for meat purposes.

8. **Reduction in Cost of Feed for Cattle/Poultry**: There is an urgent need to reduce the cost of cattle/poultry feed through grow more maize campaign as feed accounts for 60% to 70% of the cost of production. By substituting maize with other cereals, cost could be reduced and allowing free import of food grain maize, setting up of infrastructure facilities for feed milling will be helpful.

9. **Availability of Financial Assistance on easy terms :** There is a need to make available financial assistance in the form of loans on lower interest rates by banks and other financial institutions for encouraging the development of modern infrastructure of International Standards which will help meet the international market's requirements by Indian meat processors.

10. **Establishment of Cold Chains and modern storage facilities**: Adequate cold storage facilities both for domestic markets and at International Airports for exports are the important requirements in developing the country's export of hygienic and safe quality meat and meat products. Hence, there is a need to establish modern storage facilities including refrigerated transport facilities.

11. **Provision of Subsidies:** Liberal subsidies are offered by many advanced countries for production and marketing their country's products in international markets at competitive prices. Similar assistance in the form of subsidies should also be made available by the Government of India and State Governments to enable Indian exporters to effectively market their products in an effective way in international markets at remunerative prices.

12. **Packaging:** In today's competitive environment packaging of products in attractive, reliable and strong material is essential to deliver the product to the end consumer while retaining its freshness and nutritional qualities.

13. **Availability of Land on long term lease**: The Government should make available land at economic prices to the entrepreneurs along with suitable infrastructure for development of new meat processing units for increasing the country's export of meat and meat products.

14. **Social Awareness :** The consumers should be educated through effective use of media to remove their apprehensions about hygiene, sanitation and safety and quality of foods derived from the livestock and poultry sector.

POULTRY PRODUCTS

Processing of poultry products has, of late become an important adjunct to marketing of poultry. The fast-food revolution has lent a new urgency and thrust to the setting up of projects for poultry processing and ready-to-eat products to meet the growing demand for them.

However, today the wholesome chicken does not reach consumers at a reasonable price in hygienic pack. Further, processing units are being set up in cities like Mumbai and Bangalore to meet specific markets. In fact, processed poultry product has to be wholesome, hygienic, well processed and packed as per consumer needs. For added value of the product, it may be a good idea to pack it in the form of ready dishes with wide variety of easy-to-cook food to suit different tastes. It is necessary to conduct market research for identifying these tastes and variations in habits. Development of newer and more ways of eating poultry meat must be communicated for successful marketing of processed poultry products.

In recent years, consumers have become aware of the quality of food products they intend to buy, the returns they are getting for the money spent, and hygienic conditions in which they are produced, handled, marketed and distributed. To meet this requirement, standards are formulated by various quality control agencies like the Directorate of Marketing and Inspection (DMI), and Bureau of Indian Standards (BIS), (BIS was previously known as the Indian Standards Institution (ISI), (Table 20.3).

Table 20.3: Bureau of Indian Standards Specifications for Poultry Trade

Specification	Subject
IS 5558 : 1970	Chicken essence
IS 6558 : 1972	Code of practice for cold storage of shell eggs
IS 6559 : 1972	Code of practice for antemortem and postmortem inspection of poultry
IS 7049 : 1973	Code for handling, processing quality evaluation and storage of poultry
IS 4674 : 1975	Dressed chicken
IS 8539 (PTI) : 1977	Terminology of meat products and meat animals Part I (Poultry)
IS 4723 : 1978	Egg powder
IS 9800 : 1981	Basic requirement for day-old chicks (layers/broilers)
IS 9810 : 1981	Method for evaluation of quality of fresh chicken eggs (with amendment No.1)
IS 5238 : 1982	Transport of poultry-day old (part I) chick, and turkey poults
IS 5238 : 1982	Transport of poultry other (Part II) than day-old chicks and turkey poults
IS 10382 : 1982	Edible egg albumen powder
IS 10697 : 1983	Chicken canned in brine
IS 12541 : 1988	Chicken Curry
IS 12543 : 1988	Canned egg curry
IS 12561 : 1988	Pickled quail eggs

The tropical climate, absence or inadequacy of cold-storage facilities and, to some extent, resistance/ignorance of the meat-eating population towards cold, preserved and frozen meat, in general, retard the progress of marketing of dressed chicken in India. It will be much easier to introduce prices on the basis of weight once the dressed chicken makes its entry in the Indian market.

The distribution plan should aim at making the processed product available within easy reach of the present and future consumers. The future markets lie in the interiors, and therefore outlets should be planned, in a phased manner, to cover first the industrial towns, and district centers, tehsils and other important towns in that order. The infrastructure required to develop the supply lines will include refrigerated vans and deep freezers at retail outlets. In fact, development of cold chain system is unavoidable for the development of the industry. Unless almost all the dressed birds enter the cold chain route no tangible success can be achieved in the marketing field. Holding the stock during glut, diversion of the same from surplus to deficit areas and above all saving the farmers from eventualities when birds grow overweight is only possible when there is no resistance for frozen birds.

Automation in Processing

India is one of the countries which has seen growth in the field of poultry. It is not only in production that the growth has been achieved, but also in the concept of processing. No doubt that the processing industry is in its infancy. Poultry processing is still primarily in the unorganized sector. With the increased broiler production, a number of processing plants have been established in Maharashtra, Andhra Pradesh, Karnataka, Bangalore. Madhya Pradesh and West Bengal. With more money coming into food processing industry, more of processed, packed food will be seen on the shelves. The Government of India has approved investment proposals of Rs. 23,000 million in the food processing sector including deep-sea fishing, since the policy was changed in 1991. A number of tie ups have been established for Egg and Poultry Processing Plants. The details are given in Tables 20.4 and 20.5.

Future of the Industry

Integrated Operations

The Indian poultry industry is on a positive growth trend. With the open government policies, the best of the world will be available. Another reason for the foreign companies looking towards India which has to be fed and will require more eggs, more meat and more of infrastructure. It will only be possible if the efficiency of the producers is enhanced by way of better management techniques, better health cover, and producing en mass.

Table 20.4 : Egg Processing Plants in India

Name	State	Capacity	Remarks
Foods and Inns	Maharashtra	100,000	Partly owned farm (oldest plant)
Shree Warna	Maharashtra	500,000	Partly owned farm (already started)
Balaji Foods	Andhra Pradesh	1,000,000	100% EOU project to produce lysozyme and egg powder (already started)
Indo Dutch	Andhra Pradesh	600,000	100% EOU project to produce dried, liquid and frozen egg products
Ovobel Foods	Karnataka	600,000	100% EOU project
Shiva Eggs	Tamil Nadu	1,000,000	100% EOU project
SKM Feeds	Tamil Nadu	1,000,000	Egg powder, yolk and albumen

Table 20.5: Poultry Meat Processing Plants in India

Name	State	Capacity	Remarks
Venkey's Swift Foods	Maharashtra	24,000	Integrated
Shiraz Foods	Uttar Pradesh	32,000	Closed (no integration)
Shiraz Foods	Uttar Pradesh	10,000	Closed (part integration)
Agritech	Maharashtra	14,000	Integrated
Peninsula	Karnataka	10,000	Now with Godrej
Sagri	Haryana	5,000	Only processing
Nandu's	Karnataka	2,000	Further processed and cooked
Singh Poultry	Andhra Pradesh	10,000	Part integration
Bab Agro	Maharashtra	1,000	Part Integration
Arambagh	West Bengal	4,000	Part integration also direct sale through own shops
New Projects			
Oberoi	Maharashtra	10,000	Integrated
Gold Chick	Andhra Pradesh	10,000	Integrated
Golden Hill	Tamil Nadu	10,000	Integrated
Capon Foods	Uttar Pradesh	10,000	Integrated
Hind Foods	Maharashtra	16,000	Integrated
Venkey's	Haryana	24,000	Integrated

Need of the Industry

Poultry industry has reached a stage of sophistication where further innovations are needed. It calls for research and development in design of equipment by private entrepreneurs in collaboration with foreign equipment manufacturers to produce quality equipments in India which will be more effective and reduce the overheads.

Nutraceutical Eggs

Eggs are richly endowed with all essential nutrients needed for human body in an absorbable form. The high quality protein of eggs has been used for decades as a standard of high biological value against which other feed stuffs are evaluated. More than three decades ago, medical researchers began to study the relationship between diet and cardiovascular diseases. Researchers, found that human diet rich in Omega-3, polyunsaturated fatty acids as from marine fish lowered the risk of arterio sclerosis and heart attack. The work of poultry scientists in the 1930's revealed that fatty acids profile of chicken eggs could be altered significantly by changing the hens, diet. By 1990 scientists succeeded in producing greater concentration of Omega 3 fatty acids in eggs through dietary change. Chicken has the unique ability to divert increased quantities of linolenic acid into the egg from its diet.

Nutraceuticals are food or food ingredients which may enhance the health by providing physiological benefit beyond the provision of basic nutrients. The nutraceuticals likely to be included in the eggs are n-3 fatty acids, conjugated linoleic acid (CLA), tocotrienols, selenium, iodine and specific polyclonal antibodies.

Omega-3 or n-3 Fatty Acids

The pioneering discovery that n-3 fatty acid protect against heart diseases. Eskimos consuming fish has generated much interest in this field. The n-3 fatty acids in fish oil are alpha linoleic acids (LNA), Dicosahexaenoic acids (DHA) and Eicosa penataenoic acid (EPA). Steve Leeson and others at the University of Guelph in Canada found that dietary inclusion of fish oil containing Eicosapentaenoic acid (EPA) and Dicosahexaenoic acids (DHA) increased Omega-3 fatty acid concentration of eggs (Table 20.6). Consumption of Omega-3 enriched eggs produced changes in serum platelet lipid composition of human beings. The natural sources of n-3 fatty acids are flax seed or linseed rape seed, fish, algae and pearl millet.

Flax seed is a source of alpha linolenic acid, which generates Omega-3 and Omega-6 fatty acids are flax seed or linseed rape seed, fish, algae and pearl millet.

Table 20.6: Nutritive Value of Omega Eggs Compared to Conventional Eggs

Nutritional components	Omega egg (60 g)	Ordinary egg (60 g)
1. Calories	75.0	75.0
2. Proetin (g)	6.0	6.0
3. Fat (g)	6.0	6.0
4. Carbohydrates (g)	0.6	0.6
5. Saturated	1.5	1.5
6. Poly unsaturated fat (g)	1.35	0.90
Omega-3 (n-6) fatty acids (mg)	750	800
Omega-3 (n-3) fatty acids (mg)	350	60
C 18:3 fatty acids (mg)	250	40
C 22:6 fatty acids (mg)	100	20
Ratio n-6 : n-3	2.6	13.0
7. Mono unsaturated fats (g)	2.8	2.4
8. Cholesterol	180	210

Flax seed is a source of alpha linolenic acid, which generates Omega-3 and Omega-6 fatty acids at the inclusion levels in the range of 10 to 30%. Feeding of full fat flax seed or its oil increased egg yolk fatty acids from 2.3. 4.18 and 6.38% of egg yolk at an inclusion level of 5, 10 and 15% of diet. The balanced ratio of n-6 : n-3 fatty acids (2:1) becomes essential to avoid cardiovascular disease in human beings. The n-3 poly unsaturated fatty acids enriched eggs look, cook and taste the same as conventional eggs and have similar storage qualities. Consumption of two n-3 designed eggs day for 6 days in a week will have serum triglyceride level by 14 percent without increasing the cholesterol level. The new fatty acids enriched eggs from an alternative to mothers milk for pre term and orphan babies, Linolenic acid is a percursor of prostaglandin E, which is reported to be a coronary vasodilator and is one of the most potent known inhibitors of platelet aggregation.

Nutraceutical eggs are marketed in Japan as 'ISE Omega –3 eggs' in New Zealand as 'Omega' smart eggs, in Australia as 'New start eggs' in Germany as 'Omega' DHA eggs and Canada as 'Canadian designer eggs'. These eggs are sold at a price 30-130% higher than normal eggs. The higher cost of eggs is due to its higher feed costs, marketing promotion costs and profit margin incentive for the egg producers. Recently technology for large scale commercial production of Omega-3 eggs was licensed by MARDI Tech. The MARDI Omega-3 layer diet is all vegetarian containing no animal fat.

Conjugated Linolenic Acid (CLA)

The CLA isomers possess unique biological properties as powerful anticarcinogenic, anti atherogenic, anti bacterial and immuno modulator. This novel anti carcinogen can be incorporated into eggs. Studies on these areas are on and found CLA isomers enriched to the level of 1.2 percent of total fatty acids in the egg yolk and CLA content of egg peaked after five weeks of feeding. Feeding of CLA did not affect the egg production but appear to decrease feed consumption.

Polyclonal Antibodies (Igy)

The yolk of immunized chicken is a rich and inexpensive source of polyclonal antibodies (Igy). One yolk yields approximately 70-100 mg of specific antibodies. Chicken egg yolk antibodies can be administered orally for possessive immunization against infection in infants and young animals and chicks. Dried egg yolk of immunized chicken has been used to control mastitis carried by *Staphyllococcus aureus* and Streptococcus agilata in cows by feeding it for 3 weeks. Similarly, egg yolk derived antibodies prevented the piglet diarrhoea and calf diarrhoea. Salmonella infections of early ducklings were successfully controlled by the administration egg yolk antibodies through drinking water (Fulton et al 2002). The application of Igy technology to human medicine may be either by injection of pure Igy or by encapsulation of an egg yolk concentrate, so that the Igy is not destroyed by the acidity in the stomach.

Selenium and Iodine

Selenium and Iodine deficiency in human beings is prevalent in many developing countries. To enhance these trace mineral availability many formulation has been tried. One of the easy way of getting these elements into human food is through milk or eggs. Chicken eggs enriched with selenium or iodine or both would meet Recommended Dietary Allowance (RDA) of pregnant mothers and adolescent girls. Over and above these designed eggs contribute to hatchability of the eggs and better early growth of chicks.

Thus, the poultry nutritionist can make the fatty acids profile of eggs more 'heart healthy' by increasing the proportion of polyunsaturated fatty acids including omega-3 types by manipulating the hens diet. Also it is possible to increase the vitamins and mineral content, making eggs a 'functional food' or nutraceutical product which support human health and commend premium prices.

Non-conventional Poultry Products

To get a greater market in India we have to wait for the change in the food habits of the people. Food habit is changing to non-conventional poultry products such as:

Organic Farm Foods

In this sector chickens are to be reared in natural condition (not confined in the E-C controlled houses) without any antibiotic or growth promoting medicines, diet should be of G-M free cereals and grains. There is prolific demand for such chicken and eggs in US, UK and other EU countries.

Port-Folio-Diet

It is a diet of combined –plant based foods such as soy protein designed to reduce LDL-cholesterol in the blood. It includes soy foods, soy milk, tempeh (cultured soy cake), tofu, veggie bu.ger, high fibre foods e.g. oat, bran, almonds, margarine that included phytosterol, olive oil etc. This is heart-healthy diet to reduce LDL and C-reactive protein (a marker of inflammed arteries and known risk factor for CVD).

Atkins Diet

Contrary to portfolio diet, it is protein, fat, and meat heavy regimen, devised by Atkins Nutritionals, Inc. USA. This diet is obviously a boon for the poultry industry producing chicken meat and eggs. But there is some controversial arguments. A nutrition advocacy group has said this monitor the high-fat weight less approach.

Functional Foods

Any food or food component that may provide a health benefit beyond basic nutrition e.g. antioxidants. There is emerging research on this functional foods to help improve public's understanding by the International Food Information Council (IFCI). The antioxidants fact sheet contains information on the health effects and dietary source and the present research gives current recommendations. This will encourage people to balanced diet with all food items including eggs and chicken.

BYPRODUCTS

Poultry litter and poultry manure from caged layers are used extensively in feeding poultry and livestock. They are being incorporated in the feeds as protein supplement. Composition of dried poultry manure is presented in (Table 20.7). Poultry manure can be used after sterilization and dehydration. The dehydrated poultry manure can be used up to 20 and 25% in the other diet of broilers and layers respectively.

Table 20.7: Composition of Dried Poultry Manure

Composition (%)	Poultry battery	Poultry house litter	Broiler litter silage
Moisture	11.40	15.50	
Total protein	28.70	25.30	
Uric acid (NPN)	6.30	8.50	
True protein	10.50	16.60	25.80
Ether extract	1.76	2.30	
Ash	26.50	14.00	
Calcium	7.80	2.50	1.70
Phosphorus	2.20	1.60	0.38
Crude fibre	13.84	18.65	59.26

Besides their entry into the livestock and poultry feed, the manure and litter are also being used as surface dressing of agricultural fields. Poultry manure is not only a good fertilizer but it also improves the physical structure of the soil. One ton of deep litter contains 29.48 kg nitrogen (equivalent to about 136.08-147.42 kg ammonium sulphate), 20.41 kg phosphorous (equivalent to about 113.40 – 136.08 kg ordinary super phosphate, 20.41 kg potash (equivalent to about 45.36 kg potassium) together with 6.80 kg magnesium, 6.80 kg sodium and 27.21 kg calcium. Besides, poultry manure contains small amount of trace elements, especially boron, copper, iron, sulphur and zinc. The fertilizing efficiency of litter depends on its care and management. However, one problem peculiar to poultry manure is that nitrogen is too quickly available so that if care is not taken in applying if, burning occurs.

Hatchery By-Products Meal

Poultry hatchery byproducts comprise a mixture of egg shells, infertile eggs, unhatched eggs and dead as well as culled chicks, which can conveniently be converted into a meal of high-protein quality. The hatchery byproducts are cooked, dried and ground with or without removal of the fat. It contains about 18.1% calcium and 413 mg/100 g phosphorous. The hatchery by-product meal can be added up to 3-5% level in the layer ration. When used at higher level (exceeding 5%), the feed consumption was found very low; may be the meal is unpalatable or contains certain substances that depress appetite.

Inedible Eggs, Infertile Eggs or Unhatched Eggs

They result due to long storage or otherwise are suspected to be unwholesome or spoiled. They can be utilized by way of feeding monogastric animals after thermal treatment. The heat treatment makes the product sterile and prevents the spread of disease. Inedible eggs find their way in feeding pigs. The major constraint being too high a proportion of calcium in the meal. For this reason, it is recommended that the inedible eggs are broken and the shells are separated before cooking and processing.

Egg-Shell

Shells represented about 11% of the total weight of egg and are available in plenty –breaking plants. Egg shells contain approximately 94% calcium carbonate, 1% magnesium carbonate and 4% organic matter. These shells could be economically and safely used by converting them into human food and animal feed to supplement calcium, specially for poultry as it is important in maintaining eggshell quality. Besides being rich in calcium, it contributes a substantial quantity of protein as albumen residues, eggshell membrane and eggshell matrix. Poultry can utilize calcium from eggshell meal more effectively than any other calcium source.

Eggshell is prepared by drying egg shell as soon as they are collected from the source so as to prevent contamination. A temperature of not less than 80°C is used to sterilize the shells and then pulverized in a mill using 400-mesh sieve.

Egg shells can also be used as a fertilizer as a source of calcium and nitrogen.

By –Products of Dressing Plant (Processing Plant)

Irrespective of the type of poultry either layer or broiler, turkey or geese, their ultimate fate is to be converted into table chicken, and by dressing of birds different byproducts of inedible nature emit. They include feathers 6-7%, blood 3.5%, heads 3.0% feet 3.9% and intestines, lungs, pancreas and spleen 8-9% of the live weight. The natural proportion of different byproducts viz., feathers, blood and offals being 4:1:6. In addition to these, condemned chicken, racks from deboning operation and underdeveloped eggs might result during normal processing. These byproducts have a diversified use and can be processed into suitable end-products for their better utilization. There is some demand of chicken leg for soup. Poultry offal is often processed as by-product meal for feed processing plants.

Feathers

Feathers account for 6-7% of live weight and have varied uses such as livestock feed, bed, ornament, clothing, insulation, decoratives, some supporting equipments, fertilizer and as filler for chemical fertilizer. Their other possible uses include painting brush bristles, sizing agents, foaming agents for use in fire extinguishers, resin extenders and set-retarding agents for plaster, adhesive and insulating boards.

The characteristics of feathers vary according to age, sex, species and the area of the body from where they are removed. The important feathers of wing and tail are slaughtered before the carcass is scalded. The remaining feathers must be collected from under the pickers. They are being used as:

Bedding material : With the development of synthetic fibre and plastic foam, the use of feathers as bedding material has declined. Yet for good-quality bedding feathers, generally from water fowl, are still used as they are close to many natural or synthetic material.

Decorative Purpose : Shape, colour, size and plumage patterns are important when feathers are used for decorative purposes. In many cases the feathers are dyed, bent and trimmed to desired pattern.

Sporting equipment : Only selected feathers are used for sporting equipment. Sturdy feathers from mature turkeys are used for fletching arrows. Stiff feathers are used for shuttle cocks, and artificial lures for fishing require special feathers.

Manure or fertilizer : Feathers can also be used as fertilizer, as they decompose slowly and release nitrogen gradually. When used as fertilizer, they need ploughing under soil to prevent unwanted spread by wind.

Feather meal : Feather hydrolyzed with steam under high pressure, dried and ground into a meal of high-protein value are suitable as a livestock – feed supplement. Feathers are composed of a complex protein keratin – a scleroprotein which must be degraded by hydrolysis to make them digestible.

After collection from the processing plants, the feathers need to be washed off the adhering dust and blood with cold water and drained off. They are steamed and wet cooked under pressure (2.109 – 2.812 kg/cm2) for hydrolysis with constant agitation for 30 min. These feathers are further processed, viz cooked and sterilized for 2 hr to 2 hr 30 min. at a pressure of 2.109-2.812 kg/cm^2 in dry rendering cookers. They are dried, defatted and pulverized, the digestibility of feather meal is directly related to the cooking time and pressure (amount of hydrolysis). More intensive processing results in higher availability of amino acids and higher biological value. Amino acid makeup of feather meal and hatchery byproducts are presented in Table 20.8 and chart 20.1.

Table 20.8: Essential Amino Acid Makeup of Feather Meal and Hatchery Meal–
Protein (g/10 gN)

Essential amino acid	Feather meal	Hatchery byproducts meal
Arginine	7.5	6.0
Histidine	0.4	1.0
Lysine	1.3	5.5
Tryptophane		0.7
Phenylalanine	5.2	5.8
Methionine	0.5	2.7
Threonine	4.4	
Leucne	8.0	3.7
Isoleucine	6.0	4.3
Valine	8.3	4.8

Feather meal contains 70-80% digestible protein, less than 100% moisture and less than 4% fibre. Feather meal is rich in cystine, threonine and arginine but is deficient in lysine, methionine, histidine and tryptophan which are of essential nature. Therefore, whenever the feather meal is fed to monogastric animals like poultry and pigs these amino acids need to be supplemented. The practical level of feather meal in the feeds of monogastric animals is 0.5 – 1.5%. Ruminants like cattle, sheep, goats and buffaloes utilize feather meal more efficiently than monogastrics. The digestibility of feather meal can be further improved by supplementation with urea. Use of feather meal in poultry ration is limited to the extent of 4-5% because of its poor amino acid profile.

Poultry By-Products Meal

Offal meal is prepared using head, feet and inedible organs, viz. lungs spleen, intestines, windpipe, and reproductive organs of poultry. They make good livestock or pet food after suitable processing . The following processes are generally used for processing poultry byproducts.

First they are cooked and most of the moisture is removed in a dry-rendering cooker at 2.109 kg/cm^2 for 2 hr 30 min. Then the moisture is reduced to about 8% at a pressure of 2.109 kg/cm^2 for 1 hr 30 min either in the same cooker or in a separate drier. The dehydrated material is then pressed to remove excess fat (to about 10%). Finally the product is ground to a size small enough to pass through 8-12 mesh screen. Commercial meal should contain not more than 16% ash and 4% acid-in-soluble ash. It may be a satisfactory substitute for meat meal or meat scrap or fishmeal and can be used upto 5-7% in the ration. Though the processing of mixed poultry byproducts meal is different and time consuming (about 5-6 hr), it is nutritionally better balanced.

The poultry byproducts processed by rendering can be divided in 5 general categories, depending on the composition of raw materials.

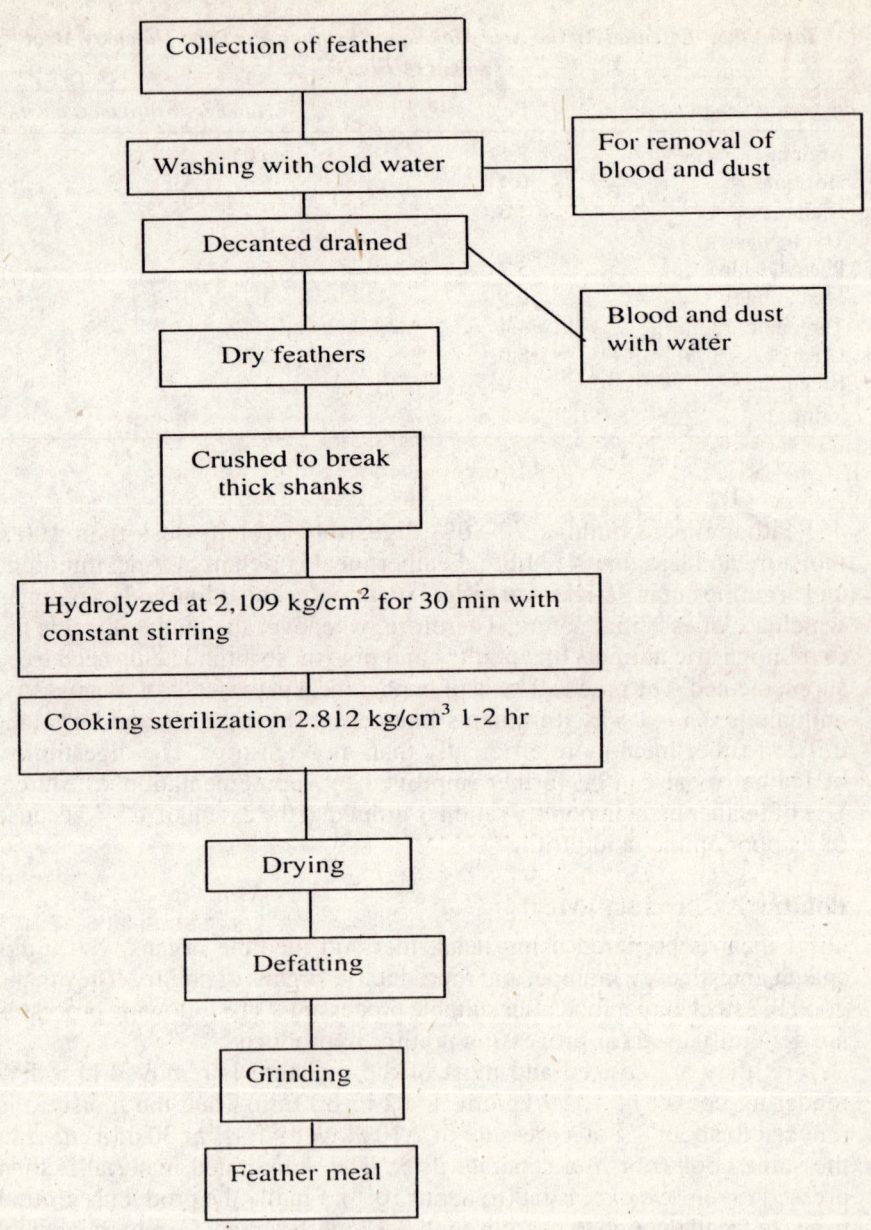

Chart 20.1

Blood meal: Blood could be collected in the larger establishments at an average rate of 3-4% from birds slaughtered and can be converted into blood meal, though not an economical proposal keeping in view the quality of blood. Blood is processed along with feathers and other inedible offals. However, blood can be converted into high quality blood meal by thermal sterilization and subsequent drying and pulverization.

Poultry – byproducts meal : The poultry byproducts meal from parts such as heads, feet, intestines but no feathers except a few which may be included in the normal processing and collection process.

Hydrolyzed feathers or feather meal : This type of meal resulted from the treatment of clean, undecomposed feathers.

Mixed poultry byproducts meal : The meal consisted of blood, offals and feathers in their natural proportion. Mixed poultry byproducts produce more balanced product nutritionally than others but it takes longer time to process, as feathers are harder to decompose.

Technical fat or poultry grease: Grease extracted from poultry offals is generally darker in colour and lower in grade than that extracted from cattle or sheep. The extracted fat is an excellent source of energy and can be used to enhance the palatability of pet foods.

DAIRY PRODUCTS

As discussed in earlier chapters, India has become the largest milk producing country in the world. The dairy business in India is currently estimated at Rs. 800 billion. With the increase of milk production, output of other milk products has also increased. More than 50 percent of the total milk production is estimated to be consumed as liquid milk and approximately 12 percent of milk is processed into value added products like casein, whey powder, & whey protein concentrated.[1] About 25 percent is processed into butter or ghee, 7 percent into paneer (cottage cheese) and other cheese, 4 percent converted into milk powder and the rest is used for other dairy products such as yoghurt (dahi) and sweet meats. In recent years, production of innovative milk products, such as, milk powder including instant milk food, malted food products, condensed milk, cheese and ice cream, is steadily increasing and the potential for such products are quite large.

North India accounts for nearly 56% of all packaged ghee sales in India, followed by Western India at half that much. The food habits of North India and its flush milk sheds make it the most profitable market for regional brands too.

Packaged Ghee Sales in India
(Share % Per Region)
Northern 56 , Southern 11, Eastern 13, Western 20

---

[1]Ministry of Food Processing: Annual Report: 2001- 2002, pp.25-26.

Reliable time series data on installed capacity, production and domestic consumption of different processed dairy products are not available. However, there are two sources, which provide some information. These include (i) Ministry of Food Processing Annual Report 2002-03 and (ii) Centre for Monitoring Indian Economy's report Industry: Market Size & Share. The Ministry of Food Processing data relate to overall production for different products at all India level for the years 1991 to 2001. CMIE publication provides information for the companies that report to them and provide data of their performance for three consecutive years or more. Their estimates cover data for the selected sample companies and total for all companies. The progress of dairy processing industry, based on these two sources of information, is discussed below.

Although Ministry of Food Processing does not give any estimates of production of butter, ghee and other fats from milk, their annual production is estimated at about 1.2 million tonnes, most of which is produced by small business enterprises and households. The conversion ratio of whole-milk (full fat) can be taken as 23 percent for butter and 20 percent for ghee. Unfortunately the time series data on production of butter, ghee and icecream are not available. Annual production of milk powder increased from 150 thousand tonnes in 1991 to 235 thousand tonnes in 2001. The annual rate of growth comes to 4.6 percent. Output of malted milk food rose from 41 thousand tonnes in 1995/96 to 68 thousand tonnes in 2000/01. This represented 5.2 percent annual increase. Condensed milk production increased by about 50 percent from 8.1 thousand tonnes to 12 thousand tonnes, while cheese output rose more than three times from a rather low base of 2.5 thousand tonnes to 8 thousand tonnes. Total production of these milk products rose by 60 percent from 201 thousand tonnes in 1991-92 to 323 thousand tonnes in 2001 (Table 20.9).

Table 20.9: Production of Milk and Milk Products: 1991 to 2001

Year	Milk (million tonnes)	Milk powder	Malted milk food	Condensed milk	Cheese products	Total milk
		...............(Thousand Tonnes)....................				
1991	55.7	150	41	8.1	2.5	201.6
1992	58.0	165	41	8.4	2.9	219.3
1993	60.6	185	32	7.8	3.1	227.9
1994	64.0	195	44	8.1	4.6	251.7
1995	66.2	200	46	8.1	5.1	259.2
1996	69.1	210	50	6.5	6.1	272.6
1997	71.9	215	55	7.8	7.0	284.8
1998	75.2	222	65	9.0	6.0	301.0
1999	78.1	225	66	11.0	5.0	307.0
2000	80.1	230	67	11.5	7.5	316.0
2001* (Estimated)	84.9	235	68	12.0	8.0	323.0

*Milk Production figures relates to the financial years (2001-02 as the last year)
Source: Ministry of Food Processing: Annual Report 2001-02: p.25

The combined annual market value of these products exceeds Rs. 100 billion. However, the organized dairy sector currently accounts for less than 10 percent of market share. Some of the constraints faced by the dairy industry are: high cost of packaging technologies for larger shelf life, lack of adequate interest by the industry, availability of poor quality of milk, low milk cattle productivity, low demand for high value added products.

The Indian dairy industry has an installed processing capacity of 20 million litres of milk per day with an estimated investment of Rs. 120 billion. About 60 percent of the installed capacity is in the cooperative sector. Along with increase in milk production, there has been a simultaneous increase in the production of milk powder including baby food, malted food products, condensed milk, etc. As a result of the liberalized industrial policy implemented by the Government in 1991, import of technology and machinery has become easier. This has resulted in the industry taking up manufacture of new products like edible casein, pharmaceutical grade lactose and whey protein concentrate and other high value products, which are export oriented.[1]

The organized milk industry in India handles only some 20 per cent of the total milk output in the country. In terms of volume of milk handled and value addition through processing and marketing infrastructure, the cooperative sector is the largest: 49 per cent; private sector : 45 per cent; and the government: 6 per cent. The products in the organized dairy sector are: processed liquid milks, butter, ghee, cheeses, condensed milk and milk powders.

The dairy industry, however, faces several constraints as the industry has traditionally been subjected to licensing and other restrictions. The Government policy in this regard has been to give preference to the establishment of milk processing plants selling liquid milk. This policy was guided by an overall shortage of milk and the national milk production falling short of nutritional requirements in the earlier years of planning era. Consequently, the processing plants manufacturing products have received a lower priority. Appropriate policy measures are needed to give fillip to this sector.

The total processing capacity of the organized sector is some 200 lakh litres per day, in over 600 milk plants, big and small. Over 50 per cent of the milk produced in the country is traded in the traditional channels, a substantial part of it going into the production of traditional products like desi butter, desi ghee, paneer, intermediates for milk sweets.

The detailed statewise information regarding installed processing capacity of the milk powder is available only for the cooperative sector. As of 31 March 2000, this capacity was 1054 tonnes of powder per day. The distribution of this capacity among different states is shown in Table 20.10.

---

[1]Government of India, Planning Commission: Ninth Five Year Plan: 1997-2002, Thematic Issues and Sectoral Progammes: vol.II, p 652.

Table 20.10: Processing Capacity for Milk Powder in Cooperative Sector as on 31.3.2000

State	Milk powder processing capacity tonnes/day	Percentage share in the total
1. Andhra Pradesh	126.0	12.0
2. Bihar	12.5	1.3
3. Gujarat	453.0	43.0
4. Haryana	25.0	2.4
5. Karnataka	37.0	3.5
6. Kerala	10.0	0.9
7. Madhya Pradesh	30.0	2.8
8. Maharashtra	60.0	5.7
9. Punjab	100.5	9.5
10. Rajasthan	60.0	5.7
11. Tamil Nadu	70.0	6.6
12. Uttar Pradesh	60.0	5.7
13. West Bengal	10.0	0.9
Total	1,054.0	100.0

The bulk of the processing capacity for milk powder is concentrated in Gujarat state, followed by Andhra Pradesh, Punjab, Tamil Nadu, Rajasthan and Uttar Pradesh. There is an urgent need to collect and make available data on total installed capacity and actual production of milk powder and other dairy products, for the cooperative as well as the private sector.

INDIAN DAIRY — CYNOSURE OF GLOBAL PLAYERS

Many global dairy companies are keen to enter the Indian dairy markets in the near future, thanks to dramatic change in their perception of Indian dairy industry and the enormous growth potential it has, according to Adrie Zwanenberg, global head, food and agribusiness, Rabo Advisory and Research, Holland. While companies like Nestle (Swiss), Sodiaal (France), Lactalis (France) and Fonterra (New Zealand) are already here, some more leading companies are expected to enter the Indian dairy market in the near future.

Among the foreign companies already present in the Indian markets, Sodiaal has tied up with Jaipuria Group, Lactalis has collaborations with two Indian companies: Karamels and L-Comps & Impex (P) Limited, and Fronterra is having ties with Britannia. Lactalis of France is also seriously looking at appointing its third distributor for south India. These companies have entered India with their value-added milk products such as cheese, icecreams, and yogurts. With changing life styles and increasing income levels, there is a growing demand for value-added dairy products. Hence, more foreign companies are expected to enter our markets to cash in on the demand for such products.

Elaborating on the reasons for the foreign dairy companies changing their perception of the Indian dairy sector, Mr Adrie felt that it's because of the steps being taken within the country for improving milk quality and the growing investments being made for improving infrastructure to handle, process and transport milk in the most hygienic way.

For instance, the National Dairy Development Board (NDDB) has launched a project for improving the quality of the milk across the country, which is having a positive impact of the Indian dairy in the eyes of the global players. In fact, Indian dairy sector needed to sell itself more aggressively to attract more attention in the future. India is the world leader producing 85 billion kgs of milk per annum of the world's 600 billion kgs per annum. However, it has failed to capitalise on this strength due to lack of aggressive marketing.[1]

Dairy Processed Products

In their study, the Centre for Monitoring Indian Economy covered data for 1995/96 to 2000/01, on Production, Sales, Market Shares and Key Statistics for sample companies and total for the following processed dairy products: (i) Milk Powder and Condensed Milk: (ii) Infant Milk Food: (iii) Malted Milk Foods: (iv) Butter, Ghee and Other Fats from Milk and (v) Icecreams.

Milk Powder and Condensed Milk

Production of Milk Powder and Condensed Milk for sample major selected companies increased from 85,809 tonnes in 1995/96 to 146,383 tonnes in the year 2000/01. The annual increase comes to 9.3 percent. Processing capacity and production of these products in the organized sector, which include companies and cooperatives, are higher than these levels. In fact, the sample covered in the CMIE publication, even some major companies/ cooperatives like Kaira District Co-op. Milk Marketing Federation, Madhya Pradesh Milk Mktg., were not included due to non-availability of data. Company-wise trends in production, sales, market share and value of domestic consumption, are shown in Table 20.11.

Based on the level of production, the processing capacity for milk powder and condensed milk varied from less than 1000 tonnes for Kwality Dairy Food to almost 10,000 tonnes for Mahan Foods. Total sale of milk powder and condensed milk increased from Rs. 4500 million in 1995/96 to Rs. 9500 million in 2000/01, registering 12 percent annual increase. Value of domestic consumption of these products, as reported by the 43-sample companies, rose from Rs. 4661 million to Rs. 8873 million during the last six years. Exports of these products which varied from one year to another, totaled 3227 tonnes in 1995/96 and 8535 tonnes in 2000/01, valued at Rs.177 million and Rs. 668 million respectively. The Market share in the total sales of these products in the year 2000/01 varied from the highest of 6.69 percent for Dynamix Dairy Industries to 1.41 percent for Ajanta Raj Proteins.

---

[1]The Economic Times, 19 February 2004.

Table 20.11: Milk Powder and Condensed Milk: Company-wise Trends in Production, Total Sales, Market Shares and Domestic Consumption: 1995/96–2000/01

Company	Production (tonnes)						Sales (Rs. Mil.)	Market share (%)
	1995/96	1996/97	1997/98	1998/99	1999/00	2000/01	2000/01	2000/01
Dynamix Dairy Inds.				5559	6864	9303	647.5	6.79
Sterling Agro Inds.				9967	8299		592.8	6.21
Continental Milkose (India)			5579	3264	6132		440.9	4.62
J K Dairy & Foods	6071	5439	6515	6170	4595	5210	440.1	4.61
Modern Dairy	5997	5831	6387	6866	6382	6105	414.2	4.34
Mahaan Foods	4546	5760	6643	6309	7085	9732	396.1	4.15
Haryana Milk Foods	6868		6519	6278	5926	5642	389.3	4.08
V R S Foods				1710	1436	1946	147.8	1.55
Milk Specialties	3090	3728	4434	3776	2461	2461	142.8	1.50
Ajanta Raj Proteins			1840	1435	1574	2353	134.6	1.41
Kisan Dudh Udyog			322	559	1561	2029	118.6	
Supreme Agrofood			1143	1427	768	784	117.2	
Kwality Dairy (India)	18	766	936	758	1826	1826	111.3	
Nijjer Agro Foods	468	1485	1648	1692	1222	1222	104.5	
Madhya Pradesh Glychem Inds.		491	849	1109	470	470	94.2	
Kamdhenu Foods					464		82.3	
Rama Food & Allied Inds.				105		1380	80.6	
Rahul Dairy 1934 & Allied Products	1081	829	1431	1518	1518		71.5	
Rama Dairy Products			545	780	1252	1610	70.4	
Premier Industry (India)	1154	953	868	720	647	750	58.5	
Total for the sample 43 cons.	63092	53506	72541	73865	76087	71972	4784.7	50.15
Total	85809	98379	94431	132928	165880	146383	9500.0	
Herfindahl Index of Concentration	0.040	0.032	0.038	0.024	0.018	0.020		
Domestic Consumption value (Rs. Million)	4661	6474	6454	9041	10730	8873		

Source: Centre for Monitoring Indian Economy: Industry: Market Size and Shares: August 2002. pp. 10-11.

The Herfindahl Index, which indicates the extent of concentration in the sector, is rather low, although it changed from 0.040 in 1995/96 to 0.020 in the year 2000/01. The Herfindahl Index, which is simple, yet sophisticated way of measuring industry concentration, is rather high in the case of infant milk food industry. It has also increased over time. The Herfindahl Index is obtained by squaring the market-share of the various players, then summing those squares and divided by a number 10,000. The Index helps differentiate between one industry in which two players have equal share and another one where one player has much larger share and a few other equal small shares. The former, which is more competitive, would have a lower Herfindahl Index. While changes in market shares would only indicate how a company has fared relative to the industry, the changes in the overall competitive intensity can be readily reckoned by computing the Herfindahl Index. A decline in the value of the Index in a specific industry would indicate that the existing players are not only losing market share, but that their pricing power is also receding. And, if the value remains constant even with the entry of several players that would indicate that the hold of the existing players has not slackened at all.

In the milk powder and condensed milk segment there is a strong competition among the three major players Amul, Nestle and Britannia. In the milk powders sector, Nestle is at the receiving end of aggressive pricing by rivals: the latest entrant, Britannia's milkman diary whitener is priced at Rs. 70 for 500 grams, against Nestlé's Rs. 80 and Amul's Rs. 70. The condensed milk price wars have been on since 1996 when Amul launched Mithai Mate. The new product was priced Rs. 10 lower than the same quantity of Milkmaid, forcing Nestle to shed Rupees five from Milkmaid price. Amul has invested Rs. 150 million to enhance production capacity of Mithai Mate at Mehsana in Gujarat form 300 tonnes to 900 tonnes. According to Nestle, milkmaid commands three quarters of the sweetened condensed milk market. Amul claims a 40 percent market share, expected to rise to 60 percent once the expansion plan and new products are lined up. The market for sweetened condensed milk is estimated at over Rs. 1000 million.

Infant Milk Food

During the last decade the dairy processing industry has expanded dramatically with the entry in some sub-sectors of several multinational companies. Data on total production of infant milk food is available only for the sample companies who reported their performance to the CMIE. Production of infant milk food for selected companies rose from 64,808 tonnes in 1995/96 to 97,971 tonnes in 2000/01. The annual increase comes to 7.2 percent during the last six years. Their total sale value and domestic consumption both increased from Rs. 5900 million to Rs. 7924 million, representing 5 percent annual growth. Less then 50 tonnes of Infant Milk Food products are exported annually by the sample companies, while these companies imported almost double these quantities in recent years.

In the Infant Milk Food sector, the multinational companies are more prominent than the milk powder and condensed milk sector. In fact, Nestle India continued to dominate the market during the last six years, with a marginal increase in its market share. It accounts for around 54 percent of the market share, and is followed by Heinz India, with market share of 27.9 and Milkfood whose market share was 1.34 percent in the year 2000/01 (Table 20.12). The overall Herfindahl index of concentration increased from 0.299 in 1993/94, to 0.380 in 2000/01.

Malted Milk Foods

Dairy processing industry has expanded dramatically during the last decade or so. Several new processed dairy products are being manufactured in India, while production of others has been expanded. According to data compiled by the Ministry of Food Processing, production of Malted Milk Foods increased from 41 thousand tonnes in 1991 to 68 thousand tonnes in 2001. However, according to the CMIE data, total production of Malted Milk Foods almost doubled, increasing from 58172 tonnes in 1995/96 to 116 870 tonnes in 2000/01, while for the sample five companies the total output was 49448 tonnes and 62659 tonnes during the two years (Table 20.13). Total value of sales of these products increased from Rs. 5,220 million in 1995/96 to Rs. 12,000 million in the year 2000/01. The total increase in value terms comes to almost two and half times, recording a fastest annual growth (15 percent) among various processed dairy products. The value of domestic consumption of Malted Milk Food is estimated to have increased from Rs. 5,024 million to Rs. 11,802 million. Export quantities have however, declined from 3035 tonnes in 1995/96 to 1.34 tonnes in 2000/01.

As regards the competitiveness in this sub-segment of the dairy processing industry, Herfindahl Index of Concentration is higher than even in the Infant Milk Food sub-section and has also increased from 1995/96 onwards. One multinational company Glaxosmithkline Consumer Healthcare held more than two-thirds of the market share in the total sale of these products, while Cadbury India (a subsidiary of another multinational company) accounted for about 11 percent of the market share in 2000/01. Glaxosmithkline Consumer Healthcare (erstwhile Smithkline Beecham Consumer Healthcare) acquired 'Health Drink Brand' (Maltova and Viva) from Jagatjit Industries in January 2000. Heinz India, one of the major companies in malted milk foods, does not provide separate information relating to this product in its annual report.

Butter, Pure Ghee and Other Fats from Milk

Butter and Pure Ghee form an essential item of household consumption in most parts of the country. According to unofficial sources annual production of butter and ghee is estimated at 1.2 million tonnes. Small businesses in the unorganized sector and household produce the bulk of this output. Total

Table 20.12: Infant Milk Food: Company-wise Trends in Production, Total Sales, Market Shares and Domestic Consumption: 1995/96 – 2000/01

Company	Production (tonnes)						Sales (Rs. Mil.)	Market Share (%)
	1995/96	1996/97	1997/98	1998/99	1999/00	2000/01	2000/01	2000/01
Nestle India	34201	32675	35726	34429	40475	36131	4264.8	53.74
Heinz India				12414	15070	15070	2212.9	27.89
Milkfood	11622	10470	10932	10485	12780	12390	858.3	10.82
Raptakos, Brett & Co.	1050	1050	1022	1036	1026	1235	261.5	3.29
Pfizer	558	524	570	639	666	722	239.2	3.01
Mahan Proteins			242	153	195	328	52.3	0.66
Modern Food Inds. (India)	2237				117			
Glaxosmithklin Pharmaceuticals				490				
Total for the sample 10 companies	49808	44718	48496	59648	70330	65883		99.41
Total	64808	58718	63496	59648	70330	97971	792.4	99.86
Herfindahl Index of Concentration	0.299	0.319	0.313	0.391	0.386	0.380		
Domestic Consumption value (Rs. Million)	5902	5636	6158	6656	7718	7934		

Source: Centre for Monitoring Indian Economy: Industry: Market Size and Shares: August 2002. pp. 12-13.

Table 20.13: Malted Milk Foods: Company-wise Trends in Production, Total Sales, Market Shares and Domestic Consumption: 1995/96 – 2000/01

Company	Production (tonnes)						Sales (Rs. Mil.)	Market Share (%)
	1995/96	1996/97	1997/98	1998/99	1999/00	2000/01	2000/01	2000/01
Glaxosmithkline Consumer Healthcare	38387	42082	45613	49693	48709	57116	8046.2	67.05
Cadbury India	4109	4171	4052	3938	4869	5539	1314.5	10.95
Jagatjit Industries	6952	7552	8174	6778	6778			
Continental Milkose (India)					123	4		
Bhole Baba Milk Food Inds.			30	68	68			
Total for the sample 5 companies	49448	53805	57869	60477	60547	62659	9360.7	78.0
Total	**58172**	**59089**	**79679**	**94573**	**106414**	**116870**	**12000.0**	
Herfindahl Index of Concentration	0.404	0.480	0.316	0.366	0.415	0.462		
Domestic Consumption value (Rs. Million)	**5024**	**5875**	**8824**	**9529**	**10299**	**11802**		

Source: Centre for Monitoring Indian Economy: Industry: Market Size and Shares: August 2002. pp. 14-15.

production of butter, pure ghee and other fats from milk for the total of 60 companies in the organized sector, which provided information in their annual reports, increased from 50,046 tonnes in 1995/96 to 65,302 tonnes in 1999/00, and declined to 56,932 tonnes in 2000/01 (Table 20.14).

The annual growth in production during the six years period (1995-96 to 2000–01) for these products in the organized sector comes to 2.2 percent. The relatively low growth is due to shift in demand away from butter and pure ghee which contain saturated fats to vegetable oils and the high price of puree ghee whose retail prices per kilogram is more than double the price of vegetable oils. Total value of sale of these products rose from Rs. 4282.5 million in 1995/96 to Rs. 5697.4 million in 2000/01. The value of domestic consumption of these products increased from Rs. 4468 million to 5838 million.. The annual increase in total sale and domestic consumption was 4.8 percent and 4.6 percent respectively. The market size and domestic consumption is larger than indicated by these figures, which pertain to companies for which information was available. Britannia Industries classified butter, cheese under "dairy products". Ajanta Raj Proteins did not disclose production and sales quantity for the years 1999/00 and 2000/01. Total sales value of Sterling Agro Industries included other products. Nestle India also did not provide separate information on butter, ghee and other fats. There seems to be a fair competition for these products with Herfindahl Index of Concentration being 0.086 in 2000/01. However, two companies viz Milkfood and Sterling Agro Industries accounted for almost 18 percent each of the total market share and next four companies' shares ranged between 5-6 percent each. Total exports of these products by the sample companies are estimated to have risen from 563 tonnes in 1995/96 to 1815 tonnes in 2000/01.

Cheese

In recent years eating habits in India have undergone a major change. Foods like pizza, which use generous amounts of dairy products like cheese, have become immensely popular. All this has meant strong growth for the domestic cheese and other milk product industries. The organized cheese market including its processed cheese, cheese spreads, mozzarella, flavoured and spiced cheese, is placed at around Rs. 3 bn. Processed cheese at 50% of the overall market is Rs. 1.5 bn. strong. The next most popular variant is cheese spread claiming a share of around 30% of the total cheese market. The market

Market Segmentation Segment Share(%)	
North	36
East	42
West	6
South	6

is primarily an urban phenomenon and is known to be growing at around 15%. The market for cheese cubes, slices and tins is growing. The flavoured cheese segment has been declining (Table 20.15 and 20.16). Cheese is regarded as a breakfast food in India and is also cooked as vegetable. Dominated by the organized sector players, the market has been growing

Table 20.14: Butter, Pure Ghee and other Fats from Milk: Company-wise
Trends in Production, Total Sales, Market Shares and
Domestic Consumption: 1995/96 – 2000/01

Company	Production (tonnes)						Sales (Rs. Mil.)	Market share (%)
	1995/96	1996/97	1997/98	1998/99	1999/00	2000/01	2000/01	2000/01
Milkfood	8016	7188	7144	6789	8674	8878	1081.7	17.81
Sterling Agro Inds.				4715	7951	9474	1062.5	17.49
Mahaan Proteins			3156	3792	3267	4165	414.3	6.82
Modern Dairies	3865	3649	4056	4339	3917	3884	373.6	6.15
Dynamix Dairy Inds.				2904	2531	4708	361.0	5.94
Haryana Milk Foods	3865		3427	4052	4176	3133	358.8	5.91
J K Dairy & Foods	3860	3135	3435	2956	2277	3065	294.1	4.84
Milk Specialties	2239	2547	3044	2592	2004	2004	226.4	3.73
V R S Foods				1644	1514	1685	176.4	2.90
Creamline Dairy Products			657	774	1462	1809	159.7	2.63
Heritage Foods (India)		202	537	757	1250	1462	133.3	
Ajanta Raj Proteins			1335	1255			110.3	
Madhya Pradesh Glychem Inds.	1	257	904	784	848	848	105.8	
Rahul Dairy & Allied Products	1035	933	602	907	990	990	104.7	
Kisan Dudh Udyog			449	894	631	1098	101.3	
Nijjer Agro Foods	295	957	891	1122	1173	1173	90.7	
Rama Dairy Products			359	820	1820	1416	76.9	
Dodla Dairy				303	621	633	56.8	
R M I Foods	4040	3116	2190	1886	1114	271	51.3	
Premier Inds. (India)	983	755	499	371	432	374	45.6	
Total 60 companies	50046	46315	54506	65311	65302	56932	5697.4	93.78
Herfindahl Index of Concentration	0.070	0.079	0.056	0.050	0.057	0.086		
Domestic Consumption value (Rs. Million)	4468	4115	5818	7285	7608	5838		

Source: Centre for Monitoring Indian Economy: Industry: Market Size and Shares: August 2002. pp. 15-16.

Table 20.15: Demand for Processed Cheese: Past & Future

Year	Rs. bn
1990-91	0.50
1991-92	0.60
1992-93	0.69
1993-94	0.80
1994-95	0.90
1995-96	1.05
1996-97	1.35
1997-98	1.65
1998-99	2.10
1999-00	2.50
2000-01	3.00
2001-02	3.45
2002-03	4.00
2003-04	4.65
2004-05	5.40
2005-06	6.30
2006-07	7.40
2011-12	15.00

Table 20.16: Market Growth Rates of Cheese

1990-91 – 1996-97	18.5%
1996-97 – 2001-02	20.5%
2001-02 – 2006-07	16.5%
2006-07 – 2011-12	15.0%
Sensitivity Coefficient	9.0%

between 15% and 20% per annum. Amul, Britannia and Dabur are the major companies in the cheese sector. Prior to the entry of Britannia, the organized market for dairy products like cheese and butter was dominated by the regional cooperatives, such as Amul, Vijaya. In recent years more regional cheese producers like Gopalji and Chaudry cheese have entered the fresh cheese market in northern states. Currently imported brands are also freely available. In the organized domestic market, Amul remains the dominant player and will continue to be a stiff competitor given its sourcing advantage and market suaveness. Amul currently produces several types of cheese. These include Amul Cheese Slice, Amul cheese powder, Amul Malai Paneer and Amul Pizza Cheese (Mozzeralla).

The domestic cheese market has been growing by more than 20 percent per annum. This is reflected in the rapid growth in domestic production of cheese that more than tripled during the last decade from 2.5 thousand tonnes in 1991 to 8 thousand tonnes in 2001. The major consumption of cheese is in the urban areas. The four metros accounted for more than 50 percent of the consumption. Mumbai is the largest cheese consuming market accounting for 30 percent, followed by Delhi at 20 percent, Kolkata at 7 percent and Chennai at 6 percent.[1]

Gujarat Cooperative Milk Marketing Federation (GCMMF) with the Amul brand continues to be the main operator in the branded cheese market in India with about 60% market share in the branded market. It pioneered the market for processed, branded cheese. What GCMMF did was to develop the technology to make cheese from buffalo milk. World over it is made from cow milk. Britannia Industries joined the fray in the cheese market in mid-1990s through an arrangement with Dynamix Dairy Industries (DDI). It was set up in 1995 by a consortium of five companies – Conwood, Indo Saigon, Hiranandani, ETA and Metro. DDI has capacity to process 500,000 litres of milk per day with an estimated investment of Rs 1500 mn. The plant designed by Valio

Lead Players	
Company	Share (%)
Processed:	
Amul	60
Britannia	33
Others: Vijaya, Verka, Vadilal	7
All cheese:	
Amul	35
Britannia	15
Dabur (Le Bon)	12
Others: Verka, Nandini, Vijaya, Vadilal	38

of Finland is run on technology tie-up with Schreiber Foods of the US. Schreiber is the largest supplier of processed cheese to fast food chains in the US with expertise in sliced cheese.

Britannia's cheese is sold in tins in the form of cubes, and in individually wrapped slices in packs of fives and tens. The slices are being promoted more aggressively worldwide, and these account for a bulk of cheese consumption. These are gaining acceptance in India as well. Amul followed Britannia in launching slices. Its cheese spread in the form of paste has been well received in the market. Britannia has been concentrating on metros and large cities. The network covers some 60,000 dairy outlets equipped with cold cabinets, refrigerators and insulated boxes. Amul covers some 500,000 retail outlets. Its market share in the branded segment is over 30%.

French cheese major, Fromageries Bel, a 10 bn French Frank outfit, has entered the Indian market with La Vache Kirit or what is worldwide known as The Laughing Cow. Its target market to start with are the two metros of Delhi and Mumbai with the distribution entrusted to Delhi based Rai & Sons, distributors for premium food brands, Ferraro Rocher and Ricola. The Bel product will be produced at Bel's facility in Poland exclusively for the Indian market. La Vache Kirit is a guaranteed vegetarian product. Fromageries Bel is expected to widen its product portfolio by launching Laughing Kirit (creamy cheese in cube form) and Babybel (semi-hard with a wax coating appropriate for sandwiches). Laughing Cow will be followed by an Austrian cheese brand, Happy Cow (which is owned by Woerle).

---

[1]Infoquest: Report on Indian Cheese market 2002.

Woerle has entered into a licensing arrangement with Veekay Foods & Beverages in Mumbai. Nestle and Kraft have been planning to make foray in the Indian market. Foreign brands in India include: Probolene, Colby, Mozzarella and Parmessan from Italy, Cheddar from Dutch, Gryueve.

The new entrants will have to compete with well-established players such as Amul, Britannia's Milkman and Dabur's Le Bon, enjoying substantial market shares in the overall Indian cheese market. The US-based Philip Morris which brought in its Kraft cheese brand earlier, has gained a significant presence in the market. The rest of the market is spread among Verka, Nandini, Vijaya and Vadilal. Dabur forayed into the dairy products market through its joint venture company, Dabon

Leading Brands
Amul, Vijaya, Verka, Vadilal, Kraft, Britannia

International, a 50:50 joint venture between Dabur India and French dairy products major, Bongrain. The company claims a product range of 20 different varieties of cheese under LeBon brand. Dabon has a manufacturing facility at Noida with an installed capacity of 12,000 tonnes per annum. Incidentally, the government has, in a move in late April 2001, barred Dabone from marketing flavoured milk and processed cheese in the country. Dabur was to launch speciality cheese like blue cheese and hard cheese. It is in the process of developing cold chains at the distributor and retail levels in the state capitals and major towns in order to increase penetration levels.

The CMIE publication unfortunately does not give any information on cheese on company-wise trends in production, sales, and market shares.

Icecreams

In rural areas, kulfis/ice creams made by/small/cottage industry are popular. The market for organized sector is restricted to large metropolitan cities. In small towns and villages, there are thousands of small players who produce ice- creams / kulfis in their home backyard and cater to the local market. Almost 45% of the ice creams sold in the country are consumed in the western region with Mumbai being the main market, followed by 30% in the north, 15% in the south and 10 % in the East. Branded products accounts for only 20 percent of the market share, while unbranded the remaining 80 percent.

Ice cream market in India is estimated to have reached the level of Rs 10 bn per annum, of which the organised sector is about Rs 6 bn. The unorganised market has been shrinking. Per capita ice cream consumption in the country is extremely low at 250 milliliter per year compared with that of the US, which is about 22 litre. The Gujarat Cooperative Milk Marketing Federation sold 16 mn litres of icecream in the year 2000-01. It represented a

Market Growth Rates	
1990-91 – 1996-97	8.8%
1996-97 – 2001-02	15.0%
2001-02 – 2006-07	14.0%
2006-07 – 2011-12	12.0%
Sensitivity Coefficient	8.8%

growth of 50%. Amul is growing at a rapid pace. HLL's sales have, however, plateaued. Sales of HLL are estimated at 24 mn litres, with a peak of 24.9 mn litres in 1998. The organised market for ice creams of about 60 mn litres, has been growing at around 15% per annum. This places Amul's share in value terms at 27% and in volume terms about 40%. The industry has grown from Rs. 3.44 billion in 1990-91 to 11.5 billion in 2001/02 and is expected to touch Rs. 40 billion by 2002 (Table 20.17) while the consumption in East India is lowest (10 per cent). West consumes 45 per cent (Table 20.18).

Table 20.17: Demand for Ice Cream: Past & Future

Year	Rs. bn
1990-91	3.44
1991-92	3.67
1992-93	3.98
1993-94	4.28
1994-95	4.66
1995-96	5.00
1996-97	5.70
1997-98	6.60
1998-99	7.55
1999-00	8.70
2000-01	10.00
2001-02	11.50
2002-03	13.20
2003-04	15.00
2004-05	17.15
2005-06	19.40
2006-07	22.00
2011-12	40.00

The ice cream industry has, in a short span of time, undergone a structural transformation. Not long ago, two brands dominated – Kwality and Gaylord. Then came a new breeds Dollops in the north, Tulika and Rollick in the east, Arun and Joy in the south and Vadilal in the west. Liberalization has brought in, through the entry of large multinational and transnational corporations, foreign investment in the dairy and domestic food industries sectors. This resulted in competition, technological upgradation and market expansion. In the face of the competition, domestic industries are gradually losing market share and thus selling their businesses to the new entrant MNCs well before the value of the brand and businesses drops further due to ongoing onslaught of multinational brands. This is happening because MNCs have much greater resources to put behind their brand and business and also have long-term vision and sustainability. Domestic industries are no comparison in this respect.

Table 20.18: Market Structure

Market Segmentation

Segment	Share (%)
North	30
East	10
West	45
South	15
Branded	20
Unbranded	80

Heinz, the world's largest Tomato Ketchup manufacturer had acquired food business of Glaxo. Due to strategic restructuring of portfolio, Glaxo decided to divest their dairy business with established brands like Complan, Glucon-D and Farex. Hindustan Lever, on the other hand, through a strategic alliance route, took control of Kwality Icecream as well as 100% Icecream brand of Jagatjit. Hindustan Lever with their own presence in dairy sectors, and with the introduction of Baskin Robbins and Walls has emerged as a dominant player in dairy segment, in general and Icecream segment, in particular. Hindustan Lever (HLL) also acquired Dollop Icecream brand from Cadburys'. HLL, however, has announced their intention to sell-off their dairy unit in UP. Icecream industry, which was previously reserved for small-scale sector, has now been in the control of multinationals through a different route. The argument that icecream is actually a frozen dessert — a nomenclature that has been accepted by both Food and Law Ministries of Govt. of India — paved the way for Hindustan Lever for this strategic acquisition. The earlier successful domestic businesses such as Dalmia Dairy, Foremost Industry and Jagatjit Industry in dairy sector were all in deep trouble — and MNCs have taken a control of this sector as well.

National Dairy Development Board (NDDB) with its strong brand Amul and with its deep root extended up to farmer's level, as a means of backward integration will of course, remain a significant force to reckon with. But nobody will deny that in branded dairy products Amul has to put up a constant fight against multinational brands. Vadilal is also a significant player in icecream but their presence is limited in Western India and for how long they will remain has to be seen. Kraft Foods, a unit of Phillips Morris, is holding a licence to set up 100% owned entity and they are expected to come and set up their operation anytime.

The Indian ice cream market was till recently reserved for the small-scale sector. It was opened to large-scale manufacturer only in 1997. Since then the market has been witnessing fierce battles and huge investments on the part of major players in cold chains and infrastructure. The overall industry has been growing at a sluggish rate of 3-4 %. But the organized sector has been growing in the region of 15 % annually over the last five years. The competition among multinational ice cream companies is growing. Several premium ice cream brands are planning to make a foray into the Indian market including international brands like Frisco, Magnolia and Nestle, Haagen-Dazs (owned by Pillsbury) and Ben & Jery's was acquired by Unilever Plc only in 2000. Apart from super-premium ice cream, other products under these brands include sorbets, yoghurt, low-fat ice creams and others. Entry of these brands would make competition fiercer in the market place.

Leading Players

The 1.34 subsidiary of HLL, Kwality Wall's has drawn aggressive plans to increase its share in the ice cream market. HLL is all set to bring out innovative flavours in its ice cream. The changeover includes introduction of new products and change in its logo.

The Kwality Wall's logo in India has been replaced with the international logo of the company in order to maintain one common visual identity all over. The new products include Tubs (in combination of Vanilla, Chocolate and Strawberry), Cornetto Snackers (to come in a convenient, snack size), Max Doodh Badam (available in both cup and family pact format and targeted at children), and Choco BikiMax. The company has plan to develop a high-impact visibility kit to carry the new logo forward through freezer stickers, glow signs, flags, umbrellas, price-board and other point-of-sales material. HLL has also entered into the softy ice cream segment by setting up softy kiosks in all the major metros starting with Chennai. Through its softy, HLL seeks to double the size of the organized ice cream market in India. HLL's share in Delhi market has increased to 48% from 44%. If pushcart sales are taken into account its share further rises to 50%. However, Mother Dairy claims to command 47% volume of the Delhi Market. The market size in Delhi is estimated at 12-15 million litres valued at Rs. 900 million to Rs. 1100 million. Delhi accounts for 12 to 1.2 of the total market.

Vadilal has also launched a low-priced range. Some products are growing at more than 30% per annum. Amul has ambitious sales target: Rs. 5 billion by 2005 and Rs. 10 billion by 2010 from a bare one billion in 2000/01. In less than a year of its launch in Mumbai, Amul ice creams were ready to face competition from Kwality-Walls. The new brand introduced with its low pricing and 'real milk real ice cream' strategy made an incisive dent in the region's market. It is commented, "What Amul was not able to achieve in chocolates, it has now achieved in ice creams." Amul seems to have made its mark by nibbling into market shares of the regional brands such as Pastonji, Dinshaw's and Joy.

Lead Players	
Company	*Share (%)*
HLL	40
Amul	27
(Kwality Walls,	
Dollops,	
Milk Food)	
Vadilal Industries	15
Mother Dairy	13

The Mother Dairy has yet no plans to expand its coverage in ice cream from Delhi to other northern cities because of sister company Amul's extensive presence. Mother Dairy has two plants in Delhi and an Amul plant at Anand. Baskin Robbins set up world –renowned Dunkin Donuts bakery chain in India in mid-2001. The company planned to take the franchise route. The new range of ice creams is to be marketed under different brand and priced 12 to 20% higher than

Product Variation	
Type	*Share %)*
Vanilla	)
Chocolate	) 75
Strawberry	)
About 200 other	
flavours	25

regular brands available in the market. The company is to set up new manufacturing units in Bangalore and Delhi. The company also plans to add a new slim range of low calorie ice creams to its range.

Leading Brands

MTR Foods, which made a quiet entry into the ice cream market in Bangalore, has been planning to reach out to consumers throughout the state. The company sells a variety of ice cream with interesting varieties like Crazy Cones, Gadbad and Chocoba. Sno Shak Frozen Foods, marketers of Blue Bunny ice creams and other diary products, was planning to enter Mumbai, Surat and Amedabad after making the debut in Delhi, Chandigarh and Ludhiana. Blue Bunney has its presence in 30 countries. The product range covers 25 varieties of icecreams, frozen desserts and novelties. It plans to import diet ice cream.

Leading Brands
Kwality-Walls, Mother Dairy, Vadilal Dollops, Amul, Gaylord, 100%, Feast, Cornetto, Arun, Joy, Rollick, Tulika, Dairy Fresh, Nax UNO, Max Joos, Max Vitameter, Bike Max, Max Rose, Frostik, Tricone, Softie.

Movenpick is a famous European brand of ice creams. Its premium coffee beans brand is Café Premium. The Movenpick launch came a few weeks after the launch of the Blue Bunny in Mumbai. Movenpick is a super premium brand as against Baskin Robbs and Blue Bunny. Movenpick is at least 30 to 40% more expensive than Blue Bunny and its pries are more than double than those of Kwality Walls products. Movenpick is launching 25 flavours in India. In Delhi, Movenpick has tied up with 25 retail outlets including supermarkets like Nanz and Modern Bazaar. The company's icecreams initially launched in 13 flavours is priced in the range of Rs. 200 to 400 a litre. Dairy Dums, a Ahmedabad-based company, which retails Yum's ice cream, has made its presence felt in Mumbai with its economical Rs. 5 per cone, challenging McDonald's cone retailing.

The ice cream market growth picked up after de-reservation of the sector in 1997. Of the total size of Rs 10 bn, around 20% is in the hands of organized sector valued at Rs 2 bn, rest of all is with the unorganized sector. Among the major players in this industry Hindustan Lever has a market share of around 40%, represented mainly by Kwality Walls brand.

Amul with an estimated market share of 27% is rapidly gaining market share while Vadilal is the player in the national market with 15% of the market share and lastly Mother Dairy accounts for 13 percent of the market share.

Growth promotional activities

The Indian government adopted the policy of liberalization regarding the **ice cream industry** also and it is since then that this sector has shown an annual growth ranging from 15 % per annum. In 1999- 00, it was estimated at worth of Rs 10 bn. The per capita ice cream consumption in India is extremely low 250 ml per year compared with that of the US, which is about 22 litre. The icecream industry had been hit by increase in excise levy year after year, six times in the last five years. From a specific levy of Rs. 2 per litre in February 1970, it had been increased to 1.2 ad valorem (equivalent to Rs. 12 per litre) in 2000/01. The icecream market is projected to continue to grow from lower base at slightly lower rates than during 1988-89. to 2001-02 (Table 20.19).

Table 20.19: Ice cream Market Demand: Present and Future: 1990/91 – 2011/12

Period	Demand (Rs. billion)		Annual growth rate(%)
	First year	*End year*	
1990/91–1996/97	3.44	5.00	8.8
1996/97–2001/02	5.70	11.50	15.0
2001/02–2006/07	11.50	22.00	14.0
2006/07–2011/12	22.00	40.00	12.0
Sensitivity Coefficient	8.8		

Types of Indian Ice Cream Market

These can be segmented in three different ways, namely, on the basis of flavours, on the basis of stock keeping units / packaging and on the basis of consumer segments. On the basis of flavours the market today has a number of flavours like vanilla, strawberry, chocolate, mango, butterscotch a number of fruit flavours, dry fruit flavours, traditional flavours like Kesar-Pista, Kaju- Draksh etc. The market is totally dominated by vanilla, strawberry and chocolate, which together account for 75% of the market, about 200 other flavours account for the remaining 25 percent.

According to the CMIE data, production of icecream for the sample 28 companies increased from 12.532 million litres in 1995/96 to 34.798 million litres. The annual rate of growth comes to 18.6 percent. In addition, Kwality Frozen Foods reported its icecream production in terms of gallons for the years 1993/94, 1995/96 and 1995/96 The respective figures being 66,929, 480,488 and 26,482 gallons. Some other companies reported their production in terms of tonnes. All these data are shown in Table 20.20.

Table 20.20: Icecreams: Company-wise Trends in Production, Total Sales, Market Shares and Domestic Consumption: 1995/96 – 2000/01

Company	Production (000 Litres)						Sales (Rs. Mil.)	Market Share (%)
	1995/96	*1996/97*	*1997/98*	*1998/99*	*1999/00*	*2000/01*	*2000/01*	*2000/01*
Hindustan Lever				6600.0	8000.0	8000.0	1639.1	44.05
" " (Tonnes)	5785	**3830**	**5090**					
Vadilal Industries		5377.0	7470.7	7470.7	8544.0	9588.8	507.8	13.65
Hatsun Agro Products							321.3	8.63
Dinshaw's Dairy Foods							316.8	8.51
Vadilal Dairy Inter.	3565.0	3127.0	2672.0	2511.0	2133.0	2002.0	118.5	3.18
Merryweather Food Products				1138.0	2059.0	2530.0	110.6	2.97
Metro Dairy					531.4	1568.9	68.3	1.83
Devyani Foods			745.6	734.6	803.6	945.8	54.8	1.47
Indus Food Products & Equp.				1070.2	894.0	894.0	43.7	1.17
Fun Cream Food (India)					57.9	245.8	18.5	0.50
Vidya Dairy					321.9	358.3	16.2	
Milkfood (**Tonnes**)	**0**	**59**	**47**	**31**	**2**	**31**	**7.3**	
Majestic Farm House,		81.0	607.0					
Kawlity Icecreams (India)			1684.4	1113.5				
Kwality Frozen Foods (**Gallons**)	686929	686929	480488	26482				
Indiana Dairy Specialties	148.0	148.0	120.2					
Goldmohur Foods & Feeds		244.9		4.6	4.6			
Dharmendra Industries	1596.0							
Total '000 Litres	12532.0	8977.9	13299.9	27910.0	31330.5	34798.2	⎫ ⎬ 3704.1 ⎭	99.54
Gallons	6868929	6868929	480488	36482				
Tonnes	61	3889	5137	31	332	388		
Herfindahl Index of Concentration	0.043	0.446	0.413	0.304	0.244	0.232		
Domestic Consumption value(Rs. Million)	1699	2099	2499	2998	3722	3720		

Source: Centre for Monitoring Indian Economy: Industry: Market Size and Shares: August 2002. pp. 17-18.

The value of total sales of ice cream of sample companies increased from Rs. 1700 million in l995/96 to Rs. 3704 million in 2000/01. Export quantities ranged between 14 and 32 tonnes, while imports varied from 27 to 291 tonnes. The value of domestic consumption increased from Rs. 1700 million to 3720 million. The Herfindahl Index of concentration which increased in 1995/96 and 1993/94, declined during the next two years, reflecting entries of three more companies in this sub-sector.

In addition to the companies listed above, K I C Food Products Private., Maharashtra Dairy Products Manufacturing Co., Private., Kwality Fun Foods & Restaurant Private., Nirula & Co Pvt., Kamaths Ourtimes Icecreams Pvt., Highrange Food Private., Snofield Food Pvt., and Sivitha Ice Creams Pvt., are among the other top manufacturers. Also due to non-availability of data, the 'Amul" brand products manufactured by Kaira Distt. Coop Milk Producers' Union and marketed by Gujarat Coop Milk Marketing Federation is not covered in the above table. Thus the icecream industry is much larger than indicted by the operations of the companies mentioned in the Table 20.19 above. Market shares are thus overstated. There are no reasonable comprehensive statistics available for this industry.

Following the merger of Brooke Bond Lipton India with Hindustan lever w.e.f. April l996, icecream business came under Hindustan Lever. Before that, Cadbury India transferred its icecream business to Brooke Bond India. Hindustan Level "icecream" includes frozen desserts also. Majestic Farm House transferred its icecream business at Parsakhera in Bareilly district of Uttar Pradesh to Vadilal Industries in September 1.34 Vadilal Industries set up a new icecream plant at Pundhara in Gandhinagar district in 1995/96 Kwality icecream stopped its manufacturing activities from 1995/96 and it is trading milk products under its trademark "Kream K-ountry" manufactured by its subsidiary Kwality Dairy (India).

THE NEXT GENERATION MILK

In its commitment to build a healthy nation, Paras group has recently launched the 'next generation milk' called Bactofuged milk. By introducing this new product based on the German technology of Bactofugation for the first time in northern India, Paras group has set a benchmark in milk technology. It claimed to be the first to use high-level technology used internationally, physically removes harmful bacteria from the milk, giving the consumers a different experience of tastier and safer milk.

Paras group, which claims to be the second largest company preparing polypouch milk in Delhi, has a mix of nutritious products in its product portfolio. From skimmed milk powder to dahi, paneer, cheese, paras group has created a niche for itself in the dairy industry. Backed by well-armed production units to cater to the market needs and a strong R and D capability, Paras is now, all set to roll out the safest possible milk called Bactofuged milk. Bactofugation has evolved as an effective process over pasteurization and sterilization, the most distinct advantage being the physical removal of harmful spores and pathogens Bactofuged milk gives the milk a better shelf life and safer milk to drink.

CONCLUSION

India has a tremendous potential for development of livestock processing industry considering the fact that it has emerged as the largest producer of milk. It has also one of the largest livestock population, apart from a long coastline of 7500 km, which makes it the seventh largest producer of fish. India is thus amongst the top-ranking nations in terms of total production of various raw material required for development of livestock processing industry. Despite all these advantages, India is nowhere in the world map in terms of processing when compared with countries like Brazil, Philippines, Thailand and Malaysia.

The Government, being well aware of the prospects for development of food and livestock processing sector, has taken various initiatives for its promotion. These include setting up of a separate Ministry of Food Processing and promotional bodies such as Marine Products Export Development Authority (MPEDA) and Agricultural and Processed Food Products Export Development Authority (APEDA). Some new measures were taken in 1997-98, e.g. dereservation of certain items including icecream. During 1991-99, for which data are available, investment in livestock processing industry totalled Rs. 164.81 billion. Of this, investment in milk and milk product processing accounted for 89.2 percent and the remaining 10.8 percent was for meat and poultry products.[1]

---

[1]Ministry of Food Processing: Annual Report 1999-2000.

21

Employment Potential of Livestock

An estimation of employment in the livestock sector is a rather tricky job. While it is primarily a part time avocation, there is no holiday, since attendance is needed every day. Before we examine the available information on the subject, it is important to have an idea of the structure of livestock in the country. The very concept of dairy, piggery or other sub sectoral development in India is quite different as compared with the developed world. The base of Indian dairying is a small holder (small and marginal farmer and the landless) with one or two milch animals raised on crop residues and byproducts with underemployed family labour-mostly female workforce. Same was more or less the position with regard to poultry till recently, when it was primarily a backyard enterprise. Having moved away from the traditional system the organised sector entered the Indian scene during the seventies and is already responsible for 100 per cent of the broiler and 90 per cent of egg production.

DAIRYING

Underemployment of agricultural workers is widespread in rural India. This is perhaps one of the important causes of poor living standard among those who do not possess basic assets such as land, farm equipment and sufficient number of cattle and buffaloes. Most families keep one or more dairy animals to supplement their income. Large land owning farmers invest in dairy animals because it is profitable, fulfills the domestic demand for milk and milk products and engage female workers of the families productively within the household. For small and medium farmers, dairy animals are an insurance against uncertainty and provide self-employment in the slack season when demand for labour is minimal.

Dairying is viewed as the most suitable subsidiary economic activity for females because it can be managed while shouldering family responsibilities. Most of the women work part-time in dairying. It suits social norms too as workers need not to go out of the household to manage dairy enterprise. Unlike cultivation, females from the land owning classes also participate in equal measure in this activity with females from small and medium households.

Information on size of holdings is available from quinquennial agricultural census and various surveys conducted by the National Sample Survey Organization (NSSO). The data collected by these two sources do not tally, but is quite sufficient to prove that India is primarily a land of small holdings. Of the total of 98 million holdings, the number of those below 2 hect. area is over 76 per cent according to Agricultural Census and around 80 per cent according to N.S.S.O. In addition, there are around 15 per cent landless rural households.

As regards the distribution of the number of animals maintained by different size of holdings, information is rather scanty. On the basis of certain regional studies, National Commission on Agriculture[1] estimated that 70 to 75 per cent of the households possessing milch cattle belong to the vulnerable category of small farmers, marginal farmers and landless agricultural labourers. Dairying, by and large, is a small man's business.

A village enumeration survey conducted by the NDDB in 1984 covering nearly six million households in 20,386 dairy cooperative villages spread over 108 milksheds in the country made some interesting revelations (Table 21.1). Nearly 60 per cent of the total rural households own generally two or three milch animals. Some 72 per cent of the families owning milch animals, are landless, and small and marginal farmers. The vulnerable group of families accounted for about 61 per cent of total buffaloes and cows in the survey area. Only the large farmers having 4 hectares or more of land holding kept more than four animals[2].

Table 21.1: Land and Milch Animal Holdings

Category	Landless	Marginal	Small	Medium	Large	All
(1)	(2)	(3)	(4)	(5)	(6)	(7)
Families (million)	2.131	1.690	1.025	0.675	0.508	6.029
	(35)	(28)	(17)	(11)	(9)	(100)
Families owning milch animals (million)	0.770	1.052	0.799	0.559	0.445	3.625
	(21)	(29)	(22)	(16)	(12)	(100)
Animals (million)	1.390	2.091	1.932	1.651	1.877	8.941
	(16)	(23)	(22)	(18)	(21)	(100)
Animals* per owner (No.)	1.8	2.0	2.4	2.9	4.2	2.5

Source: NDDB village Enumeration, 1984. A census of six million households in 20,386 dairy cooperative villages spread over 108 milksheds.

Definition of farmers according to holdings size of irrigated land: Landless: - No land; Marginal farmer: upto 1 ha; Small farmer: - 1 to ha; Medium farmer: - 2 to 4 ha; Large farmer: 4 ha or more.

*Buffaloes and cattle; male and female of all age groups. Figures in parentheses are percentages of the total.

A survey by the National Council of Applied Economic Research, 1991 found that 43 per cent of the member households of milk producer cooperative societies in 'Operation Flood' areas have only one milch animal and almost 75 per cent of the members belong to the category of landless, marginal and small farmers. Over 60 per cent of the milk output in the 'Operation Flood' areas comes from these households[3].

In the rural scenario it is a matter of common observation that the average number of bovine stock per unit of cultivated area declines sharply as the size of holding increases. Thus the overall distribution of milch cattle is much more uniform and less skewed than the distribution of land. The small and marginal farmers and the landless labourers, together with petty village artisans, rear 1-2 milch animals mainly on crop residues and byproducts with the help of underemployed and unemployed family labour, especially the female workforce. Although returns from these animals are low, they are still cost-effective. In the absence of any alternative employment opportunities, the dairy animals, therefore, could play a much greater role in the economic life of small and marginal farmers and the landless than that of medium and large farmers who derive a greater part of their income by growing crops[4].

The Indian Dairy Industry acquired substantial growth during the 8th and 9th Five Year Plans, achieving an annual output of around 85 million tonnes during 2001-2002. This has not only placed the industry first in the world, but also represents sustained growth in the availability of milk and milk products for the burgeoning population of the country. Most important, dairying has become an important secondary source of income for millions of rural families and for million more, has assumed the most important role in providing employment and income.

For purposes of employment potential, dairy industry can be divided into 2 sub sectors - household activity and the organized industry. More than 50 per cent of the total milk production is estimated to be consumed as liquid milk. About 66% of milk is procured in organized sector. Milk processing plants in cooperative sector are procuring about 28 million litres of milk per day, whereas, plants in private sector are processing 30 million litres per day. It has been estimated that approximately 12% milk per day is processed into value added products like casein, whey powder, and whey protein concentrates. Though the production of milk powder including infant milk food, malted food products, cheese, condensed milk, etc. is steadily increasing, the potential for such products is quite large.

Household Sector

Within the household sector, Operation Flood programme, which started in 1970, completed its third phase on April 30, 1996. The main thrust of the programme was to consolidate the gains already achieved, and to strengthen the dairy cooperative structure for sustainable development of the dairy industry in India. By December, 2000 about 87,000 (cumulative)

Anand Pattern dairy cooperative societies were organized involving about 109 lakh (cumulative) farmer members.

At the end of phase 3, there was a balance of Rs. 34 crore out of the EEC contribution to the Operation Flood Project. The EEC approved utilization of these funds on the following two major components:

(i) Women Dairy Cooperative Leadership Development Project; and

(ii) Strengthening of Dairy cooperatives to meet the competitive challenges of the next decade.

These components are primarily aimed at strengthening cooperatives at the grassroot level. The Programme Implementation Agreement (PIA) was signed between EEC and NDDB and was endorsed by the Government of India on August 21, 1997. Consequently, measures were initiated from September, 1997 and are still continuing.

According to a survey in Punjab, on an average, the per animal labour input works out at 619 manhours per year, which means an input of 1.7 hours per animal per day. Translated on per hectare basis, the labour employment works out at 457 man-days per hectare per annum. The operation wise labour input in 1978-79 revealed that the harvesting, transportation and chaffing of fodder accounted for as much as 58 per cent of the total labour input. The next important operation was feeding which accounted for 19 per cent of the labour input. The other operations of milking, watering, sweeping the animal shed and cleaning of animals accounted for 7 to 8 per cent of labour use each. A similar study in Rajasthan estimated a total employment of 122.54 days per hect., of which 94 per cent were females.

Usha Tuteja (Fellow, Agricultural Economics Research Center, University of Delhi, Delhi – 110 007)[5] in her study in Ambala and Bhiwani districts in Haryana state found out that the contribution of female workers in labour use in dairy enterprise was 60 per cent in Ambala district and 75 per cent in Bhiwani district on all farm sizes and it was higher than male workers in all cases. The average yearly income earned by self employment of females in dairy enterprise was Rs. 9,325 in Ambala and Rs. 11,798 in Bhiwani as against the total household income of Rs. 15,527 and Rs. 15,813 respectively from this sector.

Despite the phenomenal increase in milk output, the cooperative and the public sectors procured only a small portion of the 81 million tonnes of milk produced in 2001, the cooperative sector procured only 5.7 million tonnes and the public sector just one million tonnes. Together, they procured only 8.3 per cent of the total milk output. A large percentage - 93 per cent of the Indian milk trade is still in the unorganized sector, 6 per cent in the cooperative and 1 per cent in the public sector.

With this scenario before us, an effort is now made to calculate the employment pattern for this traditional household sector accounting for nearly 85 per cent of the available milk production. It may be added that this does not include the army of those who are engaged in the marketing of this milk in an unorganised manner either for direct consumption or processing the same into butter, ghee, khoia, cheese, etc. Nor does it include the time spent by the house lady to convert a part of the milk into ghee in her own household.

The calculation is based on a few scattered studies which have calculated the employment pattern for milk production[6,7]. By piecing together various types of scattered information, including the one from the National Commission on Agriculture, we have developed different norms for the number of animals which one person can maintain on a full time employment basis (Table 21.2). This shows that 24.6 million persons were employed in the maintenance of the bovine population during 1987 and this number is estimated to have increased to 28.2 million by the year 2000 AD.

Other Estimates

A similar exercise for other animals shows that total employment in the Livestock sector during 1987 was 30.7 million which is estimated to have increased to 35.4 million by 2000. It will not be out of place to mention in this connection that NSSO has also been giving employment estimates for the livestock sector under various rounds. Estimates of rural livestock employment given are 9.03, 10.6, 29.43 and 16.65 million during 1972-73, 1977-78, 1983 and 1987-88 respectively. Since these data, being quite inconsistant, do not make any sense, and they have not been considered.

Based on some recent studies by NDDB and earlier estimates by National Commission on Agriculture, Agriculture Division of the Planning Commission estimated that the animal husbandry sector even with the existing stock could generate employment equivalent to 86 million person years inclusive of employment in processing and marketing of milk and milk produce. Another estimate, using norms given by National Commission on Agriculture, but not including employment in processing and marketing, puts the figure for 1990-95, at 61.50 million for animal husbandry and fishery sectors, assuming a continuation of the 2.2 per cent growth of this sector experienced in the past decade. It is, however, claimed by experts that a much higher growth could be attained in this sector. Fishery sector, it is claimed, can grow as fast as 7 per cent per annum, with about two-thirds of the existing marine and inland potential unexploited. In animal husbandry sector, what is probably important is to ensure that those engaged in it, constituting about one-third of the total workers in agricultural and allied activities, are able to earn adequate levels of income. This would need to be ensured through appropriate institutional and technological support and sectoral policies[8].

Women Dairy Cooperative Leadership Programme

The project aims at nurturing leadership amongst women dairy farmers for economic and social empowerment besides ensuring their say in the governance of dairy cooperatives. The subcomponents of project activities include selection of dairy cooperative societies, selection and training of

Table 21.2: Employment Potential of Livestock Sector

Category	1987		1992		2000 (estimated)	
	Livestock Population	Employment	Livestock Population	Employment	Livestock Population	Employment
Cattle Adult						
Cross bred	7.1	2.4	9.1	3.1	13.1	4.4
Local	129.7	13.0	129.8	13.0	125.7	12.6
Cattle Young						
Cross bred	4.3	0.3	6.1	0.4	10.1	0.6
Local	58.6	1.5	59.6	1.5	58.2	1.5
Buffalo						
Adult	46.6	6.6	51.9	7.4	55.7	7.9
Youngstock	29.4	0.8	32.3	0.9	42.8	1.2
Sub-total	**275.7**	**24.6**	**288.8**	**26.2**	**305.6**	**28.2**
Sheep						
Crossbred	2.0	0.1	2.4	0.1	3.3	0.2
Local	43.7	0.8	64.4	1.2	52.4	1.0
Goat						
Local	110.2	1.5	115.3	1.6	125.0	1.7
Pig						
Cross bred	1.1	0.1	1.8	0.2	2.4	0.2
Local	8.9	0.2	10.9	0.2	11.0	0.2
Camels	1.0	1.0	1.0	1.0	1.0	1.0
Horse & Ponies	0.8	0.8	0.8	0.8	0.6	0.6
Others Poultry						
Desi	190.5	1.2	243.5	1.6	228.0	1.5
Improved	53.4	0.4	63.6	0.4	114.5	0.8
Total	**687.3**	**30.7**	**792.5**	**33.3**	**843.8**	**35.4**

resource persons for carrying out activities relating to organizing, educating and training of women dairy farmers in initiating group activities for income generation, thrift and health. Presently, the programme is being implemented by 39 milk unions and in each of these milk unions, the programme is being implemented in 25-30 village dairy cooperatives every year.

Organised Sector

The growing affluent middle class of some 300 million with increased purchasing power, the fast pace of urbanisation and the emergence of nuclear families are leading to a change in lifestyle and consumption habits. By 2000 AD, over 30 per cent of the total population was urban. Consequently, there has been a rise in the consumption of processed foods, including dairy products. Income elasticity of demand for milk and dairy products is high and estimated to be more than one. According to the National Dairy Development Board (NDDB), the domestic market for butter, ghee, cheese, dairy whiteners and icecream is growing by over 10 to 15 per cent per annum.

Presently, milk products fetch a relatively higher price than liquid milk. This has boosted production of value-added products. But the consumption pattern of milk and its products depicts a preference for liquid milk. "There is increasing awareness of health aspects of pasteurised, packed milk. This market will continue to grow." Delivery of milk to consumers, at their doorsteps, and the end-of-the-month payment for milk that is sold by the milkman has still not been matched by the organized sector. The dairy industry finds the daily receipt of lots of cash for milk an attractive proposition; very few businesses in India have positive cash inflows every day. Replacement of the traditional vendor is considered necessary by some, which is possible only if the organised sector is better in providing services of value to the customer.

Eighty per cent of the milk production is concentrated in 10 States - Uttar Pradesh, Punjab, Madhya Pradesh, Rajasthan, Andhra Pradesh, Tamil Nadu, Bihar, Maharashtra, Gujarat and Haryana. The largest milk producing State is Uttar Pradesh, followed by Punjab, Madhya Pradesh and Rajasthan. However, the milk production pattern is skewed. But this should not go against the processing of milk. After all, in the initial stages of 'operation flood' and even today, India depends on augmenting supply of its liquid milk on milk powder supplied by European Community. It may be easier for surplus regions in the north to process milk powder, which could be supplied to the deficit regions and reconverted into liquid milk. A programme of this nature will provide a further fillip to the processing of dairy products and employment in the organised sector. Employment generation for this organised sector will be in addition to rearing of the dairy animals. No estimate for this sector is available.

LEATHER INDUSTRY

Leather is one of the most important industry depending on the livestock and is a source of employment both in the organized and unorganized sectors. The processed and finished skins of Indian goats, sheep and calves fetch good prices in the international market. The leather industry in India is largely in the hands of the private sector and is all set for rapid growth during the current decade. It is all too evident that very little investment had been made either in R & D or in technology upgradation by the manufacturers of leather products. Till a few years ago dealing in leather or leather products was not considered glamorous and as a result the business was confined to the traditional families. Tanneries, for example, would not employ a leather technologist or a qualified tanner imagining that their family-held secrets would be leaked out. The government too in their political wisdom did not encourage the growth of leather industry in organised sector. For, it was considered an ideal small scale industry with the village cobbler as an essential ingredient of rural economy. Global markets or prospects of exports of leather products generating foreign exchange was beyond perception of the powers that be.

The Unorganised Indian Sector

World over, the leather industry is characterised by the predominance of small units on grounds that they can easily adapt themselves to changing fashions. In India, however, many of them are not adequately equipped with technology and manpower for high quality products. For decades, India concentrated on village shoe industry and exports of raw hides and skins - products with high demand, but lowest value-addition. Then in 1972, the Seetharamiah Committee recommended a total ban on export of all types of raw hides and skins except lamb fur. The government has now extended the ban to cover semi-finished leather too. Even export of finished leather is discouraged and the same attracts an export duty of 5 per cent.

Hides and skins are the basic raw materials for the leather industry. The livestock of a country is the potential source of supply of these raw materials. Despite India having largest livestock population in the world, one of the problems in the leather sector has been inadequate supply of raw materials, i.e. raw hides and skins. The availability of raw hides and skins is influenced, besides the population size of livestock, growth rate of different animal types, recovery of carcasses, the production and marketing chains for raw hides and skins and management practices used in the country.

According to the experts, leather is also damaged during the removal process. To educate the people involved in removal of skins and stop their move to other professions, the government has undertaken a project in Kalyani, Wardha, Athani, Muzafferpur and Lucknow. Under this project, labourers are educated in the scientific ways of removing skins from the carcass. Further, the government has already allowed the imports of raw hides and skins, semi-processed leathers and also finished leather for stock and sale without any restriction.

In 1987, the Central Leather Research Institute (CLRI) conducted an all India survey of hides and skins. The study showed a loss of nine million hides and 9.2 million skins in India due to non-recovery. Besides, nearly 200 million sq. feet of hides and skins produced in the country were inferior in quality due to many ante and postmortem defects in them. Table 21.3 shows the projected availability of hides and skins by the end of the twentieth century. Due to problems of collection and processing of skins and hides, a huge deficit is predicted. The problem is genuine because even though import of raw skins and hides is on open general list and exempt from import duty, availability is at a premium. This is because most of the other countries are also going in for domestic value addition.

Manufacturing Base & Capacity Utilisation

From the backyard tanning units to the sophisticated modern factories, the structure of the industry encompasses a wide range. The leather footwear

Table 21.3: India's Potential Availability of Bovine Hides (million pieces)

Category	Total	Fallen hides	Slaughtered Stock	Non-recovered hides
Cattle hides	28.1	10.9 (38.7%)	10.8 (38.5%)	6.4 (22.8%)
Buffalo hides	18.2	7.6 (41.8%)	8.1 (44.5%)	2.5 (13.7%)
Goat skins	81.0	6.5 (8.0%)	68.9 (85.1%)	5.6 (6.9%)
Sheep skins	35.1	3.6 (01.3%)	27.9 (10.3%)	3.6 (10.3%)

Source: Financial Express January, 31, 1994.

units which were around 19,500 in the year 1981 grew rapidly to 56,000 in the year 1991. The leather garment units and other accessories units have also a similar story to tell. Worldwide, the leather consumption per capita is increasing. Today, footwear exports account for more than 50 per cent of the $32 billion trade and the trend is likely to persist. If India wants to capture this lucrative market, quality and consistency are important. However, India's exports from this sector constitute mainly of shoe uppers rather than full shoes.

There is a considerable gap between demand and supply of leather which is expected to widen further (Table 21.4). It is estimated that nearly 30-40 per cent of leather go waste. The infrastructure for collection of carcasses is still very primitive which results in lot of wastage. Further, the religious sentiment attached with the slaughtering of cows, which leaves only buffalo skin as the only option. To check the growing deficit of leather supply, the government had set up committees which recommended the utilization of hides from fallen animals, upgradation of lower-grade hides and skins and commercial cattle farming to increase the quality.

Table 21.4: Raw Material Deficit by 2000

| Category | Requirement | | Deficit | |
	Mill/. sq. feet	Availability	Mill. sq. ft.	Mill. pieces
Hides	2,706	992	1,714	50.0
Goat skins	1,139	630	509	72.7
Sheep skins	795	210	585	83.6

Source: Financial Express, January 31, 1994.

Although the tanneries are scattered all over the country, it must be noted that the three states of Tamil Nadu, West Bengal and Uttar Pradesh account for 80-90 per cent of the total tanning capacity in all the three stages of processing of skins and hides. This unequal distribution of tanning capacity is due to historical rather than economic reasons (cow slaughter, which is banned in most of the states, continues to be permitted). Table 21.5 shows the extent of capacity utilisation in different states for the different stages of tanning process. Although the data is somewhat out-of-date, however the situation has not really changed much.

Table 21.5: Capacity Utilisation (%) In Different States – 1987-88

State	Raw to semi-finished		Semi-finished to finished		Raw to finished	
	Hides	Skins	Hides	Skins	Hides	Skins
Tamil Nadu	48.4	72.2	74.2	69.0	73.6	78.2
West Bengal	56.4	32.7	42.4	53.5	65.1	55.6
Uttar Pradesh	54.5	100.0	72.0	50.0	70.6	57.0
Andhra Pradesh	50.6	61.1	53.3	70.0	37.8	47.5
Maharashtra	-	50.0	100.0	25.2	58.5	73.1
Karnataka	71.4	54.8	81.8	78.5	39.1	-
Punjab	-	-	81.8	-	64.1	108.2
Other states	33.3	54.9	38.9	111.0	65.0	25.8

Source: Financial Express, January 31, 1994

Note: Hides include calf skins

(i) Although the livestock is evenly scattered throughout the country, tanneries are concentrated in regions of Tamil Nadu, West Bengal and Uttar Pradesh. A probable reason is that cow slaughter is banned in most of the other states. This manifests the problem of recovery due to higher transportation cost.

(ii) Tanning process is exclusively reserved for small scale sectors and this is a major factor contributing to its lack of modernisation.

(iii) Leather industry is notorious for its detrimental effects on the environment. This has been an unsurmountable problem to its on going expansion.

The capacity utilization is lowest in the stage of processing raw to semi-finished hides, which is reserved exclusively for the small sector. Regional variations show very low capacity utilisation from raw to semi-finished skins in West Bengal, semi-finished to finished skins in Maharashtra, raw to finished hides in Andhra Pradesh and Karnataka and raw material and raw to finished skins in other states.

Employment

Leather and leather goods industry is one of the biggest small-scale industries in India. It is estimated that there are at present 2 lakh cottage sector units employing 1 to 4 persons in each, 3000 small scale units employing 5 to 20 persons in each, 500 medium scale mechanized units employing 20 to 50 persons in each and 150 large scale units employing 50 persons and more in each unit. The tanneries in small and medium range are at present employing manual operations in their processes. With the change in the policy of the Government of India to export more finished leather and leather products, the tanning industry is gradually switching over to mechanization.

It has been stated above that most of the tanneries are concentrated in Tamil Nadu (379), West Bengal (233) and Uttar Pradesh (147). Footwear manufacturing units are concentrated in Agra, Ambur and Kanpur, leather goods factories in Kolkata and leather garment units in Mumbai, Bangalore and Delhi. Tanneries had not been established close to the region where animal husbandry was developed. Today, the integration of all sectors and segments of the leather industry is necessary for enhanced productivity, improved quality and added prosperity to the artisans.

More than 2000 tanneries process about 0.50 million tonnes of hides and skins annually. The industry processes skins of more than 359 million animals, including buffaloes and other cattle. The industry has recorded an eight times growth in value terms since 1980-81. Footwear, leather garments and leather accessories have been identified as the potential growth segments.

According to latest NSS estimates (43rd round), in 1987-88 there were 7.5 lakh person employed (principal and subsidiary) in the manufacturing of leather and leather products (except repair) out of whom 3.21 lakh persons were in rural areas as compared to 3.29 lakh in 1983 (38th round NSS). The decline is steeper if we take only principal status workers. Their estimated number between 1977-78 to 1983 stagnated around 3.26 lakh and had declined to 3.08 lakh in 1987-88. Among the major States. Andhra Pradesh (-72%), Gujarat (-53%), Haryana (-45%), Himachal Pradesh (-75%), Madhya Pradesh (-39%) showed sizeable decline. The decline has been partially offset by the increase in their number in States like Karnataka, Maharashtra and West Bengal, the net reduction being 0.18 lakh between 1977-78 and 1987-88.

Leather workers in the decentralised sector can be classified into three main categories i.e. flayers, tanners and manufacturers of leather products. The share of leather workers in the cottage sector in flaying, tanning and manufacturing are 100%, 86% and 79%, respectively. The cottage sector accounts for 90% of total employment in the leather industry. In order to revitalize the rural artisan sector, according to the Report of the National Commission on Rural Labour it is necessary to integrate the three categories of workers, *viz.* flayer, tanner and footwear producer. Appropriate technology for each category will have to be identified and suitably adapted to the capabilities and capacities of rural artisans. In addition, supplementary activities like meat/bone meal, tallow, horns/hoof meal could also be integrated to improve viability.

NOTE ON KAMDHENU BULLOCK DRAWN TRACTOR

Since the ages, animal husbandry has been a part of agriculture. During the last few deacdes, this integration has been broken by the introduction of the agrochemicals and agro machinery. Initially, the results were phenomenal. Of late, serious consequences have cropped up so much so that the whole sector has become uneconomic and non-sustainable.

The Planning Commission in its report on Animal Husbandry for 10th Plan made following important observations:

- Need of 80 million bullocks for agriculture and other uses;
- Improving working efficiency;
- The cost of substitution of DAP with petroleum based power also needs to be calculated rationally.

Those farmers who eschewed agrochemicals and have opted for organic methods, have been benefited by reducing costs and getting out of the debt cycle. A report by the Goverment of Punjab to Central Government, gist of which has been published in different newspapers, it is apparent that the farmers being unable to meet their obligations for loans taken for tractors, were forced to commit suicides.

Government funds of about Rs 9314 crores remained blocked. Condition of other states can well be appreciated, if this is the situation in granary of India. A few days back, while interacting with Shri Laxmi Narain Modi, Managing Trustees, BCRDF, it was a big surprise to learn that an intermediate technology was now available by the name Kamdhenu Bullock Drawn Tractor (KBDT). KBDT has been tested at Government of India Institute at Hisar and been found satisfactory. It has also been approved by NABARD and many banks for financing. Ministry of Agriculture has also included this for subsidy under Macro Management Scheme.

Some of the specialities of the KBDT are:

Two bullocks work with KBDT and the performances are even better than the job done earlier by six bullocks on traditional plough.

Each KBDT saves about 1500 litres of diesel and thus the saving to a farmer only on account of diesel after deducting the expenses for two bullocks for the whole year, works out to about Rs 15, 000/- (This figure will vary according to fluctuating rates of diesel).

KBDT comes by way of a package and include following implements:

Harrow (6 Disc) with one tyne in the centre

5 Tyne Tiller	Ridger
Desi Plough	Sub Soiler
Soil Turner	Potato Digger

Singh Patela, Improved Yoke, Halas and required ropes Spade, Sickle, Khurpi, First Aid Kit, Tool Box with Spanner and Key, Two ceramic candles, non-overflowing funnel, seeds of *tulsi* and marigold, sprouting stainless steel utensil.

A spare set of shovels is also given so that when the first set wears out, the second is available for long use without going to the market.

In addition, it also have Five Row Seed Drill, thus facilitating sowing of seeds at desired depth and distance. All tyes of seeds can be sown starting from rape seed to gram or maize.

Apart from the various accessories required, KBDT also has a package to reduce diseases and improve health with a new concept of health garden of 50-60 sq. meters alongside the farmers' houses. KBDT is so comfortable that it can easily be operated by women folk and elderly persons. Two bullocks with KBDT work more comfortably than while pulling the traditional plough since a specially improved yoke is provided which improves contact area several times and thus the chances of neck injuries are also avoided.

Farmers sit on a chair under the shade of an umbrella and having along side three litres special kind of unbreakable water bottle (provides cool water like earthen pot in hot summer) and the drudgery of walking behind the plough is eliminated which otherwise requires about 200 km walk under scorching sun, bare foot for a small plot of 100 X 100 meters.

The cost of the equipment is only about 6% of the cost of a tractor and for three of them, it will be about 18%. It has only three moving parts namely two wheels and a chain. Hence there is hardly any maintenance cost which otherwise for repairs and maintenance is phenomenally high apart from interest and instalment.

As farmers are showing greater interest to adopt organic farming, integration of bullocks with KBDT would prove to be a boon for availability of the dung and urine for manure and bio-pesticides instead kof pollution, global warming and diseases of the operators associated with a tractor.

A latest report has appeared in Outlook of November 22, 2004 that 12-Member Panchayat passed a resolution banning sale and use of pesticides in the village of Punukulas (Andhra Pradesh). On pesticides alone, they were spending Rs 8000 to 12,000 per acre. By adoption of indigenous organic method the cost came down to couple of hundred rupees pre acre while the yield remained just as good, if not better. There are several other examples in different states on the benefits derived by the farmers by integrating cattle and adopting organic farming.

CONCLUSION

Livestock play an important role in the Indian economy as a source of supplying nutritious food, draught power and employment to the vast majority of rural poor. Recently the processing industry for milk, poultry and leather has also become quite important as with urbanization and improved living standards, demand for processed products is also increasing substantially. A study of the employment potential of this sector would, therefore, involve both of these sectors.

We have tried to look into all these aspects and surveyed the available literature on the subject. One thing is very clear that hardly any reliable information is available about the employment potential of such an important sector of the economy while a large number of small/marginal farmers and landless labour (particularly their women folk) are getting part-time employment throughout the year, a proper methodology, with an empirical data base, to tackle this problem is yet to be evolved. There is otherwise no justification for such high variations in various estimates with regard to the number of persons employed in the sector.

Our estimate of 31.6 million man years relates only to the one for the maintenance of these animals. No information is available even for the household sector of the dairy industry consuming/distributing 85 per cent of the milk. What proportion of this milk is consumed by the producers and what is the marketing pattern of the surplus is not known. Whether it is the collection of milk from the small producers or hides, skins and bones of dead animals etc., even guesstimates are not available.

We have tried to put together here all the available information. We would like to stress that livestock employment, particularly under Indian conditions has its own peculiarities. There is perhaps an urgent need to look into this aspect by a multi-disciplinary team to evolve an appropriate methodology which should take note of the ground situation in the country and develop required norms. Converting the total employment into man years is not much of relevance and depicts, if at all, a completely distorted picture. The whole issue needs to be examined afresh under the following heads :-

Household Sector
1. Maintenance of animals
   a) This will include grazing, harvesting/procuring, transporting, chaffing and feeding of green/dry fodder and concentrates etc., cleaning/ sweeping of animals/sheds, watering,
       milking and conversion into butter/ghee etc.
   b) Village milk collectors/gowalas who distribute milk within or around townships.
   c) Sweet meat shops (Halwaies) who convert milk into khoia, paneer, cream etc.
   d) Men/women who maintain poultry.
   e) Those who collect fallen hides/skins and bones etc.
   f) The village slaughterer, meatshop, cobbler.

2. Organised Sector:-
   a) This will include wholetime/partime persons employed in the organised dairies, farms rearing poultry, piggery and other animals.
   b) Feed mixing plants, feed distributors, and retailers etc.
   c) Slaughter houses including other groups of people who collect/ transport the animals.
   d) Small dairies in townships etc.

3. Processing industry:-
   a) Big dairies and other processors.
   b) Poultry processing organisations.
   c) Leather processing units and their further processing into various utility products.

REFERENCES

1. National Commission on Agriculture, 1976.
2. NDDB village Enumeration, 1984. A census of six million households in 20, 386 dairy cooperative villages spread over 108 milksheds.
3. R.K. Patel, Present Status and promise of Dairying. Indian Journal of Agricultural Economics, March 1993.
4. R.S. Khanna, A Historical Perspective of Dairy Development in India, Indian Dairy Man, October 1989.
5. Tuteja Usha; contribution of Female Agricultural workers in Family Income and their status in Haryana, Indian Journal of Agricultural Economics, Vol. 55, No. 2, April-June 2000.
6. S.S. Grewal and P.S. Ranji, Economics and Employment of Dairying in Punjab, Indian Journal of Agricultural Economics, October- December 1980.
7. Usha Rani, D.L. Vyas and G.S. Jodha, Gender Differential in Work Participation in Various Operations of Crop and Livestock Enterprises in Semiarid Areas of Rajasthan, Indian Journal of Agricultural Economics, July- September 1993.
8. Planning Commission, Employment, Past Trends and Prospects for 1990s, working paper, May 1990.

22

Animal Husbandry Statistics

In the dynamic times of today one cannot take comfort in the past. The role of knowledge or intellectual capital in Policy making and Research is well appreciated. Right answers to any issue will depend on reliable database; hence the importance of Statistics. With the Livestock sector assuming an important role in the national economy, one needs to improve the present state of livestock statistics. Although considerable resources have been directed towards collecting and disseminating information on basic crops, little attention has been given to collecting, disseminating and analyzing livestock and livestock product data. Timely information on volumes produced, quantities traded, locational availability, prices and stocks is largely unavailable. They have to meet the challenges of the New Economy, the Global Economy or what we would call the 'Knowledge Economy'.

Reliable and timely data is not only a key input for informed planning and decision-making by various participants, but also for effective government policy-making and administrative decision-making. There is an urgent need to collect a comprehensive data of the livestock sector through the modern Information Technology. In view of the growing importance of livestock sector in India, it is essential to have reliable statistics on the various facets of this sector. Major heads on which data need to be collected and analyzed are given in Table 22.1.

Table 22.1: Major Heads on which Data Need to be Collected

1. Number: Cattle, Poultry, Piggery, Small ruminant, sheep, goats etc.	10. Prices
	11. Processing of livestock products
2. Production: Livestock Products	12. Draught Power
3. Consumption of livestock products	13. Foreign Trade
4. Breeding	14. Economics of Livestock
5. Feed and fodder	15. Fisheries
6. Diseases	16. Demand/Supply of major livestock products
7. Management	17. Apiculture
8. Livestock Health Care	18. Employment
9. Marketing	19. Livestock Credit and insurance Programmes

It is important to note that there is obviously a need for a comprehensive data base for proper planning and policy formulation for the development of livestock sector. The basic requirement of data relates to number and productivity of livestock and the economics of the production from livestock enterprises of different sizes. Besides, different types of related statistics/information; we also need to have comprehensive knowledge of for scientific livestock development programmes. This includes information on animal husbandry practices, feed and fodder, impact of individual inputs on the productivity of animals; inputs and output relationship in milk production, substitution possibilities as means of lowering costs and increasing the returns; balanced nutritional feed for different animals; prices of animals (breedwise); requirement and consumption of various livestock products; cost of production of milk, eggs etc.

Similarly, for any scheme for livestock insurance basic data on the productivity of animals, their life span, mortality rate and general animal health services available are needed. For the development of a good system of marketing of livestock products, the basic data needs are the prices to be paid to the producers and the prices to be received from the consumers etc. The data on prices of livestock sold in major markets/fairs need to be collected. Thus, there is an urgent need to develop a proper system of collection of information and creation of data base for livestock sector and in the Tenth Plan, due emphasis should be given in this regard.

SOURCES OF LIVESTOCK DATA

Although available data are quite scanty, there are a number of sources which supply varied types of information. Each of them is discussed in detail in this chapter and ways and means suggested to improve upon them so as to meet the present day needs of this fast growing sector of the economy. The sources are:

1. Livestock Census held quinquennially.
2. Integrated Sample Surveys.
3. National Sample Surveys.
4. Directorate of Economics & Statistics.
5. Central Statistical Organization.

We would like to add here that there are quite a large number of organizations/institutions (listed below) engaged in one way or the other in livestock activity. Each of them also generates lots of data on different aspects of livestock. A proper channel of coordination is required to be established with all such and other organisations for strengthening the livestock related data base.

1. NABARD (National Bank of Agriculture and Rural Development)
2. NDDB (National Dairy Development Board)
3. DMI (Directorate of Marketing and Inspection)
4. Ministry of Rural Development
5. Ministry of Food Processing

6. Ad-hoc/pilot surveys conducted by the research institutes and experimental stations provide information on age at first calving, calving interval, number of stillborns, abortion, conception rate, egg-laying capacity etc.
7. Reports/Returns: The periodic returns/reports from the State Department of Animal Husbandry provide information regarding veterinary dispensaries/hospitals/polyclinics and number of animals treated.
8. N.C.D.C. (National Cooperative Development Corporation)
9. ICAR (Indian Council for Agricultural Research)
10. IASRI (Indian Agricultural Statistics Research Institute)
11. NCAP (National Centre for Agricultural Economics and Policy Research)
12. Agriculture Universities and all other educational institutions dealing directly/indirectly with Livestock
13. Dairy Association of India
14. Food Processor's Association of India
15. Agro Economic Research Centers

Quinquennial Livestock Census

India possesses the largest livestock population in the world. The first livestock census was conducted in the country as early as 1919-20, followed quinquennially thereafter with expanded coverage and scope. Until the 13th Census, the scheme used to be a non-plan activity and funds for conducting it were provided from the State Budget. This used to result in delays in organizing field work, tabulation and publication of final results by the states. Hence, a Centrally Sponsored Scheme for providing assistance to states was initiated in the 7th Five Year Plan for conducting 14th Livestock Census in 1987-88. The scheme aimed at assisting the states to the extent of 50 per cent and UTs upto 100 per cent in respect of the principal components of the census i.e. primary enumeration, supervision, contingencies and support for tabulation of results of the census. In spite of this, a number of states/UTs did not conduct the census. The number of defaulting states increased from 2 (1982) to 7 (1992). What is most distressing is the fact that even a progressive state like Punjab is among the defaulting states since 1982.

Over such a long period, the scope and coverage of the livestock census have increased tremendously. At present, the livestock census covers not only livestock but includes information on fisheries, agricultural implements and machinery. The fieldwork is conduced by primary workers, who are generally patwaris in the rural areas and staff drawn from municipalities/ Animal Husbandry Departments or primary school teachers in the urban areas. Different agencies are involved in different states for conducting livestock census.

The time lag in the availability of final figures for the district level is more than 5 years and for the state level estimates it ranges from 3-5 years.

There has been no single reference date for the collection of data throughout the country in spite of best efforts and hence growth rate figures pertaining to different states are not comparable. No efforts are made to provide advance tabulation of a 10% sample of the livestock households in respect of important items and to take suitable correction if required, technically called revalidation.

Integrated Sample Surveys (ISS)

It was felt that if the estimates of individual products are to be estimated regularly and the emphasis is also to be laid on estimation of changes taking place over time (such as yearly changes or changes over plan periods) then the surveys may be planned in an integrated way. Pilot sample surveys with this concept of integrated approach were carried out in northern region comprising the states of Punjab, Haryana and Himachal Pradesh during 1969-72 and Andhra Pradesh of southern region during 1971-74 for developing a sampling technique for simultaneous estimation of all the principal livestock products in one single survey.

An essential feature of these surveys was that the stratification of each region was done on the basis of taluks important for a particular product, viz. important for poultry alone, important for sheep alone and important for both poultry and sheep. In southern region taluks important for both poultry and sheep were further divided into two substrata, viz. important for poultry and mutton type sheep and poultry and wooly type sheep. In each year one product was covered on intensive scale whereas the other product on smaller scale. Milk, poultry and egg production, wool and meat production were covered on larger scale in first, second and third year respectively. In three seasons of each year successive sampling procedure was strictly followed whereas over the years this pattern was not adopted as no independent unmatched samples were selected except in the first year. Thus, in order to obtain an improved estimates of mean of the character (say milk) per season in the first year, successive sampling methodology was used and for obtaining similar estimates for subsequent years, double sampling procedure was utilised by using information collected on large scale in the first year. The studies undertaken in these two regions demonstrated the feasibility of obtaining reliable estimates of these four products simultaneously in a single survey if we strictly use the suggested design.

At present, all the States and Union Territories are covered under the scheme for estimating the state-level estimates of production of milk, eggs, wool and meat. The Scheme is in operation since 1975-76. However, surveys for providing district level estimates of production and that of cost of production of milk and eggs are conducted on a limited scale, i.e., in a few States only. These surveys otherwise have a comprehensive coverage with 15 per cent of the total villages and for complete enumeration of livestock population (5 per cent villages for each of the 3 seasons). Scientific methods are then applied for the production of milk, egg and wool. The results are presented to the Technical Committee which releases these estimates every year.

National Sample Surveys

This is the only source which provides on a regular basis information regarding quantity and value of consumption of various livestock products – both for rural and urban areas. The Livestock Economics and Statistics Division should undertake studies to bring about a reconciliation with the production data released.

Some special surveys have also been conducted by NSSO on livestock. Thirty- Second Round (1977-78) gave a comprehensive data base on cattle mortality and various other indicators. Again 48th Round provides information on ownership of animals quality wise by size of holdings. Since the NSSO sample is very small, it is necessary that the expanded/ revised Livestock Census /Sample Survey Schedules should include such items along with others.

Directorate of Economics & Statistics

Directorate of Economics and Statistics, Ministry of Agriculture quinquennially carries out an input survey with a primary focus on agricultural inputs. This survey which covers 10 per cent of the villages and 20 households per village provides information about livestock ownership according to size of holdings. Since quite a large number of animals are also owned by landless non cultivator, the results thrown out are not of much utility. Even otherwise, contents of all-India and Statewise reports (few states publish them) differ widely. There is no uniform pattern even among the State Reports. In the light of all this the Input Survey should delete this item and should be included in Integrated Surveys.

The Directorate also brings out a weekly Bulletin of wholesale prices and retail prices of selected commodities. This includes various livestock products – milk, ghee, goat meat, fish (fresh water and marine), eggs, broilers and poultry feed – at some of the selected centers. The list is, however, not comprehensive and many more items need to be incorporated. There is also a need for larger coverage.

Central Statistical Organisation

CSO provides annual data regarding the value of output from livestock sector under the heads – (1) Milk Group, (2) Meat Group – meat, beef, mutton, pork, poultry meat, meat products, byproducts, hides, skins, other byproducts (3) Eggs (4) Wool-Hair – wool, hair & bristles (5) Dung – dung fuel, dung manure, and (6) Silk worm cocoons & honey. All calculations about the contribution of a particular sector in the national economy and its growth from year to year is being calculated only from this source. Obviously the numbers given here are assumed to be based on the unit value of each of the item listed above. Since no reliable information is available either about the quantities produced or the unit prices of the same, it is important that basic data must be improved. It is essential to reconcile these discrepancies. This type of a situation further strengthens the argument about the need for a very reliable data base of this sector.

REVIEW OF THE RECOMMENDATIONS OF THE WORKING SUBGROUP ON LIVESTOCK STATISTICS FOR THE NINTH PLAN

Continuing Schemes

To improve an efficient working of the scheme on livestock census, it was recommended to make it a central sector scheme with 100 per cent Grant-in-aid. It is a serious matter that while this part of the recommendation has been accepted and implemented, there is hardly any improvement in its efficiency. There is really some deterioration in the sense that some of the states did not start the work for 1997 census at all. Similarly under the integrated sample survey, it was recommended during the Ninth Plan that the present scheme might continue and the scope of the district level surveys for estimation of milk and egg production might be extended to cover all districts of the country and that of cost of production of milk and eggs to cover all important districts of milk and egg production.

It is really sad that the same recommendation is being repeated again and again. No action was taken during the 9th plan to improve the situation despite the fact that there would be a saving of over Rs. 2.0 crore from an outlay of Rs. 20 crores allocated under this head.

As for the new schemes, (Annex I) all of them appear to be nonstarters. A look at 9th Plan allocation and expenditure for the sector presents a dismal picture (summary Table 22.2 below) in the sense that of the total allocation of Rs. 1076.2 crores for the 9th Plan, there was a likely saving of over Rs. 580/- crore. Lack of funds cannot, therefore, be the reason for non-implementation of these schemes. It is felt that with the growing importance of the livestock in the national economy as well as within the agriculture sector, there is an urgent need to give special attention to strengthening the continuing schemes and start the new schemes as mentioned earlier as early as possible.

TENTH PLAN FOCUS AND STRATEGY

The Tenth Plan envisages that animal husbandry and dairying will receive high priority in the efforts of generating wealth and employment, increasing the availability of animal protein in the food basket and for generating exportable surpluses. The overall focus is considered to be on four broad pillars, viz. (i) removing policy distortions that is hindering the natural growth of livestock production; (ii) building participatory institutions of collective action for small-scale farmers that allow them to get vertically integrated with livestock processors and input suppliers; (iii) creating an environment in which farmers will increase investment in ways that will

Table 22.2: Allocation & Expenditure During 9th Plan

(Rs. crores)

Sl. No	Particulars	9th Plan Alloc.	1997-98 Expd.	1998-99 Expd.	1999-00 Expd.	2000-01 Expd.	BE-2001-02	Total
(1)	(2)	(3)	(4)	(5)	(6)	(7)	(8)	(9)
1.	Secretariat &Economic Services		0.67	1.31	1.62	1.67	2.20	7.47
2.	A.H. Sector Action Plan Schemes	700.45	49.59	20.01	52.75	41.93	93.95	258.23
3	Other Schemes	372.64	44.72	33.02	44.51	46.44	62.54	231.23
4.	Integrated Sample Surveys	20.00	2.54	2.62	3.35	3.84	4.40	16.75
5.	**TOTAL (A H Sector)**	**1076.12**	**94.84**	**53.03**	**97.26**	**88.37**	**156.49**	**489.99**
6.	Dairy Development Schemes	469.52	29.24	23.97	16.45	39.66	37.45	146.77
7.	Total (AH & DD Sectors)	1545.64	124.08	77.00	113.71	128.03	193.94	636.76
	Fisheries Sector	800.0	85.06	91.93	91.97	85.98	103.86	458.8
	Grand Total	**2345.64**	**209.14**	**168.93**	**205.68**	**214.01**	**297.8**	**1095.56**

Source: Basic Animal Husbandry Statistics, 2002.

improve productivity in the livestock sector; and (iv) promoting effective regulatory institutions to deal with the threat of environmental and health crisis stemming from livestock. The allocation for animal husbandry, dairying and fishery is Rs. 2500 crore during the 10th Plan.

While formulating the animal husbandry and dairy development plan, it has been recognised that currently, there is absence of lot of data like that those relating to breed/wise milk production of cattle and buffalo, egg production from commercial farms and households, cost of production of milk, egg and wool, availability of life style resources, etc. The Working Sub-Group of Livestock Statistics for Tenth Plan dealt elaborately on the deficiencies on Livestock Statistics in the country and recommended certain measures to strengthen and improving the livestock intelligence during the Plan period. The recommendations are indicated in Annexure 'II'. Acting on the recommendations, the Government proposes to establish a National Animal Health and Production Information System with the active involvement of research institutions, government departments, Panchayati Raj Institutions (PRIs), urban local bodies (ULB), private industries, cooperatives and NGOs. This will work as the national data base.

Integrated Sample Survey (ISS) Scheme for Estimation of Production of Major Livestock Products

Present Status/Progress

The scheme on 'Sample Survey for Estimation of Production of Major Livestock Products' initiated in 1975-76, had been continuing since then in the States either as a Centrally Sponsored Scheme, or as a State Sector Scheme. Since the Seventh Five Year Plan, the scheme is being implemented as a Centrally Sponsored Scheme, titled "Integrated Sample Survey for the Estimation of Production of Major Livestock Products' and the same has been continued during the Eighth and Ninth Five Year Plans.

The broad objectives of the scheme are as under:

i. Estimation of livestock numbers,
ii. Average yield per animal (in respect of milk, eggs, wool and meat) at State and National level.
iii. District level estimates of production of milk and eggs including average yield per animal.
iv. Product utilization.
v. Feeds provided to animals of different species, and
vi. Cost of production per unit of milk and eggs in the selected districts.

There are three components of the scheme:

a. Central Sector Scheme on "Strengthening of the Animal Husbandry Statistics Cell at Headquarters" in the Department of Animal Husbandry & Dairying.
b. Centrally sponsored Scheme on "Integrated Sample Survey for Estimation of Production of Major Livestock Products viz., milk, eggs, wool and meat" in States.

c. Central Sector Scheme on "Strengthening of Animal Husbandry Statistics" in Union Territories.

At present, the scheme is being implemented in all the States and Union Territories for estimation of production at State/UT level. The surveys for preparation of the district level estimates of production of milk and eggs are being conducted in all the States, while cost of production surveys for milk and eggs have been undertaken in a few selected districts of the States. The Animal Husbandry Statistics unit in the Department of Animal Husbandry and Dairying, Ministry of Agriculture, provides technical guidance and training and undertakes occasional supervision of the surveys at field level, examines/analyses the reports and coordinates the information/ statistics regarding production of major livestock products and other related aspects at all India level. The estimates of production of milk, eggs, wool and meat and other related statistics are compiled and published by the Department of Animal Husbandry & Dairying.

These surveys have a comprehensive coverage with 15 per cent of the total villages and for complete enumeration of livestock population (5 per cent villages for each of the 3 seasons). Scientific methods are then applied for the production of milk, egg and wool. The results are presented to the Technical Committee which releases these estimates every year.

Estimation of Meat Production is based on the information regarding,

(a) the total number of animals slaughtered;

(b) the average meat production per animal; and

(c) the total meat production:

The information on the number of animals slaughtered is obtained from two sources namely, (i) from the sample of households reporting slaughter of animals and from all the butchers and other agencies in the villages selected in the sample, and (ii) from records maintained at all the slaughter houses in the State.

Despite the fact that such a detailed information is collected with regard to meat production, this is not being published. Similarly, data being annually collected regarding various types of animals, feed and utilization of various products in the annual Sample Survey is also not analyzed.

The progress of physical and financial achievements under Integrated Sample Survey Scheme for the Estimation of Major Livestock Products during the Ninth Plan are given as under:

Physical Achievements

Under the Scheme, final estimates of production upto 1998-99 have been provided. For the years 1999-2000 and 2000-2001, only provisional estimates are available. The estimates of annual production of milk, eggs and wool during the Ninth Plan period are shown in the following Table 22.3.

Table 22.3: Annual Production of Milk, Egg and Wool

Year	Milk (million tonnes)	Eggs (million no)	Wool (million kgs)
1997-98	72.1	28689	45.6
1998-99	75.4	29476	46.9
1999-2000 (P)	78.8	30629	47.9
2000-2001(P)	81.4	31770	49.2
2001-2002(A)	84.6	34034	50.7

P = Provisional

A = Anticipated Achievement

Source: Basic Animal Husbandry Statistics, 2002, Department of Animal Husbandry & Dairying, Govt. of India.

Present Problems

- There is a time lag of two years for release of All India estimates of production.
- Non tabulation of all data collected in ISS due to heavy work load involved.
- Estimates of meat production from unorganized sector and poultry sector are not available on uniform basis.
- For estimating wool production, the methodology does not cover sheep shearing centers, wool extension centers and sheep breeding farms located in different states.
- Estimation of egg production from commercial poultry farms is not included in the sample.
- Cost of Production studies are not being conducted on uniform basis due to staff and funding problems.
- Efforts should be made to cover all these areas during the Tenth Plan Period.

(c) Suggestions for improvement of the scheme.

(i) The scheme should be continued with improvements in the coming years

(ii) Computerization of the work relating to data analysis, report preparation in ISS will improve the timeliness in preparation of tables and reports. This will also ensure the accuracy of the calculations involved in ISS work along with ensuring uniformity in procedures adopted by all the States. For this purpose computers along with accessories and maintenance charges are to be provided to all the States and UTs.

(iii) All the data being collected under the sample surveys – production of meat, number of animals, disposal of milk production, quantity purchased, sold, kept for conversion and consumed in the household, are collected under Integrated Sample Surveys for the estimation of major livestock products, but it is not processed and tabulated by all the States due to lack of resources. This information is required for the purpose of implementation of Milk & Milk Production Order and for developing area-specific growth strategy in terms of investment in milk procurement, processing and marketing. Same is the position regarding production and utilization of dung and feed provided to different animals, etc.

(iv) The scope of the scheme should be enlarged to cover all the districts of the country for preparation of district level estimates of milk, eggs, etc. and that of cost of production of milk and eggs to cover all important districts of milk and egg production. The Statistical Cells in the States are to be suitably strengthened, wherever necessary. Further, equipments like computers are to be provided to all the States exclusively for this work.

(v) Budget should be provided for Training of the field staff from time to time to ensure accuracy and efficiency in the field level data collection. Since supervision (both by the State and the Central teams) of field work is necessary to ensure the proper tempo needed for the field staff for performing duties in proper way, an additional component of expenditure in this regard needs to be provided in the scheme.

(vi) Since chicken production is primarily in the organized sector, the matter should be discussed with major players like Venketeshwara (Pune) and a method evolved to prepare estimates of chicken meat production. As for poultry meat in the unorganized sector, the present questionnaire needs to be revised to obtain this information from those households which are having broilers for egg. All these broilers are in any way slaughtered in the village itself at the end of their productive period of egg production which is about 18 months.

(vii) Underestimation of livestock products: There are large number of institutions which rear animals/birds for the production of milk and eggs, e.g., State/Central Cattle Breeding Farms, institutes under ICAR, State Agricultural Universities, Military Dairy Farms, big private dairy/poultry farms etc. It is believed that all these institutes/farms are not being covered under the livestock census, resulting in underestimation of number of animals/birds possessed by them and the production therefrom. This deficiency needs to be overcome urgently.

Data on Livestock Products

With regard to livestock products, the only data being released relate to milk, egg, wool and fish. This is also restricted at present to the State level. Suggestions have already been made to improve the scope of ISS, so that district level estimates can be made on a statistically viable basis for all the districts in the country.

There is at present no information available on various byproducts of the livestock industry such as (i) slaughter house wastes, offals, bones, hoofs, blood etc., and (ii) hides and skins. Research studies will have to be conducted to find ways and means for a scientific estimation of information on all such products.

Major Livestock Products – Reappraisal of Methodology

At present, all the States and Union Territories are conducting Integrated Sample Surveys under the Centrally Sponsored Scheme for estimation of production of major livestock products, viz. milk, eggs, wool and meat at State level. However, surveys for providing district level estimates of production and that of cost of production of milk and eggs are being conducted in a few States only. The type of information being collected under the Scheme includes details of livestock and poultry maintained by the householders, yield rates of livestock products, animal husbandry practices adopted, consumption of feed and fodder by the animal and their costs, number of animals died due to natural calamity and other causes, protection and treatment against diseases and disposal of livestock products and their prices, etc.

Estimation of Livestock Products

(i) Pilot Surveys: During the Second Five Year Plan, IASRI conducted a series of pilot surveys for evolving suitable sampling technique for estimation of output of major livestock products, viz. milk, eggs, wool and meat on individual basis. The regions covered for estimation of milk production were Punjab plains, Eastern Uttar Pradesh, Gujarat and coastal districts and adjoining areas of Andhra Pradesh and also the coastal districts of Orissa. For estimation of egg production, the states covered were Andhra Pradesh, Kerala and West Bengal whereas for estimation of meat production, Tamil Nadu and Haryana were covered.

(ii) Repeat Surveys: In the Third Five Year Plan period, some tracts covered during Second Plan periods were repeated to test the soundness of the techniques developed and also to study the changes in the level of output and total production of these principal livestock products. These surveys clearly demonstrated the feasibility of estimating the individual products through well planned sample surveys. However, it required a regular infrastructure to conduct these surveys regularly, if continuity of data was to be maintained. Such a system could provide yearly estimates with seasonal breakup also.

The Institute played a key role in providing guidance in improving and proper implementation of the methodology. The Institute's role in developing a sound base for technical input as well as for providing linkages with the implementing agencies through its various training and human resource development programmes. The methodology so developed is being used by different States under the Centrally Sponsored Scheme under the coordination of Department of Animal Husbandry and Dairying, Ministry of Agriculture, Government of India. In order to monitor the work under the Scheme and to provide technical guidance to the Department of Animal Husbandry and Dairying, a Technical Committee of Direction (TCD) for Improvement of Animal Husbandry and Dairying Statistics was set up during 1975-76 under the Chairmanship of Director, IASRI, New Delhi, and State Directors/Statisticians of Animal Husbandry, representatives from NSSO, CSO, IASRI, DMI, DES, etc. as its Members and In-charge, AHS (DAH & D) as Member Secretary. The Committee was made responsible to examine and approve the Statewise estimates of production of major livestock products viz., milk, eggs, wool and meat at national level. The Committee meets on regular intervals to discuss the difficulties being faced in data collection and to suggest their remedies to identify data gaps and to discuss the issues like conduct of livestock census and other related aspects.

During the last 25 years, a number of development and crossbreeding programmes have been implemented by the Government to increase the production of livestock products and accordingly a number of new breeds have come up in livestock and poultry. Besides this, livestock sector has been commercialized to a large extent due to the increasing demand of the products in the country and abroad also. The greater emphasis has been given to the poultry industry due to increasing demand of poultry meat. A number of big hatcheries have come up in the country, which cater to the need of poultry meat.

Under the Integrated Sample Surveys, the estimates of meat production do not include the meat obtained from poultry and thus has a serious data gap. There are other information which are not covered under these surveys, viz. conversion ratio of milk into different products and their cost of conversion, losses of various livestock products, prices of livestock and livestock products and their utilization pattern, etc. Similarly, for estimating wool production, the methodology does not cover sheep shearing centers, wool extension centers and sheep breeding farms located in different States. There is also a serious gap in the methodology. In order to fill up these gaps, reappraisal of the methodology is very much needed and schedules canvassed under these surveys also need modification.

The Integrated Sample Surveys include only the study on major livestock products and not livestock byproducts such as hides and skins, hair, pig bristles, bones and intestines, etc. which are utilized by other industries and thus have great economic values. The estimates of production of these byproducts are very much required by the researchers, administrators and policy makers for formulation of different policies and programmes. As regards the estimation of production of hides and skins, IASRI had undertaken a series of pilot studies in the past in different parts of the country and the methodology is now available to estimate their production.

But for other byproducts, no study has been undertaken as yet and thus requires taking up pilot studies for estimation of these byproducts.

In order to fill up these gaps, the existing methodology needs to be modified by incorporating the following information:

   (i) Breedwise milk yield of different species, viz. cattle, buffaloes and goats.

   (ii) Information of egg production from commercial poultry farms.

  (iii) Information on poultry meat included to get the total meat production.

  (iv) Breedwise wool yield from various sources like sheep and wool extension centers, wool shearing centers and sheep breeding farms, etc.

   (v) Cost of production studies on milk and eggs should be undertaken in selected districts of different States and different sampling frame be used for this study.

  (vi) Estimates for livestock byproducts should be compiled and published regularly.

LIVESTOCK CENSUS

Present Status/Progress

The Census of livestock and statistics on agricultural implements and machinery and fishery is carried out through complete enumeration. The data collected on livestock comprise cattle, buffaloes, yaks, mithuns, sheep, goats, horses, ponies, mules, donkeys, camels, pigs, dogs and poultry. The number collected is classified by species, sex, age and by purpose. From the sixteenth Livestock Census, classification by breeds has been added. However, data on broad categories of crossbred and indigenous breeds are being collected separately in respect of cattle, sheep, pigs since 1982. In case of poultry, separate information is collected for deshi and improved birds.

The first census of cattle population was conducted in 1919-20 collecting restricted information on livestock from limited zones. The second census was carried out in 1924-25, more or less on the same lines. Thereafter, each subsequent census was expanded in scope and coverage by using more refined concepts and definitions. The sixteenth census was done in 1997. The next census due in 2002 has already been initiated.

The Directorate of Economics & Statistics, Department of Agriculture & Cooperation, Ministry of Agriculture is responsible for the conduct of livestock census in the States/UTs and also for preparation and publication of the report of the census. However, the ultimate responsibility for conducting the livestock census rests with the State Governments. The census work is conducted by various agencies in different States/UTs. These are:

1. State Bureau of Economics & Statistics
2. State Directorate of Animal Husbandry & Veterinary Services

3. Department of Land Records/Revenue
4. Department of Finance
5. Department of Planning, Statistics & Evaluation

Some of the States/UTs had not adhered to reference dates in the past, leading to problems of non-comparability of the data at all India level. The scheduled date of reference for conducting the livestock census in 1977, 1982, 1987 and 1992 were not followed by a number of States/UTs. Hence many states could not conduct the 1987 census on the reference date (i.e. 15-10-87) on account of various reasons. The conduct of the Census was postponed to 1988 and for some States/UTs even to 1990. This affected the conduct of the 15th Census with 15-10-1992 as reference date as the States/UTs which conducted the census in 1990, did not think it proper to conduct the same again in 1992.

In view of the difficulties encountered during the earlier livestock census, the sub-Group on Animal Husbandry Statistics and Information for Ninth Plan had recommended that the 16th Livestock Census, with reference date 15-10-1987, should be taken up as a Central Sector Scheme. This was also agreed to by the Technical Committee constituted by the Government for advising it on conducting the 16th Census. For the first time it was decided to provide financial assistance for computerization of the work of livestock census both at the district and the State Headquarters level by providing one PC, a printer and a CVT each at a cost not exceeding Rs. 5,500/- per unit.

The 17th Livestock Census (latest in the series) will be conducted during the Tenth Plan with the following improvements: The present arrangements for conducting the Livestock Census in the States and Union Territories are not found satisfactory. Various organizations, not necessarily connected with livestock development, are handling the operations relating to the census in the States/UTs, resulting in unsatisfactory quality of data and also delays in data collection and reporting. Efforts are being made to conduct the census through a single agency. Preferably this work will be entrusted to Directors of Animal Husbandry in all States/UTs and the Department of Animal Husbandry and Dairying at the Centre. Efforts are being made to carry out the livestock census work in all the States/UTs simultaneously as per prescribed time schedule. Failure to carry out enumeration on the reference date is becoming the major shortcoming of Livestock Census data. For conducting Livestock census, a similar statutory basis as provided in the case of conducting India's Population Census may also be required. Since Livestock is a State/UT. Level

The personnel appointed on temporary basis for Livestock census must have a basic minimum qualification or experience of village conditions such as village patwari, school teacher, etc., Such primary investigators should be given proper training before putting them for actual collection of data from the households.

The format of **Sate Reports** is very comprehensive. It is, however, very unfortunate that most of the States do not prepare these Reports and even if prepared, they are not published. Every effort is made to have these reports published annually. Based on the State Reports, the Centre would bring out an All-India Report. This step will fill a major gap in the available data base. Further, there is a need to strengthen the statistical units and to introduce electronic data processing and report preparations using Personal Computers. Crude estimates may be released within two months of the completion of data collection. The final publications of Statewise and district-wise data on all the above mentioned items may be brought out within six months and a year respectively. All the data should be made available on CD Rom.

Efforts are needed to improve staff through refresher training programmes/courses involving new techniques based on computerization. Honorarium to be paid to the field investigators should be reasonable and at par with those paid for similar other primary data collection. In fact, there should be adequate incentive to carry out the assigned work sincerely and honestly. Therefore, it has been agreed to increase the present level of honorarium from Rs. 2 per schedule to Rs. 6 per schedule. Till 1997-98 the Scheme had been implemented as a Centrally Sponsored Scheme with the allocation of Rs. 11.34 crores during the 9th Five Year Plan. However, with effect from the Financial Year of 1998-99 on the same pattern as that of Population and Agricultural Census and accordingly the allocation of Rs. 11.34 crores was raised to Rs. 42.74 crores for the 9th Plan in order to meet the increased cost. However, due to economy in expenditure by Government of India, an amount of Rs. 28.49 crores was released to States in 9th Plan. A budget allocation of Rs. 1.20 crores (BE) had been provided for the 17th Livestock Census in the financial year 2002-03. The actual requirement of 10th Plan (17th Livestock Census) is estimated at about Rs. 105 crores. The outlay for conducting the 17th Livestock census during the 10th Plan period will be on 100 per cent central assistance basis.

The 17th Livestock Census (latest in the series) will be conducted during the Tenth Plan with the following improvements

The present arrangements for conducting the Livestock Census in the States and Union Territories are not found satisfactory. Various organisations, not necessarily connected with livestock development, are handling the operations relating to the census in the States/UTs, resulting in unsatisfactory quality of data and also delays in data collection and reporting. Efforts are being made to conduct the census through a single agency. Preferably this work will be entrusted to Directors of Animal Husbandry in all States/UTs and the Department of Animal Husbandry and Dairying at the Centre. Efforts are being made to carry out the livestock census work in all the States/UTs simultaneously as per prescribed time schedule. Failure to carry out enumeration on the reference date is becoming the major shortcoming of Livestock Census data. For conducting Livestock census, a similar statutory basis as provided in the case of conducting India's Population Census may also be required. Since Livestock is a State subject, it may, therefore, require a detailed deliberation at State/UT level.

The personnel appointed on temporary basis for Livestock census purpose must have a basic minimum qualification or experience of village conditions such as village patwari, school teacher etc. Such primary investigations should be given proper training before putting them for actual collection of data from the households. The format of State Reports is very comprehensive. It is, however, very unfortunate that most of the States do not prepare these Reports and even if prepared, they are not published. Every effort should be made to have these reports published annually. Based on the State Reports, the Centre may bring out an All-India Report. This step will fill a major gap in the available data base. Further, there is the need to strengthen the statistical units and to introduce electronic data processing and report preparations using Personal Computers. Crude estimates may be released within two months of the completion of data collection. The final publications of Statewise and district-wise data on all the above mentioned items may be brought out within six months and a year respectively. All the data should be made available on CD Rom.

Present Problems

- It is observed that at present, Livestock census is not being conducted in all the States/UTs as per the time schedule.
- There is a time-lag of 3-5 years in publication of the All India report of the Livestock Census (Statewise, i.e. volume-I). This time lag is much more in case of publication of district-wise data (Volume-II).
- The involvement of different agencies in this work creates problems due to lack of interest in the work, lack of knowledge about the animals and its hybrid varieties, etc.
- There are data gaps with regard to the quality of animals and, number of animals per household etc. As for poultry, the present schedule is inadequate to answer the ground situation. The present schedule collects data on items like agricultural machinery which is not related to livestock. There are also problems of varying definitions and dates of reference in different censuses limiting their comparability.
- Quality of data collected is also not upto the mark. Whatever being the coverage, there is the need to improve the quality of data collected.

Suggestions for Improvement of the Scheme

Keeping the above problems in view, following suggestions are made for the improvement of the operation of the scheme.

- The scheme of Livestock Census should be continued during the Tenth Plan with improvements in the years to come.
- The present arrangements for conducting the Livestock Census in the States and Union Territories are not found satisfactory. Various organizations, not necessarily connected with livestock development, are handling the operations relating the census in the States/UTs, resulting in unsatisfactory quality of data and also delays in data

collection and reporting. It is suggested that the livestock census may be conducted through a single agency and this work may be entrusted to Directorate of Animal Husbandry in all States and the Department of Animal Husbandry & Dairying at the Central level.

- Efforts should be made to carry out the livestock census work in all the States/UTs simultaneously as per the prescribed time schedule. Failure to carry out enumeration on the reference date is the major shortcoming of Livestock Census data. In India, the population census is a Union subject (Article 246) and is listed at serial number 69 of the Seventh Schedule of the Constitution. The Census Act, 1948 forms the legal basis for conduct of censuses in Independent India. Although the Census Act is an instrument of Central legislation, in the scheme of its execution the State Governments provide the administrative support for the actual conduct of the census. For conducting Livestock census, similar statutory basis may also be required. Since Livestock is a State subject, it may, therefore, require a detailed deliberation before making such a suggestion.
- The personnel appointed on temporary basis for Livestock census purpose must have a basic minimum qualification or experience of village conditions such as village patwari, school teacher, etc.
- Such primary investigators should be given proper training before assigning them actual collection of data from the households.
- The Technical Committee of Direction for Improvement of Animal Husbandry and Dairy Statistics, which was set up during the seventies to streamline statistical activities, to identify the data gaps and to provide guidance in statistical project may be strengthened and made active. If necessary, members may also be co-opted from private sector.

In order to overcome the problems discussed above, there is an urgent need to revise the Census Schedules before starting the 17th Livestock Census. As the census work is a complete enumeration once in five years, the coverage of data collection may be broad based. A Technical Advisory Committee may be set up to look into the revision of schedules for the census and to suggest improvements needed for the Integrated Sample Surveys. An appropriate Village Schedule may also be designed and canvassed to get information on various important issues. The revised schedule may cover additional items like (a) approximate annual livestock products in each household, (b) household income from livestock, (c) gender-wise employment from livestock, (d) common diseases and livestock health care system, (e) feed and fodder requirement together with sources of supply, (f) access to the livestock product processing industries and actual quantities sold to them.

CONCLUDING OBSERVATIONS

In order to overcome the problems discussed above, there is an urgent need to revise the Census Schedules before starting the 17th Livestock Census. As the census work is a complete enumeration once in five years, the coverage of data collection may be broad based. A technical Advisory Committee must be set up to look into the revision of schedules for the census and to suggest improvements needed for the Integrated Sample Surveys. An appropriate Village Schedule may also be designed and canvassed to get information on various important issues. The revised schedule may cover additional items like (a) approximate annual livestock products in each households, (b) household income from livestock, (c) gender-wise employment from livestock, (d) common diseases and livestock health care system, (e) feed and fodder requirement together with sources of supply, (f) access to the livestock product processing industries and actual quantities sold to them.

Poultry industry has become an important adjunct of the livestock economy. The present information being collected for poultry is most adequate for any policy decisions. In the context of today, just the total number of birds has no meaning. Distribution between broilers and layers is the first essential requirement. The investigators have to be properly guided to note that the life of a broiler is just 2 months. The former may be having 5-6 crops in a year. Separate information·also needs to be collected for cockerels and breeding stock, etc. It is recommended that variety-wise number of poultry (desi, broiler, etc.) in the organised and unorganized sectors may also be collected and compiled. Detailed information with regard to poultry feed may also be collected.

NEW SCHEMES RECOMMENDED BY THE IXTH PLAN WORKING GROUP ON LIVESTOCK STATISTICS

Informatics Development of Animal Husbandry & Dairying Sector

In order to build up a reliable data base of animal husbandry and dairying sector in the States/UTs, a comprehensive management information system for all the activities of this sector based on computerisation is needed during the Ninth Plan. In this connection a scheme of Informatics Development of Animal Husbandry and Dairying sector is recommended for implementation at district level in all the states and UTs during the Ninth Plan. Data collected from various sources like sample surveys, Census, records etc., will be fed to the computerised system. The proposed scheme would have the following three components:

(a) Animal Husbandry and Dairying Statistics and Livestock Census Information System

The system will provide reliable, timely and comprehensive information on financial/physical progress of the various schemes of animal husbandry and dairy development as well as data on livestock products such as milk, eggs, wool, meat, broiler, chicken, etc. Further, this system will facilitate the maintenance and processing of livestock census data generated on quinquennial basis in the country.

(b) Animal Disease Surveillance Information System

This system will enable timely flow of information regarding disease outbreaks such as disease name, species affected, number of animals affected, mortality etc. in different parts of States/UTs and Publication of monthly bulletin on these outbreaks.

(c) Animal Quarantine and Certification Information System

This system is proposed for four Quarantine and Certification Centres and the Department of Animal Husbandry and Dairying. It is intended to provide efficient data management and quick decision making support both at the level of Quarantine Centre and at the level of Central Government for disease management.

Network Development

A Network will be developed at various levels depending on the nature and use of the information. Normally the information would flow from district level to State level (State Animal Husbandry Department) and from State to the Centre (Department of Animal Husbandry and Dairying).

The scheme would provide hardware, necessary software, networking and functional support for computerisation of these activities to the States/UTs to cover all the districts in the country in a phased manner. National Informatic Centre (NIC) may be made responsible for installation of hardware, providing necessary software, NIC-NET connectivity and training of the concerned staff as well as for maintenance of the system.

A total sum of Rs. 40 crore will be required during the Ninth Plan under the above scheme for informatics development on NICNET in each district veterinary office and the State Directorates of Animal Husbandry (i.e. about 600 centres), of which 25% may be shared by the States.

National Animal Production and Health Information System (NAPHIS)

The Technology Mission on Dairy Development (TMDD) has proposed a project entitled "National Animal Production and Health Information System (NAPHIS)" which integrates the two schemes, viz. Animal Disease Surveillance and Sample Surveys for estimation of major livestock production. The proposed project has the following three components.

(a) Animal Production Information System (APIS) – This will provide information on the status of animal productivity and produce in the country.

(b) Animal Disease Reporting System (ADRS) – This is an active disease surveillance system providing information on occurrence, distribution and trends of animal diseases in the country.

(c) Animal Production and Health Information system (APHIS) – This will provide information on production and health profiles in animal population and economic loss due to animal disease in the country.

The proposal of TMDD is under consideration of National Advisory Committee on Control of Animal Diseases. It envisages operating project on pilot basis in limited number of districts. If it is approved by the National Advisory Committee on Control of Animal Diseases and the Deptt. of Animal Husbandry and Dairying, it could be merged with other schemes like Integrated Sample Surveys for Estimation of Major Livestock Products, Animal Disease Surveillance and Informatics Development scheme discussed in the preceding paragraphs.

Education and Training in Animal Husbandry and Statistics

It is proposed that short-term training may be provided to persons engaged in collection, computerisation and analysis of data in the States but not familiar with basic statistical technique/tools and computer based methods and also to the staff responsible for analytical studies. Such a training is necessary for improving the efficiency of the staff and quality of the data.

A sum of Rs. 3 crore will be required for the scheme during the Ninth plan as Central share.

Information System for Measurement of Milk Production and Forecasting of Milk Production and Procurement in Milk Sheds

Estimation of milk supply is a very critical input to the overall planning of activities of the dairy industry. It is felt that a system of measuring milk production be taken up in a few major milk producing milk sheds in addition to the sample data collected by State Governments. This could be done by an organised body like NDDB. A few selected union can undertake counting of total breedable cows and buffaloes once a year during the month in which number of animals in milk is approximately equal to the average number of animals in milk for the year. It will make use of individual animalwise monthly milk production data collected under progeny testing programme if the milk shed is covered under progeny testing programme otherwise it would organise milk recording in randomly selected 25 villages to estimate average milk production; and finally the milk production estimates will be worked out by multiplying number of animals in milk with average production of animals in milk. Once the system of data collection of milk production and consumption are in place the data generated through this system could be used to make forecasts of milk production and procurement for the selected districts. The programme is proposed to be implemented in 25 major milk producing milk sheds in the country. The cost of implementation of this programme for the Ninth Five Year Plan period is estimated at Rs. 8.38 crore.

Annexure II

RECOMMENDATIONS OF THE SUBGROUP ON ANIMAL HUSBANDRY STATISTICS FOR FORMULATION OF TENTH FIVE YEAR PLAN

Integrated Sample Survey Scheme for Estimation of Production of Major Livestock Products:

Recommendations for Tenth Five Year Plan to improve the scheme.

* The scheme should be continued in the Tenth Plan with improvements.

* Computerization of the work relating to data analysis, report preparation in ISS will improve the timeliness in preparation of tables and reports. This will also ensure the accuracy of the calculations involved in ISS work along with ensuring uniformity in procedures adopted by all the States. For this purpose computers along with accessories and maintenance charges are to be provided to all the States and UTs. This has to be taken care during the preparation of EFC memo for lOth Five year plan scheme. Thus will involve an additional expenditure of Rs. 55 lakhs during the plan period.

* A component needs to be added for providing Training and supervision for the field staff from time to time to ensure accuracy and efficiency in the field level data collection. A provision of Rs. 5 lakh may be kept for this purpose.

* **During the Ninth plan, an outlay of Rs. 20 crores was made under the scheme. During the Tenth Five Year Plan, estimated outlay required for the Scheme is Rs. 23.65 lakhs, to meet the increased salary expenditure and cost of additional components.**

The livestock census and suggestions for improvements.

* The scheme of Livestock Census should be continued during the Tenth Plan with improvements.

* The Scheme as at present suffers from timeliness and quantitative as well as qualitative problems. The Tenth Plan Programme intends to overcome all the issues.

* The present arrangements for conducting the Livestock Census in the States and Union Territories are not found satisfactory. Various organizations, not necessarily connected with livestock development, are handling the operations relating the census in the States/UTs, resulting in unsatisfactory quality of data and also delays in data collection and reporting. It is suggested that the livestock census may be conducted through a single agency. The Group felt that this work should be entrusted to. Directors of Animal Husbandry in all States and the Department of Animal Husbandry and Dairying at the Central level.

- During the Tenth Plan, efforts should be made to carry out the livestock census work in all the States/UTs simultaneously as per prescribed time schedule. In case of the human census which is conducted successfully; the Census Act 1948 forms the legal basis for conduct of census in Independent India. In the scheme of its execution the State Governments provide the administrative support for the actual conduct of the census. For conducting Livestock census, similar statutory basis may also be required. Since Livestock is a State subject, it may, therefore, require a detailed deliberation before making such a suggestion.

- As the census work is a complete enumeration once in five years, the coverage of data collection may be broad based. Need for an immediate setting up of a Working Group to look into the revision of schedules for the census and improvements needed for the Integrated Sample Surveys. This Group should have representatives of all stake holders in the public and private sectors to meet the present day requirements of the livestock sector. A Village Schedule may be canvassed to get information on various important issues. Annex VIII A and B of the Census Schedules calls for detailed State Reports. All the States should be required to submit these reports in time.

- Further, there is need to strengthen the statistical units and to introduce electronic data processing and report preparations using Personal Computers. Efforts are needed to improve staff through refresher training progammes/courses involving new techniques based on computerization.

- A sum of Rs. 105.45 crore, as against Rs. 42.74 crore outlay in Ninth Five Year Plan, will be required during the Tenth Plan under the scheme. The increase is mainly due to the inflation factor:

Research & Development

There are at present a large number of data gaps. The existing methodology needs to be modified by incorporating the following information.

   i) Breedwise milk yield of different species, viz. cattle buffaloes and goats.
   ii) Information of egg production from commercial poultry farms.
   iii) Information on poultry meat e included to get the total meat production.
   iv) Breed-wise wool yield from various sources like sheep and wool extension centers, wool shearing centers and sheep breeding farms, etc.
   v) Cost of production studies on milk and eggs should be undertaken in selected districts of different States and different sampling frame be used for this study.
   vi) Estimates for livestock byproducts.

Fisheries Statistics

Tentative Proposal for the Tenth Plan

For the Tenth Five Year Plan, for the Inland sector, the technical work programme will include the following:

- National inventorying and mapping of inland fisheries resources
- Census of fishers engaged in the inland fisheries sector with their socio- economic status, inventory of craft and gear, marketing and distribution
- Catch assessment through sampling techniques
- Compilation of data and estimation of results by computerization of the whole process and -creating information networking using district level NIC setup.

Against the Ninth plan allocation of Rs. 6.84 crores, tentative budget for the scheme is kept at Rs. 14 crores for the Tenth five-year plan period with the components detailed below.

NEW SCHEME: CREATION OF LIVESTOCK STATISTICS & ECONOMICS DIVISION

In view of the recommendations of the Group for increased need and demand for data on livestock, the existing AHS unit may be upgraded into a Livestock Statistics and Economics Division, with the main objective of Data Warehousing Scheme -All livestock related data will be collected/ compiled and efforts will be made to create a suitable data warehouse under DAH&D.

DONTMIS - Dynamic Online Network Transmission of Management Information System needs to be created for livestock related data. Under the scheme assistance may be provided to states to enable the exchange of data through web as per the guidelines provided by the center. There is also a need to undertake studies to create a data base for a large number of gaps. A provision of Rs. 5 crores needs to be made for this scheme.

Table 22AII.1: Outlay Proposed for the Schemes under Animal Husbandry Statistics during the Tenth Five Year Plan

(Rs. crore)

Sl.No.	Schemes	Ninth Plan Outlay	Proposed Tenth Plan Outlay
1.	Integrated Sample Survey Scheme for Estimation of Production of Major Livestock Products	20.00	23.65
2.	Livestock Census	42.74	105.45
3.	Research & Development	—	1.10
4.	Fisheries Statistics	6.84	14.00
5.	Creation of Livestock Statistics & Economics Division	—	5.00
	Total	69.58	149.20

23

WTO's Trade Reforms and Livestock Sector

The Uruguay Round (UR) of multilateral trade negotiations, completed in 1994, was historic in that it was the first successful comprehensive attempt to bring agriculture into the discipline of the General Agreement on Tariffs and Trade (GATT). The conclusion of the Uruguay Round Agreement on Agriculture (AoA) gave significant impetus to agricultural trade liberalization. It imposed disciplines on trade distorting domestic policies as well as on trade policies. It increased transparency by converting non-tariff barriers to tariffs (so-called tariffication) and placed limits on export subsidies in both value and volume terms. But protection continued to be high in many cases and trade distortions remained.

The World Trade Organization (WTO) is the successor organization to the GATT. It came into effect on 1.1.1995 after the conclusion of Uruguay Round on Multilateral Trade Negotiations. India was founder member of both GATT in 1947 and the WTO in 1995. The mandate of the WTO covers trade in goods, trade in services, trade-related investment measures and trade-related intellectual property rights. Thus, unlike GATT, the mandates of WTO have wider ramifications.

It is now generally agreed that developing countries have given more than what they have received under the Agreement on Agriculture (AOA). The WTO system seems to be tilted in favour of the developed countries. On the one hand, the developing countries were obliged to lift the Quantitative Restrictions, cut the tariffs and virtually open up their markets. On the other hand, the promised increased access to markets in the developed countries has not materialized due to the inclusion of the Agricultural regimes of the EU and the USA in the green box under the AOA and also because of various Non-tariff barriers, including sanitary and phytosanitary measures.

IMPLICATIONS OF GENERAL AGREEMENT ON TRADE AND TARIFF (GATT)

As a signatory to the General Agreement on Tariffs and Trade, India was required to:

Convert all non-tariff barriers to tariffs;

Reduce resulting tariffs by 24 percent over ten years;

Reduce export subsidies by 24 percent over ten years from a base period of 1986-90;

Reduce aggregate producer subsidies by 13.3 percent over six years and Allow minimum access of imports equivalent to three percent of domestic consumption from the 1986-88 base period, rising to 5 percent over six years. Access greater than five percent must be maintained.

Domestic support of less than 10 percent and "green box" policies are exempt from the reduction commitments.

Green box policies include general service policies (research, extension, training, direct payment to producers, income support, social safety net programmes, structural adjustment assistance, environmental programmes, regional assistance programmes and so on), and development policies (investment subsidies and agricultural input subsidies to low-income or resource poor producers). Any other form of domestic support that favours agricultural producers or "amber box" policies is subject to reduction. In addition, under GATT India could ask the Committee on Balance of Payment to impose restrictive price-based import measures on livestock and other agricultural products. Only one type of restriction could be applied to a product, and only if the government can show that increased imports will be detrimental to its balance of payment situation. In addition, the government is allowed to impose quantitative restrictions if price-based instruments do not arrest the sharp deterioration in the external payments position. India, however, had to announce a timetable for the removal of such restrictions.

Because of its balance of payment situation, India was initially exempt from GATT market access commitments on agriculture. GATT balance of payment provisions enable countries to maintain restrictive import policies for the purpose of maintaining hard currency supplies. India therefore, is exempt from reducing tariffs and from making other access commitments on agricultural products.

The GATT also provides exemptions from reductions in subsidies for developing countries with an aggregate support level of less than 10 percent on agricultural products. With a support level of less than 6 percent, India qualifies for this exemption. Thus the new trade rules will not have any impact on income support or export subsidy measures that prevail in India's agricultural sector. However, India may benefit from the increase in world agricultural prices resulting from subsidy reduction if such increases make Indian products more internationally competitive.

India's GATT tariff ceiling commitments for livestock and feed ingredients are set at extremely high levels ranging from 40-150 percent. However, current tariffs for these products have been set at levels considerably lower than the GATT tariff ceilings. The forecast of several studies which assessed the impact of the GATT on that world prices of diary products would increase by about 5 to 12 percent from mid 1980 levels while meat product prices would rise by 1 to 6 percent have not yet materialized. In fact the dairy prices had fallen to the lowest level during the first quarter of 2002. Also the international meat prices had registered a declining trend, with FAO Index of meat having fallen over the 1990-92 base by as much as 16 points during the first quarter of 2002. Despite these declines, the Indian domestic product prices remain higher than world market prices. Thus, increasing production and processing efficiency in the livestock sector is critical, if the sector is to remain competitive with imports.

Livestock Trade Policy Reforms

India initiated a policy of trade liberalization in June 1991 i.e. four years before the signing of the Uruguay Round of Multilateral Trade Negotiations. The focus of the policy is openness, transparency and globalization. The basic thrust of the reform package was an outward orientation focusing on export promotion activity, moving away from quantitative restrictions and improving competitiveness of the Indian industry including livestock industry to meet global market requirements. Since then, trade policy reforms have provided an export friendly environment with simplified procedures conducive to accelerated export performance. In 1995 the Government of India introduced a major trade policy reforms that encompassed livestock products. Trade reforms revised continuously and especially through the EXIM Policy announced for the period 1997-2001 and subsequent amendments have helped to strengthen the export production base, remove procedural irritants, and facilitate input availability besides focusing on quality and technological upgradation and improving competitiveness.

Current trade policies and duty rates/bindings on livestock products are summarized in Table 23.1. Although import tariffs were reduced for most livestock products, most commodities remain subject to restrictions (licensing and canalization). Licensing requirements act as an effective ban or at the very least serve to ration imports. Licenses are required for import of breeding stock and all consumer goods of animal origin. These major trade policy reforms had important implications for the livestock sector, especially the dairy sector. For instance, removal of quantitative restrictions on imports of large number of commodities including livestock products and lowering of tariffs have enhanced the scope of larger imports of livestock products, particularly the milk products such as powdered milk, butter and ghee. Many policy makers have therefore expressed concern about the possible adverse impact of agricultural trade.

Import Policy Reforms

With the introduction of major trade policy reforms in 1991, the dairy sector, which was reserved mainly for the cooperative sector, was delicensed in 1991 and the private sector companies including multinationals were

Table 23.1: Import Policy and Duty Rates/Bindings on Milk and Milk Products
(Milk and Milk Products fall under Chapter 4 of the
ITC (HS) Code of Classification)

Sl.No	ITC (HS) Code	Item description	Import Policy	Bound Rate	Tariff Rate
	04.01	Liquid Milk, Milk and cream, not concentrated nor containing added sugar or other sweetening matter			
1.	0404.10	Of a fat content, by weight, not exceeding 1%	Free	100%	35%
2.	0401.20	Of a fat content, by weight, exceeding 1% but not exceeding 6%	Free	100%	35%
3.	0404.30	Of a fat content, by weight, exceeding 6%	Free w.e.f. 1.4.2000	40%	35%
	0402	Milk Powder, Milk and cream, concentrated or containing added sugar or other sweetening matter			
	0402.10	In powder, granules or other solid forms, of a fat content by weight, not exceeding 1.5%			
4.	040210.01	Skimmed milk powder	Free	60% (15% within TRQ)	60% (15% within TRQ of 10,000 MT)
5.	040210.03	Milk food for babies	Free w.e.f. 1.4.2001		
6.	040210.09	Other milk and cream	Free w.e.f. 1.4.2001		
	0402.21	In powder, granules or other solid form of a fat content by weight exceeding 1.5%.			
7.	040221.00	Not containing added sugar or other sweetening matter (Whole Milk Powder)	Free w.e.f. 1.4.2001	60% (15% within TRQ)	60% (15% within TRQ)
	0402.29	Other			
8.	040229.00	Other	Free	40%	35%
9.	040229.02	Whole milk	Free	40%	
10.	040229.03	Milk for babies	Free w.e.f. 1.4.2000	40%	
11.	040229.09	Others (e.g., milk cream)	Free w.e.f. 1.4.2000	40%	35%
	0402.91	Other			

Table 23.1: *Import Policy and Duty Rates/Bindings on Milk and Milk Products (Milk and Milk Products fall under Chapter 4 of the ITC (HS) Code of Classification)* *(Contd.)*

Sl.No	ITC (HS) Code	Item description	Import Policy	Bound Rate	Tariff Rate
12.	040291.00	Not containing added sugar or other sweetening matter	Free (w.e.f. 1.4.2000	40%	35%
	040299	Other			
13.	040299 02	Whole milk	Free w.e.f. 1.4.2000	40%	35%
14.	040299 03	Condensed milk	Free w.e.f. 1.4.2000	40%	35%
15.	040299 09	Others	Free (w.e.f. 1.4.2000)	40%	35%
	04.03	Butter milk, curdled milk and cream, yogurt etc.			
16.	040310	Yogurt	Free	150%	35%
17.	040310	Other	Free	150%	35%
	04.04	Whey etc.			
18.	0404.10	Whey and modified whey	Free	40%	35%
19.	0404.90	Other	Free w.e.f. 1.4.2000	150%	35%
	04.05	Butter and other fats and oils derived from milk: dairy spreads			
20.	0405.10	Butter	Free wef 1.4.2001	40%	35%
21.	0405.20	Dairy spreads	Free wef 1.4.2001	40%	35%
	0405.90	Other			
22.	0400590.1	Butter oil	Free	40%	35%
23.	040590.02	Melted butter (ghee)	Free wef 1.4.2001		
	04.06	Cheese and curd			
24.	0406.10	Fresh cheese	Free wef 1.4.2001	40%	35%
25.	0406.20	Grated/powdered cheese	Free	40%	35%
26.	0406.30	Processed cheese	Free wef 1.4.2001	40%	35%
27.	0406.40	Blue-veined cheese	Free	40%	35%
28.	0406.90	Other cheese	Free w.e.f. 1.4.2001	40%	35%

Sources: 1. Ministry of Finance: Annual Economic Survey: From 1999-2000 to 2001-03
2. Ministry of Finance: Finance Bill for fiscal years: 1999-2000, 2002-03
3. Ministry of Finance: EXIMP Policy documents.
4. World Bank/FAO Workshop: Implications of the Uruguay Round Agreement for South Asia: The case of Agriculture: (Kathmandu: May 1996).Govt. of India, of Economics and Statistics: Agricultural Statistics at a glance: 2002, pp. 205-06.

allowed to set up milk processing and product manufacturing plants. Secondly, India being signatory to the URA of the General Agreement on Tariffs and Trade (GATT) now vested in the World Trade Organization, makes it mandatory for her to open its agricultural sector to the world markets. In April 1995, the Government of India introduced major trade policy reforms that encompassed livestock products. Import tariffs for most livestock products were significantly reduced. Tariffs for skim milk powder and pureline poultry stocks were completely eliminated. Moreover, import and export of dairy products, which were restricted through quantitative measures (canalization, licensing, quotas, etc.) and other non-tariff barriers, were brought under the Open General Licence (OGL). Import of milk powder and butter oil was decanalised and delicensed. In 1999, whole milk, yogurt, grated or powdered cheese of all kinds, blue-veined cheese, buttermilk, whey, curdled milk and acidified milk and cream were shifted to OGL list. All these developments have exposed the diary industry to open economy environment, which can have significant impact on the Indian dairy sector.

Export Policy Reforms

Trade reforms have relaxed many of the restrictions on the export of agricultural and livestock products, but GOI concerns about the welfare impact of increased exports on consumers, especially the poor, have limited the magnitude of liberalization. For example, the NDDB monopoly on diary product exports has been eliminated, but diary products remain subject to export licenses and export ceilings set by the Directorate General for Foreign Trade.

Export Incentives

Although some export incentives, such as the Cash Compensatory Support Scheme, have been eliminated, several others are available. Firms classified as export-oriented units (EOUs) and those within export processing zones (EPZs) may import, duty free, any goods – including capital goods—that they require for their manufacturing, production, or processing activities, provided that the goods are not prohibited under the negative lists of imports. In special cases an animal husbandry and poultry, the EPZ unit or EOU may sell upto 50 percent of production (in value terms) domestically. EPZs have been established in Delhi, Mumbai, Kolkata, Chennai, Vishakhapatnam, Kandla and Cochin. These firms also enjoy tax breaks and other benefits, such as concessional rents (for firms in EPZs); domestic sales that are eligible for a refund of the central government sales tax, exemption from the central excise duty on capital goods, components, and raw materials, corporate income tax exemption for a block of five years in the first eight years of operation; refund of terminal excise duty; and participation in the duty drawback scheme. To encourage investments in the agricultural and livestock processing sector, foreign equity is allowed up to 100 percent for EOUs and EPZ units (Foreign equity is limited to 51 percent for firms outside the EOU and EPZ programme).

While the establishment of the EOU and EPZs could significantly stimulate exports, the privilege given to participating agribased exporting firms to sell as much as half of their production in domestic markets provides them with an unfair advantage relative to domestic non-export-oriented firms. Given that domestic raw material input prices are higher than world market prices, the EOUs and EPZs have preferential access to lower- cost imported inputs. To create a more level playing field, the import privileges should be extended to all firms.

There are several incentive schemes sponsored by the Agricultural and Processed Food Product Export Development Authority (APEDA). The APEDA was established in 1986 to promote the export of agricultural commodities and processed foods. The authority provides subsidies to exporters, growers, trade associations, and government agencies to pursue export promotion and market development activities, strengthen market intelligence and information channels, improve export quality, develop infrastructure and human resource capacity, modernize meat processing unit facilities, and perform research and development. The subsidies range from 25-60 percent of the cost of the activities up to ceilings of Rs. 10,000 – Rs. 500,000 (US$ 300 - $ 16,000) per beneficiary.

DAIRY INDUSTRY

The dairy business in India is currently estimated at Rs. 800 billion. "Indian dairying has several in-built competitive advantages which, if exploited, would lead to manifold growth to the industry. A large bovine population, strong procurement infrastructure, skilled manpower, cheap labour and a large number of processing and allied facilities are some of the advantages which India enjoys. With the present growth rate of around 4 per cent per annum, India is expected to produce around 182 million tonnes of milk by 2030, more than one-third of the projected global production of 620 to 650 million tonnes.

Considering that the dairy market in the developed countries had reached a saturation point and emerging milk markets were expected to be in Asian and African countries. India had yet another advantage. India's geographical location is an advantage when compared with other dairying countries like the Scandinavian nations, the US, Australia and New Zealand, With increasing awareness of the importance and better values of buffalo milk, it will gain prominence at the global level. India has a vast milk procurement and distribution system with 90,000 village cooperative societies, 170 district unions and 23 state federations. With nine dairy science colleges, 31 veterinary colleges and 80 agricultural research institutes, India has large number of professionals working in the industry. One of the greatest challenges before Indian dairying is improving the quality of milk which may be attributed to lack of hygiene and sanitation at the production level. The Indian dairy industry should prioritise branded product export instead of going in for occasional exports and it requires a vigorous campaign in the international market.

World Trade

Of the total world trade of $10,000 million in milk and milk products, the share of India is a meagre $10 million only. This is despite the fact that cost of production of milk in India is the lowest in the world (about $ 21/- per every 100 litres) followed by New Zealand. Incidentally, India and New Zealand are the only two countries without any subsidy component while most other countries subsidise the production of dairy products in one form or the other. Hence, there is an urgent need for the government to look into its policy of zero duty on the import of dairy products. The conventional indices of dairy industry suggest that our domestic dairy industry cannot survive in a regime of duty-free imports. Factors such as international prices of dairy products, producer and export subsidies offered by many advanced nations, exchange rates and cost of milk are the important parameters that have an influence on the competitiveness of the industry. And, India has no control over them. India had committed zero per cent base and bound rates of duty on imports of skimmed and full cream milk powders and 40 per cent on butter fat, cheese and whey under the WTO agreement. In contrast, the bound rate of duty for fresh milk and creak buttermilk and yoghurt was fixed at 100 to 150 per cent. No other country except Singapore has agreed to zero duty. Bangladesh has tariffs on dairy products bound at 200 per cent, Pakistan at 100 per cent, Sri Lanka at 50 per cent, New Zealand at 12.8 per cent, Brazil at 31.5 per cent and Poland at 102 per cent with a weighted average base rate for 43 countries of 144 per cent.

In addition to skim milk powder and whole milk powder, which are already under the Open General License (OGL), India has shifted cheese, butter milk, whey, whole milk, curdled milk and acidified milk and cream to the OGL list. This means that subsidized exports from the advanced dairy nations of North America and Europe that depress the world market have already begun to affect Indian domestic prices, adversely affecting producers and the processing industry. Hence, it is imperative that India renegotiates base and bound rates of duty for all dairy products (SMP, FCMP, butter, butter oil and cheese in particular) on the one hand and work vigorously with those committed to free trade to reduce export subsidies by developed countries. Failure to do so would lead to slowing in the rate of growth in milk production, starting a vicious cycle where increased gaps between growing demand and supply will force India to import. As an emerging dairy nation India should press for the following in the renegotiations of the second round of WTO.

Import Duties   There is a need to renegotiate its bound rates of duty of zero per cent on skimmed and whole milk powder to about 50-60 per cent, keeping in view the global trends.

Special Safeguards (SSG)   As most of the developed nations have SSG provision for dairy products which they can impose either when prices fall below the trigger level or imports surge above a level, India should negotiate for SSG clause.

Export Subsidies   During the reference period (1986-90), export subsidies on dairy products were much higher than during the 1990s; a 36 per cent reduction in subsidies does not result in significant reduction in subsidies. Therefore, there is a need for further reduction in the export subsidies to ensure a level playing field in international trade of dairy products.

SPS Measures   Sanitary and phytosanitary measures have been used by countries as non-tariff barriers. Different countries use different scientific criteria and standards to decide about the quality and safety of the imported products. There is a need for common standards, which are not unnecessarily raised to unscientific level so as to become internationally mandated non-tariff barriers.

Multifunctional Role   Dairy for Indians is not just producing another litre of milk. A vibrant dairy industry ensures an alternative source of income to the farm families. It leads to rural socioeconomic development.

India has a zero tariff for SMP and FCMP and comparatively low tariff for other dairy products. Cheap, subsidised imports of dairy products from developed countries are a matter of great concern. There is an urgent need for India to impose import tariffs for milk powders and other dairy products. With the availability of milk at very economical prices, many large MNCs have entered into the dairy segment in India. The only thing which needs to be looked into is the basic quality of produce. Efforts are being made by the domestic dairy industry to improve the basic quality as it is going to play a major role in the competitive market. Majority of the Indian dairies are preparing to obtain quality certification like ISO and Hazard Analysis Critical Control Point (Haccp). At least nine dairy units have already succeeded in obtaining the necessary quality certification. With this beginning being made on maintaining quality, India will perhaps, be able to launch its products in other continents in a big way during the coming decades.

Quality Revolution

If we are to enter the world market, India has to move from the 'White Revolution' to the Quality White Revolution. "A litre of milk per milch animal a day and make India the number one dairying nation of the World the easy way." This catchy slogan heralding the rosy future of Indian dairying has been given by Animesh Banerjee, a top ranking dairying expert and the president of the Indian Dairy Association (IDA), the apex organisation of the Indian dairy industry. "If we are successful in realising a modest target of collecting one litre of milk per milch animal every day and process as well as value-add it, this country could easily emerge at the top of the ladder internationally". Describing Indian dairying as one "on the threshold of big opportunities" and India as a "sleeping giant" as far as international dairying scene was concerned, Banerjee gave a clarion call to policy makers and the dairy community of the country "wake up, overcome impediments and tap the comparative advantage which nature had endowed us and convert it into a competitive advantage in global market."

If India is to convert its "comparative advantage" into a "competitive advantage", the first and foremost step should be to impose self-regulation. Whether a milk producer or a private dairy or a cooperative dairy, if quality is not assured at all levels of milk production, processing or marketing, dairying cannot take a positive path. Yes, milk that is drawn by hand in India is unhygienic and sure would not be accepted by the first world consumers. Indian milk has no bacterial count. In the US, soon after milk is drawn by power-machines it is cooled within few seconds which is not true in case of India. The time span between the collection of milk and the cooling process in India is very high which results in bacterial formation. Ensuring that quality was a serious problem and it needed to be dealt with stringently by all concerned including implementation of regulatory mechanisms such as prevention of Food Adulteration Act (PFA) and the Milk and Milk Products Order (MMPO). It must be conceded that regulatory mechanisms alone may not, however, yield any positive results until and unless milk producers, processors and marketeers also took a positive attitude in discarding inferior quality milk and exposed these unscrupulous practices. Vis-à-vis the performance of Indian dairying on the export front it is agreed that though India enjoyed several competitive advantages compared to other countries it had as yet failed to make a "proper dent" in the export market. We have been adopting an easier path by going in for occasional milk exports instead of sustainable branded product exports. Whenever we have seasonal surpluses resulting out of extra production, instead of maintaining a buffer stock, we have resorted to export. Whenever we have got into shortages particularly in the summer months we have gone in for imports. Strongly advocating the prioritising of branded products export instead of occasional bulk exports, Banerjee, however, conceded that branded products export could not be just commenced. He said, a lot of campaign was required to support such exports and thus policy makers should come forward to give certain incentives. What success we have achieved has been because conditions were created where dairying became potentially remunerative for large numbers of our rural people. We did things that the mandarins of the international financial institutions and their acolytes in Delhi now feel are immoral or worse. We denied the market its role. It seems, from the record, that the dairy industries of the industrial nations are fairly well insulated from market forces. But what is good for the goose appears not good enough for the gander. We did insulate our market by channeling all dairy commodity imports through the Indian Dairy Corporation and then the National Dairy Development Board. This system has to be protected lest the goose that lays the golden egg be killed. Indian dairying has succeeded because it has deliberately evolved in a way that it is complementary and not in competition with agriculture. Dairying employs those who are underemployed. Our animals feed off the waste and byproducts of agriculture. Our milk-producing animals often produce the draught animals that till our fields. As a consequence, our dairying is energy-efficient, labour intensive and ecologically sound.

Quality assurance of milk and milk products would be the main thrust in sustaining the Indian dairy industry in the next millennium, as the international trade would be strongly regulated by WTO regime, which was farming stricter sanitary standards for regulating the quality. Processes have to be developed to produce the products that Indian consumers want and that can be sold abroad. There is a need to develop knowledge of the markets, not just the international market but the Indian one. The Indian industry has to be encouraged to produce equipment and machinery of world quality and at competitive prices. Going by recent developments at the WTO's meet to define Codex standards for International trade in milk and milk products, exports from India could be rather difficult. For one thing the minutes of the meeting stipulated that products like cheese should be derived from cows and not buffaloes (where India has a majority population). For the other, the Codex standards also spelt out that the cows should be milked by machines under covered conditions. All of which seem to guarantee the dominance in international trade of the advanced dairying nations.

Implications for Indian Dairy Industry

With agricultural trade liberalization and ushering of the new environment, as also the dairy sector moving towards less government intervention and regulation, concerns are expressed about the efficiency and competitiveness of the Indian dairy industry. However, very little effort has been made to find out the performance of Indian diary industry in terms of its capability to face the competition in the open and liberal trade framework. Furthermore, there is much criticism, without empirical evidence, about the efficiency in Indian diary processing industry, especially the cooperative sector. An attempt is made below to examine the likely impact of trade liberalization on Indian diary industry and its competitiveness, and analyze the factors determining competitiveness of this industry. These analyses can provide valuable information for undertaking appropriate measures to guide the process of globalization.

Impact of the WTO AoA on International Dairy Product Prices

Lower exports of subsidized dairy products by the European Union and the United States were expected to lead to higher world diary product market prices. The likely impact of the WTO agreement on world prices of diary products was forecast to range from 4 percent for butter to about 20 percent for cheese (Table 23.2). However, the world prices of the major dairy products in general showed a gradual decline (ranging from 3.89 percent for cheese to about 11 percent in the case of skimmed milk powder in the post-WTO period).

Table 23.2: Forecast and Actual Increase in World Market Prices for Dairy Products in Post-WTO Period

Product	Forecast Increase	Actual Change (percent /annum)*
Skim Milk Powder (SMP)	16.0	– 10.98
Whole Milk Powder (WMP)	16.0	– 7.67
Cheese	20.0	– 3.78
Butter	4.0	– 5.76

* Annual compound growth rates calculated for 1995-99 Period

Source: Sharma, Vijay Paul, and Sharma, Prittee: Implications of Agricultural Trade Liberalization for Indian Dairy Industry: in Birthal, Pratap S., et. al: Livestock in Different Farming Systems in India: (Conference Proceedings): Published by Agricultural Economics Research Association (India), 2002, pp.184.

International Competitiveness

Competitiveness is a complex term and can be defined in several ways ranging from domestic resource cost ratio concept to competitive advantage concept encompassing segmented markets, differentiated products, economies of scale and so on. The international competitiveness can be analyzed on the basis of (i) comparison of Indian and World Market prices for selected dairy and meat products: and (ii) Nominal Protection Coefficient (NPC); Effective Protection Coefficient (EPC) and Effective Subsidy Coefficient.

As discussed in Chapter 11 on Foreign Trade in Livestock, the comparison of Indian and the world prices of selected livestock products indicate that the Indian diary sector has not been competitive internationally. Although producer prices in India are significantly lower than in the United States and Western Europe, dairy product prices (butter and whole and skim milk powder) are substantially higher than international market prices. This is due to domestic processing inefficiencies. Only during mid 90's, with the devaluation of the Rupee and the sharp rise in world dairy product prices, did the gap between Indian dairy prices and world market prices narrow. In addition, fluid milk marketing margins are high in India – for example, it is about 67 percent higher than in the United Kingdom.

India also lacks international competitiveness in poultry products. Domestic price of poultry meat, in particular, is over 50 percent higher than world prices. Indian egg and broiler and day-old chick prices are only slightly above world market prices. Despite considerably lower labour and energy costs, pent-up demand and high feed costs, and marketing constraint limit competitiveness. Nevertheless, India is very competitive in buffalo meat and reasonably competitive in the production of mutton.[1] Dairy products could become internationally competitive if domestic processing efficiency were improved substantially. Improving efficiency will also require reforms of the public distribution schemes, which need to be targeted more effectively. Prices of bovine meat sector are quite competitive, but scio-cultural factors preclude strong showing in the export market. Export of mutton is constrained by domestic demand.

Analysis of global competitiveness under second method, mentioned above, is dealt with in the following sections.

Nominal Protection Coefficient of a commodity measures the deviation of domestic prices relative to world prices.

$$NPC = \frac{P^d + t^d}{P^w + t^w}$$

Where P^d is the domestic price of the commodity, P^w is the border price of the commodity in local currency, and t^d and t^w are the transport costs associated with moving commodity from the factory and border to a common consumption location, respectively. The resulting NPC represents the magnitude of direct intervention in domestic price determination by measuring the extent to which the domestic prices deviate from border prices facing the country. If the NPC is greater than one (less than one), then the commodity under consideration is protected (disprotected), compared to the situation that would have prevailed under free trade at the same exchange rate.

Effective Protection of the commodity is an estimate of the extent to which the margin between its selling price and the cost of its internationally tradable inputs has been widened or narrowed by the combined effect of the protection of the commodity and the protection (which could be negative i.e. subsidy) which is defined as the ratio of value added at domestic prices of the production activity, to the estimated value added at world reference prices. That is EPC = VA^d / VA^w, where

EPC = Effective protection coefficient:
VA^d = Value added at domestic prices
VA^w = Value added at world reference price

Effective protection coefficients are more complete indicators of the incentives to producers resulting from trade policies than NPCs, because they take into account the effects of the protection of internationally traded inputs as well as protection of commodity itself. EPCs greater than 1 represents positive effective protection at the observed market exchange

---

[1]World Bank: India: Livestock Sector Review: Enhancing Growth and Development: May 23, 1996, pp. 62-63.

rate, while EPCs less than unity represent negative effective protection and EPC = 1 represents zero effective protection.

Effective subsidy coefficient is further refinement over EPC. ESC is simply the numerator of the EPC plus the total subsidies per unit of the commodity, divided by the value-added in reference prices i.e. by the effective protection coefficient denominator.

$$ESC = (VA^d + NS) / VA^w$$

where

ESC = Effective subsidy coefficient

VA^d = Value added at domestic prices

VA^w = Value added at reference prices

NS = Net subsidies on non-traded inputs.

A value of ESC greater than one indicates that protection is being accorded to the commodity and a positive value of (1-ESC) measures the extent of its competitive strength over the relevant foreign commodity.

The NPCs, EPC and ESCs of different commodities are calculated under two alternative hypotheses: (i) the importable hypothesis, when the foreign product is an actual or potential substitute for the domestic commodity and (ii) exportable hypothesis, where the domestic product is or potentially could be exported to compete in foreign export markets. India is not a major exporter especially of dairy products but will have to face the competition of highly subsidized imports from the European Union and the United States. Therefore NPC, EPC and ESC were computed under importable hypothesis.

India is the largest producer of milk, but a minor player in the world market. India used to import milk till early 1970s. However, now it has become self-sufficient and also started exporting small quantities of skimmed milk powder, whole milk powder, ghee and butter in the 1990s. In 1997-98 India exported 1,319 tons of skimmed milk powder, 182 tonnes of whole milk powder and 455 tonnes of ghee and butter. However, the import of milk powder and butter and butter oil increased substantially in the late 1990, mainly due to zero and/or low import tariffs as a commitment to the WTO.

The global dairy market has been changing. The European Union, United States, Australia, and New Zealand are the major players in the international diary trade. The diary industry in the EU, the US and many other developed countries has historically been insulated from volatility in the world dairy market through use of various import restrictions. As a result, the domestic prices of dairy products in these regions have been supported at levels above the world price. A number of developed countries have retained the right to use export subsidies on diary products under the World Trade Organization's Uruguay Round Agreement (URA). In order to compete on the world market in early 2002, for instance the USA increased the amount of subsidy paid on exports of skimmed milk powder form US$ 386 per ton in December 2001 to US $ 864 per ton in March 2002. The latter amount constituted almost 60 percent of the world skimmed milk powder price. Over the same period, EC export subsidies on skimmed milk powder were increased from Euro 200/ton (approx. US$ 181/ton) to Euro 500/ton, and subsequently on 11 April 2002, the EC raised its subsidy to Euro 650/ton (approx. US$ 580/ton). This subsidy amounted to almost 40 percent of the world skimmed milk powder export price.[1] Such a high level of export subsidies distorts and depresses international prices. There is an urgent need for further reforms in the international agricultural policy arena in the wake of WTO agreements and other bilateral and multilateral trade agreements to reduce restrictions on trade and protection for domestic industries in dairy and meat sector, grains and other agricultural commodities. This should open the door for potentially dramatic changes in trade patterns as industries around the world adjust to the new competitive environment.

Given these potential changes, how is the Indian dairy industry positioned to compete in the world market? This is difficult but very important question, which can have a big impact on the welfare of millions of dairy farmers and processing industry. As motioned above, India will have to face the competition of highly subsidized imports from the European Union and the United States[2]. A study had been conducted to work out the NPC for major diary products like skimmed milk powder, whole milk powder and butter for the years 1995 to 1999. EPC and ESC were estimated for 1997, 1998 and 1999.

The estimates of Nominal Protection Coefficients, based on midpoint of export price (FOB) reported by the New Zealand Dairy Board worked out in the above-mentioned study are shown in Table 23.3, and Effective Protection Coefficients are given in Table 23.4.

The value of NPC for skimmed milk powder was below unity in all the years except in 1999 but showed an increasing trend. By contrast, the value of NPC for whole milk powder and butter were above unity in all the years, which indicated either higher domestic prices or low international prices. During the period 1995-99 there has been a downward trend in world prices of most dairy products due to high export subsidies given by the European Union and the United States[3], while there was no significant increase in domestic prices. On an average, the NPC of SMP was lower than that of WMP and butter.

---

[1]FAO: Global Information and Early Warning System; Food Outlook: No. 2, May 2002, p.25

[2]Sharma, Vijay Paul and Sharma, Paiteee: Implications of Agricultural Trade Liberalization for Indian Dairy Industry: in Birthal, Pratap S, et al (Eds): Livestock in Different Farming Systems in India: pp 190-195

[3]According to the FAO's analysis the international prices of most dairy products have continued to register declining trends since mid-2001 and by May 2002 they reached the levels rarely seen over the past decade: source: Food Outlook: May 2002, p.25.

Table 23.3: Nominal Protection Coefficient with and without Export Subsidies for SMP, WMP and Butter under Importable Hypothesis: 1995-1999

Year	NPC based on export price FOB 1/			NPC based on subsidy free world prices 2/		
	SMP	WMP	Butter	SMP	WMP	Butter
1995	0.853	1.092	1.074	0.853	1.092	1.074
1996	0.854	1.076	1.065	0.633	0.677	0.495
1997	0.904	1.163	0.245	0.650	0.709	0.549
1998	0.975	1.076	1.006	0.640	0.648	0.514
1999	1.086	1.221	1.250	0.674	n.a	n.a

1/ NPCs are calculated based on midpoint of export price (FOB) ranges reported by the New Zealand Dairy Board (US $/ton). 2/ These coefficients are based on FOB Export prices plus the export subsidy given by the European on diary products.

Source: Sharma, Vijay Paul and Sharma, Pritee: Implications of Agricultural Trade Liberalization for Indian Dairy Industry.

Table 23.4: Effective Protection and Subsidy Coefficients for SMP, WMP and Butter under importable Hypothesis: 1997-99

Year	SMP		WMP		Butter	
	EPC	ESC	EPC	ESC	EPC	ESC
1997	0.895	0.910	1.177	1.195	1.295	1.289
	(0.628)	(0.639)	(0.694)	(0.704)	(0.538)	(0.550)
1998	0.915	0.967	1.073	1.089	1.012	1.035
	(0.604)	(0.614)	(0.627)	(0.636)	(0.505)	(0.517)
1999	1.031	1.049	1.225	1.243	1.252	1.281
	(0.616)	(0.627)	(0.658)	(0.668)	(n.a.)	(n.a.)

Note: Figures in brackets indicate the values of EPCs and ESC calculated based on midpoint of export price (FOB) ranges reported by the New Zealand Dairy Board (US$/ ton) plus the export subsidy given by the European Union on dairy products: n.a. = data not available.

Source: Sharma, Vijay Paul and Sharma, Pritee: Implications of Agricultural Trade Liberalization for Indian Dairy Industry.

The results of nominal production indicators suggest that perhaps WMP and butter have not been efficient import substitutes, when compared with world market prices. However, the nominal protection coefficients calculated at distortion free international prices, i.e. the prices without the subsidies, came out to be well below unity for all the products. The reduction in the value of NPCs was highest in case of butter, followed by whole milk powder and lowest for skim milk powder. This is mainly due to large subsidies on fat-based products, which have low demand in the developed countries and are mostly dumped in the developing countries by giving large export subsidies. These results clearly indicate that Indian dairy industry is highly import competitive in SMP, WMP and butter, provided the developed countries remove the export subsidies.

The value of EPC was marginally higher than unity for whole milk powder and butter in 1997 and 1998 (Table 24.4). The EPC values also indicate that whole milk powder and butter are more protected than skim milk powder under the prevailing world prices. Due to low tradable inputs in overall cost structure of diary products (SMP, WMP and butter), the value of EPC do not deviate much from their corresponding NPC values.

The effective subsidy coefficient (ESC) captures subsidies on per unit basis. The ESCs are estimated by adding the value of non-traded subsidies to the ratio of the Effective Protection Coefficients. These results of ESC indicate that whole milk powder and butter are considerably more protected than SMP. However, the extent of distortion is of marginal significance, as the values of these indices differ insignificantly. Nevertheless, the values of EPC and ESC at prices without export subsidy indicate that dairy products in India are not at all protected.

Since the international prices of dairy products and exchange rates are highly volatile and are outside the direct influence of government and the Indian diary industry, the only way to increase the competitiveness of Indian dairy sector, as suggested above, is by increasing production and processing efficiency.

POULTRY AND WTO

Even as the next dose of reduction in customs tariffs has been incorporated into the 2003-04 Budget, the government has decided against lowering India's tariff bindings at WTO, especially in the case of agricultural commodities. As of now, India's tariff bindings are up to 300% in the case of certain categories like processed foods and edible oils. The bindings will be retained at the current level, according to Commerce Department sources. This means the government will retain its right to protect domestic producers with higher customs tariffs. If tariffs are bound with WTO at a lower level, the government will not be in a position to impose higher customs duties. While gradual reduction of import tariffs has no major impact on items like foodgrains, some sectors like plantations have suffered.

During the ongoing talks on agriculture, mandated by the inbuilt agenda set during the Uruguay round of WTO negotiations, India has made it clear that there would be no compromise on farm tariff. A clear message to this effect was sent out during the recent deliberations at Tokyo. Since the issue concerns the livelihood of millions of farmers in rural India, it is not feasible to open the market further. The issue of lower tariff binding on farm products will be opposed strongly since it does not make sense to do so at a time when the US continues to provide high subsidies.

How can Indian farmers compete against subsidised exports? Union Agriculture Minister said that even the recent proposal for graded reduction in tariffs over a period of ten years is not acceptable to India, The subsidies provided by the developed world have to come down first. Apart from tariffs, we do not have any other form of protection for our farmers. We do not want any surge in imports that may threaten the livelihood of poor farmers.

The US and EU are not even coming to a mutually acceptable position with regard to their respective subsidies. The current global subsidy level for agriculture is around $365 billion while the Indian farmers suffer from many drawbacks. As of now, there is no scope for lower bindings on industrial tariffs too. The official stance, however, is that India is open for discussions on all issues including agriculture and industrial tariffs. Any concession on these issues can be made only if a strong quid-pro-quo emerges. As of now, India is looking for progress in opening up of services sector which is also under negotiations as per the inbuilt agenda. On the debate over reduction of agriculture subsidies, India has adopted a flexible stand even as the United States and the European Union have locked horns. Since Indian farmers suffer "negative subsidy" and they have nothing to lose even if a cap is imposed, the government may use any offer to cut subsidies to bargain for concessions in other areas.

Subsidised Farm Exports

The Indian delegation to the Interparliamentary Conference of the World Trade Organisation (WTO) raised several crucial issues related to the international trade of agriculture produce through the "blue box" provision of the WTO. Disclosing this at a press conference, Member of Parliament Balbir Singh, who visited Geneva and Paris where sessions of the WTO, Conference were held from February 17 to 20, 2003 said that he had raised the question of highly subsidised agricultural commodities exported to developing countries by the developed nations.

US Offer to Reduce Tariffs

Bigger developed countries including the United States, European Union (EU) and Canada created a system of county-by-country quotas on the imports of textiles and apparel under so called Multi-fiber Arrangement (MFA). They also maintained unduly high customs duties, referred to as "tariff peaks", on labour-intensive products. But no agreement exists as yet on the elimination of tariff peaks.

Recently, as a part of their Doha Round offers, EU and the US have tabled proposals for far reaching cuts in tariffs on all industrial products. These products account for 70% of all developing country exports. EU has proposed that WTO members significantly reduce all tariff range within which tariff peaks and high tariffs are eliminated. The US has gone much farther by proposing that the member countries bring all tariffs on industrial products down to 8% by 2010 and to zero by 2015.

First, developing countries should be given a longer phase out so that they move to the 8% duty by 2015 and to the zero rate by 2025. Second, the World Bank and other agencies should provide significant amount of grants-in-aid to developing countries restructuring that will accompany the liberalisation. Adjustment assistance to workers who must move from declining industries to the vibrant ones is not only necessary to make liberalisation politically more acceptable but will also help make aid more effective.

India has long sought to eliminate tariff peaks against labour-intensive products in developed countries. Though top World Bank officials and many NGOs have recently raised hopes that repeated public exhortations to the effect that developed country barriers cost developing countries more than what they give the latter in aid might shame them into dismantling these barriers unilaterally, last 40 years of experience leads to a different conclusion.

UNCTAD, developing country leaders, trade and development experts and even World Bank reports have condemned the barriers against developing country export for decades. As early as 1965, developing countries had successfully deployed moral persuasion to add part IV to the General Agreement on Tariffs and Trade which explicitly committed developed countries to "accord high priority to the reduction and elimination of barriers to products currently or potentially of particular export interest to less developed contracting parties" and to "refrain from introducing, or increasing the incidence of customs duties or non-tariff barriers on products currently or potentially of particular export interest" to them.

There are at least three additional reasons why India stands to benefit big from the proposed initiative. First, our own liberalisation, to which we will be committing as a part of the deal, benefits us. We have now fully recognised this fact in our economic reforms programme with the Kelkar taskforce recommending that virtually all tariffs be brought down to 10% or less by 2006-07. All we will be doing under the proposed initiative is to bind this liberalisation with WTO and push it to its local confusion of zero tariffs by 2025. Second, with NAFTA, EU and numerous preferential trade areas between EU and its neighbours and within Latin America, Africa and even East Asia in existence, India's products face discrimination in virtually every major market. Through the zero-tariff option, in one stroke, we would have eliminated this discrimination against us. Finally, under the proposed initiative, India has the opportunity to mobilise financial aid to smooth out adjustment. These resources will have to be mobilised internally under a purely unilateral liberalisation programme.

Fears for Egg Producers

The whole infrastructure of European egg production will be undermined if rules to improve bird welfare are brought in without the introduction of protection against imports produced to lower standards, a report has revealed. This is the stark warning in an independent new report from research body, the Netherlands Agriculture Economics Research Institute, commissioned by EUWEP, the EU trade association for egg packers, traders and processors. The threat to the European industry comes in the wake of legislation to improve the welfare of laying hens, which is set to be fully implemented by the year 2012. While European producers will have to use new animal welfare-friendly systems of production, producers from outside the EU do not have these restrictions placed on them. Instead the World Trade Organisation tariffs, which help to protect the already higher standards of European producers are coming under threat. NFU poultry delegate for the region Norman Atkinson, from Blaydon, said: "When will politicians of no practical poultry experience listen to the industry, will the common sense factor ever get a foothold into negotiations? The report further points out that these regulations are being foisted upon us and are unsupported by the poultry sector. This sector does not cost the Government a penny as subsidies and we have never complained about that. However we need revised thinking from the EC and more information for consumers. Shoppers already have a choice when purchasing; come 2012 they will not have this choice. The report highlighted that birds in non-EU countries could be fed meat and bonemeal, which is banned in the EU, and could be squashed six into a cage which only measured 300 cm squared.

Canadian Poultry and WTO

The poultry and egg industries reject the paper written by WTO Agriculture Chairperson Stuart Harbinson, as it represents an attack on farmers, both in Canada and throughout the world. In particular, the paper is widely being considered a devastating blow to Canadian agriculture, when it should be the vehicle for the establishment of fair and effective trade rules. The paper, entitled, "Negotiations on Agriculture – First Draft of Modalities for further commitment", calls for significant tariff cuts and substantial increases to minimum market access commitments, both of which negatively affect supply management, while at the same time not significantly improve access for Canadian products to other countries.

The poultry and egg organisations hold that Harbinson has not recognised that failures of the Uruguay round, nor has been done anything to address the inequities that were created at that time. Instead, the gap between countries' abilities to complete in the world market is becoming more and more pronounced. The modalities being proposed by Harbinson pose a real danger to farmers throughout the world by threatening their ability to make a living in their chosen field and all but eliminating their ability to negotiate fair prices. The poultry and egg organisations concur with the Canadian Federation of Agriculture which says that the draft paper should provide Canadian farmers with the WTO disciplines to end the subsidy levels currently seen in the US.

Policy Implications and Recommendations

India is reasonably competitive in the production of eggs and mutton and very competitive in buffalo meat. However, the potential for exports of

India's main products, particularly dairy and poultry meat products, is limited by their lack of international competitiveness. Dairy products may become internationally competitive if domestic processing efficiency is improved substantially. With the liberalization of butter oil and skim milk powder in 1995 (which can be reconstituted into fluid milk), pressures to increase domestic efficiency to keep up with import have increased. Improving domestic efficiency also requires reforms of the public distribution schemes (for example, the milk schemes) which has to be targeted more effectively. Prices in the bovine meat sector are quite competitive, but sociocultural factors preclude a strong showing in the export market. Mutton exports are constrained by domestic demand.

The lifting of most import restrictions on dairy and poultry meat products since April 1995 are likely to adversely affect producers should this not be coupled with structural changes in the processing and marketing sectors to reduce marketing costs and margins. With the opening of Indian dairy industry and moving most dairy products to OGL coupled with low import tariffs, import of milk powder has increased substantially from 282 tonnes in 1995-96 to about 18,000 tonnes in 1999-2000. The inflow of cheap import resulted in lowered domestic product prices, which provided substantial benefits to the urban consumers, but might have a negative impact on the incomes of the millions of rural producers. Moreover, the world dairy sector prices are highly distorted with heavy export subsidies, which depress the domestic prices and create unhealthy and unfair competition for domestic industry. Therefore, some protection would need to be provided to Indian diary industry in order to safeguard the interest of milk producers and processors. India is the only country, which has committed zero per cent bound rate of duty for milk powders and 40 percent for butter and butter oil compared to 100-150 percent for milk and cream, which are practically not traded in the world.

Export subsidies given by EU and the US constitute the most trade distorting measures. Hence, in the next round of Multilateral Trade Negotiations governments must focus on securing (i) significant reduction in export subsidies, resulting in their eventual elimination and prohibition in dairy sector and (ii) disaggregation of all export subsidy disciplines to the 6 digit harmonized tariff level, and (iii) restriction on carry forward and roll over export provisions. The Government need to evolve a mechanism to monitor the international prices and other developments in the world market and take corrective actions such as antidumping duties, and adoption of suitable tariff rates, to protect dairy and meat industry from unfair competition.

24

Strengths, Weaknesses, Opportunity and Threat (SWOT) Analysis for Livestock and Livestock Products

General economic analysis is increasingly being used to assess the strength and weaknesses of a particular sector or subsectors. For this SWOT analysis provides comprehensive view of strengths, weaknesses and opportunities and threats that a subsector or sector is likely to face. From these analysis one can judge whether strengths and opportunities outweigh weaknesses and threats or not. Accordingly, SWOT analysis has been carried out for the Indian livestock sector and its various sub-sectors. The results are discussed below.

SWOT ANALYSIS FOR LIVE ANIMALS

Strengths

- Large livestock population — 56% of world buffalo population.
- Availability of modern and integrated meat processing facilities.
- Livestock reared naturally — free from growth promoters and hormones.
- Competitively priced.
- Proof demand in domestic market.
- Increased availability of surplus for exports.

Weaknesses

- Meat produced from aged buffalo livestock.
- Under cutting of prices by the exporters.
- Social problems against meat production.
- Quality problems — Sourcing of meat from unapproved meat plants.

Opportunities

- Increased number of modern and integrated meat production facilities for exports.

- Huge potential for exports to South-East Asia, CIS, African and East European countries.
- Rearing of male buffalo calves as meat animal.

Threats
- Discrimination by some importing countries against Indian buffalo meat. SGS inspection and restricting usage for manufacturing purpose by Philippines.
- Campaign by foreign NGOs against Indian Meat (ex PETA campaign in Malaysia).
- Export subsidies by Indian competitors.
- Aggressive marketing campaign by Indian competitors.

INDIAN DAIRY INDUSTRY

Strengths

The contribution of dairying to the nation's health and wealth is rather unique. Factors that give strength include:

- Cattle is the foundation of Indian agriculture. For the large majority of small farmers, cattle is perhaps the only tangible asset and mainstay for their socioeconomic security. Dairy farming helps directly in increasing crop production by making available draught power, manure and cash income on day-to-day basis.
- Dairying is crucial in providing employment and supplementary income to the bulk of rural families. The main beneficiaries are women who contribute over 70 percent of labour in cattle rearing.
- Crop residues and byproducts fed to the cattle on the basis of "grain saving" dairying, appropriate to the mixed farming system.
- The buffalo is India's milking machine, accounting for more than half of the country's milk production. It is notable for its efficient converter of coarse feeds into rich milk. It is preferred by dairy processors not only as a total solids (33% more than cow milk) but also for its higher fat content. Its superior whitening property renders it more suitable than cow milk for manufacture of dairy products, particularly powders.
- Cooperative dairying has spread many benefits of this sector.
- Demand profile: Absolutely optimistic.
- Margins: Quite reasonable, even on packed liquid milk.
- Flexibility of product mix: Tremendous. With balancing equipment, one can keep on adding to one's product line.
- Availability of raw material: Abundant. Presently, more than 80 per cent of milk produced is flowing into the unorganized sector, which requires proper channelization.
- Technical manpower: Professionally trained, technical human resource pool, built over last 30 years.

Weaknesses

The dairy sector is not without its share of constraints. Some weaknesses include:

- Inability to feed cattle adequately throughout the year remains the most widespread technical constraint to higher milk yield.
- Quality dairy animals are in short supply. Artificial insemination service for breeding better cattle has limited coverage, barely reaching an estimated 10 per cent of bovines.
- The animal health cover is getting increasingly neglected. In many states, over 70-80 percent of the veterinary budget is used up for staff salaries and jeeps, with little left to buy medicines and other supplies.
- Limited marketing support handicaps rural milk producers seriously. If in the case of resource-poor crop farmers "harvesting is believing", then for dairy farmers "marketing is believing". Presently urban milk supplies largely come from major milkshed districts. Dairy producers in remote areas are neglected.
- Limited investment in setting up or expansion of milk procurement network is another bottleneck. The rapid expansion in milk processing capacities has not kept pace with production and procurement.
- The immediate problem of Indian dairy industry is not just shortfall in milk availability, but poor infrastructure for transporting, processing and distributing rurally-produced milk to major consumer centres in urban areas. Improvement in raw milk by its chilling and refrigerated transport is vital for making quality products.
- The rural woman, an invisible partner, needs access to training in modern cattle management to maximise returns. Timely credit is also needed for purchase of feed/fodder and health care and other inputs.
- Perishability: Pasteurization has overcome this weakness partially. UHT[1] gives milk long life. Surely, many new processes will follow to improve milk quality and extend its shelf life.
- Lack of control over yield: Theoretically, there is little control over milk yield. However, increased awareness of developments like embryo transplant, artificial insemination and properly managed animal husbandry practices, coupled with higher income to rural milk producers should automatically lead to improvement in milk yields.
- Logistics of procurement: Woes of bad roads and inadequate transportation facility make milk procurement problematic. But with the overall economic improvement in India, these problems would also get solved.
- Problematic distribution: Yes, all is not well with distribution. But then if ice creams can be sold virtually at every nook and corner, why can't we sell other dairy products too? Moreover, it is only a matter

---

[1]UHT milk stands for Ultra High Temperature processed milk.

of time before we see the emergence of a cold chain linking the producer to the refrigerator at the consumer's home!

- Competition: With so many newcomers entering this industry, competition is becoming tougher day by day. But then competition has to be faced as a ground reality. The market is large enough for many to carve out their niche.

Opportunities

"Failure is never final, and success never ending". Dr Kurien bears out this statement perfectly. He entered the industry when there were only threats. He met failure head-on, and now he clearly is an example of 'never ending success'! New initiatives and investments to strengthen the infrastructure in animal production would lead to modernization of this long-neglected sector. It also holds promise to transform the quality of life of those most neglected in rural India. Other opportunities include:

- India has been described by one FAO expert as a "slumbering giant of the international dairy trade". For India, WTO offers exciting prospects. With the reduction in heavy subsidies that support dairy producers in the West, India's low-cost milk will become price competitive. Another plus point is India's geographical location, surrounded by milk-deficit countries in Asia, the world's fastest growing market for dairy products.
- The mass production of indigenous milk-based sweets in modern dairy plants can tap the growing demand for them. With 150 million NRI overseas, the scope for their export is promising.
- A vast scope exists to higher milk yield through better use of crop residues and byproducts by upgrading them. Emphasis must be on technologies that are simple, low-cost and easily adoptable to increase their nutritive value. Some economic incentives are needed for farmers to go in for better feeding.
- Similarly, paying attention to animal health care would minimise the economic losses caused by many major cattle diseases such as rinderpest, mastitis and FMD.
- Value addition: There is a phenomenal scope for innovations in product development, packaging and presentation. Given below are potential areas of value addition:
- Steps should be taken to introduce value-added products like *shrikhand*, ice creams, *paneer, khoa*, flavored milk, dairy sweets, etc. This will lead to a greater presence and flexibility in the market place along with opportunities in the field of brand building.
- Addition of cultured products like yogurt and cheese lend further strength - both in terms of utilization of resources and presence in the market place.
- A lateral view opens up opportunities in milk proteins through casein; caseinates and other dietary proteins, further opening up export opportunities.

- Yet another aspect can be the addition of infant foods, geriatric foods and nutritional products.
- Export potential: Efforts to exploit export potential are already on. Amul is exporting to Bangladesh, Sri Lanka, Nigeria, and the Middle East. Following the new GATT treaty, opportunities will increase for the export of agri-products in general and dairy products in particular.

Threats

Dairying is also facing threats from many quarters. These include:
- A large cattle population—200 million cattle and 76 million buffaloes—grazes on uncultivated lands, forest areas and common property resources. This imposes a heavy social cost, leading to degradation and denudation of land and loss of natural base.
- Delicensing has checked the flow of investment by cooperatives in procurement and related infrastructure in their milkshed districts. It has also affected extension services for enhanced milk production. The high cost of credit is another adverse factor that reduces the viability of dairy projects.
- Milk vendors, the unorganized sector: Today milk vendors are occupying the pride of place in the industry. Organized dissemination of information about the harm that they are doing to producers and consumers should see a steady decline of their importance.

The Indian dairy industry, following its delicensing, has been attracting a large number of entrepreneurs. Their success in dairying depends on factors such as an efficient yet economical procurement network, hygienic and cost-effective processing facilities and innovativeness in the market place. All that needs to be done is: to innovate; convert products into commercially exploitable ideas. All the time one must keep reminding oneself: Benjamin Franklin discovered electricity, but it was the man who invented the meter that really made the money!

POULTRY SECTOR

Strengths
- Strong production base (5th largest producer of eggs in world).
- High hatchability (90% as against 85% of other countries) and high productivity (300-315 eggs per bird/year).
- Availability of good and vast genetic base.
- Modern facilities for egg processing.

Weakness
- High feed cost (Maize prices Rs. 6500/- per metric tonne as against Rs. 3500 in USA, Rs. 10,000/- PMT as against Rs. 7500/- in USA for Soya bean meal).
- Lack of infrastructure facilities.
- Inadequate cargo space.

- Poor domestic demand.
- High residue problems.

Poultry Products (Costing Rs. Per Kg.)

(i)	Cost of Indian raw material/production	9.59
(ii)	Cost of processing	2.54
(iii)	Cost of Inland transportation	0.10
(iv)	Cost of freight	1.85
(v)	Import duty at destination	NIL
(vi)	Any other costs (Breakage)	0.24
	Sub Total (excluding freight)	12.37
	Realization of Exporters (in the countries in the Near East)	Rs. 9.00

Opportunities

- Reduction of export subsidies under WTO will make our product competitive.
- Reduced production expected in EU due to the legislation passed for bigger cages on animal welfare grounds.
- Huge potential for exports to EU, CIS and South East Asian countries.

Threats

- Highly subsidized exports from USA
- Declining imports due to development of poultry industry in the importing countries.

SWOT ANALYSIS FOR LEATHER

Strengths

- Strong raw material base.
- Skilled labour at competitive wage levels.
- Support of allied Industries like chemicals.
- Strong institutional backup in the areas of research and technical developments.
- Strong R & D with well-developed tanning facilities. The industry enjoys the advantages of low wage levels, liberal import of accessories, liberal industrial trade policies, and government support.

Weaknesses

- Modernization is lacking.
- Underdeveloped component industry.
- Consumers are at a great distant increasing freight cost.
- Infrastructural bottlenecks.
- Pollution control measures yet to be fully implemented.
- Eighty-five percent of the chemical needs of the Indian tanning sector is met indigenously. However, the tannery sector requires certain special chemicals that need to be imported from other countries.

- India has a shortage of skilled manpower in the product sector. Dependent on imports for accessories and modern machines. Design development and fashion forecasting are in the nascent stage. Environment pollution control is also a hurdle.

Opportunities

- Developed countries vacating the market
- Thai, Korean and Indonesian exporters troubled with problems at home front.
- Potential for new markets gradually opening up in South African and Latin American Countries.
- Need for continuous development of leather processing technology with a focus on ecofriendliness.

Threats

- Manufacturing facilities coming up at East European countries.
- Countries like Portugal and Spain have increased their productions with locational advantage.
- India is losing its competitive edge in products like footwear where imported inputs are used.
- The challenges which are becoming an integral part of the trade such as ecolabelling, child labour welfare, human rights, biodegradability, recycling, etc.
- To meet the demand for a shorter time to the global market when a number of inputs are imported and the tanning sector is unstable.
- Inadequate country image in medium and high-end market and poor unit value realisation.

SWOT ANALYSIS – GENERAL

Strengths

- India has a mega animal bio-diversity, which is manifested in the form of availability of a large number of species, and a variety of breeds even within species.
- Animal production primarily is in farm production systems, which utilize mostly straws, stovers and agriculture byproducts.
- A large professional manpower consisting of 33,600 veterinarians and 64,500 para-veterinary staff and availability of a sound animal husbandry infrastructure in terms of breeding establishment, veterinary clinics and AI outlets.

Weaknesses

- Although India has large livestock population, productivity per unit animal is low.
- Age at maturity and calving intervals are high.

- Average milk production per indigenous and crossbred cow and buffalo in milk per year is around 800, 1800 and 1200 kg respectively.
- The average carcass weight of 12 and 10 kg in sheep and goat is lowest in the world next only to Bangladesh. Wool yield during the last 15 years has been almost constant.
- Poor coverage through Artificial Insemination (15 to 20%), low conception rates (20%) under field conditions in cows and buffaloes, non-availability of quality bulls.
- Shortage of feeds and fodder.
- High losses on account of mortality and morbidity.
- Outdated health laws and regulatory mechanisms.

Opportunities

- With increasing globalization of trade, new markets are opening up.
- India has comparative advantage in meat and meat products and seafoods.
- New production technologies are increasingly becoming available.
- New techniques for genetic upgradation and preserving superior breeds and their germplasms are becoming available.
- Information technology and the Internet are generating a whole lot of information and means of communication. E-commerce is increasingly becoming the mode of trading.
- Cost of production of livestock products in India as compared to other countries is low.
- Value added processed foods production, both for internal consumption and exports, can yield higher returns.

Threats

- Inadequate price structure for milk, meat and egg is a disincentive to animal production in general and hygienic production in particular.
- Pressure on grazing or pasturelands has increased, with rise in livestock numbers.
- Conflicts between man and animal over land resources have the potential to upset the delicate ecological balance.
- Sustainable livestock development is becoming increasingly difficult.
- Poor processing and marketing facilities, and absence of cold chain are some of the major hindrances in value addition and exports.
- Heavy subsidies on both production and export of agricultural products such as dairy produce, by developed countries result in very low international prices of imports, which adversely affect the domestic producers.
- Phasing out of quantitative restrictions on a number of items has resulted in cheap imports into the country.
- Increasing emphasis on food safety issues and imposition of stringent SPS measures by developed countries is a major challenge for exporters in particular.

- These measures act as technical or non-tariff barriers and the costs of compliance with these standards are high, while the compliance assessment procedures are very cumbersome.

CONCLUDING REMARKS

The study of the **SWOT** analysis shows that the 'strengths' and 'opportunities' generally outweigh 'weaknesses' and 'threats' for most sub-sectors. Strengths and opportunities are fundamental and weaknesses and threats are transitory. Any investment idea can do well only when one has three essential ingredients: entrepreneurship (the ability to take risks), innovative approach (in product lines and marketing) and values (of quality/ ethics). Nevertheless, it is essential to stress that weaknesses will have to be overcome if the full potential of the livestock sector is to be realized and the projected demand and supply are to be achieved. Major constraints to bovine production include *inter alia* inadequate feed supply and poor quality of feed, and unremunerative prices for buffalo meat. In the case of small ruminant production, constraints relate to poor quality of most stock, weak support services and inadequate feed and fodder availability. For milk and dairy products, constraints include low prices and inefficiencies in processing.

25

Future: Constraint Analysis: A Field Survey Processing Industry

This chapter discusses the problems and opportunities for livestock product processing industry in India. Food processing industry is a nascent sector in the country, which has enormous potential. The development of the sector has so far been primarily because of the positive perception of its potential at the Central Government level and not because of interest of domestic or overseas business community. Creation of the Ministry of Food Processing Industries is a result of these positive perceptions. Notwithstanding this, there is a need for preparation of an attractive case so far as livestock based food-processing industry is concerned. The case should ideally be strong both in terms of style and substance so that both domestic and international investors find it acceptable. This is of crucial importance since radical improvement in this sector could call for substantial investment. Besides Central and State Governments, domestic and international investors must be convinced to put in their might.

Further, there is an absolute need on the part of the Government to formulate and announce proactive policy measures to dispel the general perceptions that livestock based food processing is a high risk – low return area, prone to poor capacity utilization and hence unviable as a business proposition in the long term. Needless to say, such policy measures must be framed with holistic approach and must involve all concerned Ministries and representatives of prospective investors to ensure that upstream and downstream linkages have sound basis. The existence of a large number of Panchayati Raj institutions and huge network of cottage, small and medium scale industries also points to the possibility of a bottom-up approach being more successful than a top-down approach in this matter.

The nodal concept that is being proposed is to eliminate/marginalize the role of middleman by providing a three tier structure wherein the primary producers have a preliminary storage/processing/packaging facility within twenty five kilometers of his farm and such preliminary facilities are further linked as feeder to a modern processing plant. This will not only ensure better remuneration to the primary producers, but also improve availability of hygienic quality food for the domestic and overseas market, simultaneously reducing the risk perceptions of the investors. Since the entire process would involve integration on the basis of area wise planning of sectoral programmes, for which investments are normally being made, additional investment required will not be of a very high order but the spin-off of such a process could be enormously rewarding on many counts. There is also need to pursue the following shelf of strategies: -

(i) Identification of area/location with higher prospects for vertical integration of primary producers to industrial processing units.

(ii) Creation of an interactive forum with select State Governments with higher prospects for processing industries in order to evolve a conducive policy environment for prospective entrepreneurs and to augment fund flow for the sector.

(iii) Rationalization of tax structure on fresh and processed food as well as institutional investment in campaign for hygienic food, brand formation /market promotion, activities promoting producers' organization and industrial associations, etc.

(iv) Sectoral programmes for improving raw material in target areas, creation of a dynamic database through studies and surveys at periodic intervals and dissemination of information to entrepreneurs.

(v) Prioritizing infrastructural development like roads, power, communication, cold chain, etc. in prospective areas.

(vi) Emphasis on quality control in production and processing in order to improve quality and acceptability of finished products. Adopting of Total Quality Management (TQM), Hazard Analysis and Critical Control Points (HACCP) in industrial units and extension campaign for primary producers to achieve this goal.

(vii) Adoption of appropriate technology both at the level of primary producers and at processing levels, incorporation of newer technology like remote sensing, information technology, biotechnology, etc. with concern for the environment.

(viii) Improving access to credit and transferable technology to the primary producers and promoting their own organizations will be integral part of the holistic approach.

(ix) The development of packaging technologies and harmonization of food laws to encourage reduction of high quality value added food.

(x) Assigning those roles and functions, which are necessary but cannot be performed in Government set up to non-government organizations suited to take up the same.

FIELD SURVEY OF FOOD PROCESSING UNITS

A field study was carried out to ascertain the reasons for poor capacity utilisation, potential development, and technologies used in Food Processing (including meat and milk processing) in India. The study was conducted through personal interviews with a sample of Food Processing Units as well as through a structured Questionnaire. Two of the main product categories covered were: (i) Milk and dairy Products and (ii) Meat and Meat Products. A short Questionnaire, (see Appendix I), was sent to about 30 stakeholders/ decision makers spread over the entire length and breadth of the country. In all 20 stakeholders/decision makers responded to the questionnaire. The respondents, stakeholders/decision makers, were the state government officials, mainly engaged in livestock development. State Milk Federation/Unions, non-Governmental organizations and academics, representing the main livestock producing states of the country, namely Uttar Pradesh, Madhya Pradesh, Orissa, Karnataka, Rajasthan and Haryana. The major constraints reported by the respondents are indicated in detail below. An analysis of views of the respondents is given at the end of this chapter.

The Main Constraints Reported in the Survey are as Follows

Specific problems relating to Meat and Meat Products, which emanated from the field study were:

   (i)   The limited availability of cold chain, together with its high cost was one of the major factors that affected the manufacturers of meat and meat products.

  (ii)   Meat and poultry sector is not treated as an Industry and does not therefore get any incentives and subsidies from the Government.

 (iii)   At many places poultry can only be sold in the regulated/notified market yards through the agent or a Commission Agent and not directly to the retailer making it possible for the Agents to manipulate the prices.

Constraints in the Overall Setting

 • Institutional infrastructure is underdeveloped and government effectiveness low.
 • Food processing industries are discounted as of little importance, or identified as problems not solutions.
 • Legislation on standards, production procedures are underdeveloped.
 • General lack of specific agro-industry policy and where it exists is often rudimentary with lack of continuity.
 • Lack of appropriate institutional support and poor coordination, e.g. with institutional credit supplies.
 • Absence of comprehensive strategies for phased development.
 • Capital for infrastructure projects competes with much other development needs of the governments.
 • Lack of funds for implementing adaptive R&D programmes, for accessing information and conducting long-term investigations.

- Mechanisms for identifying vital research needs and implementing the technology of transfer, need to be strengthened. (In particular concerning laboratory-to-factory or researcher-to-farmer linkage).

Backward Linkages

Livestock inputs are not well integrated or planned, resulting in supply of inappropriate inputs, low raw material quality, supply not timely etc.
- In many cases, aggregate volumes of meat input supply is inadequate, creating stranglehold on agro-industry.
- Livestock production in turn is often discouraged by exploitative conditions (very low purchase prices).
- There is lack of adequate supplier identification.

Technology and Quality Problems

- Technology used is backward, insufficient access to state-of-art technology.
- Conversely, insufficient use of well-known intermediate technology.
- Low quality output, quality fluctuation, untimely deliveries, disregard for contract obligations.
- Lack of specialized expertise and exploitative working condition (low wages).
- Inadequate project preparation (no feasibility studies are carried out).
- Lack of skilled managers and high competition for those available.
- Insufficient storage, transport, power supply, telecommunications.
- Insufficient attention paid to grading, handling, packaging, and quality standard.
- Research and development insufficient, or lacks government support.
- High capital requirements for start-up in relation to other rural financial capacities.
- Insufficient connection with trade sector.

Finance and Credit Constraints

- Cost of funding high.
- Little institutional credit and fiscal support policy.
- Low ranking of this group of industries for access to investment capital.
- Too little price protection against foreign imports at starting stage.
- Low level of value- addition by Multinationals
- High costs of attaining higher competitiveness (high prices of finishing, packaging,).

Market Constraint

- Relatively low domestic market demand due to low purchasing power.
- Small physical dimension of market restricting economies of scale.

- Lack of market information, market communication and onsourcing.
- Discrimination in access to foreign markets.
- Lack of coordination with support sectors, e.g. transport, shipping, etc.
- Lack of awareness and adaptation to market demands. Carelessness in adjusting to changing market situation.

OPPORTUNITIES

Generic Needs

- Greater use of up-to-date production technologies.
- Better use of idle installed capacity (function of raw material supply and market demand).
- Better use of available skilled manpower.
- Improved market research (mainly by government).
- Systematic examination of opportunities arising from past technical assistance.
- Greater transfer of required technology through external collaboration.
- Greater inward transfer of capital in same way.
- Better legislation for external collaboration.
- Greater intercountry coordination.
- Greater use of intermediate technology at starting stage.
- Active participation between R&D institutions and the industrial enterprises.
- Better adoption of imported technology through R&D.
- Developing appropriate low-cost Cattle -Feed Technologies to reduce cost of final output.
- Government promotional campaign and action to ensure access to international markets.
- Long-term agreements between suppliers and buyers (government intervention needed).

Specific Opportunities

- Development of water buffalo potential for dairying and meat production.
- Development of animal feed production (soybeans, mungbeans, castor beans and fermented agricultural byproducts).
- Intercounty arrangements between producers and consumers, if possible, regional arrangements.
- Upgrading of domestic abattoirs for collection of slaughterhouse byproducts.
- Adaptation of specialized production to meet world market demand for high quality products.

Livestock-Industrial Policies

Typical Livestock-industrial policy framework should include:

- Linkages policy between producers and processors.

- Credit policy taking into account the season ability, idle periods etc.
- Location policy depending on availability of infrastructure and raw materials.
- Investment policy balancing foreign investment with local entrepreneurship.
- Technology policy including issues viz., balancing of imports with encouragement to indigenous development, needs of small sector and end user.
- Regional cooperation policy in the areas of marketing and technology development.
- Marketing policy taking into consideration surplus/shortage i.e. balancing domestic needs with the need for exports and for activating demand. Support to nascent industrial units to ensure continued viability.
- Manpower policy (human resources development) whether technical education is sufficient and, if deficient, to allow for international cooperation.
- Quality improvement policy in order to ensure stability and standards of suppliers as well as output.
- Other policy consideration viz., environmental inputs, sociocultural factors (prohibitions etc.) and administrative structure is also important. The development of infrastructure must continue to be given priority attention.

Livestock-Industrial Strategies

Based on the policies defined above, the following strategies may be adopted:

(a) *Linkage Strategies:* Contract farming incorporating appropriate safeguards (legal framework) protecting interests of producers and processors.

Cooperativisation as a means of eliminating the adversarial gap between production, processing and marketing.

Foster Factory Approach for large industry to adopt small producers (suitable incentives should be given).

(b) *Credit and Finance Strategies:* Working capital norms to be specifically laid down. Collateral acceptance of agro processed products by banks. Financial needs of owners of livestock with longer gestation need attention.

Banking system in definite block allocation should make credit requirements of livestock-industry.

(c) *Location Strategies:* Primary processing in rural areas to save on transportation costs, preventing pollution, etc.

Reconstitution of repacking units in or near consumption centres.

(d) *Investment Strategies:* Long term or at least medium term and stable schemes/procedures/norms should be laid down. Tax incentive repatriation of benefits and freedom of business operations for foreign investors should be ensured.

Fiscal incentives to local entrepreneur and exposure programmes for potential entrepreneurs. Continued support to nascent industries until such industries are self-sustaining or can overcome temporary setbacks.

(e) *Marketing Strategies:* Export promotion measures should be stable (at least a medium term perspective should be considered). Marketing organisations including MNCs, could assist in view of their strength in information, access to international markets.

Information system based on market research of domestic markets to help in the identification of potential market needs. Public Sector support to popularize genetic processed products.

(f) *Quality Strategies:* Grading/Standardization for quality of inputs. Quality standards for products and inspection to enforce quality control.

(g) *Technology Strategies:* Dual promotion of small sector along with large rather than limiting growth of any one sector. Liberalized imports in areas in which countries are deficient.

Indigenous research needs greater outlays (public sector). In particular research to farmlinkages to be strengthened. Diversification into new products and processes.

Technology for increasing productivity and expanding market opportunities must continue to be assessed, adapted and/or developed. To be effective, technology for livestock-based industries must be market oriented. Technologies must also take into account comprehensive by-product utilization and control of environmental pollution. Manpower training on management skills and quality control for production workers is essential.

CONSTRAINTS OBSERVED IN MODERNISING THE MEAT PROCESSING INDUSTRY

Demand

A demand constraint for processed foods has resulted in low utilization of capacity. While a number of factors have contributed to this low demand, a major reason identified has been that production has been dictated by supply and not driven by the requirements of the market.

Technology

A majority of the units continue to utilize outdated and unsuitable production technologies, which result in high production costs as well as poor product quality. Among the small and medium scale units, the level of professionalism is low and there is very limited application of professional techniques such as feasibility studies and market research.

Raw Material Availability and Quality

Limitation of 'Feed "for the birds or animal". Cost of feed is very high and supply/ availability irregular. Frequent droughts in the country especially in cattle rich states resulting in their migration in search of fodder add to the problems of value-addition units in more than one way-high price, poor quality and irregular supply, etc.

Tax Structure

The prevailing tax structure has affected the food-processing sector adversely. The study reveals that the high incidence of excise duty and sales tax affected the viability of many units. India is perhaps the highest taxed country in this sector. There is 8-40% Excise Duty and 5-12 % Sales Tax in value-added products and 20-50% duty on Imported Machinery/ Equipment for processing and 10-40 % Excise Duty on Capital goods produced within the country, literally pricing it out in the international market.

Infrastructure

Adequate availability of electricity has been a limiting factor for higher capacity utilization. In the absence of assured electricity supply, many units utilize captive sources of power such as diesel generating sets, which adds to the cost of production.

The limited availability and high cost of using a cold chain also acts as a disincentive for storing raw materials and using them for production during off-seasons.

Technology employed by meat processing units is outdated and unsuitable/unsustainable: The quality of processed meat products manufactured is dependent to a great extent on the technology being used by the manufacturing units. The relevance of technology is critical both at the raw material stage as well as at the stage when value addition takes place through processing of the raw materials.

- Meat processing units in the country have not achieved a high degree of professionalism and continue to adopt old and outdated technologies, which result in non-optimal levels of production as well as low quality of products. A major section of the units (79.9%) studied rely solely on self-developed technology, which is essentially the knowledge of the production process acquired over a period of time through on-the-job experience.
- The study also reveals the lack of professional and scientific approach in much food processing units. These units have been started without undertaking proper feasibility study for the products to be manufactured. Nearly 70% of the units have been started purely on the basis of the entrepreneurs' feel and perception of the market demand. The absence of strategic and long-range planning has resulted in such units not succeeding in facing the vagaries of the market.

- Linkages with Indian research institutions and professional organisations engaged in the development of improved and appropriate technologies as well as in the carrying out of feasibility studies is very poor.

POLICY OF RESERVATION OF ITEMS FOR THE SMALL-SCALE SECTOR AND ITS IMPACT

- The policy of reservation of certain products for manufacture by the small-scale sector has resulted in the spawning of a large number of units with extremely small and unviable production capacities. These production units cannot therefore exploit the benefits of economies of scale. Added to this is the fact that the low technology used in the production process results in the end products being low in quality and thus having a limited market demand.
- Reservation for small-scale units can also be counterproductive if it places a restriction on the limits to growth and acts as a disincentive for upgradation of units in terms of scale and technology.
- An important finding of the study relates to the number of shifts worked by the food processing units studied. Nearly 69% of the units have reported working only one shift per day. This further reinforces the nexus between demand and low production levels.

Inability to Develop a Niche in the Export Markets

- The study of meat processing units in different parts of the country has brought out the critical fact that nearly 80% of the units do not export their products. The requirements of the domestic market remain the only source of demand for such units. This factor assumes significance because the demand for processed meat products in the domestic market is still very limited and it would take some time to change consumer perceptions and thereby generate higher demands.
- The basic premise for entering the export markets is high quality of products, price competitiveness and adherence to delivery schedules. Most of the units have not been able to meet these requirements as they operate in a limited market and are often caught in the low production-low technology-low quality trap.

A weak linkage between the Cattle-farmer and Agri-processor

- The sustained availability of raw materials has been highlighted as a major constraint. Together with the quality aspect of raw materials, this forms the single most important constraint. The study shows that 58% of the units purchase the raw materials from the open market.
- The major reason for the emergence of this constraint is the weak linkage between the cattle farmer and the agri-processor. Overall, only 10.5% of the responding units have reported a linkage with own farm production as the reason for starting the processing unit. As expected,

this linkage is stronger in the northern region and 25% of the units have reported this as a motivating factor for going in for a forward linkage of setting up of a processing unit. On a macro level, however, unlike the oilseeds sector (yellow revolution), cereals (green revolution) and milk (white revolution) neither the livestock nor its processing counterpart has been touched by any 'revolution' almost leaving it standing alone.

All these constraints are to be addressed in the proposed Policy on 'National Food Processing Industry' paving the road map for a breakthrough in the sector, befitting the size and magnitude of the livestock population, agroclimatic zones and need for diversification to generate income/ employment generation through this upcoming sector.

VIEWS OF THE STAKEHOLDERS/DECISION MAKERS – AN ANALYSIS

The responses basically, focussed on three issues, with far reaching implications, on the livestock sector. These are:
1. The Present status and prospects:
2. Policy issues, including the role of the Government
3. Export Potential

The views of the respondents on these aspects are summarized below;

Present status and Prospects

An analysis of comments from the respondents indicates that prospects of the livestock sector in the next two to three decades are bright and a revolution in this sector is in the offing. Since crop production has its own limitations, this, sector will take a quantum jump, as the demand for its products will increase with the rise in income levels and increase in population. Currently, the livestock sector is operating at the subsistence level, with traditional farming practices and suboptimum inputs/ infrastructures. It is largely confined to landless labourers and small and marginal farmers. If the input costs of the family resources like labour, feed and fodder are counted, then livestock farming becomes unremunerative. The small holder farming will continue to be an important characteristic of the Indian agrarian scenario. Intensive livestock farming, primarily, in the poultry and diary sector, will be confined only to the urban and peri-urban areas. Given the existing structure of the Indian farming system, it will not be possible to provide large capital inputs and highly productive animals, which require sophisticated management practices, health care, feed and fodder. However, there is a need to upgrade the genetic quality of the Indian livestock, retaining its inherent qualities of disease resistance and high conversion rate of roughages.

Policy Issues, Including the Role of the Government

There are divergent views on the current livestock policy regime. The views range from nonexistent livestock policy to a very restrictive policy regime.

The general consensus, however, is that the role of the government should be regulatory and acts as a catalyst, with clear-cut policies. There is also the need to develop synergies with various stakeholders in this sector, and delink many of the activities like breeding and health services from the governmental functions. Cooperatives and private sector should be involved in the key activities like veterinary health care, breeding services, processing and marketing of livestock products. Market access is an important area for growth, as the livestock is a demand driven sector. Production without market access will be "suicidal."

Export Potential

Increase in income levels, leading to improvement in the quality of life, is the aspiration of every human being: the farming sector, therefore, cannot be created in isolation. But given the present status of the farming community, it is imperative to provide the basic inputs and infrastructure in terms of processing and marketing. There is a great potential for the sale of livestock products in the domestic market itself. There is also an equally bright future for exports, especially, meat products and dairy products. However, the greatest stumbling block will be animal disease prevalent in the country. There is a need to channelise the available resources to eradicate animal diseases so that India can export livestock products, which will conform to the requirements of the importing country.

Concluding Remarks

The stakeholders, to whom the questionnaire was circulated, represented a wide cross section of decision makers and entrepreneurs involved in the production and marketing of livestock products. From the kind of response obtained, it appears that the perspective of the respondents vary widely, and sometime are divorced from reality. This underpins the need for orientation of the leaders among the stakeholders and decision makers towards a reasonably uniform perspective based on reasons as well as reality. This can only be achieved through enhanced institutional mechanism for interaction on sectoral policy framework.

Appendix I

Questionnaire for Respondents

1. What is your assessment of the prospect of livestock sector in coming 2-3 decades?
2. Do you subscribe to the idea that under the present circumstances livestock farming, in general, is unremunerative? If so, is it because of the scale of operation, or lack of inputs/infrastructure or fall out of policy initiatives in the livestock and other sectors? If not, what advantages can be drawn from the fact by the small holder?
3. Do you think intensive livestock farming will grow in the country and gradually replace extensive/semi-intensive systems? If so, can you suggest regions/locations where such intensification is likely to prosper? Do you think some sub sectors are likely to adopt intensification at a faster rate than others? If yes, brief reasons for the same.
4. Do you think current policy regime is obstructive to intensification in the livestock sector? If so, what are the major areas/policy interventions that you think are needed?
5. a) What are the most important areas (maximum four) where reorientation is required in sectoral policy.
   b) What are the most important areas (two only) in general financial policy where reorientation will help livestock sectors growth?
6. What role do you envisage for the Government in coming years? Can you suggest some areas/functions from where Government should direct particular attention or areas/functions from where Government should withdraw?
7. Do you think sectoral programmes for livestock development will have better impact on the livelihood of rural masses than programmes for empowering the masses encouraging farmers own institutions?
8. What is likely to have a more favourable impact on the sector – introduction of sector specific technologies or general infrastructure development?
9. Can you place the following focus of activity covering livestock sector in order of priority:
   (i) Improving productivity, (ii) Improving processing and value addition, (iii) Improving marketing access, (iv) Income supplementation, (v) Employment generation, (vi) Food security, (vii) Environmental protection and conservation of bio diversity.
1. What are the expectations of livestock farmers, how much of these are reasonable? Who, other than the Government can meet these expectations?
2. Are there specific groups who never benefited most from Livestock Development Programmes? If so, briefly describe the nature of beneficiary groups.

3. Do you think the current livestock population exceeds the current carrying capacity of the land? If so, what are the most probable solutions to the problem?

4. a) Do you think the country has very good prospect of international trade in livestock and livestock products which is not being realized? What are the major constraints and what are the likely solutions?

   b) In the context of global trade and emerging diseases of livestock, particularly BSE (Mad Cow Disease) do you expect changes in the livestock industry in developing countries? What prospect does it hold for India?

26

Livestock Revolution – The World Scenario

Livestock production is important for the majority of farmers in developing countries, especially for small farmers in more marginal conditions where land cannot be used for other purposes. Smallholders keep livestock for food, fibre, fertilizer, fuel, draught power, as a buffer in case of crop failure, and also for social and cultural functions. Increasingly, livestock is also produced for cash, which is the main objective of specialized livestock production systems. This type of livestock production strongly depends on the dynamics of the global markets.

Two-thirds of the world's livestock are found in 'developing' countries. Most farmers in these countries practice multiplepurpose, nonintensive methods of animal production. Animals are critical for their livelihoods, cultures and social status. Many of these animals graze areas not suitable for crops or scavenge freely, often consuming garbage and harmful insects. Small farms that combine livestock and crops use the land relatively sustainably: crop residues are fed to animals; manure provides good fertilizer and fuel; and animal draught power reduces the need for fossil fuels. Smallholder livestock production makes a substantial contribution to the economy.

In India, for example, livestock contributes about 30% of the total farm output, and 80% of livestock products come from small farmers with 3-5 animals and less than 2 ha. of land (Rangnekar 2001). It is estimated that one-quarter of the world's total land area is being used for grazing livestock, including extensive grazing systems. A further one-fifth of the world's arable land is used for growing cereals to feed livestock. This makes livestock production the largest user of land in the world.

THE 'LIVESTOCK REVOLUTION'

Livestock production systems in the developing countries are changing fast, due to the so-called 'Livestock Revolution'. The global demand for meat is expected to be more than double over the next twenty years, creating an increased demand for cereal feed. Southern countries are expected to become the main producers of meat and animal products with increasing dependency on imported grain. It is expected that there will be a shift from livestock being kept for multiple purposes and local food supply to animals being raised under factory farming conditions for export. Many small-scale farms will be out-competed and replaced by large-scale industrial farms (Delga o, et. al., 1999).

This Livestock Revolution will provide new opportunities for agriculture in the South. But, who will benefit from it, what will be the cost to small farmers, food security, the environment, farm animal genetic diversity and farm animal welfare? Compassion in World Farming Trust (CWFT), a research-based farm animal welfare organization that investigates the development of factory farming at an international level, recently studied the effects of the rise in factory farming on Southern countries, their farmers and farm animals (Cox and Varpama 2000). An overview of the results is given below.

Small Farmers are Loosing

The leading agencies working on hunger alleviation admit that rural small farmers are being pushed out of business by factory farming. Farmers in the UK, US and Europe have already experienced the painful consequences of the so-called 'vertical integration' of livestock production, in which specialized enterprises such as feedlot farms, animal feed traders, and meat packers, all merge under one giant company. This leaves very limited market opportunities for small, independent farmers, many of whom have been forced to leave the business altogether. According to the US Department of Agriculture, there were 5.7 million farms in the USA, in 1950. Today, the number has decreased to about 2 million farms.

This same pattern is quickly taking hold in Southern countries. Brazil's poultry industry is a good example. Between 1970 and 1991. Brazil's poultry industry grew from small backyard farmers to a multinational mechanized industry, becoming almost entirely vertically integrated. Originally, small family farmers were given day-old chicks by major companies and were paid to raise them. Sadia is an example of a family-owned company, which employed 14,000 smallholder farmers to raise chickens on their mixed farms with a clear benefit to these farming families. The chickens were brought back to Sadia, who processed and distributed them to consumers.

Unfortunately, this system began to change four or five years ago, due to financial troubles of family owned companies, such as Sadia, which were taken over by financial interest groups and foreign companies. Now, Sadia is raising, providing feed for, and processing its own chickens in large production units. Certainly, most of the 14,000 mixed farmers, who once raised chickens for the Sadia industry, do not benefit from this new 'development' initiative.

By following a more holistic, ecological approach many farmers seem to come closer to their own 'gut feeling' of how they should manage their farm, which is also more in line with the way their parents thought about it. The problem is, however, to get other players such as researchers, policy makers and educators involved in this approach to form (inter) national networks and local platforms for change. Although, increasingly, these players are aware that there is something wrong with the conventional approach to livestock production, they have to make quite a change in attitude and thinking to take a different stand. For example, animal science as taught in Latin American Universities and farming schools is focused in reaching the maximum productivity per animal, limited to the animal species used in industrialized livestock keeping, especially cattle, pigs and chicken. The absence of the essential elements of family-level livestock keeping and basic principles of integrated ecological livestock production in the curriculum is reflected in the frequent failures of livestock projects and the negative impact of livestock production on the environment.

Although integrated livestock systems have considerable potential to improve livestock production, the changes of small farmers competing with industrial livestock production will remain weak as long as research, policies and education systems do not change.

Harm to Import-Dependent Developing Countries

There are many examples that support the view that the introduction of industrial livestock rearing not only harms the individual small-scale farmer but also the developing countries as a whole. As a consequence of industrial livestock rearing, these countries have become more import-dependent. Grains, tractors, fuel, fertilizers and special animal units and processors are required for intensive livestock rearing, none of which a developing country starts out by making itself.

Over the last decade, Asia has begun to import large amounts of grain to feed its industrially-produced farm animals. Likewise, machinery, oil and production units are being imported and subsidized by the government. The Asian economic crisis of 1999, that raised prices of imported feeds and depressed urban demand, proved that being an import-laden economy can be disastrous and unsustainable.

Threat to Food Security

A *World Poultry* study (Gueye 2001) done in sub-Saharan Africa indicates the importance of family-level poultry rearing for food security, poverty alleviation, environmental health and genetic diversity. While the one or two breeds of broiler chicken used for chicken meat in factory farms are generally imported, 85% of rural families keep several species and breeds of poultry of indigenous types. The products of these local breeds are often preferred to those from exotic breeds by local consumers. Furthermore, the local breeds are better adapted to local diseases, pests and climate.

Poultry are usually raised in extensive systems, while some families specialize in semi-extensive and small-scale intensive poultry systems.

In extensive production (backyard) systems, birds are reared with little land, labour or capital, can be accessed by even the poorest social communities in rural areas, and are of great importance for women, especially in female-headed households. The study indicated that an average flock of 5 chickens enabled a women in Central Tanzania to earn an additional US $ 38 per year or a 9.5% increase in income. Poultry raising has contributed to the "greater empowerment of women by improving their financial status, if sociocultural and religious environments allow it". As such, the loss of family farming to industrial farming could seriously affect women and children.

Painful experiences in the North teach us that this development towards 'factory farming' will put enormous pressure on natural resources, food safety, animal diversity and welfare, as well as threaten the income generating possibilities of small farmers. In reality these systems are very inefficient and the hidden environmental and social costs of the livestock industry are enormous. Also, to meet food needs in 2050, it is necessary to increase human food production considerably. But, the "Livestock Revolution" will compete strongly with human food production. Presently, livestock industry already consumes almost 50% of world cereal grain supplies. It is therefore very important to develop livestock production systems, which do not depend on cereal grain. The Animal Welfare Review in 1998, therefore, raised the all-important question: "should this type of intensive livestock production continue to be encouraged globally or should alternatives be sought?"

Effects on the Environment

Factory farming was developed in Europe with the aim of ending food shortage after the 2nd World War. Science and technology were promoted, farmers were given subsidies to encourage production increases, and consumers were given cheaper food. But, these policies of production at all costs can no longer be supported. As far back as 1997, the chief of the FAO's Asian Pacific Regional office declared that it was time to move away from the 'Green Revolution' livestock model, as the environmental problems of this approach were already obvious.

Industrial animal farming has proved to have detrimental effects on the environment both in the short and the long term (Haan, et al 1998). For example, the production of cereals for the livestock industry often takes place far away from where the animals are raised. This is leading to depletion of soil fertility where cereals are produced, and pollution at the other end of the trading spectrum where cereals are used for animal feed. Soya and maize are major products of the US supplied to industrial animal farms around the world. Such monoculture systems, though strongly promoted by governments, have unintended consequences for soil and water quality. Thirty percent of the total cropland in the United States is now eroding at excessive rates, according to the Soil and Water Conservation Society (http://www.swcs.org/).

Globally, farm animals produce 13 billion tonnes of waste per annum (Turner 1999). Animals on industrial farms consume high-protein feeds and produce waste that is extremely environmentally damaging. Industrial animal farming contributes 5-10% of the total of greenhouse gases in the world, accelerating climate change. Moreover, large amounts of water and fossil energy are required to grow, process and transport industrial farm animal feed and treat the animal waste (Pimentel, et al 1997).

Even without the "Livestock Revolution", livestock keepers already have enough ecological problems, for example, due to overgrazing and burning. Research has developed technology mainly for intensive and industrialized livestock production systems. But, many modern technologies do not fit the reality of low-input livestock systems.

Enhancing the Quality of the Whole System

To optimize the performance of farming, it is important that management practices enhance the ecological functioning of the 'web' of all living organisms within the production system by influencing the interactions between climate, soil, vegetation, animals and farmers. Traditional farmers often have mixed systems in which the production of crops, animals and natural resources are integrated, products are of multiple-use, and a waste products of one subsystem are used as inputs in other subsystems. Within this integrated system, depending on needs, opportunities and risks, farmers may follow different strategies: keep many different animal species under low input management system, or combine this with the intensive production of one specific species. Traditional systems can be relatively productive, while making optimal use of the available natural and human resources. Presently, influenced by modernization and globalization, most of these traditional systems are loosing their economic and social coherence.

The awareness that agro-ecological systems are complex and integrated, and that the quality of all parts of the system, including its social and cultural dimensions, is important to optimize the performance of the whole system, has been lost in more modern agriculture. Intensive livestock production in the Netherlands, for example, strongly focused on high input/high output relations and profit making, forgot about the environment. Two environmental associations of dairy farmers, rediscovered the importance of the quality of the whole system. They found that the quality of the cow manure influences the quality of the soil, which, determines the quality and quantity of the pasture and fodder crops, the feed for the animals, which is important for animal health and the quality and quantity of their products. They have developed a new way of feeding their milk cattle with lower protein and higher fibre contents by using less concentrates and fertilizers, which reduces nutrient losses while maintaining milk production at the same level.

Loss of Genetic Diversity

The FAO (2001) reports that the greatest threat to the world's domestic animal diversity is the export of specialized breeds of farm animals from developed to developing countries. Crossbreeding with and eventual replacement of local breeds has resulted in a situation that around 1,350 domestic animal breeds (30% of all domestic breeds) are at risk of extinction. Every week, two breeds of farm animals disappear.

One of the greatest misjudgements of the 'Livestock Revolution' is to deny the importance of genetic diversity for food security. For example, in 1996, some 942,000 inseminations have been carried out in the Netherlands alone, with semen from a single Holstein Friesian bull, named Sunny Boy. In that period the Dutch dairy sector averaged 1.7 million milking cows! (Compas Magazine, Oct. 1999, p. 26). Semen of this bull was also used in many other countries. Nearly 12,000 years of domestication and breeding under different environments have resulted in some 4000 breeds of farm animals. The genetic diversity of these breeds has made it possible for humans to thrive in all corners of the globe, facing a range of environmental challenges including varied climates, diseases, parasites and pests. Unlike imported industrial breeds, local farm animals in given environments have developed resistance or adaptations to these challenges.

For example, in Rajasthan, India, nonindustrial breeds of farm animals have benefited human food security even in a harsh desert climate, where temperatures can rise to 50°C. This region counts 7 local breeds of cattle, 8 breeds of sheep, 4 breeds of goats, as well as camel and horse breeds. Through these local breeds Rajasthan significantly contributes to the national milk and wool output. Marginal lands can contribute to food security only by working with farm animals adapted to the local climatic conditions (Rathore, et al 2001).

Government interventions in Rajasthan have focused on 'improving' local breeds by crossbreeding them with exotic breeds from other climates. Not surprisingly, the crossbreeding of local sheep with exotic sheep has failed to achieve any improved yield, mainly due to high mortality and problems with feed supply. In the case of cattle, the government has realized the detrimental effects of crossbreeding, and in 1998 revised its policy to protect and improve local breeds.

Negative Impact on Farm Animal Welfare

Another negative impact of industrial farming is its impact on farm animal welfare. As recognized by the Treaty of Amsterdam, farm animals are living creatures capable of feeling pain and suffering. Industrial animal farming often closely confines the animals indoors, without light and with little or no exercise. This inhibits the natural behaviour of animals, and is known to create aggression, stress and injuries in animals. Industrial animal farming also carries out standard practices of mutilation: the hen is debeaked, so that she can no longer peck her cage mate, and the pig is tail-docked, so that his bored pen mates can no longer bite its tail.

Measure to benefit the poor to better compete with the livestock industry (LID 1999)

- Access to credit (to allow for the purchase of animals);
- Access to appropriate (community based) animal health services and simple preventive measures such as vaccinations and improved hygiene;
- Secure grazing rights and access to water;
- Access to markets;
- Trade policies and frameworks that allow smallholders and pastoralists to compete with industrial animal production. For example: support to cooperative, levying taxes from animal producers based on their ecological and social impacts;
- Improve feeding to increase the performance of local breeds (Haan, et al 1998);
- Support livestock production based on local resources (feeds, breeds, indigenous knowledge and institutions) and integrated farming systems;
- Stop subsidizing intensive animal production in the North and the South;
- Stop export of subsidized products of the livestock industry to developing countries.

German NGO Forum Environment and Development
Am Michaelshof 8-10, D-53177 Bonn.
Fax: +49 (0)228-359096;
E-mail: gura@foromue.de;http://www.forumue.de

The surroundings of industrial animal farms can be dirty and poorly ventilated, leading to poor animal health. Moreover, selected breeding for large muscles and fast growth, especially in pigs and chickens raised for meat, leads to leg problems, cardiovascular inadequacy, increased risk of mortality and poor welfare.

Learning from the Mistakes of the North

In superficial economic calculations, industrial animal farming is considered the cheapest and most productive form of animal production. But, these calculations do not include the 'total costs' of this production system. Industrial animal production looks viable only when selected aspects of the production – consumption system is viewed. In reality, the hidden costs of industrial animal production for future generations are enormous. It is therefore very important that policy decision makers examine questions such as: Is it acceptable to cause job losses by putting small-scale farmers in poverty stricken populations out of business? Is it acceptable to cause ecological degradation, environmental pollution, climate change and increased ozone layer depletion? Is it acceptable to cause unnecessary pain and suffering to farm animals?

The UK, for example, has been struck by diseases such as foot and mouth disease and mad cow disease (BSE) that has brought the industrial animal farming system under serious questioning by the public. Food poisoning connected with eating animal products is also higher than it has ever been in the UK, leaving consumers to doubt the safety of industrial animal products. More and more consumers are turning away from the products of industrial animal farming towards the products of more sustainable systems such as organic and free-range. The governments in Europe are now beginning to recognize this situation and the value of more quality-driven livestock production. The Netherlands government, for example, has recently begun to subsidize organic pig production by 30%. An editorial comment in World Animal Review in 1998 raised an all-important question: "Should this type of livestock production continue to be encouraged globally, or should alternatives be sought?".

Policy makers must now support more sustainable and humane forms of animal farming and realize that industrial animal farming holds no future for Southern and Northern countries alike.

Chain Management and Weak Links

An increasing number of organizations are working towards livestock development. NGO interventions in improving the livelihoods of people dependant on livestock is increasingly becoming popular with activities spread over a range of aspects that include training local youth as animal health workers, conservation of livestock as well as fodder species, production of herbal medicines and dissemination of local technologies. Alternative means of reaching the rural masses by building capacities of rural youth through training, as paratechnicians are also being successfully promoted by KVKs in collaboration with local NGOs.

Often there is a weak link in the production chain, which could strongly inhibit the overall performance of the system. Strengthening of weak links may have unexpected results. Unlike in the intensive systems in the Netherlands, mentioned earlier, in extensive systems, for example, animals often get too little proteins or lack specific minerals (e.g. phosphate, calcium, magnesium or cobalt). Integration of leguminous or other protein-rich crops and trees into the system and feeding of protein-rich concentrates with added minerals could contribute a lot to improve animal health and production.

In Kenya, Luo farmers had a lack of manure to fertilize the crops. By adopting "zero-grazing" they succeeded in strengthening the livestock component of their integrated crop-livestock system, which then brought the whole system to a higher level of production. However, intensification of indigenous farming systems, e.g. by introduction of zero grazing, has to fit local perceptions, needs and opportunities.

References

- Cox J and Varpama S, 2000. **The 'Livestock Revolution' development or destruction? A report into factory farming in 'developing countries'**. Compassion in World Farming.
- Delgado C, Rosegrant M, Steinfeld H, Ehui S, and Courbois C, 1999. **Livestock to 2020. The next food revolution.** Food, Agriculture and the Environment Discussion Paper 28. IFPRI, FAO and ILCA.
- FAO In: Reuters, 19 Sept. 2001 **Biodiversity shrinks as farm breeds die out.** http://enn.com/news/wire-stories/2001/09/09182001/reu_farm_45000.asp.
- Gueye EF, 2001. **Marketing of family poultry products in Africa to be improved.** World Poultry. Volume 17, No.5.
- Haan C de, Steinfeld H and Backburn H, 1998. **Livestock & the environment: Finding a balance,** FAO, World Bank, USAID.
- LID 1999. **Livestock in poverty focused development.** Livestock in development, Crewkerne, UK.
- Pimentel D, et. al., 1997.**Water resources: agriculture, the environment, and society. An assessment of the status of water resources.** Bio Science Vol. 47, No.2.
- Rangnekar DV, 2001. **Livestock production in rural systems and expected impacts of free trade.** In Vision 2020: Food security from the grassroots perspective. Forum Umwelt and Entwicklung, Bonn, Germany.
- Rathore, Singh H and Kohler-Rollefson I, 2001. **Indigenous institutions for managing livestock genetic diversity in Rajasthan (India)** In Experiences in Farmer's Biodiversity Management. Forum Umwelt and Entwicklung, Bonn, Germany.
- Turner J, 1999. **Factory Farming & The Environment.** A Report by Compassion in World Farming Trust.

27

Fisheries – An Overview

Fisheries deal with aquatic organisms management and procurement from open and with farming of aquatic organisms under control conditions. Aquaculture is the farming of aquatic organisms including fish, molluscs, crustaceans and aquatic plants such as sea weeds. Fisheries and aquaculture production comes from rivers, reservoirs, ponds, oceans, seas, estuaries. Techniques of their biological harvesting and post harvesting have no parallel with any other farming system in the world.

Fisheries fall under two main categories: capture and culture (commonly known as aquaculture). Capture fisheries in the open water are very complex involving different fish population density, their interaction, feeding, breeding, and migration in relation to oceanographic, seas and rivers variables and to the pressure on natural and human exploitation as a common resource. Aquaculture on the other hand is farming of aquatic organisms under controlled conditions to a certain extent and with ownership right. Its productivity is governed in general by the principle of "as you sow so you reap" and its management is highly labour and input dependent.

The method of culturing shrimps/prawns from post-larvae phase into fully grown ones in controlled condition is also known as aquaculture. The term 'shrimp' is used for the variety grown in brackish water and the 'prawn' is used for the variety grown in fresh water. The culturing of shrimps was originally discovered in mid-seventies and this was encouraged in India in the early 1980s as wasteland development in coastal areas. Aquaculture in India has assumed importance as a source of food for fish production and also as a foreign exchange earner. The harvest from the Indian seas has been dwindling over the past several years. Culturing of freshwater fishes, shrimps, prawns and other crustaceans has received a big boost in recent years in the coastal as well as the inland states of India. It has rich and diverse inland water resource. Also, the brackish water areas including estuaries and backwaters have the potential to sustain many of the economically important cultivable species. The landlocked states are becoming more and more important. The future increase in fish production would be mainly in the aquaculture sector.

Fishery sector is also classified as inland fisheries and marine fisheries. For each of these two sub-sectors, there are three major components, viz. capture fisheries, culture fisheries and culture-based capture fisheries. Culture fisheries group included all the activities of raising fish production through human efforts. Under reservoir fisheries stocking of fry or fingerlings in large tanks, reservoirs, and lakes is done to increase fish production for future capture. This chapter gives a broad outline of fisheries sector highlighting the role of the Government in developing fisheries, focus and strategies in the Tenth Five Year Plan, policy issues, role of cooperatives, the economics of rural aquaculture and export prospects of fish and fish products.

FISHERIES RESOURCES

India holds big potential in the fishery sector. The aquatic resources of Indian waters are varied and abundant. The country is endowed with 8,000 kilometers of coastline and 2.02 million square kilometers of perennially clear, mercury free water within the Exclusive Economic Zone (EEZ). The marine resources of the EEZ are comprised of shrimps, lobsters, crabs, tuna, squid, pomfret and most of other varieties of fish. The estuarine resources (2.7 million hectares.) are also substantial with extensive backwater, tidal estuaries, lagoons, and swamps along the entire coastline. In the inland sector, the country has 45,000 kilometers of rivers, 126,334 km network of canals, reservoirs and lakes covering 3.3 million hectares and fresh water ponds and tanks, which are nearly 2.4 million hectares (Tables 27.1 & 27.2). Development of inland fisheries is particularly significant for the rural economy of States such as West Bengal, Bihar and Orissa. The natural resources available for development of marine fisheries are also large and varied. The continental shelf has an area of 0.16 million hectares in the form of narrow belt. Statewise details for Inland Water resources are given in Annexure I.

India now is the 3rd largest producer of fish and second largest producer of fresh water fish in the world.

The fish production during 2002-03 is estimated at 6.05 million tonnes consisting of 3.15 million tones Inland fish and 2.9 million tones Marine fish.

A network of 429 Fish Farmers Development Agencies (FFDAs) have covered all the potential districts in all the States and Union Territory of Pondicherry.

During Ninth Plan about 1.11 lakh hectares of water area was brought under scientific fish farming through FFDAs.

About 6.50 lakh fish farmers/fishermen were trained in improved practices during Ninth Plan.

India has vast and varied fisheries resources both marine and inland. After China, Peru and Japan, as already stated, it is the fourth largest producer of fish in the world and second in inland fish production. The fishery sector provides gainful employment to about 5.96 million full-time

Table 27.1: Inland Fishery Resources

Resources	Area (million hecs.)
Ponds and tanks	2.52
Oxbow lakes & derelict water bodies	1.3
Reservoirs	2.16
Rivers	45,000 km
Canals	1,26,334 km
Estuaries	2.7
Brackishwater	1.69

Table 27.2: Marine Fisheries Resources of India

Sl. No.	State/union territory	Continental shelf ('000 sq. kms)	Number of landing centres	Number of fishing villages	App. length of coast Line (KMS)
1.	Andhra Pradesh	33	508	508	974
2.	Goa	10	88	72	104
3.	Gujarat	164	190	190	1600
4.	Karnataka	27	29	221	300
5.	Kerala (P)	40	226	222	590
6.	Maharashtra	112	184	395	720
7.	Orissa	24	67	589	480
8.	Tamil Nadu	41	362	591	1076
9.	West Bengal	17	65	652	158
10.	Andaman & Nicobar Island (P)	35	57	45	1912
11.	Daman & Diu (P)	-	7	31	27
12.	Lakshadweep (P)	4	11	10	132
13.	Pondicherry	1	28	45	45
	Total	508	1822	3571	8,118

(P) – Provisional

Source: State Governments/Union Territories.

or part-time fishermen. In addition, another 6 million people are engaged in fishery and aquaculture related ancillary activities.[1] Contribution of fisheries sector to Net Domestic Product at current prices increased from Rs. 400 million in 1950/51 to Rs. 201.7 billion in 1998/99. The value of output of the inland and marine fisheries increased from Rs. 650 million and Rs. 680 million in 1950/51 to Rs. 105.9 billion and 152.9 billion respectively in 1998/99.[2] The contribution of this sector to Gross Domestic Product of the country is approximately 1.2 percent.

---

[1]Government of India, Planning Commission: Ninth Five Year Plan (1997-2002), Vol. II: Thematic Issues and Sectoral Programme, p.466. and also NABARD; Development of Fisheries Sectors in India. Website on internet.

[2]Central Statistical Organization: National Accounts Statistics: 2000 and 2001.

Fisheries sector, especially its marine component, has tremendous export potential. According to the recent study carried out by the Policy Research Penang-based Centre, India is expected to boost its foreign exchange earning by seafood exports in the future. The world consumed 130 million tonnes of fish in the year 2000, accounting for 7 percent of global food supplies and providing people with their primary source of animal protein, calcium and vitamin. Globally, fish production is projected to grow around 0.4 percent annually, while the world population is expected to reach 8.5 billion by 2025, compared with 6 billion currently. The study concludes that India will be in a position to increase its exports because its domestic consumption is not likely to grow that fast and that other Asian countries are not expected to be exporters by the year 2020. The study indicated that India is likely to post net exports of 400,000 tonnes annually by the year 2020, slightly less than China's expected exports of 500,000 tonnes.[1]

Growth of Fisheries Sector in India

Share of agriculture and allied activities in the GDP is constantly declining. It has been observed that agriculture sector is gradually diversifying towards high value enterprises including fisheries. It is evident from the contribution of fisheries sector to the GDP, which has gone up from 0.46 per cent in 1950-51 to 1.1 per cent in 1999-2000 (at current prices) (Table 27.3). The share of fisheries in Agricultural GDP (Ag. GDP) has increased more impressively during this period from mere 0.84 per cent to 4.19 per cent. This is largely due to a sustained annual growth rate of well over four per cent in the fisheries GDP during the last five decades. The fisheries sector has recorded faster growth as compared to the agricultural sector in all the decades. The growing production of fish suggests that fisheries sector is booming and contributing to the economic growth of the nation. More than 6 million fishermen and fish farmers are totally dependent on fisheries for their livelihood in India.

Table 27.3: Contribution and Growth of Fisheries Sector in India

Period	Percent contribution to		Percent annual growth	
	GDP	Ag GDP	Fisheries GDP	Ag. DGP
1950-51	0.46	0.84		
1960-61	0.54	1.18	5.63	2.68
1970-71	0.61	1.37	3.92	1.50
1980-81	0.73	1.98	2.86	1.72
1990-91	0.93	3.00	5.11	2.89
1999-00	1.16	4.19	4.75	3.12

Source: National Accounts Statistics, Central Statistical Organization, Government of India.

---

[1]The Economic Times: Fish Exports to Become Major Foreign Exchange Earner for India: 4 Novemebr, 2002.

Fish Production: Structure and Trend

The fisheries production in India during 1950s was more pronounced in the marine fisheries and it remained the major contributor till early 1990s (Table 27.4). Its share in the total fish production was more than 70 per cent in 1960s, but thereafter it started declining and came down to about 62 per cent in 1970s and to 59 per cent in 1980s. In the mid-nineties, the fisheries production witnessed a significant change. The share of inland fish production became almost half of the total fish production in 2000. It seems that marine fisheries production has reached a plateau and at best, it can register only a marginal increase in the near future. On the other hand, inland fish production was on constant rise and its share rose to 38 per cent in 1970s to 41 per cent in 1980s and jumped to over 45 per cent in 1990s. This rise in inland fish production is attributed to the development of aquaculture in our country.

Table 27.4: *Changes in the Structure of Fish Production in India*

(In million tonnes)

Year	Marine	Inland	Total
1950-51	0.53 (71.01)	0.22 (28.99)	0.75
1960-61	0.88 (75.86)	0.28 (24.14)	1.16
1970-71	1.09 (61.85)	0.67 (38.15)	1.76
1980-81	1.5 (59.12)	0.89 (40.88)	2.44
1990-91	2.30 (59.96)	1.54 (40.04)	3.84
1995-96	(2.71 (54.70)	2.24 (45.30)	4.95
1999-00	2.83 (50.09)	2.82 (49.91)	5.66

Figures in parentheses indicate percentage to total.

Source: Hand Book on Fisheries Statistics (2000), Ministry of Agriculture, Government of India.

The growth trends in fisheries production in India during 1980-81 to 1999-2000 is given in Table 27.5. Since 1980-81 fisheries production in India has been increasing at a rate of 5.12 per cent per year. The inland sector has shown a better performance with an annual growth rate of 6.22 per cent. A disaggregated view of the pattern of growth shows that growth in inland fisheries production has accentuated in the 1990s while marine fish production witnessed deceleration. The latter slowed down from 3.73 per cent in the 1980s to 2 per cent in the 1990s. the share of culture fisheries in both freshwater as well as brackish water in the inland sector has increased tremendously in recent years. Within the culture fisheries, the major contributor has been the freshwater aquaculture. The policy for fisheries development has also been given a tilt towards inland fisheries particularly aquaculture in recent years.

Table 27.5: Growth Trend in Fish Production in India

Source of fisheries	Annual compound growth rate during different periods (%)		
	1980-81 to 1989-90	*1990-91 to 1999-00*	*1980-81 to 1999-00*
Marine	3.73	2.01	4.23
Inland	5.14	6.34	6.22
Total	4.30	4.03	5.12

Source: Hand Book on Fisheries Statistics (2000), Ministry of Agriculture, Government of India.

Strategies for Sustainable Fish Production

Intensification of practices, recycling of abundant organic material, comprehensive environmental management, development of genetically superior fish breeds, systematic measures against fish diseases, community aquaculture and financing are prominent strategies to increase fish production. Some of the important approaches for sustainable fish production from freshwater aquaculture sector are:

- Need to develop complete package of technology for different levels of fish production i.e. two tonnes, five tonnes and 100 tonnes per hectare.
- Production of balanced feeds for different stages of finfish and shellfish.
- Demonstration of listed technologies in farmers ponds in different agroclimatic zones.
- Greater role of human resource development and extension with emphasis on training to farmers, entrepreneurs and state fisheries officials.
- Diversification of culture systems with culture of unconventional species like chanos, lates, mugil, anabas, aallago, clarias and singhi need to be promoted.
- Establishment of freshwater prawn hatcheries, especially in west coast of India and also in saline soil belt of inland states.
- Integrated Fish Farming (IFF), practiced in different forms mostly in the East and Southeast Asian countries, is one of the important ecologically balanced sustainable technologies. The technology involves a combination of fish polyculture integrated with crop or livestock production. On-farm waste recycling, an important component of IFF, is highly advantageous to the farmers as it improves the economy of production and decreases the adverse environmental impacts of farming. In order to have sustainable development of brackishwater aquaculture more emphasis has to be given for modified extensive and semi-intensive culture systems with the following measures.
- Geographical Information System (GIS), a system known to integrate geographically referenced spatial and non-spatial data acquired at

different scales, times and in different formats, can be usefully employed in the identification of suitable locations/sites for aquaculture. The criteria for site selections are to be mainly based on physicochemical properties of soil, land use pattern, water quality parameters, species and habitat types.

- Marking of buffer zones between farms to provide enough space for developing discharge systems and sufficient accessibility to sea, drinking water wells etc.
- Identification and demonstration of location specific culture systems.
- Development of economical and eco-friendly feeds.
- Health monitoring, prevention and control of diseases with emphasis on seed certification and quarantine measures.
- Environmental Impact Assessment (EIA) needs to be carried out with a view to promoting eco-friendly technologies.
- Diversification of culture activities involving alternatives species to tiger shrimp like *P. indicus*, *P. merguinsis*, Chanos, mullets, lates, pearl spot, crabs etc.
- An integrated approach utilising knowledge and technology available on quarantine measures, immunostimulants, chemoprophylaxis, genetic resistance of shrimp to disease, Specific Pathogen Free (SPF) shrimps, used together in conjunction with good husbandry and specific farm management appear to be the answer for environmentally and economically sustainable aquaculture.

FISHERIES IN SUCCESSIVE PLANS

The outlay for fisheries sector as percent for the agricultural sector over the Five Year Plans has been increasing continuously (Table 27.6). It increased from 1.74 percent in the First Five Year Plan to about 6 percent in the Ninth Five Year Plan. This shows that greater importance in terms of higher allocation of funds to fisheries sub-sector within agriculture has been accorded. Its share in the total outlay during different plans has been hovering between 0.26 and 0.52 percent. Unfortunately, in the Tenth Five Year Plan separate allocation for the fisheries sector is not given.

The development plans for India's fisheries sector were aimed at increasing the fish production, improving the welfare of fishermen, promoting export and providing food security. The main objectives of the fisheries and aquaculture development progammes under successive Five Year Plans are summarized as follows.

(i) Enhancing the production of fish and the productivity of fishermen, fisherwomen, fish farmers and the fishing industry:

(ii) Generating employment and higher income in fisheries sector:

(iii) Improving the socioeconomic conditions of traditional fisherfolk and fish farmers;

(iv) Augmenting the export of marine, brackish and freshwater fin and shell-fishes and other aquatic species;

Table 27.6 : Outlay for Fisheries Sector During Five Year Plans

(Rs. crores)

Five year plan	Total outlay	Outlay for agricultural sector	Outlay for fisheries sector	Share of fisheries sector (%)	
				Total outlay	Agricultural outlay
First	1960	294	5.13	0.26	1.74
Second	4600	529	12.26	0.27	2.32
Third	7500	1068	28.27	0.38	2.65
Fourth	15902	2728	82.68	0.52	3.03
Fifth	39332	4302	151.24	0.38	3.52
Sixth	97500	6609	371.14	0.38	5.62
Seventh	180000	10524	546.54	0.30	5.19
Eighth	434100	22467	1232.82	0.28	5.49
Ninth	859200	37546	2069.78	0.24	5.51

Source: Government of India: Ministry of Agriculture: Hand Book of Fisheries Statistics (2000).

(v) Increasing per capita availability and consumption of fish;

(vi) Adopting an integrated approach to fisheries and aquacultures, taking into account the need for responsible and sustainable fisheries and aquaculture;

(vii) Conservation of aquatic resources and genetic diversity.

Review of the Ninth Plan

During the last five decades, fish production has increased with an annual growth rate of 4.1 per cent. Fish production touched 5.66 mt in 1999-2000 and was estimated to have remained at the same level in 2000-01. It was assumed to have reached a level of 6.12 mt by the end of the Ninth Plan, which was much below the target of 7.04 mt. This was because of slow progress in the fish production to the extent of 1.44 per cent per annum [marine: (-) 1.32 per cent and inland: 4.87 per cent] during the first four years of the Ninth Plan. At present, resource-wise (reservoirs/rivers/ponds/ tanks etc.) data on fish production and productivity are not available in the country. In the absence of any major initiative for strengthening of infrastructure, fish seed production remained almost static (16,000 million fry per annum) during the first four years of the Ninth Plan.

Inland Fish Production

The share of inland fishery sector in fish production, which was 29 per cent in 1950-51 (0.22 mt), increased to about 50 per cent in 1999-2000 (2.82 mt.) In spite of this, the present level of fish production in the country is about 67 per cent of the estimated potential of 8.4 mt. There is enormous scope both for augmentation of production potential as well as enhancement of productivity in the inland fishery sector. The 429 Fish

Farmers Development Agencies (FFDAs) have covered about 5.67 lakh ha. (inclusive of 1.70 lakh ha. in Ninth Plan). But the average productivity from waters covered under this programme remained almost static at about 2.2 tonnes/ha./year during the Ninth Plan period. States like Andhra Pradesh, Punjab and West Bengal have shown better response and faster development. The highest productivity of about 5 tonnes/ha/annum from FFDA ponds/ tanks has been achieved in Punjab. About 6240 ha. was brought under brackish water aquaculture activities during the Ninth Plan through 39 Brackish Water Fish Farmers Development Agencies (BFDAs). The performance of the programme has also been affected due to litigation.

Marine Fish Production

Marine capture fisheries play a vital role in India's economy. The sector provides employment and income to nearly two million people. Marine fish production eves had risen from 0.53 mt in 1950-51 to 2.81 mt in 2000-01 with a growth rate of 3.43 per cent. Most of the major commercially exploited stocks are showing signs of over exploitation. Problems of juvenile finfish mortality and bycatch discards in with the intensification of shrimp to Plateauing of catches and overfishing a centers and inter sectoral conflicts in the belts have highlighted the need for caution management of coastal fishery resources suitable enforcement mechanisms like uniform ban on fishing during monsoon which is considered the breeding season for majority of commercial species, regulation on craft and gears etc. are the priority issues in the sector to allow for its rational exploitation. The development of the deep-sea fishery industry is of concern to the entire marine fishery sector because it would have considerable impact on the management of near-shore fisheries, shore-based infrastructure utilization and post-harvest activities both for the domestic market and exports. With the growing demand for sea food, it becomes imperative that the current level of marine fish production from the exploited zone to be sustained by closely monitoring the landing and the fishing effort and by strictly implementing the scientific management measures.

Infrastructure

The existing fishing harbours and infrastructures need to be modernized to meet minimum international standards necessary for fish quality assurance. Under the Fisheries Extension & Training Programme 28 training centers and 15 awareness centers were established for the benefit of fishermen and fish farmers during the Ninth Plan. Research projects in the area of aquaculture and marine biotechnology are supported to strengthen the gap in the areas of fish health and disease diagnostics, transgenic aspects, cell and tissue culture, intensive prawn culture, carp-culture, feed and seed production, bio-active compounds and development of culture technology in non-conventional species etc. by the Department of Biotechnology.

Tenth Plan Focus and Strategies

Development of Fisheries

The major thrust during the Tenth Plan will be on integrated development of riverine fisheries, habitat restoration and fisheries development of upland waters, development of upland waters, development of reservoir fisheries, management of coastal fisheries, deep-sea fisheries with equity participation, vertical and horizontal development of aquaculture productivity, infrastructure development and improved post-harvest management, policy intervention including monitoring, control and surveillance. The Tenth Plan has proposed a fish production target of 8.19 mt. envisaging a growth rate of 5.44 per cent per annum (marine 2.5 per cent and inland 8.0 per cent).

Development of Aquaculture

In the recent years, there has been a spurt in the growth of aquaculture in the country. The inland fisheries sector has registered an impressive growth rate of 6.55 percent per annum in the 1990s. However, in spite of the vast resources of culturable water bodies as well as availability of proven technology for aquaculture, the levels of production and productivity are not adequate and there is a large gap between the potential and actual yields. Therefore, increase in productivity and production of fish/shrimps from freshwater and brackish water areas under ongoing programmes would continue during the Tenth Plan. The present production level of about 2.2 tonnes/ha. /year from fish farming will be raised considerably by adopting existing advance technology. Programmes will be devised to develop fisheries in fallow derelict water bodies, waterlogged areas, saline waters, lakes, beels, etc. for enhancing fish production. Aquaculture activities will also be taken up for development of cold-water fisheries in the hill areas of the ecologically fragile zone. On the basis of experience of pilot projects taken up for fisheries development in reservoirs during the terminal year of the Ninth Plan, programme to enhance fish production will be formulated on a large scale during the Tenth Plan. An integrated approach to marine and inland fisheries, designed to rational exploitation and to promote sustainable aquaculture practices, will be adopted. Biotechnological applications in the field of genetics and breeding, hormonal application, immunology and disease control will receive particular attention for increased aquaculture production.

Seed and Feed Development

Seed and feed are critical inputs required for the development of fisheries and aquaculture for enhancing production and productivity. Research and development (R & D) programmes will be taken up for production of quality fish/shrimp seed and feed. The present level of fish seed production of 16,000 million fry will be raised to 25,000 million fry by the end of the Tenth Plan at an 8 per cent growth rate per annum. Diseases-free and diseases-resistant fish/shrimp seed will be ensured with strict quarantine measures. Besides, adequate infrastructure will be required for increasing production and productivity of other commercially important fishes/ prawn such as freshwater prawn, catfish, sea bass, grey mullet, grouper snapper, chanos, etc. for diversifying fishing activities during the Tenth Plan. The Research Institutes under the ICAR like Central Institute of Fisheries Education (CIFE), Mumbai, Central Marine Fisheries Research Institute (CMFRI), Kochi, and Central Institute of Fresh Water Aquaculture (CIFA), Bhubaneswar, have developed technology for pearl culture, which needs to be taken up on a commercial basis through concerted efforts for further development during the Tenth Plan period.

> Enhancing Productivity and Production from Inland Waters. Technical and financial support for enhancing production and productivity. R & D programmes for enhancing production of quality Fish/Shrimp Seed and Feed. Diversification of Activities for Development of Fisheries and Aquaculture. Improving post harvest management by processing, value addition, setting up of cold chains and packaging. Creation of health and sanitary check facilities to ensure quality of products as per international standards. Integrated Approach for Sustainable Development of Fisheries and aquaculture.

The Path Ahead

The main thrust for fisheries development during the Tenth Plan would be to utilize the full potential of inland fishery resources as well as deep seas to increase per capita consumption to a substantial level from the present level of 9 kg. per head per annum. Special emphasis will be given on[1]:

- Increasing the depth of fishing harbours especially for small fishermen using dredgers and the upgradation of hygienic conditions there.
- Strengthening of data base and information networking in the fisheries sector for standardization of methodologies and estimation of catch from diverse aquatic resources.
- Aquaculture and development of capture fisheries of inland water resources.
- Measures will be taken to increase fish production from the deep sea marine sector.
- Infrastructure development, post harvest management for marketing by setting up of model fish markets and establishment of cold chain through viable fishermen cooperatives.
- Popularisation of pearls developed by CIFA, CMFRI etc. and value added products developed by the Central Institute of Fisheries

---

[1]Government of India: Planning Commission: Tenth Five Year Plan: 2002-2007: Sector Policies and Programmes: Vol.II: pp. 579-580.

Technology (CIFT), Kochi and Integrated Fisheries Project (IFP), Kochi made out of low value fish with suitable credit/subsidy support.

- Welfare measures for fishers will be strengthened to ensure their safety at sea etc. and also to involve more women in fisheries sector.
- Research & technology needs in fisheries institutes to be upgraded to meet the growing demands.
- Formulation of a comprehensive deep sea fishing policy and passing of the Aquaculture Authority Bill in Parliament to be expedited for rational exploitation of deep sea fishery resources and sustainable aquaculture development.
- Strategy for an effective enforcement mechanism is needed to prevent poaching in the EEZ and thereby safeguard our resources.
- Suitable mariculture programmes needed to be undertaken for commercially important fin/shell fish species for replenishment of resources in our seas.
- Setting up of disease control laboratories and quality certification centers to ensure international standards for fishery products.
- Technologically improved fishing boats with proper communication network etc. to be introduced for the benefit of small fishermen.

Policy Issues

The national policy on fisheries development generally stresses on optimal utilization of natural resources through their rational exploitation, the concept of giving a better deal to socially backward communities, providing more and better employment opportunities, and increasing aquatic productivity on a sustainable basis.

The national development programmes include organization of necessary infrastructure for fish production, storage and distribution, and mobilization of manpower at various levels for production and marketing, thereby accruing maximum assured benefits to the producer and consumer, reducing middle level involvement to the minimum. Earning of foreign exchange through export of fishery products, without adversely affecting domestic requirements is also an integral part of national programme.

Production programmes for inland fisheries include collection/production of spawn, distribution of fry and fingerlings, establishment of nursery areas, reclamation of derelict water areas for fish farming and development of reservoir fisheries. Programmes were also launched to bring a large area under intensive pisciculture and stocking of big area of brackish water with suitable species. In the marine sector, the most important programme related to the mechanization of boasts, introduction of trawler and large fishing crafts for deep sea fishing, establishment of deep sea fishing stations and procurement of survey vessels. Other programmes included provision of landing and berthing faculties, both at major and minor harbours. Under various Five year plans, under the public sector progammes, composite refrigeration plants, ice plants and cold storages were set up and refrigerated rail vans introduced. In the field of research a number of ICAR institutes were strengthened and a number of All-India Coordinated Research Projects under the supervision of Indian Council of Agriculture Research were launched.

One of the serious handicaps in the development of fisheries has been the absence of a proper marketing system. In various plans measures were taken to review the role of the Central and State Fisheries Corporations and where necessary these organizations were strengthened. Cooperative fishermen's federations were promoted enabling to play a more important role.

DEVELOPMENT OF INLAND FISHERIES AND AQUACULTURE

Thrust Area

Fishery is a State subject and as such the primary responsibility for development rests with the State Governments. The major thrust in fisheries development, as stated above, has been on optimizing production and productivity augmenting, export of marine products, generating employment and improving welfare of fishermen and their socioeconomic status.

Under the successive Five Year Plans special efforts have been made to promote extensive and intensive fish farming activity in the inland sector through modernization of coastal fisheries, and by giving encouragement to deep-sea fishing through joint ventures, etc. For exploitation of the fishery resources from the sea, the country has a fleet, which includes 181,000 country boats, 35,000 mechanized boats, nearly 400 purse-seiners and 174 fishing vessels including a few tuna long liners. A quantum jump in marine fishery production in recent years was possible through speedy modernization of traditional fishing craft with added incentive provided for reimbursement of central excise duty on high speed diesel oil used by the mechanized boats and introduction of larger vessels besides banning of bulk trawling of chartered foreign fishing vessels. Landing and berthing facilities were increased and constant efforts were being made to build infrastructure and promote exports. Lately, the country has embarked upon a big programme to develop brackish water fishery. When fully developed, this may also cover an area of about 1 million hectares.

During the last few plans tremendous development has taken place in the fishery sector. In the inland fishery sector, fish farmer development agencies have been created and the inland fish production has increased. The introduction of a World Bank Project covering five states helped in developing inland fisheries, particularly the seed production. Of the total inland fish production estimated at 2.85 million tonnes, about 60 per cent is contributed by the pond culture sector. The country has launched a big programme to develop brackish water fishery. Special emphasis has been put on riverine fisheries, reservoir fisheries, wetland fisheries, and estuarine fisheries.

Scheme of motorization of traditional craft was launched during the VII Five-Year Plan. Initially a subsidy of Rs. 7,500 given per outboard motor (OBM) was subsequently increased to Rs. 10,000 and later to Rs. 12,000 per inboard motor (IBM). The Centre and the State governments equally shared the subsidy. Out of about 2,10,000 traditional crafts in the country at present, nearly 33,000 have been motorised so far ever since the inception of the scheme during the 7th Five Year Plan. The total Central share of subsidy provided under the scheme so far is Rs. 16.63 crores. The evaluation of the scheme through the Tropical Fisheries Consultancy Services (TFCS), New Delhi revealed that the scheme had been a boon for traditional fishermen. The subsidy was enhanced to Rs. 30,000 for diesel run OBM and Rs. 25,000 for kerosene OBM.

A new component of chemical treatment of Catamarans has also been incorporated in the revised scheme with a subsidy of Rs. 4,800 per unit, the scheme has been revised with a total cost of Rs. 38 crores including Rs. 10.64 crores as central subsidy to motorize about 12,000 additional crafts.

The vision statement of DAHD (Dept. of Animal Husbandry and Dairying) envisages motorizing 60 per cent of the traditional craft in the next ten years and to cover 15 per cent of the existing craft with communication equipment.

A National Welfare Fund for fishermen established during 1984-85 promotes housing scheme, water supply, health, recreation, education and old age pension in selected villages.

For achieving accelerated growth and enhancing production and productivity of fish and marine products, 17 plan schemes were implemented during Ninth Plan. The two schemes namely, Assistance to coast Guard and World Bank Aided Project on Shrimp and Fish Culture have been discontinued during 10th plan on the recommendation of the Planning Commission. It has been decided to merge the remaining schemes into six major schemes for Tenth Plan as a sequel to the Zero Based Budget Exercise for convergence/merging macro-management and on the recommendations of the Working Group on Fisheries. National Scheme on Welfare of Fishermen and Central Sector Scheme on Training and Extension are now being implemented. The Scheme on Inland Fisheries Statistics is being revised for the Tenth Plan. The existing schemes on Development of Freshwater Aquaculture and Establishment of Fishing Harbours and Fish Landing Centres, which are being merged with other components under macro-management mode, are also being continued.

In the Ninth Five Year Plan the ongoing scheme of Development of Freshwater Aquaculture and Integrated Coastal Aquaculture were combined with four new programmes, viz. Development of Cold water Fish Culture; Development of Waterlogged Areas and Derelict water bodies into Aquaculture Estate; Utilization of Inland Saline.

Alkaline Soil for Aquaculture and Programme for Augmenting the Productivity of Reservoirs. This scheme has two components – Aquaculture and Inland Capture Fisheries. The details of the various subcomponents are as under.

Aquaculture – It has following subcomponents:
(a) Development of Freshwater Aquaculture
(b) Development of Brackishwater Aquaculture
(c) Development of Cold Water Fisheries and Aquaculture in Hilly Regions
(d) Development of Waterlogged Areas into Aquaculture Estates
(e) Utilization of Inland Saline/Alkaline Soils for Aquaculture

These schemes are also being continued during the Tenth Five Year Plan period.

Development of Freshwater Aquaculture

In recognition of the increasing role of inland fisheries in overall fish production, the Government of India has been implementing two important progammes in the inland freshwater sector since the Fifth/Sixth Plans. These are the Fish Farmers' Development Agencies (FFDAs) and the National Programme for Fish Seed Development. A network of 429 FFDAs is currently functioning covering all potential districts in the country. A large water area has been brought under the intensive fish culture through the efforts of these FFDAs. Under the national programme for fish seed production, more than 50 fish seed hatcheries have been commissioned. It has led to a marked improvement in the production of fish seed. Their production having increased from 409 million fry in 1973 to about 20000 million in 1999/2000. Some Brackishwater Fish Farmers Development Agencies (BFFDAs) have also been established in the coastal areas of the country; these provide a compact package of technical, financial and extension support to shrimp farmers.

Generally production targets set in different plans have not been achieved. For instance, as already mentioned, fish production at the end of Ninth Plan (1997-2002) was likely to reach 6.12 millions tonnes, which was much below the target of 7.04 million tonnes. This was because of slow progress in fish production to the extent of 1.44 percent per annum (marine (-) 1.32 percent and inland: 4.87 percent) during the first four years of the Ninth Plan. At present resource-wise (reservoirs/rivers/ponds/tanks/etc.) data on fish production and productivity are not available in the country. In the absence of any major initiative for strengthening of infrastructure, fish seed production remained almost static (16 billion fry per year) during the first four years of the Ninth Plan.

During 2001-2002 about 32,544 hectare of water area was brought under scientific fish farming through FFDAs. These agencies have trained 48,296 fish farmers/fishermen in improved practices during the same year and scheme has benefited about 59,937 persons. During 2002-03, through assistance to FFDAs an additional area of 30,000 ha was expected to be brought under scientific fish culture. About 20,000 fish farmers were expected to have been trained in improved practices of fish farming by FFDAs during the year.

Programmes for Development of Marine Fisheries

The programmes for development of marine fisheries as envisaged in different Five Year Plans include: (i) intensive surveys particularly of exclusive economic zone (EEZ), on marine fishery resource assessment, (ii) optimum exploitation of marine resources through a judicious mix of traditional country boats, mechanised boats and deep-sea fish vessels by completing the ongoing construction of major and minor fishing harbours, (iii) intensifying efforts on processing, storage and transportation, (iv) improving marketing particularly in the cooperative sector and (v) tapping the vast potential for export of marine products. The major developments include construction of 30 minor fishing harbours and 130 fish landing centres apart form five major fishing harbours, viz., Cochin, Chennai, Visakhapatnam, Roychowk and Paradip. The Government also provide subsidy to poor fishermen for motorizing their traditional crafts, which increases the fishing area and the frequency of operation with a consequent increase in catch and earnings of fishermen.

Welfare Programmes for Fishermen

This scheme has the following three components:-
   (i) Development of Model Fishermen Villages
   (ii) Group Accident Insurance Scheme for Active Fishermen
   (iii) Saving-sum-relief Scheme

Development of Model Fishermen Villages

The objective of the component is to provide basic civic amenities such as housing, drinking water and construction of community hall for fishermen villages. A fishermen village may consist of not less than 10 houses. There is no upper limit for the number of houses to be constructed in a village, which would depend on the number of eligible fishermen in that village. The village would be provided with tube wells at the rate of one tube well for every 20 houses. As recreation and common working place, a fishermen village with at least 75 houses is eligible to avail financial assistance for construction of a community hall. Unit costs under the scheme have been revised from 2000-01 as Rs. 40,000/- for houses, Rs. 30,000/- for a tube-well (Rs. 35,000 for North Eastern Region) and Rs. 1,75,000 for community hall. The expenditure is shared equally between Central and State Government. In case of Union Territories, the expenditure is fully borne by the Centre.

Group Accident Insurance Scheme for Active Fishermen

The objective of this component is to provide insurance to cover fishermen engaged actively in fishing. Such active fishermen are insured for

Rs. 50,000/- for one year against death or permanent disability and Rs. 25,000/- for partial disability. The upper limit for insurance premium is Rs. 15/- per head. The 50% of the annual premium is subsidized as grants in aid by the Centre and remaining 50% by State Governments. In case of Union Territory 100% premium is borne by the Government of India. A single policy has been taken in respect of all those States/Union Territories who are participating through FISHCOPFED.

Saving-cum-Relief Scheme

The objective of this component is to provide financial assistance to fishermen during lean fishing season. Under this component, beneficiary has to contribute a part of their earning during non-lean months. The monthly contribution of marine fishermen is Rs. 75 for eight months, while that of inland fishermen is Rs. 50/- for nine months. A matching amount is provided with equal contribution from Central and State Governments and the accumulated amount is distributed back to fishermen in four/three equal instalments at the rate of Rs. 300/- per month to marine/inland fishermen. In case of UTs, entire matching share is borne by the Central Government.

Programmes with International Aid

Several international organizations, including the World Bank, UNDP, FAO, DANIDA, NORAD, ODA (UK and Japan) provide aid to India for the development of fisheries sector. Under the Bay of Bengal Programme (BOBP), started in 1979, assistance was provided for the development of small-scale fisheries and enhancing the socioeconomic conditions of the fishing communities. ODA (UK) provided technical aid for the prevention of post –harvest losses in marine fisheries. The FAO has launched a scheme for providing technical assistance to implement Hazard Analysis Critical Control Points (HACCP) in seafood processing industries. A shrimp and Fish Culture Project was started with the assistance of the World Bank in May 1992 and it continued for a period up to December 1999. The states of Andhra Pradesh, Bihar, Orissa, Uttar Pradesh and West Bengal were covered under this project. Six sites covering a brackish water area of 797 ha have been developed for shrimp culture operations. A total of 101 reservoirs and 22 oxbow lakes have been developed for fish culture

Environmental Issues

Loss of productivity and of water from fallow ponds is of great concern in India. With the availability of adequate sunlight, aquatic ecosystem has the potential for a sustained rate of assimilation as high as 4 to 8 g biomass/m^2/day or about 30 tonnes of dry weight/ha/yr. If this productivity is not optimally utilized through aquaculture, it disrupts the aquatic environment and with continued nutrient run off from the catchment, results into obnoxious weed infestation. It is important to note that animal waste in the form of urine and excreta of large number of cattle, buffalos, goats, pigs and poultry, continually find their way to aquatic ecosystem in the country.

Aquatic ecosystem shows first sign of disruption when the amount of its oxygen production does not keep pace with its requirements. Scientific fish culture management improves the oxygen imbalance, otherwise, reduction stage sets in the ecosystem and considerable amount of hydrogen sulphide and methane are produced.

Gradual appearance of aquatic weed form submerged to emergent variety normally shows highly distressed condition of ecosystem. Because of such weeds, increasing amount of silt is trapped, adversely affecting the total volume of the ecosystem and its carrying capacity. The most noxious weed like water hyacinth starts flourishing. In India 60-70 percent of inland water is presently infested with aquatic weed predominantly by water hyacinth.

Considering the capacity of growth and regeneration of water hyacinth, loss of water from the ecosystem is enormous. It registers 5 percent gain in weight every day. Two parent plants produce about 30 offspring in 23 days resulting in 12, 000 plants, with a total weight of 470 tons in 4 months. At least 80 percent of the plant body constitutes water, i.e., 376 tonnes of water is contained in 470 tonnes of water hyacinth. Added to this, loss through transpiration is also considerable and many-folds of their normal evaporation from the aquatic system.

Although India is not among the 26 countries of the world, which have been declared water stressed, it cannot afford to lose such an amount of freshwater from the ecosystem. In fact, it faces the challenges of water scarcity, the per capita availability of water in the country is l/3 compared to two decades ago. Also in many places the water table has gone down from 8 meters to 48 meters now.

Because of poor productivity management and eutrophication, aquatic ecosystem to a large extent are stressed and disrupted in the country. Wherever fish culture is taken scientifically, it improves and maintains the oxygen balance, which is the lifeline of the ecosystem. Thus fish is to be viewed as a major ecological player and fish culture as a major tool to improve and restore the aquatic ecosystem.

Environmental Consequences of Brackishwater Aquaculture

Loss of Mangrove

A great concern has been shown towards loss of mangrove in India because of shrimp farming. A rough estimate indicates that in Andhra Pradesh, the maximum loss of mangroves towards shrimp farming is 8,000 ha, accounting for about 40 percent. Whereas Orissa and Tamil Nadu have lost about 4,000 ha (26%) and 4, 000 ha (26%) respectively. In West Bengal, a total of about 5,000 ha out of a total of 420,000 ha i.e. about l.25 percent of mangrove areas in the Sunderbans have been cleared for shrimp farms.

Loss of Biodiversity

The shrimp culture industry initially relied heavily on wild seed, which resulted in a very serious threat to the natural populations of fish and shellfish in estuaries and rivers. It has been estimated that 18 post larvae of other species of shrimp and fish are sacrificed for every post larva of *P. monodon* collected from the wild. In West Bengal, total annual harvest of wild shrimp seed was around 400 million, causing destruction of billions of other fish and shrimps. This is a colossal loss of biodiversity. However, now the situation is improving fast because of the establishment of shrimp hatcheries.

Conversion of Agricultural Land

No detailed survey is yet undertaken to see the trend of conversion of agricultural land. But a rough estimate indicates that in Andhra Pradesh, about 4, 000 ha (about 1.5 percent) of paddy fields have been converted into shrimp farms. This is followed by 2,000 ha (0.5 percent) in Orissa and 800 ha (0.8 percent) in Tamil Nadu. The trend of such conversion is not very desirable, however it should not be viewed as an alarming situation particularly when the total coastal saline soil of the country amounts to 3.1 million ha. Further, there are reports that about 800–1,200 ha of saltpans have also been converted into shrimp farms in the State of Andhra Pradesh.

Salinization of Potable Water

Salinization of fresh water has been reported because of heavy consumption of ground water for shrimp farming. Freshwater wells have been reported to have turned saline in Nellore, Krishna and west Godavari districts in Andhra Pradesh.

Nutrient Loading

Nutrient loading is yet another problem which has been encountered in semi intensive and intensive culture mainly because of high protein food. As much as 7.5 percent of N and 80 percent of P from feed are wasted and enter the environment. A rough estimate puts it as one tonne of *P. monodon* production results in a loading of 57.31-118.1 kg of N and 13.0-24.4 Kg of P in the pond, causing unmanageable self-pollution.

Study undertaken by the National Environmental Engineering Research Institute (NEERI), Nagpur, on the socioeconomic condition of the farmers in Andhra Pradesh and Tamil Nadu, suggested that the cost of the ecological and social damage had exceeded the benefits that had accrued to the farmers due to adoption of shrimp aquaculture activities. The validity of the findings needs proper evaluation. Many seriously doubt such inference. Some fisheries experts have clarified many of the points raised regarding pollution being caused by shrimp farming. However, the Government of India acted immediately and formulated guidelines for sustainable aquaculture and also created a regulatory and monitoring body known as Aquaculture Authority of India to regulate and oversee the desirable development of aquaculture.

It is important to note that paddy-shrimp culture and extensive system of shrimp farming are environmentally compatible. The problems start with intensification and multiplication to the farms without giving serious thought of the implications.

Loss Due to Sub-Optimal Production

Loss due to suboptimal production becomes very important in the context of rural aquaculture. It should be viewed seriously and all attempts should be made to improve the productivity under traditional culture. For example, about 33, 000 ha. in West Bengal is under the traditional method of shrimp cultivation, with production range of 70-215 kg./ha/yr., average 186 kg/h/yr. This is about 714 kg/ha/yr less than the production obtained in Kerala under traditional culture, i.e. 900 kg./ha. Considering the total bheri area available in West Bengal this low average production amounts to loss of 23, 562 tonnes equal to financial loss of Rs. 4, 712 million.[1]

Similarly, in the States of Karnataka, Maharashtra, and Gujarat the average production is in the range of 100-340 kg./ha/yr. Taking into account the area available in three States, the production revenue loss is very significant. Thus, there is a strong justification to raise the shrimp production level under the traditional culture system in these States, so as to reach 900 kg/ha/yr as in Kerala.

Environmental Impact Assessment

The aquatic resources management and exploitation, except marine resources, are under the state governments control. The Central Government, however, provides overall guidance and suggestion for impact analysis of all the projects having an impact on the natural resources or on people's habitat. Aquaculture projects should not violate any customary right and rights guaranteed by the constitution particularly about water resources. The people can challenge the execution of projects on grounds of violation of fundamental right guaranteed under Article 19(1) (g) of the Constitution. Environment assessment (EA) is not yet mandatory for all aquaculture projects. The Ministry of Environment, Government of India, on a case basis examines individual project on its merit to determine whether EA will be required. Certain states have Land Use Board or their own Environment Department, which review the project environmentally. But the Aquaculture Authority of India requires EA of large aquaculture projects.

In many areas of the world, aquaculture development is constrained due to increasing aquatic pollution from various industries such as distilleries, rayon, rubber, paper and pulp, textiles, tanneries, chemicals, fertilizers and thermal plants. The farmers use antibiotics indiscriminately causing nutrient deficiency. Taking advantage of the present situation, some unscrupulous businessmen are gearing up to purchase the prawns at low prices. The

---

[1]V.R.P. Sinha: Rural Aquaculture in India: RAPA Publication 1999/21, p.

Marine Production & Export Development Authority (MPEDA), which is supposed to protect the interests of aqua-farmers, is also in a helpless condition. The white spot viral infection has crippled aquaculture in many states. The farmers have not recovered from the heavy loss. The viral infection has become a perennial problem.

In Andhra Pradesh, the deadly disease affected the booming aquaculture for the first time in 1994-95, killing the shrimp population on a massive scale. The ponds became lifeless overnight with dead prawns floating on the surface. The situation worsened with the stoppage of foreign exports. The mother prawns imported from Taiwan and Malaysia were suspected to have transmitted the virus vertically to the offspring.

It is learnt that some merchants had exported substandard prawns to other countries recently, which were promptly rejected, throwing the industry into the crisis. India mainly exports prawns to USA, Japan, Singapore and European countries. Aquaculture doesn't adversely affect the environment. In fact, aquaculture merges and interacts with the environment. It utilizes the resources and causes only slight environmental changes. Most interactions have beneficial effects. The demand for good-quality water for aquaculture may encourage the prevention of pollution from other sources.

Experts say that compared to other industries, pollution from aquaculture is negligible. Reclamation of fallow lands for aquaculture may also be beneficial to human health by serving to eliminate many disease vectors, especially mosquitoes which flourish in such unutilized swamps. Some states have initiated measures to mitigate the impending ruin. Among the measures considered are restricting the shrimp crop to one in a year and curtailing the size of the crop to 50,000 shrimps per hectare.

The twin measures are intended to reduce the incidence of infection, as a long gap between crops would prevent horizontal transmission of the disease through water.

The Andhra Pradesh government has drafted a legislation that will empower the fisheries department to take punitive action against those who sell infected mother prawns. Priority should be given to identification of suitable locations/sites for aquaculture. It should be based on physicochemical properties of soil, land use pattern, water quality parameters, species and habitat types. Development of economical and eco-friendly feeds is also important. Environmental impact assessment should be carried out with a view to promoting eco-friendly technologies.

ROLE OF FISHERIES COOPERATIVES IN INDIA

Cooperatives are the shield of the weak and in India fishermen are among the weakest sections of the community. Illiteracy, poverty, and lack of knowledge of latest fisheries technology are contributing factors. This vicious circle is further strengthened by lack of institutional support, both in infrastructure and finances. Consequently, the middlemen, who act as moneylenders, traders and contractors, exploit fishermen.. A number of factors have hampered the growth of cooperative societies, the more important of these being: (a) fishermen do not generally own boats, nets and other fishing equipment. In consequence, middlemen, who provide credit, bind fishermen to work on their boats. For allowing the use of the boat, as much as 50 percent of the net sale proceeds is recovered as charge for hire; and (b) cooperative societies which are previously engaged in providing credit, did not make adequate efforts to develop production and market.

Fishermen discovered cooperatives could spare them from exploitation and improve their socioeconomic conditions. Formation and running of fisheries cooperatives formed an important aspect of fisheries development under the various Five Year Plans. However, efforts made in this direction though have yielded good results in some areas, but the overall picture of fishery cooperatives is not encouraging.

The fishery cooperative movement in India began in 1913 when the first fishermen's society was organized under the name of 'Karla Machhimar (Fishermen) Cooperative Society' in Maharashtra. The state of West Bengal was the next to organize cooperative societies in the fishery sector in 1918. In the same year, Tamil Nadu also organized one cooperative society. Revitalization of the existing fisheries cooperatives and their further development and linking up with marketing and processing cooperatives was an important task carried out under the development Five Year Plans. Thus, the cooperative structure grew over years into multifunctional units at the primary level, federations at district/regional, state and national levels. Currently the following Federations and Primary Societies are operating. The membership at the primary level is 0.95 million.

- National Level Federation   1
- State Level Federations   17
- Central (District/ Regional
- Level Federations   108
- Primary Societies   9,369

A study conducted by the Council for Social Development confirmed the suitability of the fishery cooperatives as a tool for promoting the interests of fishermen. The study also emphasized the need for, "organizing active fishermen into cooperatives and for strengthening and encouraging the fishermen's cooperative societies for performance of multipurpose functions and social interest of their members". To ensure that a well-knit structure of fishery cooperatives is created in the country, the study recommended that, multifunctional primary cooperatives could be retained.

In some of the states, the fishery cooperative movement is working very effectively and a number of evaluations have confirmed the efficiency of these organizations. One evaluation confirmed that arrangements of marketing made by the fishery cooperatives in the states of Maharashtra save the members from exploitation. A number of fishery cooperatives in the country are helping their members and their family members to the extent of providing complete marketing infrastructure for the sale of the catch at remunerative prices.

National Federation of Fishermen's Cooperatives

National Federation of Fishermen's Cooperatives Ltd., (FISHCOPFED) began in 1982. Its goal is to facilitate the fishing industry in India through cooperatives. Within a short period of its active functioning, FISHCOPFED carried out a number of activities, both business and promotional, including organizing conferences, supporting training initiatives, facilitating exchanges, demonstrating new technologies, introducing marketing techniques, liaising with member organizations, and providing health care and insurance programmes.

Problems and Solutions in the Fishery Cooperative Sector[1]

The fisheries cooperative sector in India faces many crucial problems. Existing cooperative law does not support fisheries cooperative development. Countries like Japan and South Korea have special enactments, which guarantee allotment of fishing waters to fisheries cooperatives and ensure membership of genuine active fishermen.

In most of states special provisions in the Cooperative Societies Act or a separate Act for Cooperative Land Development Banks (now known as Agricultural and Rural Development Banks) exist. In order to promote fisheries, the State Governments should formulate separate provisions for fisheries cooperatives within the Act or enact separate legislation to allot water bodies and avoid overlapping operation, finances, and structural linkages among fisheries cooperatives in the state.

Those states, which have not yet organized a federation of fisheries cooperatives, should begin one with sufficient equity to take up business and promotional activities for fisheries cooperatives in the state. Existing state level federations must be activated.

At the regional level, the gap is very wide in these states. In light of the establishment of fish farmer development agencies inland and brackish water fisheries, it is necessary to organize regional/district level fisheries cooperative federations to provide inputs, operational inputs, harvesting and marketing support to the members of primary fisheries cooperatives and fish farmers.

At the primary level in most states fisheries cooperatives overlap. This results in unhealthy competition between them, particularly for water bodies. State governments should take necessary steps to correct this, and to

---

[1]Mishra, B.K.: Fisheries Co-operatives in India: Co-op Dialogue, vol.7, No.2, May-August, 1997: p.28.

organise/re-organise the existing primary level fishery cooperatives. They should also issue clear-cut instructions to allot water bodies to reorganized cooperatives so that they may have necessary fishing water to provide employment to their members.

In the marine sector, the primary fisheries cooperatives should be strengthened with infrastructure facilities like landing centres, market yards, roads, transport facilities. Fisheries cooperatives should be given necessary support to pull their catch and have access to strong export infrastructure with qualified staff.

The National Cooperative Development Corporation has revised its pattern of assistance to fisheries cooperatives. Poverty in fishing communities in the country necessitates liberalization of norms for fisheries cooperatives and provide support through low interest rates.

Women play a very important role in fisheries cooperatives. Once the fishermen bring in the catch, their job begins. Cooperative law does not allow membership of both husband and wife, which prevents women from participating in the management of the fisheries cooperatives. Women involved in the fishery must participate in the management of fisheries cooperatives. The Ardhanareeswaran Committee has recommended joint membership of husband and wife in cooperatives. This should be implemented.

Cooperative banks and other financial institutions have not helped to develop fisheries cooperatives in most of the states. Financial aid is often not available where it is needed, like payment of lease money, welfare and credit. NABARD should take immediate steps to encourage cooperative banks to provide credit to fisheries cooperatives where it will be most effective.

To market fish profitably, ensuring a fair price for both producers and consumers, cooperative marketing in India must be strengthened. For this purpose, marketing infrastructure must be developed. Funding for infrastructure should be provided by central, state and local bodies, then handed over the management to fisheries cooperatives.

There is a need for coordination and cooperation between the Government of India and state governments to achieve continued growth in the fishery cooperative sector, which is so vital to the economy and poor people.

ROLE OF NATIONAL BANK FOR AGRICULTURE AND RURAL DEVELOPMENT

In view of the importance of the sector in the national economy, the National Bank for Agriculture and Rural Development (NABARD) has played a pivotal role in the development of the sector. The Bank has so far provided refinance assistance to the tune of Rs. 6,132 million. All the activities subject to their techno-economic feasibility are covered under NABARD's refinance assistance. An illustrative list is given below.

I. Marine Fisheries
A. Capture Fisheries -
Traditional boats: Motorization of traditional crafts: Mechanized fishing vessels: and Deep sea fishing
B. Culture Fisheries
Mariculture in coastal waters: Open sea culture in cages, etc.

II. Inland Fisheries
A. Capture Fisheries -
Crafts/gears for fishing in reservoirs/rivers:
B. Culture Fisheries:
Composite fish culture: Fish seed hatchery: Culture of air breathing fishes Culture: of trout integrated fish culture: Sewage fed fisheries: Running water fish culture: Ornamental fish breeding : Fresh water prawn hatchery: Monoculture/polyculture of freshwater prawn & fish : and Tilapia culture.

III. Brackish water fisheries:
Shrimp farming in traditions/improved traditional/extensive/modified extensive system shrimp hatchery: Culture of other finfishes like pearl oyster, edible oyster, and mussels.

IV. Ancillary activities (as individual schemes or as integrated units with any of the above activities):
Ice plants and cold storages: Processing and value addition: Ice plants: Feed mill and Net making units.

FISH PROCESSING AND EXPORTS

The preservation and processing infrastructure include 372 freezing plants with capacity of 52.5 tonnes per day, 148 ice making plants with about 1, 800 tonnes capacity per day, 450 cold storage having capacity of over 80,000 tonnes and 15 fish meal plants with about 330 tonnes capacity per day. There are also 900 registered prawn-peeling sheds with a capacity of 2,684 tonnes, which form the preprocessing centres. The capacity utilization of the processing plants at present is hardly 25 percent, mainly because of the shortage of raw materials. Most of the processing factories are old and only a few meet the criteria of the European Union Certification for imports to Europe.

The stringent import policies of many importing countries have also influenced the type and quality of products being exported. Out of the total marine fish landings, only about 15 percent, including cephalopods and crustaceans, is exported. Finfishes constitute the single largest commodity in the seafood export market with major varieties are ribbonfish, pomfrets, seerfishes, mackerel, reef cod, snappers and tunas. The surimi based products; pasteurized crabmeat and live fish (crabs, groupers, lobsters) also offer an immense scope for development. Fresh and frozen mussels are also exported to countries like UAE, Germany and Republic of South Africa. Exports to European countries require certification of the water bodies used for mariculture and the appropriate authority issuing such certificate has to be decided. Production of value added fishery products is also being done, although it is highly capital intensive and advanced processing and packaging technologies are currently insufficient in India.

Quality assurance in fishery has been introduced since 1995 with pre-shipment inspection scheme (Export Quality Control and Inspection Act) and the In Process Quality Control (IPQC) was implemented in early 1978, prescribing the minimum requirements for raw materials, manufacturing processes, end product testing, preservation and packaging of final products. The Hazard Analysis Critical Point (HACCP) with stress on safety was introduced in 1995 and it is the responsibility of the processors to ensure proper hygienic conditions and observe the prescribed standards for seafood exports.

The steps taken by the Government of India to relax the policy on trade and convertibility of Indian Rupee into foreign currencies have resulted in an increase in exports of fish-fishery products. The MPEDA is also conducting numerous promotional efforts, which have benefited exporters of fish and fishery products. In view of the rigorous quality requirements of the European countries, the quality of vigilance and compliance to attain the required international standards are being stepped up. Irradiation process (radurization) for the expansion of shelf-life of fresh fishery products and improvement in microbial safety have been standardized in India and many other countries and would pave the way for the reduced post-harvest losses.[1]

---

[1]Shamsundar B.A. (2001): Fish Processing. In: Sustainable Indian Fisheries, (Pandian, T.J. ed.): National Academy of Agricultural Sciences. Pp. 250-271.

Annexure 1

INLAND WATER RESOURCES OF INDIA

Sl. No.	State/UTs	Rivers & canals (Kms.)	Reservoirs (Lakh Ha.)	Tanks & ponds (Lakh Ha.)	Flood plain Lakes & derelict water (Lakh Ha.)	Brackish water (Lakh ha.)
1.	Andhra Pradesh	13891	2.34	4.63	-	1.50
2.	Arunachal Pradesh	2000	-	2.50	2.00	-
3.	Assam	4820	0.02	0.26	1.27	-
4.	Bihar	2000	0.06	0.64	0.40	-
5.	Chhattisgarh	3573	0.84	0.63	-	1.47
6.	Goa	250	0.03	0.03	-	-
7.	Gujarat	3865	2.43	0.71	0.12	3.76
8.	Haryana	5000	0.09	0.10	-	0.30
9.	Himachal Pradesh	3000	0.42	0.01	-	-
10.	Jammu & Kashmir	27781	0.07	0.25	0.06	-
11.	Jharkhand	1200	0.94	0.29	-	-
12.	Karnataka	9000	2.11	2.90	-	0.08
13.	Kerala	3092	0.30	0.30	2.43	2.43
14.	Madhya Pradesh	17088	2.27	0.60	-	-
15.	Maharashtra	16000	2.79	0.59	-	0.10
16.	Manipur	3360	0.01	0.05	0.04	-
17.	Meghalaya	3194	0.08	0.02	Neg.	-
18.	Mizoram	1750	-	0.02	-	-
19.	Nagaland	1600	0.03	0.50	Neg.	-
20.	Orissa	7219	1.96	1.16	1.80	4.18
21.	Punjab	15270	Neg.	0.07	-	-
22.	Rajasthan (P)	6802	1.20	1.80	-	-
23.	Sikkim	900	1.20	-	0.03	-
24.	Tamil Nadu	7420	0.52	2.56	0.07	0.56
25.	Tripura	1200	0.05	0.13	-	-
26.	Uttar Pradesh	28500	1.38	1.61	1.33	-
27.	Uttaranchal	2686	0.20	Neg.	Neg.	-
28.	West Bengal	2526	0.17	2.76	0.42	2.10
29.	Andaman & Nicobar Islands	115	0.01	0.03	-	0.37
30.	Chandigarh	2	-	Neg.	Neg.	-
31.	Dadra & Nagar Haveli	54	0.05	-	-	-
32.	Daman & Diu	12	-	Neg.	-	Neg.
33.	Delhi	150	0.04	-	-	-
34.	Lakshadweep	-	-	-	-	-
35.	Pondicherry	247	-	Neg.	0.01	0.01
	TOTAL	**195567**	**21.61**	**25.15**	**9.98**	**16.86**

(P) – Provisional

Source: State Governments/Union Territories.

28

Inland Fishery

Inland fishery is defined as inland culture plus aquaculture. The inland fishery system consists of both flowing water (rivers, estuaries and swamps), which is also called freshwater culture fisheries and still water resources (reservoirs, lakes, ponds and brackish water). The inland fishery can therefore be divided into four groups: (a) Freshwater culture fisheries: (b) Reservoir fisheries; (c) Riverine fisheries and (d) Brackish water culture, estuaries, lakes, and swamps. Still water, being within confined area, is more amenable for adoption of culture technology and, therefore, the scope for increased production through development of still water resources is higher. Inland fisheries production subsystem is indicated in Fig. 28.1.

Capture fisheries have been the major source of inland fish production till mid-eighties. But the fish production from natural waters like rivers, lakes, canals, etc., followed a declining trend, primarily due to proliferations

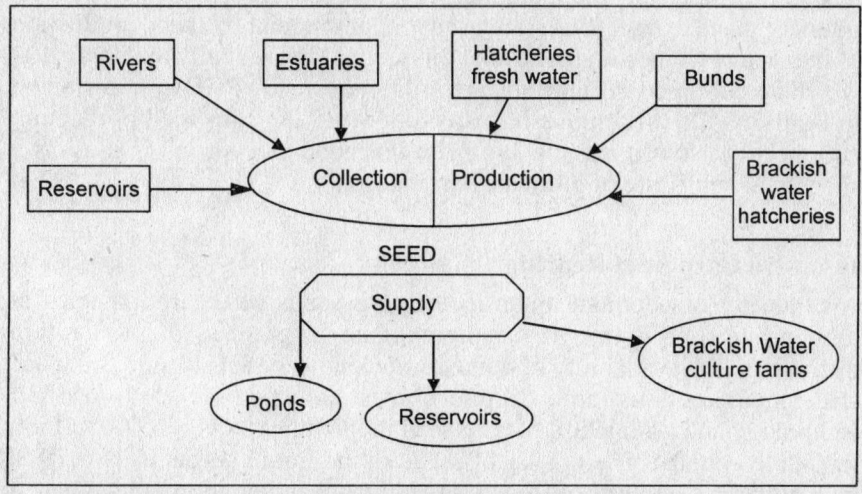

Fig. 28.1

of water control structures, indiscriminate fishing and habitat degradation. The depleting resources, energy crisis and resultant high cost of fishing, etc., have led to an increased realization of the potential and versatility of aquaculture as a viable and cost effective alternative to capture fisheries. During past one and half decade, the inland aquaculture production has increased from 0.51 million tonnes to 2.38 million tonnes, while for inland capture fisheries the same has declined from over 0.59 million tonnes to 0.40 million tonnes. The percentage share of aquaculture has also increased sharply from 46.36 percent to 85.65 percent. It is primarily because of tremendous 4.5 fold increase in freshwater aquaculture. Its share in total inland fish production has also increased from 27.95 percent to 66.4 percent. Still, it has considerable scope for enhancing fish production.

PROGRAMMES FOR DEVELOPMENT OF INLAND FISHERIES

Key Freshwater Aquacultural Technologies

The aquaculture technologies got momentum only in seventies at Central Inland Fisheries Institute (CIFRI), Barrackpore under All India Coordinated Research Project on Composite Fish Culture, Air Breathing Fish Culture, Riverine Seed Prospecting and Fisheries Management of Freshwater Reservoirs. Later, a new coordinated project on brackishwater was framed and implemented. The aquaculture technologies may be categorized into technologies for fish seed production and production of table size fish.

Fish Breeding and Seed Production Induced Breeding

The development of indigenous technique of hypophysation has revolutionized the seed production of major carps. The eco or circular hatcheries, based on the technology of induced breeding of carps with pituitary gland extract (PGE) are used for commercial fish seed production of Indian and Chinese carps. Under this technology sexually mature fishes, which do not breed in captivity, are bred in ponds by PGE to spawn them in captivity. This technique has revolutionized the carp seed production enormously. Nowadays, the synthetic hormone "Ovaprim" is used as a successful substitute of pituitary hormone.

Intensive Carp Seed Rearing

Availability of adequate quantity of carp seeds of desired species at appropriate time is one of the prerequisite for success of aquaculture operations. The availability of standard stocking materials in time and space still remains a constraint, despite domestication of induced breeding technology and production of carp seed to the tune of over 16,500 million fry in the country. The raising of seeds in the initial stages is associated with high rates of mortality due to several management problems. Thus, it is essential to follow standardized package of practices for higher growth and survival in intensive seed raising at higher stockings densities, leading to hypoxic conditions and competition for food space. The technology for intensive seed production includes:

- Eco or circular hatchery or collection of spawn from natural abode;
- R ising the spawn to fry in nursery ponds; and
  Rearing of fry to fingerlings in ponds.

First Farmers Development Agencies

Increasing role of inland fisheries in overall fish production, the Government of India (GOI) has been implementing two important programmes in the inland freshwater sector since the Fifth/Sixth Plans. These are the Fish Farmers' Development Agencies (FFDAs) and the National Programme for Fish Seed Development. A network of about 429 FFDAs is functioning today covering all potential districts in the country. The water area brought under the intensive fish culture through the efforts of these FFDAs was 0.46 million hectares (ha) up to 1997-98. The agencies have trained 0.6 million fish farmers in improved practices. Additionally, about 0.07 million ha. area has been developed for shrimp culture. Some Brackishwater Fish Farmers Development Agencies (BFFDAs) have also been established in the coastal areas of the country; these provide a compact package of technical, financial and extension support to shrimp farmers. Under the national programme for fish seed production, more than 50 fish seed hatcheries have been commissioned. It has led to a marked improvement in the production of fish seed. Their production has increased from 409 million fry in 1973-74 to about 20000 million in 1999-2000.

Fish Breeding

Fish seed is the critical input for successful culture operations and till the sixties a major part of the seed required for culture was being collected from riverine sources. A breakthrough achieved during the fifties in induced breeding through hypophysation gave the thrust to mass production of quality spawn in a controlled environment thereby reducing the dependence on natural seed collection.

Further, the use of various synthetic formulations including the ovaprim, has largely replaced the use of pituitary, making the technology of induced breeding much more farmer-friendly. Improvements in this regard include the administration of a single dose of ovaprim against double dose of pituitary extract reducing the stress on fish as well as the costs. From earthen pits to double-walled hapa hatcheries and associated modifications, carp hatcheries have come a long way from running water glass jars or circular hatcheries. These eco-hatcheries have not only provided the scope to produce and handle mass quantities of eggs during hatching but to a great extent reduced the requirements of water, manpower and economy. Further, the technology of multiple carp breeding has prolonged the normal breeding season of carps and resulted in a quantitative increase in seed production levels.

The development of hatchery technologies of catfish species such as magur (Clarias Batrachus) and singhi (Heteropneustes Fossilis) along with freshwater prawns (Macrobrachium Rosenbergii and M. Malcolmsonii), has opened up possibilities for further expansion of grow-out culture systems. The growing demand for the seeds of these varieties is indicative of the potential of diversification of the freshwater aquaculture industry.

The present and future contribution of inland fisheries, in particular of subsistence fisheries, to food security, while probably under reported, is very significant. In many developing countries including India, in particular, there is a significant scope for enhancing contributions of inland fisheries and aquaculture to food supplies and poverty alleviation. Enhancement techniques in inland fisheries offer good prospects, and small reservoir fisheries have the potential to develop as community-based management initiatives become more widely accepted. However, most fishermen still lack access to adequate technical information as well as institutional and technological support required improving their practices to increase production. One of the greatest threats to the sustainability of inland fisheries resources is environmental degradation and deterioration of wild resources. Public concern about increase in aquatic pollution, destruction of fish habitats, water abstraction and impacts on aquatic biodiversity is high and these trends must be reversed. More information and guidance is urgently needed on protection of living resources in inland waters.

The extensive network of Indian rivers and canals constitute one of the major inland fishery resources of the country besides being the source of the original germplasm. The present day riverine fishery is below the subsistence level with average yield of 0.3 tonne per km, which is only about 15 per cent of their actual potential. Reservoirs form the most important inland open water fishery resource in the country. However, at the present level of management and utilization, the average field yield is only 20 kg/hectare/yr. The three pronged strategy of reservoir fisheries development comprising enlargement of mesh size, balanced fishing effort and sustained stocking support has been paying rich dividends and a production of 50-100 kg/hectare/yr can be realised from large (> 5000 ha) and medium (>1000 to <5000 ha) reservoirs.

The vast floodplain wetlands in the form of oxbow lakes (mauns, chaurs, jheels, bheels – as they are called locally), especially in the states of Assam, West Bengal, Bihar and Eastern Uttar Pradesh, occupy an important position in the inland fisheries resources of India because of their magnitude as well as their production potential. These water bodies are rich in nutrients, as reflected by rich organic carbon and high levels of nitrogen and phosphorus in their soil. The yields of floodplain wetlands can be increased to average one tonne of fish per hectare from the present average yield of 200 kg/ha/yr by following appropriate culture practices. The practices of pen culture are an ideal operation, for exploitation of these resources. The other approaches for sustainable fish production from inland capture fisheries sector include cage culture, ranching of fish seed for higher production, provision of fish passage for migratory species and endemic gnome conservation through fish sanctuaries.

In India there is a considerable scope for increased production of fish through development of still water resources. However, the question of further development depends on the existing unexploited potential of still water resources.

CULTURE PRACTICES

Over the years, the country has standardized a number of culture systems to suit input availability in the region as well as the investment capacities of the farmers. The introduction of scientific composite carp culture technology has virtually revolutionized the aquaculture sector of the country raising the freshwater pond productivity from a subsistence level of 500-600 kg/ha/yr to a national mean level of about two tonnes/ha/yr.[1]

For the resource-poor marginal farmers, a host of culture system involving low levels of inputs have been standardized, such as composite carps culture (4-6 t/ha/yr), sewage-fed fish culture (3-5 t/ha/yr), biogas slurry-fresh fish culture (3-5 t/ha/yr). Further, the integration of poultry, ducks, pigs and other farm animals as also horticulture crops along with fish culture has shown its potential with production levels of 3-5 tonnes of fish/ha/yr, solely with the use of their byproducts.

The development of intensive culture technology with production levels of 10-15 tonnes/ha/yr during recent years is another breakthrough, showing the potential for the vertical expansion of the sector. Given a production estimate 5-6 t/ha/yr during the next decade, the country is expected to increase at least 2-3 folds even with the present area under farming. Further, with the potential perceived by other non-conventional farming practices like cage and pen culture and running water fish culture with production level as high as 100-150 tonnes/ha/yr, freshwater aquaculture provides great scope for industrial enterprises.

The fresh water aquaculture resources in the country comprise of 2.52 million hectares of ponds and tanks, 1.30 million hectares of bheels and derelict waters, 2.05 million hectares of lakes and reservoirs as also 0.12 million kilometers of irrigation canal, and 2.3 million hectares of paddy field. Similarly, brackishwater resources are also vast and varied. The country has a number of lakes, most important of which are the Chilka and Pulicat Lakes and Vemband backwater. An estimated potential area of 1.42 million hectares is available for brackishwater aquaculture. In addition, nearly 2 million hectare salt affected soils exist, having potential to be used for aquaculture.

There is a vast potential available in still water as well as in flowing water resources in India. Aquaculture production has increased three times

---

[1]Ayyappan, S. Fresh Water Aquaculture: Focus on future growth. The Hindu Survey of Indian Agriculture, 1999

during the last decade. Though aquaculture has made very good progress during the last five decades, it is still a very small sub-sector of agriculture. Considering the country's vast potential for aquaculture (both freshwater and coastal), the recent achievements in R&D on various aspects of aquaculture, and the public and private interest in the sub-sector, the future of aquaculture as an economic activity is promising. A Ten-year Brackishwater Shrimp Farming Development Plan with the aim of developing 0.1 million hectares of shrimp farms has been prepared. Similarly, a Five Year National Freshwater Aquaculture Development has been developed with a view to doubling the freshwater aquaculture production to over 3 million tonnes.

Most of the aquaculture activities in India could be regarded as rural aquaculture. Freshwater aquaculture in village tanks and ponds follow the improved traditional or semi-intensive composite culture/polyculture system and they serve the household needs for fish and generate some additional income for the family. Only in recent years, commercial pond fish culture has become very successful in the States of Andhra Pradesh, West Bengal, and Punjab, etc. In brackishwater aquaculture more than half of the total area (l00,000 ha) under shrimp culture is made of small farms following the traditional/improved traditional/extensive system of culture and as such they are considered as rural aquaculture.

Freshwater Aquaculture

Indian freshwater aquaculture has evolved from the stage of domestic activity in West Bengal and Orissa to that of an industry in recent years with States like Andhra Pradesh, Punjab, Haryana and Maharashtra taking up fish culture as a trade. With technological inputs, entrepreneurial initiatives and financial investments, pond productivity has gone up from 600-800 kg/ha/yr to 8-10 tonnes/ha/year in several parts of the country with the national average being around 2000 kg/ha/year.

While carps form the mainstay of Indian freshwater aquaculture, a host of other produce like catfish, fresh water and molluscs for pearl culture are being brought into culture systems. A range of technologies such as pen culture, cage culture, running water fish culture, sewage-fed fish culture, rice-cum fish culture and integrated farming systems have made freshwater aquaculture increasingly popular across the country.

Being mainly organic-based, freshwater aquaculture practices are also able to receive and treat a number of organic wastes, including domestic sewage, enabling eco-restoration. It is significant that the freshwater aquaculture sector contributes 23 per cent to the total fish production of 5.66 million tonnes in the country with an annual growth rate of over 5 per cent and a production potential of 4.5 million tonnes.

Dramatic Growth

During the last 50 years fisheries production in India increased from about 0.75 million tonnes of fish and shellfish in 1950/5l to over 6 million tonnes in 2002/03. The Inland fisheries increased from 0.22 million tones in 1950/51 to 3.15 million tonnes, whereas marine fisheries rose from 0.53 million tonnes to 2.90 million tonnes (Table 28.1). Aquaculture development in the country has been phenomenal with the quantity increasing from 0.79 million tonnes in 1987 to 2.2 million tonnes during 2001. The value rose from $827 million to $2380 million. The share of the inland sector, which was 29 per cent in 1950-51, exceeded 53 percent by 2000-01 and the percentage share of aquaculture in the total inland fish production increased from 18 per cent to 68 per cent during the same period. Two specific aqua produce, carps in fresh water aquaculture and shrimps in brackish water aquaculture, have contributed to the growth of the sector.

Table 28.1: Fish Production in India during 1950-51 to 2000-01

(Million tonnes)

Year	Marine	Inland	Total
1	2	3	4
1950-51	0.53	0.22	0.75
1960-61	0.88	0.28	1.16
1970-71	1.09	0.67	1.76
1980-81	1.56	0.89	2.45
1981-82	1.45	0.99	2.44
1982-83	1.43	0.94	2.37
1983-84	1.52	0.99	2.51
1984-85	1.70	1.10	2.80
1985-86	1.72	1.16	2.88
1986-87	1.71	1.23	2.94
1987-88	1.66	1.30	2.96
1988-89	1.82	1.33	3.15
1989-90	2.28	1.40	3.68
1990-91	2.30	1.54	3.84
1991-92	2.45	1.71	4.16
1992-93	2.57	1.80	4.37
1993-94	2.65	1.99	4.64
1994-95	2.69	2.10	4.79
1995-96	2.71	2.24	4.95
1996-97	2.97	2.38	5.35
1997-98	2.95	2.44	5.39
1998-99	2.69	2.57	5.26
1999-2000	2.85	2.82	5.67
2000-01	2.81	2.85	5.66
2001-02(P)	2.83	3.13	5.96
2002-03 (P)	2.90	3.15	6.05

(P) Provisional

Source: Department of Animal Husbandry and Dairying, Ministry of Agriculture, New Delhi

The world scenario is similar with the aquaculture sector increasingly contributing to the total fish production over the years. It has shown a growth rate of over 9 per cent in the last 10 years. The major increase in global aquaculture production in the last decade has been witnessed by India, China, and Southeast Asia using systems that have already proven to be sustainable. Recognizing the exhaustible nature of marine and inland fisheries, the concepts of stock replenishment and ranching are being discussed to bring in sustainability in these areas. In this context, aquaculture holds great promise for both substantiating and sustaining the fish production levels.

Asian countries continue to be the global leaders in shrimp production, contributing to 80 per cent of the total farmed shrimps. China was the leading country in the 1980s, but later gave way to Thailand, which now produces 155,000 tonnes from an area of 60,000 hectares.

The global market for shrimps increased at 14 per cent per annum between 1984 and 1997, totaling about 941,000 tonnes of shrimps and prawns valued at $6.1 billion, /cultured shrimps and prawns accounted for 27 to 29 per cent in 1991, which increased to 49 per cent by 1999.

Thailand was the world's largest shrimp producer with a output of 266,000 tonnes in 1994, declined to around 215,000 tonnes in 1997 due to disease outbreak, but stabilized in 1998. India emerged as the second largest exporter of shrimps and prawns in 2001-02 recording 127,576 million tonnes of exports, relegating Indonesia to third position. Three-fourth of global shrimp production is located in Asia.

The freshwater aquaculture resources in the country as already discussed above, are immense. India being basically a carp country, indigenous and exotic carps (catla, rohu, mrigal, kalbasu, silver carp, grass carp, common carp) account for 82 percent of the total production. Several other medium and minor carps such as *Labeo fimbriatus*, *Labeo ganius*, *Labeo bata* besides *Oxygaster spp.*, *Rasbora spp. Cirrhinus cirrhosa*, *Puntius kolus*, *Puntius carnaticus*, *Puntius sarana*, *Puntius sophore*, *Puntius ticto and Amblypharyngodon mola* have high regional demand.

While large non-air breathing catfishes such as *Wallago attu, Mystus seenghala, Mystus aor, Pangasius, Rita pavimentata* are in great demand in northern and northwestern States, the smaller varieties of both air breathing (*Clarias Batrachus, Heteropneustes Fossils*) and non-air breathing fishes (*Ompok Bimaculatus, Ompok Pabda*) are considered delicacies are considered delicacies in eastern and north eastern States. Murrels (*Channa marulius, Channa punctatus*) are also potential species for culture. The freshwater prawns, *Macrobrachiium rosenbergii and Macrobrachium malcolmsonii* receive attention with regard to the establishment of hatchery and grow-out systems. Molluscan culture is gaining emphasis in the context of production of cultured freshwater pearls through nuclear implantation in the bivalve, *Lamellidens spp.*

Apart from the water resources that can be used for fish culture the other resources that can be recycled into culture systems are organic materials such as domestic sewage, 321 million tonnes of agro-residues, animal wastes in the form of urine and excreta and a host of agro-based industrial effluents. The aquaculture systems not only utilise the wastes as nutrient inputs but process and treat a large number of wastes as no other farming system.

Considering the increasing demand of fish to meet the nutritional requirements of the growing population in the country and the potentials of the fisheries sector in general and freshwater aquaculture in particular with regard to their contribution to the country's food basket, several technologies have been developed and evaluated for different agro-ecological situations for increasing fish production in the country. The freshwater prawn has been gaining popularity as an important candidate species for farming in view of its disease resistance, faster growth rate, capacity to adjust to varying environmental conditions and ready acceptability of artificial feeds.

Inland fishery is practiced in all states and Union Territories. West Bengal tops the list. It contributed 31 percent of total inland fish production of 2.85 million tonnes in 2000/01, followed by Andhra Pradesh (14 percent), Bihar (8 percent) and Uttar Pradesh (7 percent)

PRODUCTION SYSTEMS AND SPECIES

Unlike the development of monoculture of common carp (*Cyprinus carpio*) in Europe and elsewhere, culture of Indian major carps originated automatically as polyculture of catla (*Catla catla*) rohu (*Labeo rohita*) and mrigal (*Cirrhinus mrigala*). This was mainly because culture operation entirely depended on the wild mixed seeds of carps, which are collected from the rivers during monsoon when they bred and farmers had no means to segregate them. Over the years, farmers have learnt better husbandry practices; and scientific research and extension services helped further improvement of culture practices.

Introduction of three other Asiatic carps namely grass carp (*Cteno-pharyngodon idella*) silver carp (*Hypophthalmicthys molitrix*) and common carp in India as the component of Composite Fish Culture (Polyculture of Indian and Chinese carp) has resulted in enhancing the productivity of rural aquaculture. Carps are the main output of freshwater pond aquaculture production system, which is photosynthesis dependent, most suited to poor resource farmers. The other most prevalent system is trapping and holding system in paddy field, which results in carp, catfish, prawn and shrimp harvest. Integrated production system of crop-livestock-fish has been very old but because of lack of good management skill and ready market of all the products it has not developed as expected (Table 28.2).

Table 28.2: Aquaculture and Capture Fishery Production: 1961–2001

(Tonnes live weight)

Year	Aquaculture			Capture fishery			Total Production
	Inland water	Marine area	Subtotal	Inland water	Marine area	Subtotal	
1961	49,359	...	49,359	228,041	683,600	911,641	961,000
1962	54,368	...	54,368	275,232	644,300	919,532	973,900
1963	59,927	...	59,927	330,473	655,400	985,873	1,045,800
1964	66,096	...	66,096	393,804	861,700	1,255,504	1,321,600
1965	72,947	...	72,947	434,153	824,200	1,258,353	1,331,300
1966	80,561	...	80,561	396,939	889,700	1,286,639	1,367,200
1967	89,022	...	89,022	447,778	863,600	1,311,378	1,400,400
1968	98,471	...	98,471	523,229	863,900	1,427,129	1,525,600
1969	109,321	...	109,321	583,879	911,800	1,495,679	1,605,000
1970	121,651	20	121,671	551,249	1,085,580	1,636,829	1,758,500
1971	136,647	50	136,697	554,953	1,161,350	1,716,303	1,853,000
1972	153,848	110	153,958	513,752	971,390	1,485,142	1,639,100
1973	172,830	250	173,080	577,470	1,210,150	1,787,620	1,960,700
1974	191,897	424	192,321	593,102	1,471,568	2,064,670	2,256,991
1975	213,121	696	213,817	571,966	1,481,409	2,053,375	2,267,192
1976	236,741	1,382	238,123	565,650	1,373,323	1,938,973	2,177,096
1977	263,042	1,906	264,948	603,221	1,446,534	2,049,755	2,314,703
1978	292,331	2,523	294,854	527,691	1,487,164	2,014,855	2,309,709
1979	324,958	3,124	328,082	526,362	1,488,848	2,015,210	2,343,292
1980	361,312	3,868	365,180	529,362	1,550,795	2,080,157	2,445,337

Table 28.2: Aquaculture and Capture Fishery Production: 1961–2001 (Contd.)

(Tonnes live weight)

Year	Aquaculture			Capture fishery			Total Production
	Inland water	Marine area	Subtotal	Inland water	Marine area	Subtotal	
1981	401,832	4,790	406,622	601,731	1,439,989	2,041,720	2,448,342
1982	447,006	5,933	452,939	494,827	1,421,554	1,916,381	2,369,320
1983	497,387	7,346	504,733	491,889	1,511,976	2,003,865	2,508,598
1984	562,000	10,000	572,000	523,136	1,779,383	2,302,519	2,874,519
1985	620,250	13,000	633,250	471,900	1,734,157	2,206,057	2,839,307
1986	672,260	14,000	686,260	534,266	1,716,944	2,251,210	2,937,470
1987	773,310	15,000	788,310	454,836	1,678,739	2,133,575	2,921,885
1988	873,330	20,000	893,330	445,995	1,786,637	2,232,632	3,125,962
1989	976,500	28,000	1,004,500	405,065	2,231,124	2,636,189	3,640,689
1990	982,136	35,000	1,017,136	592,378	2,190,208	2,782,586	3,799,722
1991	1,185,261	40,000	1,225,261	471,566	2,353,167	2,824,733	4,049,994
1992	1,348,644	46,800	1,395,444	373,287	2,470,815	2,844,102	4,239,546
1993	1,354,702	62,000	1,416,702	575,905	2,486,807	3,062,712	4,479,414
1994	1,436,628	82,900	1,519,528	552,874	2,704,733	3,257,607	4,777,135
1995	1,588,799	70,008	1,658,807	608,378	2,656,862	3,265,240	4,924,047
1996	1,688,330	70,409	1,758,739	633,425	2,814,529	3,447,954	5,206,693
1997	1,795,987	68,335	1,864,322	641,775	2,881,673	3,523,448	5,387,770
1998	1,823,899	84,586	1,908,485	692,439	2,681,053	3,373,492	5,281,977
1999	2,054,991	79,823	2,134,814	696,083	2,776,067	3,472,150	5,606,964
2000	1,844,236	97,968	1,942,204	955,620	2,786,676	3,742,296	5,684,500
2001	2,098,447	104,183	2,202,630	974,710	2,787,890	3,762,600	5,965,230

Source: FAO Fisheries Database

Table 28.3 gives a general picture of different aquaculture systems prevalent in rural India; the rate of production is directly dependent on the extent of input supply and the degree of management.

In order to enhance the natural productivity, pond water is fertilized with organic and inorganic fertilizer or wastewater is fed to the pond. Sometime biogas slurry is put in the water. The fish is normally fed with rice bran and oil cake. Formulated feed is given for higher production and pond water is also aerated or changed to support a very high biomass. But normally feeding with formulated feed or aerating the water are beyond the means of common farmers. Polyculture of Indian major carp along or together with exotic carp as Composite Fish Culture are most popular which are undertaken with or without fertilization and feed.

Package of practices has been standardized for wastewater-based system, biogas slurry based system, and aquatic weed-based system. Cage culture, pen culture and running water fish culture are still in the infancy.

Extent of Rural Aquaculture

The whole system of production is a continuum and it is very difficult to strictly divide in different categories like extensive, semi-intensive and intensive culture systems mainly on extraneous feed supply or off-farm agro-industrial inputs. Similarly, it is difficult to segregate rural aquaculture from entrepreneurial aquaculture, which normally concerns with the intensive cultivation. In fact, many farmers who have been involved in subsistence level production increased their production over the years, with more inputs and better management skill, resulting in enlarging their resource base and gradually becoming entrepreneurial. For example, a farmer who used to stock fry in unprepared pond because of not knowing the technique of pond preparation and usefulness of fingerlings stocking, when came to know, followed the technique strictly and got better harvest and more income. Thus, over a period of few years he could afford more inputs and intensified his management and became entrepreneurial. In fact, it is most desirable that rural aquaculture should be evolved ultimately into entrepreneurial aquaculture and makes resource poor farmers entrepreneurial farmers. Such evolution is already taking place in rural India particularly in freshwater sector.

Subsidy and Bank Loan

The landless and rural poor have also practically no asset to offer for collateral as security for obtaining institutional finance, which howsoever directed toward social goal of raising the lots of the poor, serves by and large a commercial concept of lending. It is therefore, necessary to develop mechanisms to provide institutional finance without physical collateral. Perhaps farmers' certificate of successful completion of training in fish culture from a government institution or their actual knowledge of fish culture could be considered as collateral.

Table 28.3: Aquaculture Production Systems with Varying Degree of Management and Range of Estimated Output

S.No.	System	Species	Prevalence	Seed	Feed	Fertilizer	Aeration	Production range (Kg./ha/yr)
1.	Polyculture	Indian major carp	Very common	Fry	-	-	-	100-300
2.	-do-	-do-	Very common	Fry	-	-	-	300-600
3.	-do-	-do-	Common	Fingerling	-	Little	-	600-1000
4.	-do-	-do-	-do-	-do-	-	Little	-	1000-2000
5.	-do-	-do-	-do-	-do-	Rice bran & oilcake	-do-	-	2000-3000
6.	-do-	-do-	-do-	-do-	-do-	Adequate	-	3000-5000
7.	Composite fish culture	Asiatic carp	-do-	-do-	-do-	-do-	-	3000-10000
8.	-do-	-do-	Not common	-do-	-do-	-do-	Plenty	10000-15000
9.	Air breathing fish culture	Anabus testudineus	-do-	High rate of fry stocking	Rice bran oil cake, fishmeal	-do-	-	1000-2000
10.	Prawn culture Mono culture	M.rosenbergii. M.Malcomsonii	-do-	Post larva ed Feed	Forumlat- -do-	-do-	At Times	1000-2000
11.	Carp and prawn polyculture	-do- Asiatic carp and prawn	-do-	Carp fingerling and prawn post larvae	-			1300-500 of prawn300-500 of fish
12.	Rice-fish culture in freshwater	Carp or/and catfish	-do-	Wild	-		-	100-300 of fish 1—10% increase of rice
13.	Fish & Livestock	Carp and pig	-do-	Fingerling 30-40 pig/ha	-			5000-6000 of fish and 1500-2000 of pork

Table 28.3: Aquaculture Production Systems with Varying Degree of Management and Range of Estimated Output (Contd.)

S.No.	System	Species	Prevalence	Seed	Feed	Fertilizer	Aeration	Production range (Kg./ha/yr)
14.	Fish & bird	Carp and duck	—do—	Fingerling & Duck raising 200-300/ha	-	-	-	3000-4000of fish and 18000-18500 eggs and 500-600 kg of duck meat
15.	Rice-fish culture in brackish water	Prawn & mullet and other brackishwater fish	Common	Wild auto Stocking—	-	-	-	700-0900 of fish and prawn
16.	Shrimp culture	P.monodon P.indicus	Common	Post larva	Little	Little	-	1000-1500
17.	—do—	Increasing number	—do—	Adequate formulated feed	Adequate	Adequate	Adequate	3000-4500
18.	—do—	—do—	Not Common	Very high density	—do—	—do—	Plenty	10000-20000

Source: FAO, RAPA: Rural Aquaculture in India: by V.R.P. Sinha, RAP Publication 1999/20

Under the FFDA scheme the subsidy for tank reclamation and inputs, farmers get 25% subsidy whereas banks give 75% loan. But the amount of subsidy and loan are inadequate and farmers normally do not have the means to do adequate improvements or to buy required inputs. Procedural delay in obtaining this amount also creates problems to the farmers and at times they get frustrated and discouraged. The financial institutions also require that the Government release the subsidy before they release the loan and any delay in releasing the subsidy also delays the sanction of the loan and thus adversely affects production.

Lease of Water Bodies

Short duration lease of water bodies has been one of the main constraints. A study undertaken by the Indian Institute of Management, Ahmedabad (IIMA) has shown that at the all India level 87.5% of the ponds were leased out for 5 to 10 years and 9.4% for less then 5 years. Merely 3% of ponds were leased out for more than 10 years. Individuals (30%) and partners (70%) took lease.[1] Uncertainty attached to short duration lease discourages the farmers to undertake major renovation of the ponds and in the last year of the lease they normally do no spend on the inputs also. Banks normally hesitate to lend money in such cases.

Marketing

It is interesting to note that during 1970s carps from Bangladesh were seen being sold in Kolkata markets but now fish from Andhra Pradesh are being sold in Bangladesh. Indian major carps are sold in the U.K. markets, particularly in those places where Indian population is sizable. However, secondary and tertiary markets for carps are emerging all over India. Yet, strictly speaking poor farmers have to sell their produce in the local market at a very cheap price or to middlemen. Proper mechanism is still inadequate to collect and disseminate information about the prices and markets. Wholesalers and commission agents have the key role in marketing fish for the farmers. However, the farmers' share some time is as high as 88% of the sale price of the local sale. In the outstation sale the producers get about 60% of what consumers pay.

It is important that proper infrastructure is created for efficient marketing of aquaculture products. Government should invest more and also encourage private sector investment in market infrastructure development. Also creation and expansion of small-scale credit and saving institutions are necessary to facilitate development of aquaculture trading, transportation, and processing enterprises.

---

[1] IIMA (1991): Report on Performance of FFDA Programme for Freshwater aquaculture, National Workshop on Performance of FFDA Programme for Freshwater Aquaculture: Ahmedabad.

Supply Change in Inland and Marine Sectors

The stakeholders involved in the supply chain of inland fish catch and marketing includes the fishermen, 'mandali', wholesaler, dealer, retailer and consumer. The inland catch in some areas is sold to the 'mandali' (fishermen cooperative society). The 'mandali' has yearly contract with the wholesale sellers. Wholesale sellers collect the fish from 'mandali' and dispatch it to the big markets mainly in north India and West Bengal by trains or refrigerated vans. In certain cases, it was observed that most of the small fishermen sell their catch in the local retail market or in the markets of nearby villages.

In the marine sector, the supply chain is almost similar except that the processor is involved in the marine sector (Fig 28.2). Most of the catch is purchased by the commission agents directly from the fishermen and then sold it to the processors or wholesale sellers. Some fishermen even directly sell their catch to the processors or consumers. The processed fishes are sold mainly in the export market, where they get a good profit margin for the value addition. The processed fish is also sold in the domestic markets through the wholesale-seller-retailer chain.

CULTURE-BASED FISHERIES IN RESERVOIRS AND LAKES IN INDIA[1]

Most nations are reported to be exploring the possibilities of utilizing inland lakes and reservoirs to improve or commence culture-based fisheries. This should be attractive to most environmental groups as it entails little or no manipulation of the environment. The social relevance of culture-based fisheries is equally important. Unlike intensive aquaculture systems, culture-based fishery is practiced in community or common property regimes, where the benefit accrued from the increased productivity is more equitably distributed.

In India growth in the marine sub-sector has slowed down considerably over the years while the share of inland fisheries has increased. Nearly one million tonnes of inland fish production in India is attributed to culture-based fishery and other forms of enhancement practiced in reservoirs, small irrigation impoundments and floodplain wetlands.

Reservoirs

In broad terms, the small reservoirs are managed as culture-based fisheries, while medium and large reservoirs can be considered as more akin to stock and species enhancement. However, there cannot be a thumb rule to differentiate the two systems on the basis of reservoir area alone (Table 28.4). Fishing conditions, shallowness of the reservoir and natural recruitment are major factors that determine whether capture or culture-based fishery is followed.

---

[1]Based on article prepared by Dr. V.V.Sugunan.

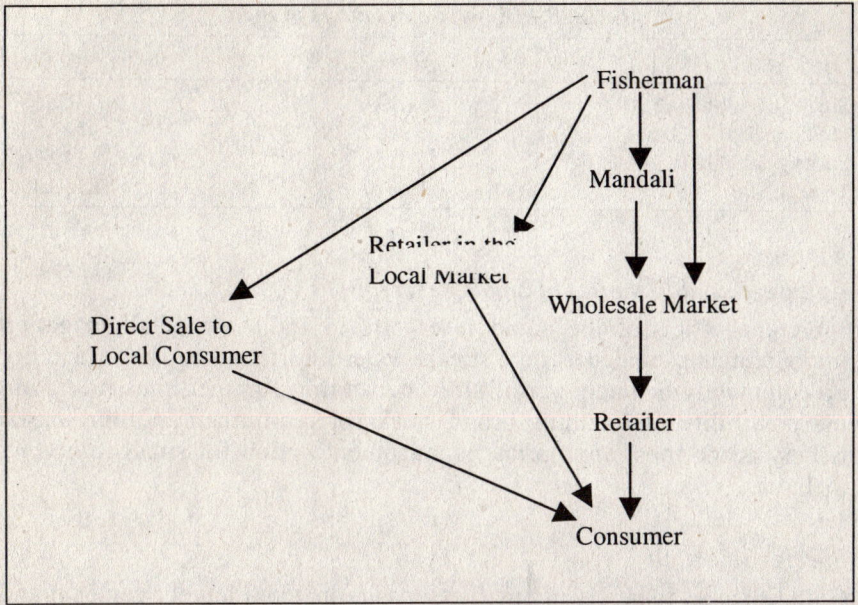

Fig. 28.2: Profile of Fishermen Households Inland

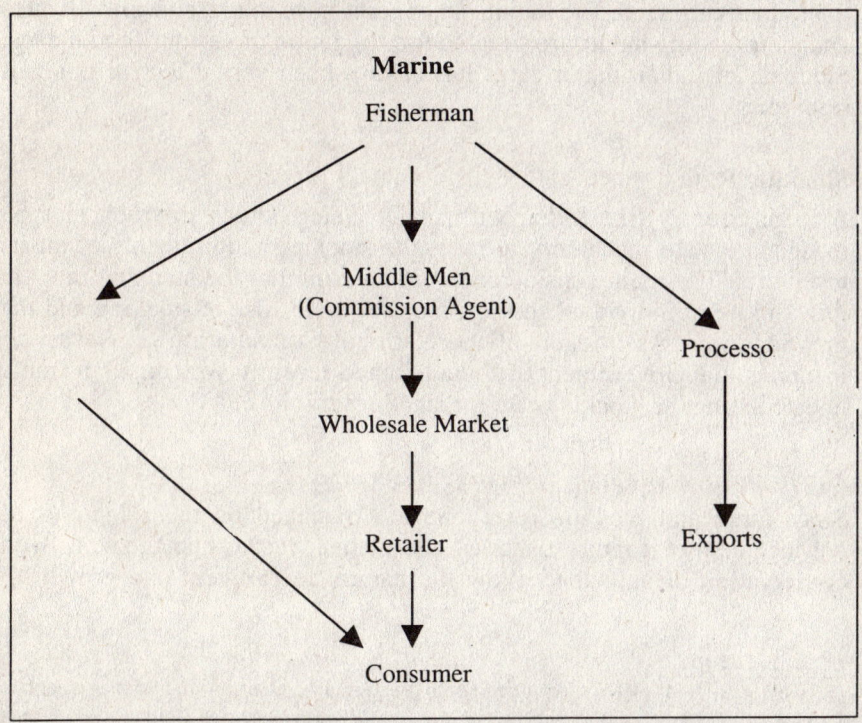

Fig. 28.3: Profile of Fishermen Households

Table 28.4: Reservoir Resources of India

Category	Number	Area (ha)
Small (<1000 ha)	19,134	1,485,557
Medium (100-5000 ha)	180	527,541
Large (>5000 ha)	56	1,140,268
Total	19,370	3,153,366

Culture-Based Fisheries of Small Reservoirs

More than 70% of the small reservoirs in India are small irrigation impoundments created to store stream water for irrigation. They either dry up completely or retain very little water during summer, thus ruling out the possibility of retaining brood stock for recruitment. Culture-based fishery is the most appropriate management option for small reservoirs in India.

Species Selection

Culture-based fisheries of small reservoirs in India largely center round the three species of Indian major carps—*Catla catla, Cirrhinus mrigala* and *Labeo rohita*—because many Indian States have the technical capability to produce carp seed. The Indian major carps have impressive growth rates and their feeding habits are suitable for utilization of various food niches. Stocking of Indian major carps has always been very effective in small reservoirs.

Stocking Rate

A large country like India, with many water bodies to stock, has an inadequate state machinery to meet the stocking requirements of all its reservoirs. The main considerations in determining the stocking rate are growth rate of individual species, mortality rate, size at stocking and the growing time. As a result of the National Consultation on Reservoir Fisheries, the Government of India adopted recently Welcome's formula in calculating the stocking rate for small reservoirs.[1]

Management of Medium and Large Reservoirs

Since large and medium reservoirs are managed on the principles of enhancement of capture fisheries, the main focus of management is on conservation of habitat to allow the natural recruitment and growth of

---

[1]Welcome, R.L. (1976): Approaches to Resource Evaluation and Management in Tropical Inland Waters, Proceedings of the Indo-Pacific Fisheries Council. Food and Agriculture Organization of the United Nations, Colombo , October 1976: pp 500.

the target species. Stock monitoring is achieved through the maneuvering of fishing effort and following mesh size regulations. Introduction is undertaken to correct imbalances in the species spectrum, while stocking is done as a temporary measure to compensate for recruitment failure.

Stock Enhancement

Stocking attempts made in medium and large reservoirs were successful when the stocked fishes bred and propagated themselves. In a number of reservoirs, even repeated stocking for more than 10 years did not make any impact because the fish did not breed. The increase in fish production due to recapture was not enough to recover the expenditure involved in stocking. Thus, the main aim of stocking efforts in medium and large reservoirs should be stock enhancement rather than recapture (unlike the culture-based fisheries).

Species Enhancement

Species enhancement aims to augment the species range by adding fish species from outside. These introductions colonize all the diverse niches of the biotope. The three Indian major carps, *Catla catla, Labeo rohita and Cirrhinus mrigala*, were being stocked in the peninsular reservoirs for the last five decades. This was done despite the fact that the peninsular rivers have habitats distinctly different from those of Ganga and Brahmaputra where fishes are indigenous. In some of the south Indian reservoirs, they have established breeding populations. The hallmark of the Indian policy on stocking (introductions in the case of peninsular reservoirs) is heavy dependence on Indian major carps.

Introduction of Exotic Species

The government policy clearly disallows stocking of exotic fish in reservoirs to prevent any adverse impact on the biodiversity. However, tilapia (*Oreochromis mossambicus*), silver carp (*Hypophthalmichthys molitrix*), grass carp (*Ctenopharyngodon idella*), and three varieties of common carp (scale carp, cyprinus carpio communis, mirror carp *C. carpio specularis,* and leather carp *C. carpio nudus*) have gained entry into Indian reservoirs either by accident or deliberate stocking. A spectacular performance of silver carp is recorded in the Gobindsagar reservoir (Himachal Pradesh) where, after an accidental introduction, the fish formed a breeding population and brought about a phenomenal increase in fish yield. Silver carp was instrumental in enhancing production of Gobindsagar from 160 tonnes in 1970-71 to more than 1,000 tonnes at present. However, this high yield was at the cost of Catla catla. Moreover, as the people did not accept the exotic fish, this resulted in social and economic problems.

Fish Production

The average national yield from culture-based fisheries of small reservoirs in India is nearly 50 kg/ha[1], which is low compared to other countries in Asia and Latin America such as China (743 kg/ha), Sri Lanka (300 kg/ha) and Cuba (100 kg/ha).[2] Even a modest increase in yield can push up the production of small reservoirs to at least 0.15 million tonnes, against the present level of less that 0.07 million t. Similarly, the medium and large reservoirs can add another 0.13 million t. Producing 0.2 million t of fish from aquaculture would entail creation of 100,000 ha of new ponds at a cost of Indian Rupees 20 billion (US$ 440 million). Considering that this yield enhancement can be achieved at a much lower cost, on sustainable and eco-friendly terms, reservoirs should receive adequate priority in future plans for inland fishery development in India.

One of the reasons for the low yield is under-stocking. There are 900 hatcheries across the country producing more than 18,000 million fry of Indian major carps annually. However, most of the fry produced in the hatcheries go to aquaculture managed by the private sector. The government and cooperative societies, which manage the reservoir fisheries, do not have enough infrastructures to produce the required number of fingerlings.

Recent Trends

Efforts made by the Central Inland Capture Fisheries Research Institute (CIFRI) in many small reservoirs across the country have demonstrated the efficacy of culture-based fisheries. For instance, in Aliyar reservoir (Tamil Nadu) fish yield increased from 35 kg/ha to 194 kg/ha. Successful stocking has also been reported from a number of small reservoirs in India.

A World Bank-assisted reservoir fisheries development project in India confirmed the validity of using Indian major carps in the culture-based fisheries of small reservoirs. The project, covering 78 reservoirs (24,613 ha) in three states, involved erection of pen nurseries in the reservoirs to ensure that the fish seed was reared to at least 100 mm in size before stocking. Loan was provided to cooperative societies to buy boats and nets. A perceptible relation between stocking and yield was obtained.

Floodplain Wetlands

Wetlands located at the floodplains of major rivers form an important fishery resource in the northern and northeastern states of the country. Known as beels, boars, pats, and chaurs, they spread over more than 200,000 ha of

---

[1]Sugunan, V.V. and M. Sinha (2000): Guidelines for Small Reservoir Fisheries Management in India: Bulletin No. 93. Central Inland Capture Fisheries Research Institute, Barrackpore, pp. 31.

[2]Sugunan, V.V. (1997): Fisheries Management of Small Water Bodies in Seven Countries in Africa, Asia and Latin America: FAO Technical Circular No. 933: Food and Agriculture Organization of the United Nations, Rome: pp. 149.

surface area in the eastern and northeastern regions of the country. Studies conducted by the CIFRI in the past 15 years have shown that fish yields from the floodplain wetlands of West Bengal can be raised to 1,000-1500 kg/ha/yr from its present level of only 100-150 kg/ha/yr by adopting culture-based fisheries.[1]

There are two kinds of floodplain wetlands, namely, *open and closed*, depending on their connection with the parent river. They have different patterns of community metabolism.

Fisheries of the Open Lakes

The open type of floodplain wetlands is a typical continuum of rivers, where the management strategy is essentially akin to riverine fisheries. In capture fishery management, the basic approach is to allow recruitment by conserving and protecting the brooders and juveniles. Therefore, an insight into population dynamics including recruitment, growth and mortality is very much essential. Identification and protection of breeding grounds, free migration of brooders and juveniles, and protection of brood stock and juveniles through conservation measures are important. Common strategies followed are summarized as:

- Increase the minimum mesh size to catch fish at the size of at least 500 g:
- Increase or decrease the fishing effort to maintain maximum sustainable yield :
- Observe the close season (usually during the southwest monsoon) to protect the brood stock:
- Maintain the diversity of the gear that comprise a number of indigenous designs (fish aggregating devices, traps, lift nets, dip nets, cast nets, etc.) :
- Selective augmentation of stock, only if unavoidable:

Culture-Based Fisheries of the Closed Lakes

Culture-based fishery is most suitable for closed lakes. In culture-based fishery, growth depends on stocking density and survival depends on the size of the stocked fish. The growth varies from one water body to another depending on the water quality and food availability. The management parameters are:

- Stocking density
- Size at stocking
  - Fishing effort
  - Size at capture
  - Species management
  - Selection of species

---

[1]CIFRI (2000): Ecology and Fisheries of Beels in West Bengal: Bulletin Central Inland Capture Fisheries Research Institute, Barrackpore. pp.82.

Closed lakes are ideal for practicing culture-based fisheries for the following reasons: First, they are very rich in nutrients and fish food organisms, enabling the stocked fishes to grow faster to support a fishery. Growth is achieved at a faster rate than in reservoirs. Second, the floodplain wetlands allow higher stocking density because of better growth performance and high yield. Third, there are no irrigation canals and spillways unlike in small reservoirs, which cause stock loss. Also, the lack of effective river connection prevents entry of unwanted stock. Stocking of detritivores is allowed as the energy transfer takes place through the detritus chain.

Culture and Culture-Based Systems

There are systems that can combine the norms of culture and culture-based fisheries. The marginal areas of the lakes are cordoned off for culture systems either as ponds or as pens and the central portion is left for culture-based (or capture) fisheries. Floodplain wetlands also can be part of an integrated system.

Pen culture in Floodplain Wetlands

Culture of fishes and prawns in pen enclosures is a very useful option for yield enhancement in floodplain wetlands, especially those infested with weeds and harvesting is a problem. Pens are barricades erected on the periphery of lakes to cordon off a portion of the water body to keep captive stock of fish and prawn. They can be constructed in any shape and size using a variety of locally available material. CIFRI has standardized the methods for culture of freshwater prawn (*Macrobrachium rosenbergii*) in pens. Pens made of bamboo are stocked with juvenile prawns at the rate of 40,000/m², which are given locally made feed with 38% crude protein. The required feeding rate in the pens was very low (as low as 1-2% body weight) due to the rich natural fish food resources in the lake. The rate varies according to the scale of operation and availability of natural food. At the end of a 90-day growth period, prawns grew from 4 to 65 g (average) with a survival rate of 60%, resulting in a yield of 1,560 kg/ha of pen area. Reservoirs and floodplain wetlands in India can make substantial contributions to fish harvests through the adoption of culture-based fisheries.

CONCLUSION

Rivers, estuaries and lagoons, being threatened with environmental degradation, are not expected to play a major role in meeting the additional requirements of inland fish production. Intensive aquaculture entails high cost and its unchecked growth may lead to many new environmental, social and legal issues. Therefore, any substantial increases in inland fish production may have to come from the development of culture-based fisheries in small reservoirs and lakes. Various kinds of development technologies in medium and large reservoirs need to be applied on priority basis.

The inland fish production in India has gone up from 0.22 million tonnes in 1951 to 2.85 million tonnes in 2001, due largely to the contribution of newly developed technologies. Aquaculture production alone now constitutes about 72 percent of the inland fish production. Though the newly developed aquaculture technologies have helped in raising fish, prawn and shrimp production and income of the farmers, the small and marginal farmers are still largely practicing the traditional methods and operating at or little above the subsistence level. Modern methods of scientific aquaculture have been adopted either by educated or rich farmers, as the extension efforts have remained confined to urban or semi-urban areas.

29

Marine Fisheries

Since time immemorial, sea fishing has been an important occupation with the people of India living in coastal areas. However, fishing operations largely remained near the shores venturing out into the open sea only a few kilometers from the base up to distances which could easily be covered by sailing craft. However, later on, the major thrust was given on motorization of traditional craft and introduction of intermediate craft (trawlers) of 12-166 metre size for exploiting offshore resources. The occupation of fishing in general, was earlier considered low in society and this, coupled with the prohibition of travel on the sea, in common parlance it was 'kala pani', prevented the induction into it of capital and organization from more resourceful communities. As a result, the industry remained solely with the traditional community of fishermen for centuries. During the pre-independence period, fisheries, which in the maritime states had reached considerable proportions, was viewed principally as a source of revenue, and barring notable exceptions like the erstwhile Madras Province, precious little support was received from the government towards its development. Considering the circumstances under which the community of marine fishermen had evolved different techniques of fishing, built various types of craft and gear and successfully applied indigenous methods of preservation, it can be stated that the industry had reached a high degree of viability by the time of Independence. However, when compared with the contemporary status of marine fishing in industrially advanced maritime countries, India's progress was quite tardy. A meaningful move towards a modernized marine fishing industry was made with Independence, considering the vastness of its resources and the need to apply tools of research and mechanization for its development.

In the development of marine fisheries, the Government initially considered broadly four categories of tasks: (i) improvement of fishing methods, (2) development of deep sea fishing, (3) the provision of fishing harbours, and (4) the organization of fish transport, storage, marketing and utilization of fish. Emphasis was also laid on the provision of research support to the industry which was fulfilled by establishing the Deep sea Fishing station at Bombay (now Mumbai) in 1946, the Central Marine

Fisheries Research Institute (CMFRI) at Mandapam in 1947 and the Central Institute of Fisheries Technology (CIFT) at Kochi in 1957, each having respective field stations at selected centers along the coast. These research stations including the field stations undertake research on problems of marine fisheries, including estimation of fishery resources, the rate of present exploitation, the possibilities of increasing production and utilization and measures of conservation. Impetus to development is given through the fisheries schemes in the five year plans, which include loans and subsidies for several activities, mainly channelised through the fishermen's cooperatives as a step towards socioeconomic progress of fishing communities.

The progress attained till the 1970s undoubtedly raised the status of the industry by its recognition as a promising arena of economic growth. The apathy of the earlier years was replaced by all round interest including the induction of capital and management not only from individuals but also from highly organized corporate sectors in other industries. However, such developments have also led to over exploitation of stocks reaching beyond the unsustainable production limits in many regions.

PROFILE OF INDIAN MARINE FISHERIES

The Indian marine fisheries sector is characteristically an open access one with free and common property rights. The multispecies fishery comprise over 200 commercially important finfish and shellfish species. Being a multigear fishery, fishing practices vary between different regions, depending on the nature of the fishing grounds and the distribution of the fisheries resources. Pelagic stocks like mackerel, sardines, whitebaits, ribbonfish, carangids, seerfishes, coastal and oceanic tunas; demersal groups like croakers, threadfin breams, silverbellies, catfish, lizard fish and goatfish; crustaceans like penacid prawns, crabs, lobsters and stomatopods and cephalopods like squids and cuttlefish are common. The abundance of these stocks varies from region to region with large pelagics like tunas being more abundant around Island Territories and small pelagics like sardines and mackerel supporting a fishery of considerable magnitude along the southwest and southeast coasts. The Bombayduck (*Harpadon nehereus*) and non-penacid prawns form a good fishery along the northwest coast, while perches (pigface breams, groupers and snappers) are dominant in the southwest and east coasts, especially in the Gulf of Mannar, Palk Bay and Wadge Bank areas.

Among gears, gillnets, drift nets and bag nets of varied mesh sizes are widely employed by traditional fishermen along both the coasts, while ring seines, purse seines and mechanized gillnets are confined to the southwest coast. Bottom trawls up to 13 m OAL are operated along the entire coast, while the second generation large trawlers 13-17 m are operated from selected harbours along both the east and west coasts. Currently, 2251 traditional landing centers, 33 minor and six major fishing harbours serve as bases for 2,08,000 traditional non-motorized crafts, 55,000 small scale beach landing, motorized crafts, 51,500 mechanized crafts (mainly bottom trawlers, drift gillnetters and purse seiners) and 180 deep sea fishing vessels of 25m OAL (Anonymous 2001).

The growth of the fleets shows that the artisanal fleet (including the motorized) increased by about 110 per cent from the 1960s to the 1990s and the mechanized fleet by about 570 per cent during the same period (CMFRI 1997) and resulted in an overdeployed fleet operating in the inshore waters (Table 29.1). The pattern of marine fish landings in India during the past fifty years (Figures 1 and 2) clearly reveals that the contribution by the artisanal sector to the total production was significant up to 1960s while presently, the contribution by the mechanized and motorized sector accounts for 91 per cent of the marine fish catch and the rest by artisanal gear (CMFRI 2000). The development of harbours and landing jetties, motorization of artisanal crafts and the rapid expansion of mechanized fishing have contributed towards a significant increase in fish production, employment generation and revenue earnings.

Table 29.1: Optimum and Existing Fleet Size, 1996-97 (in number)

Fleet	Existing (number)	Optimum (number)	Excess percent	Contribution to total catch (percent)
Mechanized	46918	20928	55.0	67.0
Motorized	31726	12832	60.0	20.0
Non-mechanized	159481	31059	81.0	13.0

Total catch: 2.41 million tones (1996-97)

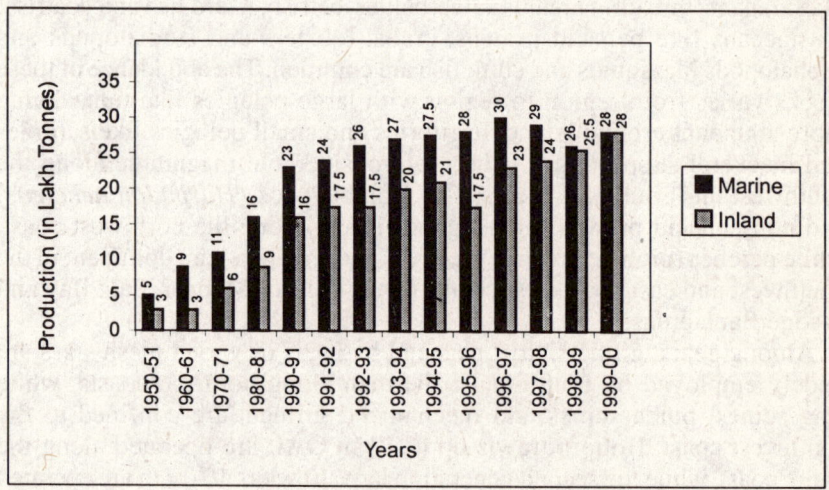

Fig. 29.1: Fish production in India

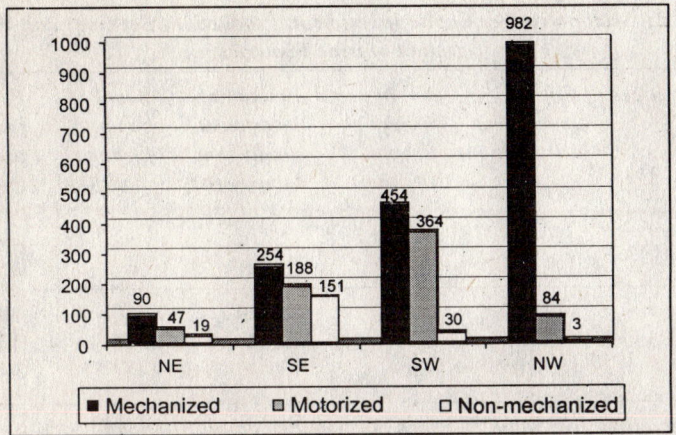

Fig. 29.2: Fish production in India

Socio-Economic and Demographic Features

Currently, one million active fishermen are engaged in marine fishing in India, of which about 0.2 million are engaged in the mechanized sector, 0.17 million in the motorized sector and the rest in the artisanal sector. Among those engaged in the mechanized sector, 75 per cent work in trawl fisheries and 25 per cent in the fisheries operating gillnets, bag (dol) nets, purse seines and deep sea vessels. In the case of the motorized sector, 60 per cent are engaged in the ringseine fishery alone, which is predominant on the southwest coast and the rest in various other forms. In the artisanal sector, of the total 0.63 million active fishermen, 41 per cent are engaged in the operation of catamarans, 31 per cent in plank built boats and the rest in the dugout canoes and others (Devaraj *et al.* 1998). Only 30 per cent of the fisherfolk posses some sort of ownership of fishing implements, while a large number (70 per cent) of them work as labour force. The annual income of labourers working in a mechanized boat was estimated to be Rs. 34,200, while in motorized boat it has Rs. 15,200 and in artisanal unit Rs. 8,000 during 1995 - 96 (Table 29.2). This wide disparity in income between those engaged in the different subsectors results in clashes and conflicts (Sathiadhas 1996).

Diverse Fisheries

Species diversity is the hallmark of Indian marine fisheries. There are nearly 1,570 species of finfish and about 1,000 species of shellfish. Capture fisheries employ various types of craft and gears for the exploitation of the commercial stocks of these species. The abundance of these stocks varies from region to region. Development activities helped increase the harvest from about 0.53 million tonnes in 1950 to 2.81 million tonnes in 2000, showing an average annual growth of 3.4 per cent.

Table 29.2: Sector-wise Per Capita Investment, Production, Earnings and Wages in Indian Marine Fisheries

Sectors engaged	Capital investment (Rs. million)	No. of per fishermen fishing (million)	Percapita investment production labour (Rs.)	Annual percapita of fishing labour (kg)	Per capita production per kg labour per working day (kg)
Mechanized	17,710	0.2	88,550	7,550	38
Motorized	3,380	0.17	19,888	2,588	13
Artisanal	8,810	0.65	13,440	437	2.4

Sectors engaged	Av. Value realized by fishing of fish (Rs.)	Income generated fishing .labour/ trip (Rs.)	Percapita earnings of fishing labourer per trip (Rs.)	Annual wages* of Labourer (Rs.)
Mechanized	45	1,710	171	34,200
Motorized	35	455	76	15,200
Artisanal	25	60	40	8,000

*Assuming 200 fishing days per annum
Source: Sathiadas, et al 1999

However, the annual growth rate declined from 6.5 per cent during 1950-60 to 2.3 per cent during 1960-70, increased to 4.3 per cent during 1970-80 and to 4.8 per cent during 1980-90, and declined to 2 per cent during 1990-2000. This fall in growth is reflected in the annual catch attaining the optimum levels in the inshore fishing grounds extending up to the 50 m depth of about 180,000 sq. km.

Currently 1.91-lakh non-mechanised craft (including 35,000 motorised craft), 47,000 small mechanised craft and 180 large fishing vessels operate in the Indian EEZ. The fleet size referred to above is in excess of the optimum by 55 per cent, 60 per cent and 81 per cent respectively. The contribution from the mechanised sector to the total catch is 67 per cent, motorised 20 per cent and non-mechanised 13 per cent. The alarming fleet capacity warrants the imposition of stringent fishing practices and proper codes of conduct for sustainable growth in this sector.

Marine fishery is carried out in thirteen states. These include Andhra Pradesh, Goa, Gujarat, Karnataka, Kerala, Maharashtra, Orissa, Tamil Nadu, West Bengal, Andaman and Nicobar, Islands, Daman Diu, Lakshadweep and Pondichary. Among these Gujarat state is the largest producer, which accounted for 22 percent of the total marine output in 2000/01. This was followed by Kerala (20 percent), Maharashtra (14 percent) and Tamil Nadu (13 percent).

Inland fishery is practiced in all states and Union Territories. West Bengal tops the list. It contributed 31 percent of total inland fish production of 2.85 million tonnes in 2000/01, followed by Andhra Pradesh (14 percent), Bihar (8 percent) and Uttar Pradesh (7 percent) (Table 29.3.)

Table 29.3: State-wise Fish Production in 2000-01 (in tonnes)

States/UTs	2000-01		
	Marine	Inland	Total
1	*2*	*3*	*4*
Andhra Pradesh	182502	407186	589688
Arunachal Pradesh	—	2500	2500
Assam	—	158620	158620
Bihar	—	222160	222160
Goa	67328	4240	71568
Gujarat	620474	40261	660735
Haryana	—	33040	33040
Himachal Pradesh	—	7020	7020
Jammu & Kashmir	—	17510	17510
Karnataka	175906	127468	303374
Kerala	566571	85234	651805
Madhya Pradesh	—	48844	48844
Maharashtra	402838	123266	526104
Manipur	—	16050	16050
Meghalaya	—	6179	6179
Mizoram	—	2860	2860
Nagaland	—	5500	5500
Orissa	121086	138556	259642
Punjab	—	52000	52000
Rajasthan	—	12121	12121
Sikkim	—	140	140
Tamil Nadu	367855	113560	481415
Tripura	—	29420	29420
Uttar Pradesh	—	208286	208286
West Bengal	181000	879230	1060230
A & N Islands	27618	66	27684
Chandigarh	—	82	82
D & N Haveli	—	43	43
Daman & Diu	16382	0	16382
Delhi	0	3980	3980
Lakshadweep	12000	0	12000
Pondicherry	38950	4350	43300
Chattisgarh**	—	43386	43386
Uttaranchal**	—	9074	9074
Jharkhand**	—	43600	43600
Deep Sea Fishing@	30000	—	30000
Total	2810510	2845832	5656342

**For the period December 2000 to March 2001, @ Estimated, Note: Figures are provisional.

Source: Ministry of Agriculture, Directorate of Economics and Statistics: Agriculture Statistics at a Glance 2002.

Fishery Environment

The total area of EEZ of India is estimated at 2.02 million sq.km against its land area of about 3.2 million sq. km. The continental shelf area between 0 and 50 m depth is estimated at 191.97 thousand sq.km and that between 0 and 200 m depth as 452.06 thousand sq.km. There are general topo-hydrographical differences in the features of the coastline and adjacent seas, distribution and abundance pattern of the species and their fishery characteristics along the west and east coasts.. The primary and secondary productivities are higher on the west coast compared to the east coast, mainly due to the strong upwelling process, which therefore supports a more abundant fishery. The northwest coast (15°-23° N latitude) has extensive fishing grounds and the sea bottom is generally muddy while the southwest coast (8°-15°N latitude) has a narrow continental shelf with less extensive fishing grounds. The southeast coast (10°-15° N latitude) is characterized by coral and rocky grounds while the sea bottom of the northeast coast (15°-21°N latitude) is predominantly muddy and suitable for bottom trawling.

The northern Indian Ocean, together with its two major bays, the Arabian Sea and the Bay of Bengal, is landlocked in the north by the Asian continent which separates the northern Indian Ocean from the deep-reaching vertical convection areas of the Arctic seas and the cold climate regions of the northern hemisphere. This geographic separation is a major factor, which determines the oceanographic conditions of the northern Indian Ocean. Circulation of waters in the Arabian Sea and Bay of Bengal is influenced by the pattern of winds associated with the summer and winter monsoons and comprise the monsoon current, the equatorial current and the equatorial counter current (Varadachari and Sharma 1967; Pillai et al. 1997). The monsoon current which is westerly during the northeast monsoon period (October-December) and easterly during the southwest monsoon season (May-October) has significant impact on the coastal fisheries. Average salinity value ranges between 34 and 37% in Arabian Sea and 30-34% in the Bay of Bengal. Both sea and land breezes are common in this area except during the southwest monsoon (along the west coast) and the northeast monsoon season (along the east coast).

In the Arabian Sea, temperature ranges between 23 and 29°C and in the Bay of Bengal, it is 27 to 29°C. With regard to vertical distribution of temperature in the Bay of Bengal, the thermocline is usually below 50-55 m occasionally going down to 100-125 m while in the Arabian sea, if fluctuates a great deal, showing definite seasonal trends (Rao 1973). Coastal upwelling occurs in varying intensities along the west and east coasts of India, corresponding with the southwest monsoon and determines the seasonal productivity patterns. During the months of strongest monsoon winds, coinciding the upwelling, linear banks of greenish, highly organic and mobile mud (chakara) form inshore in many areas between latitudes 8 and 10°N (Bristow 1938) and support a seasonal fishery mainly consisting of sardines, whitebaits, mackerel and prawns.

Fish Marketing System

The estimated first sale value of marine fish landings in the year 2000 was Rs. 102 thousand million with seafood exports earning Rs. 63 thousand million during 2000-01. the post-harvest fisheries including processing, product development, transport and marketing generate more employment than the harvesting sector, which, due to increasing demand and price of fish in both domestic and export markets, keeps growing. While the infrastructure for fish marketing is still principally oriented towards the export market, vast improvements in handling technologies and quick transportation facilities have led to increased market penetration of fresh iced fish to interior markets also. Currently, 50 per cent of fish is consumed fresh in an around producing centers, 43 per cent in centers up to 200 km interior to the coast and 5 per cent beyond 200 km limit (Sathiadhas *et al.* 1994). It is estimated that 44 per cent of fresh fish is auctioned off by fishermen themselves and the rest by involving intermediaries like wholesalers and retailers. Fisherman's share can be as high as 95 per cent in case of direct sale to the consumers (Devaraj 1987) and 30-68 per cent otherwise, with the wholesalers receiving 5-32 per cent and retailers 14-47 per cent of the consumer's rupee for different species of marine fish (Devaraj *et al.* 1998). Earlier, hardly 5 per cent of fish in the internal marketing ,system was marketed through cooperatives but the recent significant development of fisheries cooperatives has helped in reducing the high costs of marketing through integration of marketing and credit, establishing links with consumer cooperatives and introducing modern machinery and labour saving gadgets in all stages of marketing (Singh 2000). Fisheries associations are also coming up which will take up not only fishing but also direct selling of the catches to the consumers, thereby eliminating middlemen traders. At present, about 30 per cent of the total landings are processed after they become unsuitable for fresh consumption (Devaraj *et al.* 1998) and hygienically processed and packed dried fish for domestic consumption in interior towns and canned fish in cities and defence establishments offer a good scope.

Maladies of Open Access and Aftermath

Marine fishing activity in India is an example of uncontrolled exploitation in the initial phase followed by subsequent inefficient management. The growth in marine fisheries production reaching 2.7 million tonnes in 2000 and its plateauing thereafter marks a series of crises that this sector is facing today.

The sector that has enjoyed free access to the resources is not prepared to face stringent restrictive management measures. Hence, regulation of common property rights and introduction of the concept of responsible fishing pose problems. Resources management is not being considered seriously or where it is considered has failed to restrain the fisherman from exploiting the wild stock beyond sustainable levels leading to increasing scarcity of fish, and conflicts between different economic or ethnic groups of end users. Population pressure and commercial considerations, working in tandem with inadequate fisheries management regime, have failed to prevent massive overcapitalization in fishing capacity.

The per capita production has declined, as each fisherman continues fishing as long as his average cost of fishing equals average returns. There are about 2 lakh artisanal fishing units landing catches to the tune of 9 per cent of the total landing, 32,000 motorised units (about 26 per cent) and 52,000 mechanised units (about 64 per cent). Average annual production per active fisherman is 332 kg for those operating non-mechanised craft and 9880 kg for mechanised craft. The active fishers' population increased from 234,478 in 1961-62 to about one million in 1996-97. This implies less fishing area per fisher. The number of active fishers per unit area in the inshore fishing grounds extending to a depth of 50 ml increased substantially from 1961 onwards.

The present fisheries situation along many parts of the Indian coasts falls under any of the following: (1) the decrease in abundance which is reflected as decline in catch rates, (2) the yield per recruit and the recruitment decreases, (3) fishing mortality equals or exceeds natural mortality and (4) deviations from the normal characteristics of landing including over dominance of juveniles in catch.

Challenges

The marine fisheries sector has the following options to meet the challenges in the next two decades: (1) management of the exploited stocks to realise sustainable yields through responsible fishing, (2) exploiting and monitoring the deep sea fisheries resources, (3) increasing production substantially through coastal seafarming and mariculture, and (4) addressing the socioeconomic, environmental and conservation needs.

Capture fisheries: The focus in this regard should be on bridging the gap between the current production of 2.81 million tonnes and the potential of 3.9 million tonnes from the EEZ. This would require: (1) Intensifying the exploitation in the offshore grounds by mechanised vessels that can be operated from marina-type berths along the numerous fishing villages in the coastal waters, (2) Enhancement of coastal stocks through sea ranching, (3) Creation of artificial fish habitats in the inshore grounds, (4) Limited entry, effort rationalization and closed fishing seasons, (5) Gear, area and temporal restrictions and mesh-size regulation to prevent growth overfishing and recruitment overfishing (6) Fishery forecasts linked to biotic and abiotic factors, (7) Tuna longlining and oceanic squid jigging, (8) Monitoring ecosystem health, (9) Utilisation of bycatch by conversion into value-added products like IQF and Surumi, (10) Further development of production, post-harvest and market infrastructure, optimum utilisation of existing capacity of freezing plants, canning plants and fishmeal plants, (11) Human resource development, (12) Creation of environmental awareness, (13) Organised extension programmes and (14) interinstitutional linkage for R & D between the various organisations in the sector (Devaraj, 1999).

Fishing Regulations

Until 1970s, the emphasis of fisheries management in India was on increasing the fish production through improved fishing technology, infrastructure (harbours, roads, processing and market facilities) development and incentives and subsidies to the fishermen. These paved the way for increasing the marine fish production from 0.5 million tonnes in 1950 to 2.7 million tonnes in 2000. However, during the 1980s and 1990s, serious concerns were expressed for the unrestricted growth of the fishing industry which might become counterproductive (Devaraj and Vivekanandan, 1999) and therefore, the management strategy started aiming at sustaining the fisheries. Marine Fisheries Regulation Acts (MFRA) were promulgated in the 1980s with the focus on controlling the fishing area, fishing gears, enforcing mesh size regulations and closed seasons.

Options for Sustainability

The issues pertaining to marine fisheries in India are not unique to the country but common to most of the tropical developing countries. Under the present scenario, there is a need for policy support on:

- Effective implementation of the regulatory measures for optimising the exploitation of the fishery resources in the inshore waters.
- Exploitation of the deep-sea and oceanic resources in the EEZ and beyond.
- Effective prevention of third country fishing in the Indian EEZ.
- Increasing the pace of motorisation of artisanal craft to improve their capabilities.
- Monitoring and regulating fishing effort in the inshore waters.
- Improvements in the system of data generation as well as quality of data on exploited stocks.
- Protection, conservation and sustainable utilisation of marine biodiversity.
- Improvements in domestic and export marketing through value addition.
- Manpower development in R & D, fishing and processing sectors.
- Development of linkages between stakeholders as well as between stakeholders and Governmental Institutions.
- Development of Marine Fisheries Information System.
- Development of infrastructure – fishing harbours – berthing facilities, capacity utilization of post harvest infrastructure.
- Stock enhancement through artificial reef habitats, fish aggregating devices and sea ranching.
- Development of and adhering to a National Code of Conduct for Responsible Fisheries.

Deep Sea Fishing Policy

To increase fisheries production from the outer continental shelf, the Govt. of India introduced the Deep Sea Fishing Policy (DSFP) in 1991, which allowed for chartered and leased vessels and joint ventures with foreign fishing vessels to operate in the Indian EEZ. But, due to protests from the fishery sector, this policy was scrapped and has adversely affected the exploitation of offshore resources. The lack of harvesting infrastructure and expertise on onboard processing of offshore resources is a serious bottleneck in developing the deep sea fishing sector.

MOLLUSCAN CULTURE

Edible Oyster Farming

The first attempt to develop oyster culture in India dates back to 1910 by James Hornell. Since 1970s, the CMFRI has taken up R & D programmes on all aspects of oyster (Crassostrea madrasensis) culture and has produced a complete package of technology, which is presently being widely adopted by small scale farmers in shallow estuaries, bays and backwaters all along the coast.

In the adopted rack and ren method, a series of vertical poles are driven into the bottom in rows, on top of which horizontal bars are placed. Spat collection is done either from the wild or produced in hatcheries, on suitable cultch materials. Spat collectors consist of clean oyster shells (5-6 Nos.) suspended on a 3 mm nylon rope at spaced intervals of 15-20 cm and suspended from racks, close to natural oyster beds. Spat collection and further rearing is carried out at the same farm site and harvestable size of 80 mm is reached in 8-10 months. Harvesting is done manually with a production rate of 8-10 tonnes/ha. Oyster shells are also in demand by local cement and lime industry and culture production has increased to 800 tonnes in the year 2000.

Mussel (*Perna viridis, Perna indica*) Farming

Raft method (in bays, inshore waters), rack method (in brackishwater, estayrues)or longline method (open sea) are commonly adopted for mussel farming. Mussel seeds of 15-25 mm size collected from intertidal and subtidal beds are attached to coir/nylon ropes of 1-6 m length and enveloped by mosquito or cotton netting. Seeds get attached to rope within a few days while the netting disintegrates. The seeded ropes are hung from rafts, racks or longlines. A harvestable size of 70-80 mm is reached in 5-7 months and production of 12-14 kg mussel (shell on) per metre of rope can be obtained Attempts to demonstrate the economic feasibility of mussel culture has led to the development of groupfarming activities in the coastal communities (especially rural women groups) with active support from local administration and developmental agencies like Brackishwater Fish Farmers Development Agency (BFFDA) and State Fisheries Department. Cultured mussel production has increased from 20 tonnes (1996) to 800 tonnes (2000) mainly through the rack system in estuarine area. Molluscan culture technologies and their economics are given in Table 29.4.

Table 29.4: Molluscan Culture Technologies and Economics

Technology	Edible oyster farming	Mussel farming	Pearl oyster culture
Species	Crassostrea Madrasensis	Perna Viridis, P. indica	*Pinetada* fucata
Farming method	Rack and Ren (30 x 10m)	Raft(8 x 8 m)	Cages Suspended from rafts racks
Culture period	8 months	5-7 months	12-15 months
Unitarea	300 sq.m	64 sq.m	Open sea; 6 rafts and 600 box cages
Economics (USS)			
Initial Investment	371	203	10,000
Recurring cost	139	357	4,419
Total cost	510	560	
Production	5.83 tonnes shell-on (0.48 tonne meat)	0.81 shell on	
Revenue	736	934	Depends on percentage pearl production and market value of pearls
Profit	226	303	30% (at 25% pearl production)

Source: ICAR 2000.

Pearl Oyster Farming and Pearl Production

In India, the marine pearls are obtained from the pearl oyster, *Pinctada fucata*. Success in the production of cultured pearls was achieved for the first time in 1973 by CMFRI, Raft culture and rack culture in nearshore areas are the two methods commonly adopted for rearing pearl oysters and recently attempts have been made to develop onshore culture methods.

Shell bead nucleus (3-8 mm) implantation is done in the gonads of the oyster through surgical incision while graft tissues are prepared from donor oysters of the same size and age group. Implanted oysters are kept under observation for 3-4 days in the labs, under flow through system and then shifted to the farm in suitable cages for rearing. Periodic monitoring is done and harvest is carried out after 3-12 months. Pearls are categorized into A,B and C types depending on colour, luster and iridescence 25 per cent pearl production has been successfully demonstrated in a series of farm trials at various locations along the Indian coast. Research is also directed towards development of a technology for in vitro pearl production using mantle tissue culture of pearl oyster.

The technology for mass production of pearl oyster seed and pearl production has paved the way for its emergence as a profitable coastal aquaculture activity at certain selected centers along the coast. Village level pearl oyster farming and pearl production, through direct involvement of small scale fishermen have been carried out successfully as part of technology transfer programme along the Valinokkam Bay on the east coast (Table 29.5). Pearl oyster farming has already generated income worth US $ 26,000 and several young women who are trained in pearl surgery in pearl farms are finding ready employment in this developing industry. The CMFRI also imparts training on pearl culture to trainees in neighbouring Asian countries, and various Memorandum of Understanding (MoU) have been signed with entrepreneurs, desirous of pearl culture since 1996.

Table 29.5: *Economics of Pearl Culture Programme at Valinokkam Bay–A Group Farming Success*

Number of oyster implanted	9414
Total expenditure incurred, US$	1571
Rate of Return %	56.7
Total Pearls Harvested	1849
Revenue earned from sale of pearls, US$	2178
Pearls distributed to fishermen	250
Revenue earned from sale of pearls	US$ 2178

Expenditure incurred (as percentage of total)

Raft	Cages	Pearl Oyster (for implantation)	Pearl Oyster (for graft tissue)	Shellbead nuclear	Labour	Miscellaneous
24	18	24	2	17	6	9

Source: APAARI 2000

VARIOUS FISH CULTURES

Clam Culture

Package of clam culture practices has been developed for the blood clam *Anadara granosa and Paphia malabarica*, where production of 40 tonnes/ha/6 months and 15-25 tonnes/ha/4-5 months have been achieved in field trials. Induced spawning and larval rearing to setting of spat has been perfected for clams like *P. malabarica, Meretrix and Marcia opima*.

Sea Cucumber Culture

More than 200 species of sea cucumbers are found in Indian waters mainly in the Gulf of Mannar, Palk Bay and Andaman and Nicobar Islands. The most important commercial species is *Holothuria scabra*, whose continuous exploitation has led to depletion of natural population (James 1999). Seed of *H. scabra* was produced in the hatchery for the first time in India in 1988 through induced spawning using thermal stimulation (James 1989) and has been used widely since then to produce seed for stock enhancement programmes. Water quality is the most important parameter in hatcheries with ideal conditions being temperature, 27-29°C, salinity 26.2, 32.7 ppt, dissolved oxygen 5-6 ml/l; pH, 6-9; and ammonia content, 70-430 mg/cubic metre (James 1999). Larvae require different diets at different developmental stages and algae like *Isochrysis galbana, Chaetoceras calcitrans, Tetraselmis chuii and Sargassum* are used. Seed produced in hatcheries are grown in velon screen cages (2 sq.m area), neilon cages (1.65 sq.m area, 5 mm mech net), concrete rings (70 cm dia x 30 cm height) and also at the bottom of prawn farms. Artificial diets prepared with soyabean power, rice bran and prawn head waste is used for feeding juveniles and results are encouraging. Juveniles have been stocked a 30,000/ha and grown along with shrimps (*P. monodon*) in farms (James 1999). Sea cucumbers being detritus feeders, feed on waste shrimp feed and organic matter on the pond bottom, reducing organic pollution load in the farm. Being an eco-friendly practice, which also provides an additional income to the farmer, it is expected to become popular among farmers who have been facing problems of shrimp disease outbreaks in the recent past.

Marine Finfish Culture

In the area of marine fish culture, the country is still in the experimental phase only. Attempts are being made to develop suitable hatchery and farming technology for mullets (*Mugil cephalus, Liza macrolepis, V.seheli*), groupers (*Epinephelus tauvina*), seabass (*Lates calcarifer*), milkfish (*Chanos chanos*) and pearlspot (*Etroplus suratensis*). The Central Institute of Brackishwater Aquaculture (CIBA) has developed an indigenous hatchery technology for seabass using captive broodstock which were stocked in large RCC tanks (12 x 6 x 2 m) with 70-80 per cent water exchange daily. Maturation process was accelerated using LHRH hormone injection and larvae were maintained with rotifers and *Artemia* nauplii. Cooked and minced fish meat is used for nursery rearing and survival rates up to 14 per cent in larval rearing phase and 84 per cent in the nursery phase have been recorded.

Ornamental Fish Culture

There are a wide variety of ornamental fishes in the vast water bodies and coral reef ecosystems along the Indian coast, which if judiciously used, can earn a sizeable foreign exchange. Hatchery technology for clownfish (*Amphiprion chrysogaster*), damsel fishes (*Pomacentrus caeruleus. Neopomacentrus nemurus and N. filamentosus*) and the sea horse (*Hippocampus kuda*) has been developed, which can be scaled up for mass production of these species.

Seaweed Culture

Around 60 species of commercially important seaweeds with a standing crop of one lakh tonne occur along the Indian coast, from which, nearly 880 tonnes dry agarophytes and 3,600 tonnes dry alginophytes are exploited annually from the wild (Kaladharan and Kaliaperumal, 1999).

OVEREXPLOITATION OF COASTAL RESOURCES

A major emphasis need to be placed on positive and purposeful checks on over exploitation of resources in the near shore areas through appropriate regulations on the number of fishing vessels, their operational areas, ban on monsoon fishing/close season, mesh size, use of the right type of fishing gear and other such restrictions to prevent uneconomic and oversize fishing.

Exclusive Economic Zone

Exploitation of offshore resources in the EEZ may be considered in terms of both the resource available and the infrastructure. Along with the absolute right on the EEZ, India has also acquired the responsibility to conserve, develop and optimally exploit the marine living resources within this area. Efforts may be made to exploit fishery resources in the EEZ on a priority basis. Satellite-assisted Vessel Monitoring System (VMS) will be helpful in the EEZ for both Indian and foreign fishing vessels. This would ensure the safety of fishers and vessels, and also provide emergency help whenever required. This would also help in the collection of fishery-related technical data as well as determining the number of fishing vessels required in a particular area for exploiting the available fishery resources.

Efforts are also needed to maintain World Trade Organization (WTO) catch levels by rational exploitation of our resources and to counter measures taken by neighbouring countries like Pakistan in collaboration with USA which is resulting in the over-exploitation of resources in the adjoining areas and there by curtailing our rights in these areas. Besides it should also be ensured that suitable measures are taken to exploit resources beyond the EEZ so that we put our due stake in the international water along with other countries.

Investment

Increasing public/private investment is needed for strengthening infrastructure for diversifying fisheries and aquaculture activities enhancing fish production and productivity. Enhanced public investment is also required in research programmes, strengthening infrastructures for training, post-harvest, marketing etc. Setting up of minor fishing harbours and creation of common facilities for maintenance and usage of dredgers by the Government should be given priority for improvement of infrastructure facilities in the marine fishery sector. Product developed by the value addition of low quality fish and development of products like chitosene out of wastes like prawn shells, products out of fish bladder etc. need to be encouraged. Private sector investment in fisheries may also be encouraged particularly in seed and feed production adopting existing technologies for higher production, human resource development, post-harvest management and marketing. For sustainable development of coastal areas, establishment of agro-aqua farms along coastal regions, linking ecological security with livelihood security may be encouraged by States/NGOs. Such farms involve concurrent attention to culture and capture fishery and forestry and agro-forestry programmes. Besides, conservation of fisheries resources, these farms may also be used for demonstrations. Besides, conservation of fisheries resources, these farms may also be used for demonstrations of diversifying activities of different techniques to be used for fishing operations. Emphasis may also be given for technological upgradation of the traditional fishing sector with improved motorized crafts and gears for the development of coastal fisheries and for the introduction of new generation of fishing vessels, for development of offshore fishing with modern communication equipments to ensure safety of fishermen while out at sea etc. Proper credit and technological support for standard bankable projects and ventures by small fishermen groups in the inland sector and setting up of cooperative marketing network in marine sector should be ensured through institutional finance from the National Bank for Agriculture and Rural Development (NABARD) and National Cooperative Development Corporation (NCDC).

CONCLUSION

The fisheries production in India during 1950s was more pronounced in the marine fisheries and it remained the major contributor till early 1990s. However, their share became almost half of the total fish production in 2000. It seems that due to overfishing, the marine fisheries production has reached a plateau and in future its share in the total production may further decline. But the persistent growth in fish consumption is very likely continue in the decades ahead and the major supply may come only from inland aquaculture. Further enhancement of marine fish production requires diversification of fishing activities not only in the offshore oceanic regime but also in deep sea fishing which is capital intensive and risk prone. There have already been strong protests in India against foreign equity participation in deep sea fishing and the government had to rescind its Deep Sea Policy in March 1997. In fact, any substantial growth in capture fisheries may not be feasible, given widely held pessimism as to the sustainability of capture fisheries. Utilization of marine resources by catch and fishing for unconventional fish species may not be economically viable initially.

Although capture fisheries production may not grow much overall, technology to prevent it from shrinking further in EEZ of the country may be in considerable demand, technologies that permit better fisheries management are foremost among these, including information technologies that permit easier, most sustainable, and more easily documented fishing. Mechanization programme in marine fishing, no doubt, initially helped in increasing the fish production, but it also led to, in many cases, switching over from the species hitherto important to some others for which good international market has emerged. With the introduction of mechanization, seasonality and variability of capture fish have been reduced drastically. Solutions of such problems will have to be found in a combination of technologies and policies directed at the same problem. Appropriate institutional arrangements may also be necessary to play a level playing field among the different categories of marine fishing operators and to facilitate use of new technologies for the purposes of the common good.

REFERENCES

1. Anonymous, 2001, Report of the Expert Group for Formulation of Comprehensive Marine Fisheries Policy. Ministry of Agriculture, Department of Animal Husbandry and Dairying, New Delhi, 27 pp.
2. Bristow R.C. 1938. History of Mudbanks, Government Press, Cochin, 37 pp.
3. CMFRI, 1997. Vision 2020-CMFRI Perspective Plan (ed. Murty, V.S.) Central Marine Fisheries Research Institute (ICAR) Cochin, 70 pp.
4. CMFRI, 2000, annual Report 1999-2000, Central Marine Fisheries Research Institute, Cochin, 148 pp.
5. Devaraj, M. 1987, State of Act of Marine Fisheries in India. Proc. Nat.Symp. Utilization of Living Resources of the Indian Seas. National Academy of Science of India: 101-114.
6. Devaraj, M., Murty, V.S.R., Sathiadhas, R. and Joshi, K.K. 1998. The New Economic Policy and Perspective for Marine Fisheries Research and Development in India. Fishing Chimes (18(5): 18-29.
7. Devaraj, M: Marine Fisheries-Regaining the Momentum: The Hindu Survey of Indian Agriculture, 1999.
8. Devaraj, M. and Vivekanandan, E. 1999. Marine capture fisheries of India: Challenges and opportunities. Curr.Sci., 76(3): 314-332.
9. James, D.B. 1999. Hatchery and culture technology for the sea cucumber Holothuria scabra jaeger, in India, NAGA, the ICLARM Quarterly, 22(4): 12-17.
10. Sathiadhas, R. 1996. Economic evaluation of marine fisheries of India for sustainable production and coastal zone development. Naga the ICLARM Quarterly, 19(3): 54-56.
11. Sathiadhas, T., Narayanakumar, R. and Sehara, D.B.S. 1994. Exploitation of marine fisheries and their utilization.
12. Proc 4th Swadeshi Science Congress, Swadeshi Science Movement, Kerala, Kochi, pp. 20-25.
13. Sathiadhas, R. Reghu, R. and Immanuel, Sheela 1999. Human resources utilization, productivity and earnings in Indian marine fisheries. Seafood Export Journal, XXX(4): 51-55:
14. Singh, S.K. 2000. Role of fisheries cooperatives in reducing the high cost of marketing involved in fisheries sector. In: Symposium of Ecofriendly Mariculture Technology packages- An undate (pillai, P.P. ed.) (Abstracts) 25-26th April, 2000. MBAI, CMFRI, Mandapam Camp.

30

Future Policy and Recommendations

The key issue for future development of livestock is whether India can address her major weaknesses while remaining true to the basic principles that have been the foundation of this success. In the answers to this question lie the international competitive advantage that will take our farmers and our industry well into the 21st century. The task before us is not to become the biggest - but the best. The building blocks of our success are well known, if not well understood. First is the partnership of farmer with the professional. The wisdom and energy of the farmers, combined with the knowledge and skills of the professional have created the conditions of confidence and strength that enabled our farmers, mostly women, to achieve a miracle.

The second block consists of the Indian consumer. Whichever be the region, whether urban or rural, rich or poor, our people consume milk and dairy products. The world's largest domestic market is the strong foundation of our industry. Third is our system of dairying. The traditional farming systems that have evolved in our country depend on the livestock that produce our draught power, our manure and our milk. Our animals survive on residues and the byproducts of our agriculture. This gives our industry an enormous competitive advantage in terms of energy efficiency. Quality is the bedrock of success for any enterprise: there is no substitute for consistent, superior quality. Our system has not yet provided built in quality at every stage from the udder to the consumer. Until India achieves world standard quality, it will not only find limited markets abroad and will be vulnerable to challenges at home. Productivity is the key to growth. We have no option but to raise the productivity of our national milch herd through breeding, feeding and management, the goal is no longer the farmer's share of the consumer's rupee-it is significant and sustained increase in farmer's income.

The core business of the dairy industry is sale of fluid milk to millions of our fellow citizens whose health and welfare depend on it. We cannot risk raising prices to the point where milk becomes a luxury, available only to the elite. Meeting the needs of our domestic consumers requires that we expand and achieve superior economics in production, transport, processing and marketing. The answers of 1990 may no longer work today, much less tomorrow. We must brutally dissect and rebuild our total system to achieve the highest standards of efficiency. In so doing, we must innovate solutions uniquely appropriate to our own environment. Our infrastructure, though strong and widespread, is aging and too often poorly used. The cost of traditional dairies is increasing. Our research and design must provide new answers to new questions. Our support to clients must help raising significantly their efficiency and economy. The future of dairy industry rests not only on the farmer, but on the scientist, the technologist and the professional. We must equip a new generation to compete head on with the best human resources of the advanced dairying nations.

On the macro level, the livestock sector in India looks bright and is steadily marching to prepare itself for the challenges in the next millennium. In India the land-man ratio is low and the distribution of land is skewed; diversification of a crop-based rural economy into an animal husbandry mixed farming system must be encouraged for rapid economic development and generating equitable income and employment in the country. Technological change embodied in better breeds, improved health, nutrition and processing must be accorded high priority along with credit, marketing and organization of producers to farther this trend.

The livestock sector's future performance will be significantly influenced by its international competitiveness. As trade protection is cut back, the sector needs to improve efficiency and low costs. As mentioned in the earlier chapters, the underlying current trends in livestock production systems present tremendous challenges. However, they also offer opportunities. Despite some intensification in livestock production, especially among dairy and poultry producers, the sector is still dominated by low-input production systems operating at significantly lower levels of intensification. Intensification of production is further constrained by sociocultural factors, which prohibit the slaughtering of cows. Large cow populations are one of the main factors contributing to overgrazing.

Output increase in the dairy sector will have to come from improvements in the quality of the animals and not, as in the past, from increases in the animal population. The future policy will have to lay emphasis on the use of improved buffalo and high producing crossbred cows. In the small ruminant sector, increased meat production will have to come in the short term from an increase in herd numbers. But in the long term it is essential to make genetic improvement of local breeds. Also, the development of intensive feedlots for sheep fattening will offer an important means of increasing total meat production. The poultry sector, provided its competitiveness improves, will be able to maintain its spectacular growth. Growth will come from the expansion of intensive production systems, mainly operated by the private sector.

The most crucial factors governing these trends will be the availability of high quality and low-priced feed. This will in fact determine the feasibility of stall-feeding. The low productivity and poor nutrition of most domestic livestock contribute to low yields per animal. It is of utmost importance to balance livestock sector growth and feed and fodder supply. The current status of feed and fodder system and the future policy direction on this front are already discussed in Chapter 16 entitled "Consumption and Supply of Feed and Fodder"

As regards livestock marketing system two key areas needs to be addressed. These include marketing efficiency and the environmental problems associated with livestock processing. The government's role in the new and more open market would be to ensure that fair competition in the market persists. Public sector enforcement of hygiene and sanitary standards would also become more critical and require more resources. Identification of real marketing bottlenecks through an improved livestock information system would facilitate government policy formulation and more efficient public sector resource allocation. Improved market information would be critical in promoting market competition.

RESEARCH POLICY AND PRIORITIES

As mentioned above, the past growth in many livestock products has largely been population driven. Therefore, technology will be a key factor in sustaining the growth momentum. While the research resources are limited to meet the emerging challenges, these underscore the need for a critical and objective evaluation of livestock research priorities at national and regional level. Livestock research receives about 19 percent of the agricultural research resources. This however, has witnessed considerable variation over time. In 1970s, share of livestock research was 27 per cent, higher than the relative contribution of livestock sector to agricultural GDP. The emphasis during this period was to strengthen research infrastructure. The share of livestock research fell drastically (14 per cent) in 1980s, but increased in 1990s. Yet, it remained low compared to its contribution to Agricultural GDP. Currently, India has well-developed research infrastructure with species/commodity orientation.

An assessment of priorities with the sole objective of accelerating growth suggests highest priority in the future should be given to Uttar Pradesh, followed by Maharashtra, Punjab, Madhya Pradesh, West Bengal, Andhra Pradesh, Rajasthan, Bihar, Gujarat and Haryana. These states contribute considerably to the national value of livestock production. The consideration of equity, sustainability and export promotion clause is the tradeoff in regional resources allocation. As regards the species of livestock, at the national level, buffalo research appears as the main priority demanding a share of 40 per cent in the livestock research resources. Cattle research comes next with 38 per cent. About 10 per cent of the livestock research resources need to be allocated to poultry and 7.5 per cent to goat. Share of these species is in the range of 1-2 per cent.[1] A comparison of the existing pattern with the one suggested here indicates substantial under-investment in buffalo and cattle research. This needs to be corrected in the future allocations. Cattle and buffalo have long gestation interval compared to small ruminants and monogastric, and thus the research of these animals is long-term and capital intensive.

Research on goat should focus on meat production (57 per cent), and followed by milk production (33 per cent). Investment in sheep research should be mainly for meat production (67 per cent). Wool production shares only 11.4 per cent. Poultry research resources should be allocated to meat and eggs in the ratio of 2:1. Meat production should be the main concern of pig research. For camel and equine, research should focus on improving their draughtability.

Most of the livestock species are widely distributed cutting across agroclimatic boundaries, but in varying density depending on their relative utility in provision of food and other products and services. The species priorities therefore vary across regions. Cattle research should target mainly the western region (Madhya Pradesh, Rajasthan and Maharashtra). Uttar Pradesh, Bihar, West Bengal, Orissa, Tamilnadu, Assam and Gujarat should be other target domains for cattle research. Most of these states are rainfed and have sizeable number of cattle for both milk and draught supplies. Buffalo research activity should concentrate in Uttar Pradesh in the north, Madhya Pradesh, Rajasthan and Maharashtra in the west. Andhra Pradesh in the south and Bihar and West Bengal in east that together require about 43 per cent of the national goat research resources. Andhra Pradesh and Maharashtra are the main candidates for incremental poultry research resources. Pig research should focus on northeastern states, while Bihar and Uttar Pradesh ranks highest in priority for equine research. The regional distribution of species-wise research resources thus indicates the necessity of taking into consideration the regional distribution of different livestock species and their relative utilities in the process of allocation of research resources.

Need for Livestock Policy

Budgetary allocation of the sector has further declined to 0.62 percent of the total budgetary resources for the Tenth Plan and 1.1 per cent during the Ninth Plan. The Centre will shortly unveil a national livestock policy which will lay down the road map for putting the sector on a high growth trajectory and make the sector more competitive in the WTO regime. Despite the potential in the livestock sector remaining under exploited, the contribution of this sector of the GDP has been continuously growing at 6 to 8 percent

---

[1]Birthal, Pratap S, Joshi, P.K., Kumar Anjani: Assessment of Research Priorities for Livestock Sector in India: National Centre for Agricultural Economics and Policy Research (ICAR): Policy paper 15.

as against the 2 percent growth rate in crop production. In addition, despite the highest milk production of 85 million tonnes during the year 2002, the per capita availability of milk in the country is low at 221 gm per day as against the world average of 285 gms per day. Available estimates indicate a deficit of 61 per cent in green fodder and 22 per cent in dry fodder with frequent droughts further compounding the problem. Immediate measures need to be taken to protect Indian producers from cheap imports. The cooperative sector has to play an active role in the poultry sector and it is important to establish an extensive marketing network of cooperatives.

Livestock Support Services

The Indian livestock sector's ability to achieve its potential growth in productivity and output will be greatly influenced by the quality, availability, and accessibility of livestock services. However, livestock services do not have to be supplied exclusively by the public sector. The role of the state governments in the Indian livestock services sector must be adapted to market realities. The private sector can efficiently and effectively provide those services classified as private goods or toll goods.

Future policies should strengthen the capacity of central and state agencies to manage tasks that remain in the public sector, such as basic research and most agricultural extension activities. Policies should limit public sector involvement with these tasks as the private sector becomes more established.

BREEDING POLICY

Majority of cattle and buffalo in India being of poor quality, the future livestock policy has to give high priority to 'breeding'. The perspective and relevant strategy documents have been prepared with expertise provided by the Swiss Agency for Agriculture and Cooperation. Separate institutional arrangements are to be set up to monitor the project. The proposed project is designed to help augment milk production in the country. Centre had initially conceived of this project for ensuring doorstep delivery of breeding services, including artificial insemination and total coverage of breedable cows and buffaloes within a span of five years. The experts, however, opined that it was not possible to cover 100 percent artificial insemination within this short period of five years without compromising the quality. They have suggested that the programme should be for a period of 10 years and be conducted with a combination of artificial insemination and natural service in difficult areas using both quality semen and quality bulls. Castration of scrub bulls should also be taken up. It is agreed that there should be no compromise over the quality of bulls and microbial quality of semen. There is the need for a national and integrated approach for development of infrastructure, stepping up supply of liquid nitrogen through standby loans, funding arrangements, technology transfer, monitoring health cover, feed and fodder and marketing. The National Bull Programme and

Extension of Frozen Semen Technology Programme will be integrated to support the project.

Buffalo

A two-pronged strategy has to be adopted for sustainable production of buffaloes. There is a need for genetic improvement of buffaloes using selective breeding amongst the descript breeds. These breeds should be further used to improve the breed of nondescript buffaloes so as to develop buffaloes with average production of 1800 litres of milk per lactation. High yielding elite buffalo breeds must be identified so that their male progeny could be procured and raised optimally to meet the requirements of superior bulls. High yielding buffalo population should be stabilized at a sustainable 50 million level.

As regards the utility of buffaloes as a milk, meat and draft animals, not much scientific attention has been paid so far. Although, buffalo meat exports had increased from 59.14 thousands tonnes to 157.57 thousand tonnes, there is a need to expand the trade further. Male calves must be saved from early death for conserving germplasm. A systematic nutrition studies on fattening of animals should be carried out. About 86 per cent of the world buffalo meat comes from Asia, mostly from old and culled animals. According to an estimate, about 10 million male buffalo calves are born annually; but mortality rates are high due to poor nutrition and care. India has a rich genetic resource of buffalo. Potential of milk production from buffaloes has only been partially tapped as 80-85 per cent of them are nondescript and yield on an average is only 1.5 litres of milk a day. There is the need for intensive research on various aspects of embryo transfer to salvage superior genetic females. Also the proven buffalo bulls are in short supply. As against the requirement of 3500 bulls, the Central and State governments annually produce only around 400.

The fate of Haryana's pride, the Murrah buffalo, is uncertain. It could be under serious threat of extinction, animal husbandry experts feel. Each year nearly two lakh young high quality buffaloes, the top 20 per cent of the best genotypes, leave the state for metro cities and after lactation, almost all end up in slaughter houses. These leave no offsprings. The fate of the "Haryana" breed of cows and bullocks is equally bad. This dual purpose breed of cattle - good milk yield and good bullocks known for standing to adverse weather conditions has been the pride of the state since time immemorial. According to experts cows and oxen also end up in slaughter houses in the big cities.

One micro level survey conducted in Mumbai showed that 70 per cent of the Murrah buffaloes were of Haryana origin. These, after one to three lactations, finally end up in the slaughter houses. So far nearly 60 lakh buffaloes and 20 lakh cows have ended their lives in this fashion, the experts calculated. The ever expanding markets for milk in the metro cities in the country exert a vicious pull on the high-yielding milch animals in Haryana, especially the Murrah buffalo.

All these have made the experts sit up and think of ways and means to save the Murrah breed. A project now under implementation envisages strengthening of artificial insemination network, converting them from stationary to mobile, strengthening of the semen production stations and semen banks, investing on a streamlined liquid nitrogen storage and delivery system; and setting up of a centre of excellence for northern region for quality assurance at all levels.

A two pronged strategy has to be adopted for sustainable production of buffaloes. There is thus the need for genetic improvement of buffaloes using selective breeding amongst the distinct breeds. These breeds should be further used to improve the breed of 'nondescript' buffaloes to develop buffaloes with average production of 1800 litres of milk per lactation. We must identify High Yielding Elite Buffalo breeds so that their male progeny could be procured and raised primarily to meet the requirements of superior bulls. We also need for extensive use of multiple ovulation and embryo transfer for faster production of superior bulls which are in short supply. High yielding buffalo population should be stabilised at a sustainable 50 million level.

The reason for South-East Asian tardiness in recognising the buffalo's economic potential goes back to the 1960s and 70s when the frenzied era of development and modernisation first hit the Third World. Everything new, especially foreign, was in and everything old, especially if it was indigenous, was out. Water buffalo - the mainstay of Asian agriculture for a millennia became an embarrassment and an all too-visible symbol of low-tech, even no-tech, represent backwardness, apathy and rural poverty. There would be no progress, ran the arguments, until farmers replaced the offending beast with modern machinery.

Farmers and officials have now discovered that the water buffalo is not merely a work animal, but a dependable producer of milk and meat needed for an expanding international market. A recent report by the US Department of Agriculture (USDA), written with American tastes in mind demolishes much of the negative buffalo dogma. The USDA compared the nutritional value of water buffalo meat with beef and chicken. This shows that Asian buffalo meat has 41 percent less cholesterol, 92 per cent less fat and 56 per cent fewer calories than traditional meat, the report says. It also has a good flavour and texture, can be a substitute for beef in practically any American recipe, and stores well. Overall, the report says, buffalo can be regarded as a delicacy for health-conscious Americans.

In south-East Asia, buffalo meat generally sells for 40-50 per cent less than cow beef, because it comes from animals worked until old age. Their meat is, therefore, tough and stringy. But when the buffalo is raised as a meat producer one gets a completely different quality. The meat becomes succulent and tender, at least as tasty as beef and many would say more so. Pakistan, with about 20 million buffalo, has built a flourishing industry on the slaughter of male calves for high quality veal. Non-vegetarian Hindus in India and Nepal have no qualms about eating buffalo meat, though cow meat remains taboo.

In Hong Kong, three-quarters of the beef served in restaurants is buffalo meat bought at knockdown prices from South-East Asia. Buffalo milk accounts for three quarters of all Indian milk consumption, and in Italy - home to half a million prime quality buffaloes - it is used to make mozzarella cheese. Today, Australia's buffalo meat and milk industry is so high-tech that buffalo roundups are often carried out by helicopter. It also earns good money exporting prime breeding stock to a growing number of countries outside Asia, including Brazil, Bolivia, Mexico, Central America and even the USA. Outside Asia, buffalo herds are growing by 2.6 percent a year, compared to the much lower Asian rate of 1.5 percent.

Rohtak: This historical town of Haryana, has developed over the years an important centre for the famed Murrah breed of buffaloes. A large number of high milk-yielding buffaloes of this breed are not only supplied to various parts of the country but are also exported to several countries. Perhaps, this is one reason why this town is also called the "city of dairies' in northern India.

The town has over 124 dairies involved in the sale and purchase of milch cattle. About 60 to 80 buffaloes and cows are loaded or unloaded here every day and over 2500 persons, including about 150 commission agents, are working full-time in this business. The Dairy colony is spread over several acres and has been a source of milk and milk products to the town and nearby areas. Hundreds of litres of milk are supplied from here.

At least 200 to 225 head of cattle of the Murrah breed can be purchased at any time as the dairies have ready supply while dairy owners or commission agents charge rent for keeping the animals here for sale, some of the agents contact the farmers or the owners to purchase the buffaloes from them and supply these to markets outside. The commission agent usually charges 1 per cent commission from the seller and Rs. 100 from the buyer for each cattle during the transaction. There are at least four varieties of the Murrah breed and these are charged as per the variety and demand. For example, the demand from the western region is different from what is sought by the traders from the eastern region or U.P.

Extension Service and Globalisation

The focus of agricultural extension efforts is mainly on achieving higher productivity, whether in the field of agriculture, animal husbandry or dairy. Taking stock of the infrastructure today, we would see that extension services are largely in the public sector, while other operators (NGOs, etc.) remain at the periphery without having clear policy enunciation or institutional support. The services also operate largely in an interpersonal mode with select contact farmers–mostly men–without planned and optimum utilization of the media and other modes.

There is very little involvement of farmers in the technology development and dissemination process. The top-down approach leaves little scope for localized planning and action. The extension services are also manned by functionaries with low morale, knowledge level and incentives, with limited exposure to recent developments in communication technology.

DAIRY

The dairy business in India is currently estimated at Rs. 80,000 crore. "Indian dairying has several in-built competitive advantages which, if exploited, would lead to the manifold growth of the industry. A large bovine population, strong procurement infrastructure, skilled manpower, cheap labour and a large number of processing and allied facilities are some of the advantages which India enjoys. With the present growth rate of around 4 per cent per annum, India is expected to produce around 182 million tonnes of milk by 2030, more than one-third of the projected global production of 620 to 650 million tonnes.

Considering that the dairy market in the developed countries had reached a saturation point and emerging milk markets were expected to be Asian and African countries, India had yet another advantage. "India's geographical location is an advantage when compared with other dairying countries like the Scandinavian nations, the US, Australia and New Zealand,' With increasing awareness of the importance and better values of buffalo milk, it will gain prominence at the global level. India has a vast milk procurement and distribution system with 90,000 village cooperative societies, 170 district unions and 23 state federations. With nine dairy science colleges, 31 veterinary colleges and 80 agricultural research institutes, India has large number of professionals working in the industry. One of the greatest challenges before Indian dairying is improving the quality of milk as presently there is lack of hygiene and sanitation at the production level.

Increasing efficiency in the dairy-processing sector is critical, especially as dairy trade is increasingly liberalized. Effective competition would not be achieved if barriers to entry and protection embodied in the amended MMPO are maintained. The key measures suggested in the chapter on Dairying and Environmental aspects need to be tackled properly. The trade liberalization should be coupled with government action that induces the needed structural changes in the processing and marketing sectors. Such changes require reevaluating existing financial and technical assistance programmes to the rural poor in order to achieve more efficient use of rural resources. Necessary social safety nets may be needed for the poorest farmers.

Policy

The key issue is whether India can address the significant weaknesses while remaining true to the basic principles that have been the foundation of this success. In the answers to this question lie the international competitive advantage that will take our farmers and our industry well into this century. The task before us is not to become the biggest - but the best. The building blocks of our success are well known, if not well understood. First is the partnership of farmer with the professional. The wisdom and energy of the farmer, combined with the knowledge and skills of the professional have created the conditions of confidence and strength that enabled our farmers-mostly women - to achieve a miracle. The second block is the Indian consumer. Whatever the region, whether urban or rural, rich or poor, our people consume milk and dairy products. The world's largest domestic market is the strong foundation of our industry. Third is our system of dairying. The delicate farming systems that have evolved in our country depend on the livestock that produce our draught power, our manure and our milk. Our animals survive on residues and the byproducts of our agriculture. This gives our industry an enormous competitive advantage in terms of energy efficiency.

Milk Policy and Cow

Poor genetic potential is an inherent character in our milch animals, which limits their productivity and fertility. It takes generations to improve it by selection and intercrossing. The process can, however, be accelerated by induction of superior exotic germplasm. However, even a high-genetic – potential cow or buffalo would not be able to express it fully in terms of milk production without proper production environment and nutritious feeding, concepts of which Indian farmers are virtually unaware at present. These two major factors inhibit the profitability of milk production.

The economies of nutrition has to be fully understood vis-a-vis productivity. Our buffaloes have poor genetic potential and fail to qualify as economic milk producers in spite of their high fat content in milk as milk production has to compete with cash and commercial crops. They calve for the first time at 4.5 years and their average lactational yield is 1,300 kg only. Their lactation is hardly for 210 days. The inter-calving period is 15-18 months, which means the dry period is 270 to 330 days. The maintenance cost during this unproductive period raises the cost of milk production.

Unfortunately, no better genetic material is available anywhere in the world for improving their productivity. Buffalo, thus remains the poor man's animal, which can be sustained on crop residues and grass under semi-starved and unhygienic conditions. The genetic potential and performance of our cows is equally unsatisfactory. In spite of the fact that we started crossbreeding long back, the outlook of the Directorate of Animal Husbandry has not gone much beyond health cover for animals. That is why several schemes like the "key village" programmes or the intensive cattle development projects did not lead to great success.

We continue to rely on mopping up milk from an ever-increasing number of villages, while the quality of animals has degraded. Ironically, crossbred cows with high exotic breed do not find a place in the prevailing pattern o milk production. This is so because we have not been able to educate our consumers that the nutritional value of milk is not in its fat content, rather in its solids-non-fat (SNF) and that its yellow colour makes it richer in vitamins. There is also no rational milk pricing policy for encouraging dairy farming with crossbred cows. There is valid criticism that crossbred cows are a failure because of inefficient health and artificial insemination services and their being more susceptible to diseases. We have to be globally competitive, and in that context our policy makers should redefine the policies for increasing the quantity of milk as a source of proteins and calcium (SNF).

We need a new policy, strategy and approach for the production of cow milk in higher quantity and quality. This requires a class of progressive farmers with means to invest in quality production environment, including nutritional feeding. Al present the average lactational productivity level of Punjab's crossbred cows is 3,000 kg. This can easily be raised to 7,000 kg in five years by introducing a hi-tech milk production programme. A villager should maintain cows and buffaloes only if it makes economic sense. To expect the rural poor to be in milk production merely out of tradition is to perpetuate the present. Unsatisfactory socioeconomic situation. Most milk producers carry on cattle rearing despite low returns because of the ready cash-flow factor. The real issue whether milk producers can optimize their herds to become dairy farmers with a decent income from milk production as an independent profession.

All dairy countries of the world have evolved their own breeding indexes, taking into consideration the international standards for cost-effective milk production. India should also work for attaining in five years a breeding index at hi-technology satellite dairy farms (with 20 or more animals) as under:

- Inseminate selected crossbred cows with semen from high-productivity – proven sires (with over 10,000 kg lactation) out of the 10 HF strains identified by the FAO of the United Nations.

- Rear female calves for early maturity to attain a weight of 250 kg at the age of 11-13 months for becoming pregnant and calving before they are 24 months old.

- After normal calving, cows come in heat every 21 days. Watch them for heat on the 21st and 42nd days after calving, failing which they should be treated. Ensure that they get inseminated on the third heat, or 63 days after calving, and become pregnant. During summer, cool the cows and inseminate in shade. Inseminate twice with an interval of 2/3 hours for ensuring a better conception rate.

- Cows must have a longevity and persistency of lactation, extending over 3000 days.

- Dry period of the cows should not be more than 65 days, which means a calving interval of only 12 months.

- Prefer heifers that get pregnant with one or two shots of insemination in a heat and cows that conceive on or before completing 84 days from calving.
- Discard "leaky teats" cows, as they are more prone to mastitis.
- During summer, cool the cows before milking.
- By adopting proper farming technologies, increase fodder production from an acre of land to meet the green fodder requirement of five crossbred cows as against the present of three cows only and take to silage making from summer fodder crops in a big way.

POULTRY

The cost of broiler meat production in India is lower than that in most countries, even as compared to USA and Brazil, where the price of maize, which is the main chicken feed ingredient, is lower than that in India. Under the WTO Agreement if the bound rate on import duty on poultry products is enforced, dumping of leg meat (which is sold very cheap in the US), into the Indian market may be difficult. Opening up of the industry to outside competition is fine as long as it is fair, but this free import of chicken legs has already killed domestic industry in Russia and Sri Lanka and may kill our industry as well.

Developed countries have the benefit of huge subsidies that give them an unfair price advantage over developing countries. Under the WTO agreement, developed countries are not required to withdraw these subsidies totally. It is only essential for them to cut production subsidies by 20% and export subsidies by 36% over 10 years, which indicates that subsidies will still be at high levels after 10 years. It has been advocated by the governments that if developed and developing country farmers are to compete in the same markets then the $ 280 billion annual subsidies that developed countries provide to their farmers should be reduced to the negligible amounts that developing countries provide. Otherwise, developing countries should be allowed to increase both their subsidies and their tariffs to protect their markets from the highly subsidized exports of the developed countries. Developed countries should eliminate the tariff escalation on product chains of interest to developing countries. If the WTO continues to force all countries down the liberalisation path, the protected sectors in the US must also be liberalised to open up new export markets for developing nations.

Poultry industry today is at cross roads. It seems to be ridiculous that in one news, NECC asks poultries to cut egg production at least 20 per cent on account of less market demand and also to save feed ingredient during this scarcity period, in another news there were inauguration ceremonies of new hatcheries in some parts of north India. Cutting of egg production and saving of feed ingredients involve reduction of layers tremendously by way of random culling of birds above one year as well reduced production of layer chicks. It is just like in war where sometimes retreats become necessary for ultimate gain and win in the battle. When we are retreating for some gainful purpose in our poultry industry why there is some advancement at the same time! Does it not foil the very purpose? Hatcheries are started for production of broiler and layer chicks and not for mere showcase in the public. This industry had already suffered over production few years back and millions of chicks as well as hatching eggs were destroyed sustaining a tremendous loss to our nation. There is no parity and correlation between the market demand and production, and this hapless, disorganised industry faces, tremendous problem everytime. If we consider right from the Grand Parents (GP) operation up to the grass root level of production, we will see aimless and disorganised activity everywhere. The breed is highlighted by some GP operators in such a way that hatcherymen are overwhelmed for a single factor. Hatchery operators have more of the orientation towards earning profits by selling day-old chicks to the poultry farmers, and are only interested in the number of chicks obtained from the parent stock. They do not bother about other factors like Feed Conversion Ratio (FCR), dressing yield, meat conversion ratio, which are not taken into account although these traits are the key factors towards evaluation of production cost. Due to poor FCR there is obviously a wastage of feed ingredients thus causing a set back to the economy.

As to the Indian meat industry, it is highly undeveloped and disorganised as compared to that of other countries as, much of the focus is on the production aspect with little or no inroads into marketing and distribution of processed chicken to the end consumers. Markets and segments are fragmented with only new integrated players. Processing which is the nucleus of value chain is not fully developed as the customers preference goes to the live chicken (about 95%) rather than processed chicken (5%). There is lack of effort towards creating food awareness amongst the consumers unlike the customers of developed countries where some organisations and food laws have been formed for the special type of consumers preferring some different kind of products much like organic chicken and organic eggs. Our industry is getting a great jolt due mainly to the disorganised marketing system specially in the broiler industry. After going for the broilers, these are sold to the suppliers in the live market and ultimately these intermediaries, sell at a high margins to the end customers.

In India, most of the entrepreneurs are having stand alone business and the broiler producing units have grown like mushrooms without control having no market assessment and study. As a result, broiler being a perishable product, requires immediate marketing with no other alternative than to depend on any middle man trader who spares no time to utilize this situation and opportunity of exploitation. This type of present unbridled activity, it is expected, will no longer remain and a revolution is required in the ensuing days. The first and foremost attitude will be towards integration of hatcheries, feed mills, broiler growing and processing. The breeds will be selected on the basis of economic traits and not only on hatchery level, just to produce more numbers of chicks. All small and marginal producers (both in egg and meat sector) should come under contract of the large integrators to avoid both risk and the middlemen. Farmers should follow biosecurity and should be calculative for FCR, dressing yields etc. in addition to good management. Due to increased customer awareness towards quality and hygiene, demand for such products is expected to grow fast. There is a huge potential in the untapped rural market as the consumption of poultry products is limited to 25% of the total population only due to many social and religious taboos, orthodox ideas and superstition.

India is running behind other developed countries due to non-application of new-technologies in the poultry sector and as a result the industry suffers a penalty. So, like America we require to form a National Chicken Council that will have three functions: (1) To represent the government with all types of industry problems; (2) To create awareness to the consumers regarding all problems so that suggestions may come from them; and (3) To bring all the small farmers under one roof by giving membership to all of them. The challenge with the EU countries and with WTO at the present moment has to be met by adopting new technologies in the field of poultry production, with emphasis on the feed problems, cold storages for the processed products, and transport system in our country. It is also necessary to give proper attention in chicken processing, gradation, quality control and labeling in addition to animal welfare, health care and the environment.

The Deputy Director, CII Mr. Dilip Chenoy expressed his views on the National Poultry Policy and advised to keep pace with the advancement of the poultry industry in other countries. The poultry world is changing rapidly and we are to keep our eyes open on this aspect. In India, on the other hand, 97% of the chicken are slaughtered in the roadside wet shops and the customer preference is more on fresh chicken rather than hygienically dressed chicken in the processing plant. Till now we could not reach the interior villages with our products. As regards maize problem, that import tax on maize should be exempted to make it available cheaper. The vegetarians should know the benefit of egg consumption. Today anti snake venom drug may be prepared from the eggs laid by a genetically modified hen. To increase egg consumption the Midday Meal system in schools should be introduced.

India has the immense potential for its advancement in this field of poultry production. Still India lags behind due to want of proper data which are very essential to achieve success in future programme. We are still behind other countries because we are unable to take bold steps in the modernisation of broiler rearing, poultry meat production and other changes in the industry. Our poultry policy should be changed by enforcing food safety measures, increasing quality standards including packaging, labeling, etc. like developed countries. The government should take an advanced step to help this industry so that we can be successful in changing our policy matter discarding all the old and indigenous methods in the field of poultry production. We should give special stress on marketing so that we are able to find out market for our processed products. IT sector can help a lot in opening new markets with information of different market rates of the world. This IT sector in the poultry industry would be of great help and solution to most of the problems in the industry.

Broiler Cooperatives

Poultry farmers of the northern region are all set to form cooperative societies to achieve the twin objective of making fresh chicken available at an affordable price as well as reducing malpractices in the trade. Though Bromark - All-India Broiler Farmers Marketing Cooperative – has already evoked good response from both poultry farmers and consumers in Andhra Pradesh, Maharashtra and a few other states, it will soon be spreading its operations in Chandigarh, Punjab and Haryana.

If one looks at the price at which a poultry farmer sells a bird and the rate at which a consumer buys it, one will find the difference unacceptably high. For example, the prevalent rate that farmers get is Rs. 32 to Rs 35 a kg, while in the retail market it is sold for Rs. 75 to Rs. 80 per kg Chandigarh is a big market. The average consumption is about 15,000 birds a day. If we make chicken available at an affordable price, say Rs. 60 to Rs. 65 a kg, it will push up sale and help both producers and consumers. The idea is that both farmers and consumers should benefit and prevent trade malpractices. Once this cooperative movement is in place, the market scenario will improve. Such cooperative should have its won outlets so that consumers are assured of quality as well as affordable price. One of challenges facing the poultry industry is establishing credibility. Because of the big variation in the price of chicken, at times consumers get the impression that they are being supplied diseased or dead birds.

The endeavour of the new cooperative federation would be to build credibility and promise consumers that they would get healthy birds. All outlets will have a standard design and each outlet will have to maintain hygiene and cleanliness standards. Regarding low prices, the increase in consumption will offset the decreased margin of profit of traders and retailers. The idea is not to replace the existing trade channels in any manner, but to ensure quality products at affordable price.

The new concept is modelled on the National Egg Coordination Committee (NECC), which ensures that the egg prices are remunerative to the producer and fair to the consumer. With its various activities and promotional campaigns, it has been successful in keeping the gap between the farmgate price and the consumer price at not more than 30 per cent. In the present-day chicken industry, the difference is 100 to 110 per cent. Once farmers join the cooperative, things would change.

PIGS

After poultry, turkey and ostrich, it is now the turn of lowly pigs. With the USA witnessing a dramatic switchover in food palate, ushering in an unprecedented explosion in the demand for pigmeat, it is a matter of time before pig factories emerge as a major agri-business enterprise in India. Such is the rapid growth of the pig industry that international banks and financial institutes are vying with one anther to increase funding for a sector which was never considered to be credit worthy. Realising that the US pigmeat industry is poised to expand in search for international markets, pig farming is turning into specialized activity. But with the strict environmental regulations slowing down the development of the pig industry, already shifting the production base to relatively less populated areas in southwest America, the dirty and unhygienic enterprise is sure to be translocated to India. And like the boon in floriculture, "pig factories" will also bring in a highly environment- unfriendly production activity to India in return for hard currency.

In North America, the outlook was for a continued increase in pig production till the year 2001. Much of it coming after strong price increase for slaughtered pigs following the mad cow disease related demand shifts since 1996. An ample indication is available from the export projections. From 4,26,000 tonnes of carcass weight equivalent achieved in 1996, the USA was able to double its exports to over 9,40,000 tonnes in 2001. With the consumption of meat products continuing to increase in Asia, the industry is targeting the two populated giants - China and India. And as it normally happens, India's infant agri-business industry blindly looks up to and draws inspiration from such developments in the Western markets.

At least, four multinational food giants have found cassava, the staple food of some 350 million Africans; to be a money - spinning commodity after it was discovered that it could be suitably modified as pig feed. Unlike the inhabitants of George Orwell's Animal Farm, the pig factories are huge industrial complexes, with over 1,00,000 pigs crammed in the pigpens. And like the poultry farms, pigs are cramped in stalls in such a way that it leaves no room for any manoeuvre. The most popular "bacon bin" system of housing pigs, provides for 500 individual cages, each measuring not more than seven square metres of living space. Every pig spends his entire life cramped into a space less than one-third of the size of a twin bed. Pork engineers feel that the "bacon bin" is advantageous as it ensures that pigs don't burn calories in useless' activities like walking and playing. And still worse, these pigs never get to see daylight.

The high intake of hormones and pesticides results in environmental contamination. Already, high pesticides residues in pig droppings have contaminated the ground water supplies in the Netherlands to such an alarming extent that public protests is forcing the government to look for alternatives. Since the pig droppings cannot be dumped into the sea, Holland had unsuccessfully tried to ship it to India, With the World Bank seal of approval and with huge subsidies available from the European Union, Holland is now banking upon the World Trade Organisation (WTO) to pave the way for unhindered export of pig droppings and dung to developing countries.

If the USA and other countries of the OECD find it to be a profitable enterprise irrespective of the ethical, religious and environmental considerations, the Indian agri-business industry must faithfully follow. Considering the dubious role of agricultural scientists and planners in promoting the controversial bovine somatotropin (BST) hormonal drug for cattle, coastal aquaculture and floriculture at the cost of sustainable farming practices, Indian Council of Agricultural Research (ICAR) and APEDA would possibly prepare a research and development blueprint for putting pigs on the industrial map.

FISHERIES

The Marine Products Exports Development Authority has been engaged in export of marine products since its establishment. Its valuable contributions have enabled generation of employment potentiality as well as good foreign exchange reserves, which have no doubt, played an important role in the economic development of the country. India exported 424470 MT of seafood valued at Rs. 5957.05 crore equivalent to US$ 1253.35 million in the year 2001-02. As seafood processing and marketing have become competitive, a multi-pronged attempt is required, right from techno-economic appraisals to technical support, farm technology upgradation to total quality management and farm market intelligence for market penetration.

The 1.3 billion dollar export seafood sector has to focus on issues related to increasingly strict hygiene standards of the western bloc, the value-addition scope and potential, the need for conservation of fishery resources, the rich untapped resource of waste hinterlands for aquaculture and the much-needed financial support package needed by the industry. We have to offer an opportunity to the foreigners to understand the technological improvements made by the industry in India and offer scope for discussions on future potential in the Indian subcontinent on various segments of the marine product industry, which is expected to play a key role in the export plan of the country. International trade in fish and fishery products should be conducted in accordance with the principles, rights and obligations established in the World Trade Organisation (WTO) and other relevant international agreements. We should ensure that our policies, programmes and practices related to trade of fish and fishery products do not result in obstacles in the trade but to enhance our exports in the competitive international market.

All the stakeholders should make all possible efforts to adopt the national and international standards of trade to enhance exports in the competitive international market. We should take full advantage of the modern technologies in vogue in developed countries in the world to increase fish production, specially reducing pressure on depleted fish stocks and preserve our fishing grounds from over fishing and pollution, etc. Natural resources are to be maintained for future generation. We have to learn to coexist with nature and on playing effective role in securing the sustainable development of this resource. Now is the time that direction be determined and policy be amended. Fisheries sector has great scope for expansion like other sectors contributing to the economy. Fisheries have also potential for increasing food for domestic and international demand, value-added fishery products export can also contribute to the foreign exchange earnings. The code of conduct for responsible fisheries need to be fully adopted for sustainable development.

Desired objectives in fisheries sector cannot be achieved until and unless we ensure proper implementation of code of conduct for responsible fisheries at the grossroot level. Marine fisheries resources, although renewable, they are subject to over exploitation, depletion and to the influence of environmental factor. Marine fisheries resources therefore need to be managed scientifically and such management should be understood not as a constraint upon rational exploitation but as an essential tool for sound and sustained development. There is a need today for identification of suitable development schemes for the improvement of on board fish handling practices and close coordination with processing plant owners and exporters and promotion and dissemination of the objectives and implementation of the code of conduct for responsible fisheries to create awareness of its benefits to all stakeholders and existing laws to be amended to reduce the catching of juvenile fisheries resources. Further, there is the need to improve fisheries data system and better coordination among all stakeholders and human resource capacity of provincial fisheries departments and to ensure the strict enforcement of the existing laws regarding destructive fishing gear, ban during breeding season and handling of fishery products, in letter and spirit. This also calls for providing loan to fishermen on soft-terms for the upgradation of their boats and for developing shrimp aquaculture and improving harbour management.

HIGH QUALITY LEATHER

As the Centre mulls over a proposed ban on cow slaughter, a nationwide assessment indicates that a well-developed network of fallen carcass recovery system can not only help in adding about Rs 300-400 crore of rural income but also create jobs for 300,000 people. Scientists at the Chennai-based Central Leather Research Institute have shown that it is possible to convert low-grade hides from old and dead animals to obtain high quality leather. Their work had caught the attention of then HRD Minister M.M. Joshi, who also handled the Department of Science and Technology. Joshi was so gung-ho about the new technology that he had asked for a proper feasibility study.

The proposal is that the government should go in for a 'cow care mission' to ensure that cattle-heads are taken care of by villagers, who use cow-dung as an alternative source of energy. When the animals die naturally they would be taken to low-cost technology centres for recovery of hides and other biowaste. In other words, it is still possible to get good leather from animals without killing them. Recovery centres were set up as part of leather technology mission of CLRI at 31 locations. According to CLRI Director, Dr T. Ramasami, scientists have demonstrated the viability of the technology in Kanpur, Lucknow, and Unnao. Each centre, using quick collection system of dead animals, earned between Rs. 22,550 and Rs 91,000 in 25 days. Even byproducts in the form of hides, meat meal, bone meal, horn powder, tallow and other products became economic activities even if each centre was not able to collect three animals a day.

EXTENSION SERVICE

Agricultural and livestock extension in India is at the crossroads. New opportunities (and threats) for trade in international markets join older concerns of supporting the rural economy where agricultural and livestock production and employment support the livelihoods of many of the poorest in society. The shortcomings of public sector extension arrangements in India are well documented and some reform measures have been implemented. But unfortunately, planning and evaluation of such programmes are based on a very narrow view of the proper role of extension, equating it to an agency for technology dissemination. This is certainly a role which extension can play. However, it is widely acknowledged that there are other important facilitating functions that it could perform to help create a stronger livestock development system adapted to evolving rural economics and the agenda of stakeholders, especially the poor.

To remain relevant, Indian agricultural and livestock extension has to reinvent itself. This will require considerable institutional and organizational changes in both the public research and extension arena. This policy brief explains the restrictions that a technology dissemination focus places on the debate of extension reform and provides a more holistic viewpoint to help reconsider critical policy questions India's public research and extension organisations. For the last 30 years the practice of extension has been guided by the all-pervasive, "diffusion of innovations" tradition. Thinking on the nature of the agricultural and livestock technology development and promotion process has, however, advanced in the last 20 years. This includes the recognition that: technological innovations come from multiple sources, including farmers[1]; and that the way the agendas of different stakeholders are represented affects the "appropriateness" of new technologies developed. Farmer participation in technology development and participatory extension approaches have emerged as a response to such new thinking. This has often failed, however, to challenge the wider institutional and political context in which "participation" takes place.

During the last decade, the extension literature has been notable for holistic ideas such as the Agricultural Knowledge and Information System (AKIS)[2]. This recognizes a wider set of information sources and the value

[1]Biggs, S.D. (1990) A Multiple Sources of Innovation Model of Agricultural Research and Technology Promotion, World Development (18) 11, pp 1481-1499.

[2]Roling, N.G. (1990) The Agricultural Research-Technology Transfer Interface: a Knowledge System Perspective. In D. Kaimowitz (ed), Making the Link: Agricultural Research and Technology Transfer in Developing countries, Westview press, Boulder.

of creating systems that assist in the generation and dissemination of knowledge, especially in the context of sustainable agriculture and progress towards an ecological knowledge system. More recently the notion of extension as part of a wider system has emerge. For example the "interdependence model"[1] and the innovation system framework[2] offer more inclusive way of thinking about the actors and the institutional context in which the generation, diffusion and use of new knowledge takes place. This system of actors and process not only includes research and extension, but also technology users, private companies and nongovernmental organisations and supportive structures such as markets and credit.

The innovation system framework, in particular, places emphasis on the importance of learning processes as a way of evolving new arrangements specific to local contexts. The political economy in which these processes and activities take place is viewed as a key contextual element, where investigating and managing stakeholder agendas can help address the asymmetry of conventional research-extension-farmer relations. The advocates of the approach suggest that its use for the evaluation and planning of technology development and promotion activities is the only way to build locally adapted, collective operational capacities where institutional concerns such as a poverty focus can be monitored and sustained[3,4]. Although these various "systems" concepts of technology development and promotion provide significant policy insights, none of them has yet found mainstream operational uptake in agricultural and livestock extension system.

A paradigm shift is required from production-oriented extension service to "knowledge/information" — based extension that is relevant to market demand and supply, pricing trends (inputs/outputs), weather forecast and is situation-specific. It must also enable farmers to adopt "coping" strategies for livestock management and profitability. With the changing role of farmers' wives in decision-making at home/farm and women taking part in village institutions the next generation of extension services shall also have to be oriented towards them as well in respect of home management, education of girl child, health, nutrition etc. as part of the government endeavor to empower women. It is time to reorient this service for dissemination of farm/home science information and knowledge from

[1]Bennet, C (1992) A New Interdependence Model-Implications for Extension Education, University of Illinois, Office of International Agriculture, Interpaks Digest, Vol 1, Fall, 1992

[2]Lundvall, B.A. (ed) (1992) National Innovations System: Towards a theory of innovations and interactive learnings, Printer, London.

[3]Biggs, S.D. and G. Smith, (1998) Beyond Methodologies: Coalition Building for Participatory Technology Development, World Development 26 (2): 239-248.

[4]Hall, A.J, M.V.K. Sivamohan, N. Clark, S. Taylor and G. Bocket (2001) Why Research partnerships Really Matter: Innovation Theory, Institutional Arrangements and Implications for Developing New technology for the Poor, World Development 29 (5): 782-797.

laboratory to land in tune with the world farm produce/product market or the WTO regime or to reinvent extension education teaching Agricultural University in the interest of farmers and their wives.

The World Bank has also taken cognizance of this aspect of agriculture and livestock development. Its rural strategy backgrounder series, "rural extension and advisory services" report shows a roadmap to reorient state extension service and reinvent university's extension education system, which it expects to be adopted. The analogy of the World Bank extension service system is that agriculture together with livestock has to act as an "engine of growth" for integrated rural development, which is the key to meeting global challenges of poverty reduction, economic growth, food security and environment conservation. The bank has provided some $3.07 billion in direct support of extension, while mobilizing another $2.54 billion from governments, beneficiaries and other sources in the past 20 years.

In Punjab, one of most advanced agriculture states in India, ever since Agriculture Inspectors got designated as Agriculture Development Officers (ADO) by using political influence as a fulcrum, extension service has been neglected and ignored. At present while ADOs' links have snapped with farmers, particularly small, marginal and medium, who own up to four hectares and are the backbone of agriculture, their interaction, relation and equation have become more pronounced with "dealers/ahrtiays" of farm inputs. Today, an ADO is "equal" in status to a Chief Agricultural Officer. This has severed the chain of command and control in the districts, as even transfer/posting of an ADO is now done at a higher level. Insofar as ADOs' functions and responsibilities, less said the better. As catalysts of change, ADO' are to distribute mini-kits to farmers for trial run of new crops, establish "demonstration" plots, showing application of recommended agronomic practices, supervise quality production, collect samples to check sale of spurious inputs (fertilizer, seed, insecticides etc.) and ensure timely supply of farm inputs. But it is best left to ADOs to spell out how "honestly" they discharge these functions and who their real clients are.

Weaknesses

The following administrative weaknesses in the transfer of technology programmes may be identified:

- The top–down administrative system continues to govern the rural/agricultural and livestock development work with the result that rural people have merely been passive recipients of benefits rather than being active participants in the development process.

> Globalisation of agriculture poses the challenge of identifying a suitable extension approach that can provide continuous, relevant and modern technology to commercial minded and export-oriented farmers.

- Lack of adequate incentives to attract and retain good extension functionaries in the villages.
- Lack of short- and long-term training programmes for upgrading extension functionaries in their professional background and technical qualifications.
- Indifferent attitude of the field-level functionaries towards extension work.
- Non-availability of trained staff, delay in recruitment, frequent transfers and diversion of ill-equipped staff to extension projects.
- Lack of transport facility for the extension staff.

Corrections Needed

Globalisation of agriculture throws the greatest challenge to identify the suitable extension approach that can provide continuous, relevant, modern technology messages to commercial minded, export-oriented farmers by making use of the latest information technology. Many state governments have opted for one or more of the following solutions to strengthen the extension systems:

- Improving the modus operandi of the existing structure of extension services.
- Administrative decentralization of services.
- Devolution of functions of regional development authorities that work free of government regulations.
- Transferring responsibility of advisory services to private or quasi-public organizations.

Globalisation

Agricultural and animal husbandry farming in global environment has brought its on requirements. Farmers have to be trained to be made aware of GATT and its implications. Export-oriented technologies will have to be generated for different agroclimatic zones and enterprises. The present extension system will have to be reoriented to suit the small farmers. Farmers should be taught to become more competitive. They also need to be trained in agro-processing and livestock products processing. The farm education services should also advise farmers on maintaining quality standards of their products.

Farmers should be provided indirect subsidies and extension personnel should see to the equal and proper distribution of the subsidy amount. Infrastructure facilities like transportation, communication, storage, processing, packaging and marketing, etc., have to be strengthened. Cooperative village management has to be promoted, i.e., the management of village affairs by the local people themselves under the aegis of certain associations or cooperative societies.

Privatisation

Extension services, which were mostly public worldwide until a decade ago, are increasingly being transferred to the private domain. The inability of governments to fund the extension machinery is the real reason behind the search for alternative approaches such as cost sharing and privatisation. In India, the increasing costs of providing services and the government's unwillingness to give full support forced research organizations (ICAR and SAUs) and training organizations (KVKs) to identify the services that could generate resources.

Services, such as a soil testing, input cost of field demonstrations, consultation, etc. are now starting to be charge for. There is a new concept of livestock-clinic emerging, meant to provide timely advisory services to farmers in respect of both crop production and marketing aspects on payment. Since these agri-clinics operate at the grass root level, farmers–specific problems can be tackled properly.

Recommendations for Development of Livestock Sector

Based on the discussion and analysis given in various chapters, major recommendations for the future policy are summarized below:

(i) Bringing animal husbandry in the concurrent list, under which both the Central and State Government can pass legislation. However, in case of conflict or disagreement, the central law will prevail. This would enable more coherent policy framing and implementation.

(ii) Initiation of legislative measures to amend laws concerning cooperatives.

(iii) Elimination in phases of subsidies in other sectors which are prejudicial to Livestock sector.

(iv) Adoption of National Livestock Policy with broad outlines of policy-strategy-programme framework.

(v) A rejuvenated waste land development programme with a fresh look on the carrying capacity concept in the light of recent development.

(vi) Creation of an institution on the line of Commission on Agricultural Cost and Prices, in order to have dynamic studies on cost of inputs concerning livestock products.

(vii) Livestock resources mapping in line with "Food Insecurity Map of India" conceptualized by World Food Programme is needed. This Livestock Atlas will enable zone specific planning for future. This will also cause a shift from the current species/discipline based programmes in the livestock sector to area specific programmes.

(viii) Restructuring of government departments, both at the Centre and the States, fostering new institutions and synergies of emerging players-setting up Pashu Vigyan Kendras (Livestock Research Centres).

(ix) Coordination mechanism among government agencies on areas of converging interests like fodder.

(x) Augmenting fund flow
   (a) tapping resources from multi-disciplinary schemes (rural development, watershed development, etc.)
   (b) imposing cess on large processing capacity for milk, meat, wool, etc. and using the same for sectoral development.
   (c) Disinvestments of government infrastructure that can be used for commercial purposes (land, livestock farms, sperm stations, vaccine production centres, milk plants, etc.)
   (d) Cost recovering of goods and services from consumers.

(xi) Policy on containing animal number and animal slaughter.

(xii) Major programmes towards containing important communicable diseases.

(xiii) Improving access to credit technology and information including market information. Massive upgradation of information network for livestock and assimilation of new methods of creation of a dynamic database concerning production economics.

(xiv) Privatization of livestock extension services and vet health services to the extent possible – bare foot doctors (Tamil Nadu and Maharashtra).

(xv) Setting up of Universities of Veterinary, and Animal Sciences – Two such Universities have already been established.

Concluding Remarks

The key issue for future development of livestock is whether developing countries including India can address major weaknesses while remaining true to the basic principle that have been the foundation of this success. In the answers to the question lie the international competitive advantages that our farmers and our industry will get in 21st century. The task before us is not to become the bigger but the best. In this respect we have no doubt a few strength which are we have already stated at the outset. These are: (i) a strong partnership between our farmers and the professionals; (ii) a very large domestic vibrant market; (iii) a very efficient system of livestock farming contributing to crop farming with competitive advantage in terms of energy efficiency and at the sometime without competing with humans in foodgrain sharing; and (iv) quality of products. However, application of more intensified science and technology is a prerequisite for achieving further improvement in quality and diversification of livestock products.

Productivity is the key to growth. We have no option but to raise the productivity of our livestock through scientific breeding, feeding and management, the goal is no longer the farmer's share of the consumer's rupee. It is significant and sustained increase in farmer's income and employment. Quality is the bedrock of success for any enterprise and there is no substitute for consistent, superior quality. Our system has not yet any built-in quality at every stage from the udder to the consumer. Until we achieve world-standard quality, we will not only find access to markets abroad limited and difficult but will continue to be vulnerable to challenges even at home. The wisdom and energy of the farmers combined with the knowledge and skills of the professionals would create the conditions of confidence and strength that has already brought out many success stories and instances of miracles.

It may be reiterated that there is a need for expansion and adoption of superior economics in production, transport, processing and marketing to meet the growing domestic consumer demand. It is also essential to restructure our production system, if necessary, abandoning the older ones to confront the present day and future challenges.

Our infrastructure, though widespread, is too often poorly used. The cost of traditional livestock based enterprises is increasing. Our research and design must provide answers to emerging questions. Our support to end-users must help raising significantly their efficiency and economy. The future of livestock sector rests not only on the farmers, but on the scientists, the technologists and the professionals. We must equip a new generation to compete head on with the best human resources of the advanced nations. In this backdrop, it becomes difficult to remain divorced from the personnel and organisational structure, which is to formulate policies and execute programmes for the development of the animal husbandry sector.

Efforts have been made to control major livestock diseases namely Rinderpest, Foot and Mouth, Haemorrhagic Septicemia, Black quarter and Anthrax over the years. Although Rinderpest has been eradicated, the other diseases continue as major impediments in animal production. Some of the emerging diseases like Peste des petits ruminants (PPR), Bluetongue, Sheep Pox, Classical Swine Fever, Contagious Bovine Pleuropneumonia, New Castle etc. are causing substantial economic losses. National/regional programs for control of some of the important livestock diseases need to be taken up on priority: Strong disease diagnosis network and efficient disease monitoring programs would be critical to our effort in controlling livestock diseases.

Small ruminants which are reared by the poorest of the poor have been neglected by the planners and kept mostly out of development plans. In spite of these, sheep and goat continue to grow at around 0.5 and 3% even after a slaughter rate of 35-40% and high mortality of 10-20% per annum. But the fine wool production in the country is only around 4 million kg as against the demand of around 35 to 40 million kg.

Pig husbandry is the most important activity of tribal people in North Eastern Region which has around 25% of the country's pig population. The bulk of pig population is indigenous type which have poor growth rate and productivity. Both research and development efforts are needed to make pig production and processing an economic and attractive proposition. Meat production is largely a by-product system of livestock production utilizing spent animals at the end of their production life. This is more so in bovines, which contribute about 60% of the total meat production.

Export earnings from livestock and related products rose from about Rs 17 billion in 1994-95 to Rs 35 billion in 2000-01, an increase by 107%. Leather and leather products accounted for around 50% while meat and meat products accounted for nearly 40% of the total export. As the potentiality for export of livestock products is immense, we need to strengthen SPS regime to harvest the export potential. Programs to support clean and hygienic milk and meat production need to be strengthened. A cess on leather, leather goods, carpets and meat exports should be imposed and these resources ploughed back to improve the related industries at farmer's level. In order to encourage exports, all licensing controls for processing of livestock products/by products should be repealed and restriction, if any, on the export of livestock and their products need to be removed. The minimum requirements for export are: creation of disease free zones, value addition, cold chain, organic farming, etc. These should be created in selected areas having large marketable animal products.

Most of the livestock services like AI, vaccination, deworming, etc. are time sensitive which Government institutions are not able to deliver due to financial as well as organisational constraints. This necessitates for providing efficient and effective decentralized services in tune with demands emanating from users. Such services should be delivered at farmer's doorstep and linked with cost recovery for economic viability. However, limited Government involvement should be continued for people below poverty line who are vulnerable, mostly illiterate and unable to integrate with the mainstream. Sustainable rapid growth and development in livestock sector can only be ensured if the owners, service providers, veterinarians and planners become knowledge based and acquire the ability to assimilate and adopt the spectacular development that has taken place in the veterinary sciences and related technologies. A massive program encompassing village schools, veterinary colleges and universities should be taken up to improve the skills and competence of all the stakeholders.

Livestock extension is presently a part of agriculture extension. Livestock extension is primarily based on providing services and goods and is different from crop related extension activities that are based on transfer of knowledge. Animal husbandry extension worker is basically a service provider. Panchayats, Cooperatives and NGOs should play a leading role in generating dedicated band of service providers at the farmer's doorstep.

Public sector lending in livestock is abysmally low and such inadequate credit support leads to poor capital formation. The livestock farmers are mainly dependent on the informal financial intermediaries and end up paying an exorbitant interest rate. NABARD and other leading institutes should ensure that at least 30% of the total agriculture sector lending is reserved for Animal Husbandry and Dairying schemes and that financing should be done against model projects that have demonstrated their economic viability. A conducive climate through favourable price and trade regime to promote farmer's own as well as private sector investment need to be created. Resource mobilization has to come through institutional financing, capital market and private investments, which are to be tapped as a major drive to put the infrastructure in place.

The issue of animal welfare and managing livestock during natural calamities and disaster calls for special attention. Suitable programmes need to be developed since such asset loss can drive the poor into destitution. The issues of animal suffering due to ill designed carts and implements, etc. also need to be looked into and integrated in the Production System.

SAARC Poverty Commission Report in 1990 had made two significant points. It warns that open economy and the free markets were alright only so long as they could carry along the poor. South Asia, which is home to nearly half of the world's poor could not leave them to fend for themselves. The developmental process in the countries of this region can proceed ahead only if it stands on its own legs. The second important point that the Poverty Commission made was that it is not necessary to make the poor dependent on the governments handouts, if they have to survive. All what is needed is to make it work. What they need are some strategic inputs such as micro-credit, some basic training, access to technology underwriting, easy access to market and ways designated to incorporate them into the development process. They have the capacity to realize their productive potential if only they could be provided certain basic inputs and some economic space to operate in. In practical terms, that takes into account decentralized, grassroot organisations and relatively meagre financial inputs. This is essentially the basic bedrock of this report. The demand driven livestock revolution can easily be brought in and activated in a manner that the small and marginal farmers and landless labour who own livestock can move from the present nonviable occupation to a financially viable entrepreneurship. They could thus participate directly in the growth process and come out of the poverty net through the provision of some organisational help, micro credit; training and access to technology underwriting by a service provider.

Index